ROSENBLOOM
& MORGAN'S

# VISION
## and
# AGING

# ROSENBLOOM & MORGAN'S

# VISION and AGING

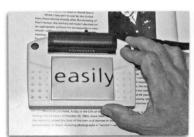
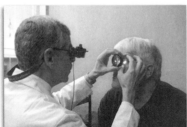
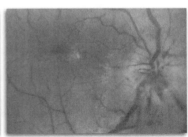

*Edited by*

## Alfred A. Rosenbloom, Jr., MA, OD, DOS

Founder and Chair Emeritus, Low Vision Service
The Chicago Lighthouse for People Who Are Blind or Visually Impaired
President Emeritus and former Dean, Illinois College of Optometry
Adjunct Professor, Department of Ophthalmology & Visual Sciences,
University of Illinois Medical Center
Assistant Professor of Ophthalmology, Rush University Medical Center

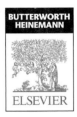

BUTTERWORTH
HEINEMANN

ELSEVIER

**BUTTERWORTH
HEINEMANN**
ELSEVIER

11830 Westline Industrial Drive
St. Louis, Missouri 63146

ROSENBLOOM & MORGAN'S VISION AND AGING

ISBN-13: 978-0-7506-7359-4
ISBN-10: 0-7506-7359-1

---

### Notice

Knowledge and best practice in this field are constantly changing. As new research and experience broaden our knowledge, changes in practice, treatment and drug therapy may become necessary or appropriate. Readers are advised to check the most current information provided (i) on procedures featured or (ii) by the manufacturer of each product to be administered, to verify the recommended dose or formula, the method and duration of administration, and contraindications. It is the responsibility of the practitioner, relying on their own experience and knowledge of the patient, to make diagnoses, to determine dosages and the best treatment for each individual patient, and to take all appropriate safety precautions. To the fullest extent of the law, neither the Publisher nor the Editor assumes any liability for any injury and/or damage to persons or property arising out or related to any use of the material contained in this book.

The Publisher

---

**Library of Congress Cataloging-in-Publication Data**
Rosenbloom & Morgan's vision and aging / edited by Alfred A. Rosenbloom, Jr.
     p. ; cm.
  Includes index.
  ISBN 0-7506-7359-1 (pbk.)
 1. Geriatric ophthalmology. 2. Vision disorders in old age. 3. Eye—Aging.
I. Rosenbloom, Alfred A. II. Morgan, Meredith W. III. Title: Rosenbloom and Morgan's vision and aging. IV. Title: Vision and aging.
  [DNLM: 1. Eye Diseases. 2. Aged. 3. Vision Disorders. WW 620 R813 2006]

RE48.2.A5.R67 2006
618.97'77—dc22                    2006047504

*Publishing Director:* Linda Duncan
*Senior Editor:* Kathy Falk
*Senior Developmental Editor:* Christie M. Hart
*Publishing Services Manager:* Patricia Tannian
*Project Manager:* Claire Kramer
*Designer:* Teresa McBryan

Printed in the United States of America

Last digit is the print number:  9  8  7  6  5  4  3  2  1

*Dedicated to the memory of*

**Meredith W. Morgan**

*an academic leader in optometry without peer, a superb teacher,*
*a gifted author, an accomplished researcher, and a dear friend.*
*He has inspired and guided me*
*throughout my professional career.*

# Contributors

**Ian L. Bailey, OD, DSc, FBCO, FAAO**
Professor of Optometry and Vision Science
School of Optometry
University of California
Berkeley, California

**R. Norman Bailey, OD, MBA, MPH, FAAO**
Clinical Professor
College of Optometry
University of Houston
Houston, Texas

**Edward S. Bennett, OD, MSEd**
Director, Student Services
Co-Chief, Contact Lens Service
University of Missouri
College of Optometry
St. Louis, Missouri

**Paige Berry, BS, MS**
Clinical Assistant Professor
Rehabilitation Counseling
Virginia Commonwealth University
Richmond, Virginia

Coordinator
Senior Adult Program
Helen Keller National Center
Richmond, Virginia

**Norma K. Bowyer, OD, MS, MPH, FAAO**
Public Health/Health Education Consultant
Morgantown, West Virginia

**Barbara Caffery, OD, MS, FAAO**
Private Practice
Toronto, Canada

**Richard E. Castillo, OD, DO**
Professor of Optometry
Consulting Surgeon
Oklahoma College of Optometry
Northeastern State University
Tahlequah, Oklahoma

**Jack A. Cohen, MD, FACS**
Associate Chairman of Education
Program Director
Rush University Medical Center
Department of Ophthalmology
Chicago, Illinois

**Walter I. Fried, PhD, MD**
SureVision Eye Center
Gurnee, Illinois

**Michael J. Giese, CD, PhD**
Professor
School of Optometry
Ohio State University
Columbus, Ohio

**James Goodwin, MD**
Director, Neurological Service
Department of Ophthalmology & Visual Sciences
University of Illinois Medical Center
Chicago, Illinois

**Gunilla Haegerstrom-Portnoy, OD, PhD**
Professor of Optometry and Vision Science
Associate Dean for Clinical Sciences
Department of Optometry
University of California
Berkeley, California

**Suzanne M. Hagan, MA, OD**
St. Louis, Missouri

**Sohail J. Hasan, MD, PhD, FRCSC**
Vitreoretinal Surgeon
Illinois Retina Associates
Assistant Professor of Ophthalmology
Rush University Medical Center
Chicago, Illinois

**Siret D. Jaanus, PhD, LHD(hon)**
Professor of Pharmacology
Southern California College of Optometry
Fullerton, California

**Robert J. Lee, OD**
Assistant Professor
Southern California College of Optometry
Fullerton, California

**Joseph H. Maino, OD, FAAO**
Clinical Professor
Department of Ophthalmology
University of Kansas Medical Center
Kansas City, Kansas

Adjunct Professor, School of Optometry
University of Missouri
St. Louis, Kansas

**Gary L. Mancil, OD, FAAO**
Chief, Optometry Service
Hefner VA Medical Center
Salisbury, North Carolina

**John Mascia, AuD**
Executive Director
E.H. Gentry Facility
Alabama Institute for Deaf and Blind
Talladega, Alabama

**†Meredith W. Morgan, OD, PhD**

**Lyman C. Norden, OD, MS, FAAO**
Chief, Optometry Section
Birmingham VA Medical Center

Adjunct Associate Professor
School of Optometry
University of Alabama
Birmingham, Alabama

**Alberta L. Orr, MSW**
Consultant, Specialist in Aging and Vision Loss
New York, New York

**Melvin J. Remba, OD, FAAO**
Chief Emeritus, Optometry Section
Cedars Sinai Medical Center
Los Angeles, California

**Alfred A. Rosenbloom, Jr., MA, OD, DOS**
Founder and Chair Emeritus, Low Vision Service
The Chicago Lighthouse for People Who Are Blind or
    Visually Impaired
President Emeritus and former Dean, Illinois College
    of Optometry
Adjunct Professor, Department of Ophthalmology &
    Visual Sciences, University of Illinois Medical Center
Chicago, Illinois

**Earl P. Schmitt, AB, MA, OD, MS, EdD, DOS**
Emeritus Professor of Optometry
Northeastern State University College of Optometry
Tahlequah, Oklahoma

**Melvin D. Shipp, OD, MPH, DPH**
Dean and Professor of Optometry
Ohio State University
College of Optometry
Columbus, Ohio

**Bernard A. Steinman, MS**
Research Assistant
Ethel Percy Andrus Gerontology Center
University of Southern California
Los Angeles, California

**Rod Tahran, OD, FAAO**
Vice President, Professional Relations/Clinical Affairs
Essilor of America, Inc.
St. Petersburg, Florida

**Gale Watson, MEd**
National Blind Rehabilitation Specialist
Rehabilitation Strategic Health Group
Veterans Health Administration
Washington, DC

Certified Low Vision Therapist
Atlanta VA Medical Center Eye Clinic
Decatur, Georgia

**Barry A. Weissman, OD, PhD, FAAO (DipCL)**
Professor of Ophthalmology
Jules Stein Eye Institute
David Geffen School of Medicine
University of Southern California
Los Angeles, California

**Bruce C. Wick, OD, PhD**
Private Practice
Vision Rehabilitation and Research
Houston, Texas

Professor Emeritus
University of Houston
College of Optometry
Houston, Texas

**Shelley M. Wu, OD, FAAO**
Central Valley Eye Medical Group
Orinda, California

---

†Deceased.

# Foreword

It is with great pleasure that I recommend to the reader's attention *Rosenbloom & Morgan's Vision and Aging* by Dr. Alfred A. Rosenbloom. The volume is arguably overdue, coming as it does fully 12 years after *Vision and Aging,* second edition, by Dr. Rosenbloom and the late Dr. Meredith W. Morgan. Indeed, significant progress has occurred in the fields of vision assessment and vision care in the intervening years. As never before, the burgeoning numbers of aged people are offered the opportunity to age successfully, that is, to adapt actively and creatively to the diminishments of age. Such adaptations are increasingly available in the fields of optometric and ophthalmological assessment and care. This volume, because it provides thorough discussions of the key aspects of vision-related and foundational knowledge that must be present and marries these with reports of the state-of-the-art assessment and care for older people, is therefore an important contribution to both fields.

Of the 21 chapters in this volume, 11 have been updated from *Vision and Aging,* second edition, to reflect the most current knowledge and clinical practice. The remaining 10 chapters present new material, not discussed in earlier publications. For example, the volume deserves plaudits for bringing together up-to-date chapters on age-related systemic diseases in the older adult. The focus on neurological diseases is particularly relevant to vision care of older adults. This book also includes a new chapter on auditory impairment in the older adult. The volume is unique in its recognition of public health aspects of vision and aging, which should be of interest to both public health professionals and professionals working in the vision field. In addressing assessment and care in the clinical setting, the volume includes separate chapters on the use of vision-assistive technology with the older adult and the provision of vision rehabilitation services through the "aging network." Impressively, there is a new chapter on vision care for the older driver. Studies show the incidence of accidents among older drivers strongly suggests the need for the consistent implementation of a more comprehensive vision evaluation standard. Finally, the new chapter on ethical issues in care of the older adult brings to vision professionals an area of focus that cannot go amiss in any discipline.

It has been said that at least 50% of the primary care physician's caseload is made up of older adults, and the same must be true of primary care optometrists and ophthalmologists. That being the case, I believe this volume should be required reading for every practicing ophthalmologist and optometrist and every student and resident training in the practice of ophthalmology or optometry. If the level of knowledge and sophistication about patient care requirements and treatment options envisioned in this book is achieved by the field as a whole, then the vision needs of older American adults will indeed be well served.

**Linda L. Emanuel, MD, PhD**
Buehler Professor of Medicine
Director, Buehler Center on Aging
Feinberg School of Medicine
Northwestern University, Chicago, Illinois

# Preface

During the past decade, there has been a veritable explosion of scientific literature in virtually every aspect of geriatric vision care. Present demographic trends indicate an ever-increasing number of elderly patients with unmet vision and health care needs. It becomes increasingly imperative that optometry and ophthalmology meet the challenges of providing high-quality vision care in an efficient and cooperative environment that encourages each provider to function at his or her highest level of expertise and training.

To that end, the purpose of this text is to give both practitioners and students clinically relevant knowledge based on sound scientific principles. In keeping with this goal, this text presents important chapters that reflect a broader scope of relevant geriatric topics often expressed within an interdisciplinary frame of reference.

The framework of this text is based on several guiding principles. One of these principles is the concept that aging is *not* a disease—even though there are physiological, psychological, sociological, and visual changes with time. A second principle is the concept that diversity rather than homogeneity becomes the norm with increasing age. Physiological indicators, for example, show a greater range of differences in persons older than 65 years than in any other age group. On the basis of such evidence, it becomes increasingly clear that *norms,* as performance guidelines, cannot be established with any certainty. The application of these principles demands that this volume, even more than its predecessors, serves as an overview to understanding the many complexities of providing effective primary vision care to the older adult. The overriding goal continues to be an emphasis on the improvement of the quality of life for the older person, fostering goal-directed activities and an independent lifestyle. Espousing this point of view stresses the importance of seeing the aging person as an integral part of total society.

My sincere appreciation and gratitude go to the outstanding work of not only those authors who have contributed for the first time but also those who have contributed to previous publications. Their expertise and commitment have made this book possible. I also acknowledge the helpful advice and expertise of Bruce Rosenthal, OD, and Mark Wilkinson, OD. Their review of selected chapters has been exceedingly helpful.

Science, it has been said, lives in the details that are universally valid. The purpose of *Rosenbloom and Morgan's Vision and Aging* is not only to report past and present knowledge, but also to bring into perspective new insights that will better serve all aging individuals.

**Alfred A. Rosenbloom, Jr.**

# Contents

1 *Primary Vision Care in Geriatrics: An Overview,* 1
EARL P. SCHMITT, RICHARD E. CASTILLO

2 *Normal Age-Related Vision Changes,* 31
GUNILLA HAEGERSTROM-PORTNOY, MEREDITH W. MORGAN

3 *Age-Related Systemic Diseases,* 49
WALTER I. FRIED

4 *Age-Related Neurological Diseases,* 73
JAMES GOODWIN

5 *Anterior Segment Diseases in the Older Adult,* 93
MICHAEL J. GIESE, SHELLEY M. WU

6 *Posterior Segment Diseases in the Older Adult,* 105
SOHAIL J. HASAN, JACK A. COHEN

7 *The Optometric Examination of the Older Adult,* 133
IAN L. BAILEY

8 *Factors That Complicate Eye Examination in the Older Adult,* 163
LYMAN C. NORDEN

9 *Auditory Impairment in the Older Adult,* 179
PAIGE BERRY, JOHN MASCIA, BERNARD A. STEINMAN

10 *Pharmacological Aspects of Aging,* 189
SIRET D. JAANUS

11 *Vision Corrections for the Older Adult,* 201
ROBERT J. LEE, ROD TAHRAN

**12**  *Contact Lenses and the Older Adult,* 215
EDWARD S. BENNETT, BARRY A. WEISSMAN, MELVIN J. REMBA

**13**  *Functional Therapy in the Rehabilitation of Older Adults,* 241
BRUCE C. WICK

**14**  *Care of Older Adults Who Are Visually Impaired,* 267
ALFRED A. ROSENBLOOM, JR.

**15**  *Assistive Technologies for the Visually Impaired Older Adult,* 285
GALE WATSON, JOSEPH H. MAINO

**16**  *Older Drivers,* 299
MELVIN D. SHIPP

**17**  *Nutrition and Older Adults,* 333
BARBARA CAFFERY

**18**  *Delivery of Vision Care in Nontraditional Settings,* 347
GARY L. MANCIL, SUZANNE M. HAGAN

**19**  *Public Health Aspects of Older Adult Patient Care,* 365
NORMA K. BOWYER

**20**  *Ethical Issues in the Care of the Older Adult,* 381
R. NORMAN BAILEY

**21**  *The Vision Rehabilitation Field and the Aging Network,* 393
ALBERTA L. ORR

*Index,* 401

# CHAPTER 1

# Primary Vision Care in Geriatrics: An Overview

## EARL P. SCHMITT and RICHARD E. CASTILLO

## DEMOGRAPHICS

In 1830 Thomas Malthus probably was the first to formally voice concern about the possible social and economic impact imposed on a nation as a result of a constantly expanding population.[132] Although research and technology have dispelled many of Malthus' original anxieties, these same scientific and innovative discoveries have given rise to a problem that was not debated seriously in the early nineteenth century, namely an increase in the average life span of both men and women. The United States is currently experiencing this trend. A growing number of older adults comprise an ever-increasing percentage of the American population. One result of this demographic realignment is significant stress on the various health care systems and providers who are charged with the responsibility of keeping the general society as well as possible, but in particular maintaining the soundness of mind and body of older adults. Although this challenge is recognized, it is far from being resolved.[86]

To illustrate, at the turn of the century a typical American's life expectancy averaged only 47 years. Currently a white male born in the year 2000 can look forward to a life span of some 77 years, with women living longer than men; this tendency toward longevity continues. Today more than 12% of U.S. inhabitants are aged 65 years or older. By the year 2030 this group is predicted to account for 20% of the total American indigenous population.

Although geriatric individuals encompass only approximately one eighth of the census, they consume approximately 30% of the health care dollars spent annually in the United States. One third of all hospital beds are occupied by persons aged 65 years or older, one fourth of all prescription medications are used by older adults, and the nation's nursing homes are virtually filled with older citizens. Fortunately only 5% of older adults need institutionalized care, which means that 95% of these older citizens remain in their communities. Sadly, approximately one fifth of the indigent population (defined as having an annual income at or below the government's established poverty level) is composed of geriatric individuals.

Over the past several decades the most rapidly expanding segment of the American population has been those who are aged 60 years and older. Demographers have acknowledged this trend, and although it has continued into the twenty-first century no single definition of the term *geriatric* satisfies everyone.[60,85] Nor has a universally accepted theory of the cause of the aging process been developed.[30,151,186]

Specifically, not all sociologists and demographers agree as to just when to begin considering a person an older adult. Although the rather arbitrary age of 65 years and older generally is accepted when referring to the geriatric population, this is merely a convenient point of reference. As a figure, age 65 years is commonly found in many publications when referring to older adults,[57] but data from the U.S. Census Bureau sometimes start at age 60 years.

A significant but often overlooked aspect of the aging population is the health care needs of the increasing number of older inmates who are incarcerated in state and federal correctional institutions. Approximately 14,000 male and 2000 female penitentiary inmates aged 65 years or older were incarcerated in the United States in 2000. At the same time, within this age cohort (and as a related category), 401,000 men and 1,157,000 women were residents of nursing homes. Another 13,000 older citizens were housed in mental hospitals and various psychiatric wards throughout the country.[180] Some evidence shows that that this patient group has been neglected, yet when provided vision care many seem capable of responding favorably to training in selected daily activities.[163]

Indigenous changes in population figures worldwide have occurred in remarkable fashion during the twentieth century, with the most dramatic demographic shifts taking place within the last 50 years.[73] By 1982 an estimated 48.9 million adults in the United States were in the 55 years and older age bracket, a figure that represented 20% of the national census. Of these, 32,000 were centenarians.[173] Despite susceptibility to illness, accidents, physiological dysfunctions, and the general ravages of time, in 1984 approximately 5000 American adults turned 65 years each day. Allowing for losses from all sources, this resulted in a net daily increase of some 1400 to 1500 individuals in the 65 years and older age bracket.[62,98] This trend continues to the present day.

By 2020 older adults will reach a total population of 52 million.[14,136] In 2030 the post–World War II baby boomers will begin to enter the older adult category, increasing the number of older Americans to 65.6 million, a figure that will embrace 21.8% of the entire population. By 2080 those aged 65 and older in the United States will comprise 24.5% of the country's residents.

This growth will seriously affect future tax-supported expenditures by the federal government on programs for older adults. Projected government spending in this area will rise from what now amounts to 8% of the gross domestic product to 21% in 2075. By 2100 this share of the gross domestic product will reach 24%.[113]

Government figures, based on the 2000 census, showed the total population of the United States to be 281,421,906 persons. Of these, 12.4% (34,896,316 individuals) were aged 65 years or older. Florida had the greatest representation of older citizens (17.6% of the total number, or 6,141,752 persons) and Alaska had the smallest (5.7%, or 1,989,090 individuals). Such trends persist, with Florida having gained the most older adults in the year 2000, followed by Arizona and then California.[114] These same reports estimate that the U.S. population should have grown to a total of 288,368,698 by July 2002. Those aged 65 years or older would have reached a count of 35,601,911 persons.[180]

The most significant growth in numbers among older adults has taken place within what has been termed the "old" cohort, those between the ages of 75 and 84 years, and in the "old-old" group, or persons aged 85 years and older.[1] In 1982 fewer than 5% of Americans were aged 75 years or older. This percentage will double by 2030. Between these dates individuals who are subcategorized as being "old-old" will grow in numbers as well. In 1982 individuals who were aged 85 years and older represented a mere 1% of the country's entire population. By 2050 this cohort will be 5% of the total, will number 16 million individuals, and will constitute the single most rapidly expanding population segment in the nation.[14,173]

That the majority of older Americans will be female has been foreseen.[136] In 1999, 24.7 million men and 30.6 million women were aged 55 years or older in America. The gender ratio was 81 males to 100 females, a figure that decreases steadily as the groups become more mature. For those in the 55- to 64-year-old cohort, the numbers were 92 to 100, whereas in the 85 years and older segment the ratio was 49 to 100. Obviously, as the population ages, an increasing number of older adults will be female.[93]

## TERMINOLOGY

As mentioned, the term *aging* is difficult to define, primarily because its meaning varies with the individual. Students of the subject have claimed that several categories must be considered when trying to identify anyone who might be considered "aged." Developmental changes often are the most obvious, including irreversible physical and physiological consequences occurring with the passage of time such as normal and expected alterations in growth patterns, sexual maturation, loss of skin elasticity, facial wrinkles and creases, and the graying of hair color. Precluded are instances of abuse, misuse, disuse, or disease that might induce comparable changes in the human organism.

Physiological changes include gradual variations in such functions as breathing and heart rates, changes in body weight, and alterations in muscle tone. Maturational changes occur in such areas as bone mass and density, stamina, and intellectual ability. Although these are not absolute differentiations, they suggest the complexity of variables that can influence the process of aging.

Other unpredictable events have an affect on how aging can be defined and how the individual responds to these inevitable influences. Chronologically, the mere passage of time can affect how one perceives himself or herself as a member of society. Social aging is a critical facet that describes how individuals continue (or fail) to interact with society and the various other population groups within the community and family circle. Psychological changes are unavoidable and include adjustments to the realities of retirement, the gradual loss of friends and companions, and the dwindling influence often experienced as a result of the withdrawal from more active roles within the community. Finally, the economic aspects of aging must be considered. The loss or reduction of income and discretionary spending resources, the lack of contact with former business and professional colleagues, and the resulting lowered self-esteem, all contribute to the cumulative effect known as "aging."

## PRIMARY CARE ISSUES

Primary care has been described as largely an ambulatory service activity, initiated for the most part by self-referral. The primary care practitioner is usually the first professional contacted within the health care delivery system by the patient. The primary health care provider then evaluates the patient's health status, discovering, categorizing, and prioritizing the dysfunctions as they become known. Those situations that can and should be treated immediately are done so by the provider, and condi-

tions that fall beyond the scope of the primary care practitioner are referred for secondary or tertiary care.[188]

Comanagement begins when such referrals are made. The comanagement of health problems may be as simple and routine as the regular monitoring of a patient's blood pressure[71] or as complex as the referral and management of obscure conditions such as Behçet's disease.[140] Secondary care often is conducted on a hospital or medical outpatient basis. The appointment for such care can be made by the primary level practitioner and represents one means of controlling the patient's progression through the health delivery system. Tertiary care consists of more intensive and extensive service, often requiring multidisciplinary, hospital-based expertise but still incorporating the primary care practitioner's controlling judgment regarding the referral process.[188]

The primary care practitioner is responsible for the total health scene of his or her patients, from infancy through maturity. Brown and Hawkins[26] list 11 specific areas of primary health care concern that the primary eye care practitioner should be ready to address. Among these are several issues particularly applicable to older adults, including detection and appropriate referral of ocular and systemic diseases, the amelioration of refractive and binocular dysfunction, the maintenance of a satisfactory health status through proper diet and exercise regimens, and the analysis of environmental factors that might adversely affect health and sensory mechanisms or job and recreational performance.

People become more diverse as they grow older. Moreover, profound differences exist regarding the availability of professional care for selected groups in American society. In particular, rates of blindness and visual disorders are significantly higher among black populations than among whites. Such problems as age-related cataracts and open-angle glaucoma are leading causes of vision loss within minority groups, yet both conditions can be managed successfully by a primary eye care practitioner. Other health issues common to black Americans, such as hypertension and diabetic visual complications, likewise can be monitored appropriately by the primary care practitioner.[22]

## Overview of Primary Aging

*Primary aging* refers to the anatomical and physiological changes associated with the aging process, irrespective of any concomitant or coexisting disease mechanism. The process that causes aging to occur is largely unknown. Indeed, a demonstrable decrease in functional cell mass occurs in virtually every organ system. Also, physiological functions diminish in these systems as a consequence of aging. These changes begin at approximately age 30 years and continue steadily thereafter. Fortunately, nature has imbued the human body with tremendous reserves that make these gradual losses insignificant for most individuals until the age of approximately 65 years is reached.

Yet aging is much more complicated than simply the loss of cells in various organs. For example, proper nutrition, reasonable exercise, and the maintenance of a proper mental outlook are all known to have a positive effect on the process of aging.

In "normal" primary aging every organ of the body loses function. This functional loss seldom becomes a problem until approximately age 65 years unless associated secondary age-related complications are present. Most of the body organs reach a peak of efficiency and reserve at approximately age 20 years and remain relatively stable then until approximately age 30 years. Thereafter a steady and gradual decline is experienced in functional activity and ability. At about age 75 or 80 years, most physiological structures have lost approximately 50% of their original functional capabilities. The good news is that most organs and organ systems have much more than a 50% reserve, so adequate life-support activities remain but the reserve capacities dwindle. For instance, the liver and kidneys have a 90% reserve capacity at age 20 years and so should remain viable and perform adequately when a person reaches the seventies or eighties under normal conditions.

The main problem resulting from the primary aging process is that of a diminishing reserve potential in the bodily organs. This means that a serious disease or injury is tolerated less well and that recovery time for most debilities and dysfunctions becomes longer and is less satisfactory in many cases as human beings grow older. The goal in health care should therefore be to minimize these primary aging changes and control those factors that accelerate the entire aging process.

Currently aging cannot be prevented, but some evidence exists that the process may be slowed. The general consensus is that dietary and caloric restriction unarguably is the only intervention capable of slowing aging and maintaining health and vitality in mammals. Although such paradigms have been recognized for more than 60 years, their precise biologic mechanisms and applicability to human beings remain unknown. Possibly the best antiaging medicine is exercise, properly done and conducted within the individual's physiological limits. Eating behavior, regular physical activity, cigarette smoking, alcohol consumption, and environmental conditions can potentially affect the health and functional capacity of older people. A regular exercise program can mediate, to a large extent, many of the declines in cardiovascular and metabolic functions experienced with aging. Although the exact mechanics by which physical conditioning contributes to longevity are not known, systemic exercise and resistive strength training programs can have important and positive medical and socioeconomic benefits for the health and well-being of aging Western populations.[70]

Resistance exercise seems to be particularly useful because it improves strength, enhances cognition, and decreases depression. Yet although the concept of antiaging therapies is intriguing, no medically based regimen has been proven to be effective in the long run. Health care providers should recognize this reality and not support without reservation any of the antiaging therapies currently on the market. More to the point, antiaging medicines do not work and may be dangerous. The physiological aging process cannot be reversed. The reality is that antiaging nostrums and ostensibly related health care practices are part of an industry intended to make money for those selling these products.

Butler et al[28] endorse this viewpoint and suggest that "instead of 'antiaging medicine' the term 'longevity medicine' should be considered by the scientific community, and that it should apply to all means that would extend healthy life, including health promotion, disease prevention, diet, exercise, and cessation of tobacco use, as well as advanced medical care and new discoveries that result from basic research."

## Secondary Aging

*Secondary aging* is defined as the aging process that has been accelerated because of otherwise controllable or preventable circumstances. These conditions arise from treatable diseases or disorders, social problems, psychological difficulties, and economic stresses. Chronic diseases have replaced acute illness as the leading cause of death in older adults. Often an acute illness such as pneumonia results from long-standing terminal diseases or events from which the older adult is dying.

The leading maladies associated with secondary aging include cardiovascular diseases, cancer, cerebrovascular disease, diabetes, and rheumatic disorders. In addition, smoking, poor nutrition, excessive use of alcohol, and a lack of proper exercise also accelerate the aging process.

Preventive health care must be at the forefront of all health care programs. This is especially true for older adults. Screening programs to detect diseases associated with secondary aging are important. Obviously, appropriate patient education and referrals into the health care system are vital if screening programs are to be effective in getting better control of these diseases associated with secondary aging.

## Major Organ Systems
### Cardiovascular

Coronary artery disease caused by atherosclerosis is the single most common event leading to death as a result of cardiovascular complications. It is estimated that 40% of Americans older than 65 years will die of some form of cardiac disease. Aging changes noted within the cardiovascular system are manifested as deterioration of the overall capacity of the heart to pump blood, distribute blood to the tissues, and maintain adequate tissue perfusion. Aging is further accompanied by progressive increases in both systolic and diastolic blood pressure. Risk factors associated with acceleration of this process include lack of exercise, smoking, and hyperlipidemia.[133]

The incidence of hypertension and cardiovascular disease in general, which is approximately 10% in adults aged 65 years, approaches 40% in patients older than 80 years. Ophthalmic manifestations of these conditions include visual field defects (e.g., homonymous hemianopsia), hypertensive retinopathy, and amaurosis fugax. The incidence of orthostatic hypotension and syncope is also increased. The latter may be related to poor or declining nutritional habits.[121]

Primary care providers are urged to monitor blood pressure of their adult patients and to feel comfortable about recommending modifications in lifestyles or to make referrals to medical specialists as appropriate. Kogan et al[102] review the latest thinking in this area, citing authorities that emphasize that eye care practitioners have an important role to play in their patients' general health status. For example, blood pressure has become an important part of the general eye and vision examination. Many people enter the health care system as a result of primary eye care. Optometrists and ophthalmologists therefore have an important responsibility in the delivery of health services.

The most common symptom of hypertension is *no* symptom at all. Early detection of elevated blood pressure therefore is critical. Although "there is ample evidence that treatment of hypertension reduces morbidity and mortality, current management of hypertension is characterized by underdiagnosis, misdiagnosis, undertreatment, overtreatment, and misuse of medications."[177] All primary health care providers must routinely take and record blood pressure readings for their patients so that those who might be at risk can be discovered and a prompt and appropriate referral can be made.

Finally, a carefully balanced diet can lower blood pressure in those with hypertension.[152] Limiting the intake of salt, typical in diets of American and northern European adults, also reduces blood pressure. In this regard, the amount of salt in the diet probably should not exceed 5670 mg per day.

### Gastrointestinal

Gastrointestinal transit time increases with advancing age. Prolonged transit time results in incomplete absorption of some nutrients and medications.[110] Excessive water reabsorption caused by prolonged transit time through the alimentary canal can lead to dilated colon, rectal fissures, and hemorrhoids.[137] Decreased force and coordination of smooth muscle contraction in the colon are also observed.[138]

The incidence of metabolic and nutritional derangements increases in older adults. As previously mentioned, of special concern is the gradual inability to absorb vitamin $B_{12}$, a deficiency that leads to the development of pernicious anemia and certain neurological deficits. This is just one dietary variable that must be kept in mind when caring for older adults. Again, hepatic function diminishes by approximately 50% by the end of the eighth decade of life. The liver does have an approximately 90% reserve capacity when at its peak, so under normal circumstances this age-related loss does not pose any threat unless an associated secondary aging problem is present that affects the liver, such as excessive use of alcohol.

*Endocrine*

Endocrine changes attributable to advancing age include a decrease in the circulating hormones responsible for repair and maintenance of cellular tissues, such as human growth hormone and testosterone. Decrease in secretion of endogenous insulin or a decrease in insulin receptors with a resultant decline in the effectiveness of circulating insulin also occurs with increased age. Furthermore, the immune response, both cellular and humeral mediated, declines in effectiveness with age.

Hyperthyroidism is common among older adults and may occur with or without Graves' ophthalmopathy. Of those patients with Graves' ophthalmopathy, 15% to 25% are older than 65 years. Thyroid disease may be iatrogenically precipitated by iodine-containing contrast, as in dye administered in preparation for contrast-enhanced computer tomography. One subgroup of older patients with a particular form of hyperthyroidism (apathetic thyrotoxicosis) may present with depression and apathy.[94]

*Immunological*

The immune system experiences a loss of efficiency as a byproduct of the aging process. Cellular immunity appears to be affected more significantly than does the humoral antibody system, however. This decrease in immunological functioning accounts in large part for the severity of and the increased susceptibility for infections among geriatric populations. An important responsibility of the cellular immune system is in cancer cell rejection. This documented decline on the part of the cellular immunity mechanism may contribute to the incidental increase in cancer that is noted among older adults.

*Renal*

Kidney function declines by approximately 50% between the ages of 20 and 75 years. This decline is generally attributed to a progressive loss of glomeruli, or functional renal units. Fortunately the kidneys have an approximately 90% reserve at age 20 years, so seldom does the slow wasting of renal function become a problem when no associated secondary aging complication is present.[25]

*Respiratory*

As the individual ages, the pulmonary system experiences a decreased compliance or elasticity of the lung tissues that interferes with the ability to expand on inspiration. Rib cage mechanics are also altered with age, leading to loss in muscle strength and flexibility with corresponding restriction of pulmonary potential. Pulmonary function is reported to decline approximately 60% by age 80 years. Additional pulmonary parameters that decline with age include vital capacity, maximal voluntary ventilation, expiratory flow rate, and forced expiratory ventilation.[176]

Pulmonary diseases such as tuberculosis are more common in older adults (25% of active cases).[87] Tuberculosis may cause anterior or posterior uveitis and present with neuro-ophthalmic signs and symptoms. Antituberculosis therapy (e.g., ethambutol and isoniazid) may produce toxic optic neuropathy.[119] Importantly, 60% of deaths associated with respiratory disease occur in patients older than 65 years.[135]

*Skin*

The skin is dramatically affected by the aging process. Primary aging leads to decreased dermal elasticity, so-called bagginess and wrinkles. Wrinkling always occurs at right angles to the pull of underlying muscles, which accounts for the radial pattern around the mouth and eyes. Patchy skin pigmentation and vascular ectasia are part of primary aging. A major potential problem in primary aging of the skin is the loss of dermal appendages such as the sweat glands. The associated decrease in the ability to thermoregulate as a result of sweat gland losses makes older adults susceptible to heat prostration and heat stroke during hot weather. The decrease in oil and sebaceous gland function leads to skin dryness and itching, which tend to become worse in the winter when air humidity both inside and outside is low.

Secondary aging is a major problem for the skin. Excessive exposure to the sun significantly accelerates and contributes to this process. Additionally, skin cancer is not uncommon in older adults and is directly related to total sun exposure. The most common form of cutaneous cancer among the aged is basal cell carcinoma, but the incidence of squamous cell carcinoma and malignant melanoma is also increased in this population group.

### Musculoskeletal

Bone is a two-component system with an organic and an inorganic phase. The organic phase (osteoid) consists of a matrix of collagen, glycoproteins and phosphoproteins, mucopolysaccharides, and lipids. The inorganic phase (hydroxyapatite) consists of an insoluble calcium-phosphate mineral. Three types of bone cells exist: osteoclasts, which resorb bone; osteoblasts, which form bone; and osteocytes, which maintain bone structure and function. The outer portion of bone (cortical bone) comprises 80% of total bone volume and consists of less than 5% soft tissue. The inner portion of bone (trabecular bone) is more porous and includes 75% soft tissue.

Bone is metabolically active. It continually remodels itself throughout life along lines of mechanical stress. Bone mass peaks in the third decade of life. With advancing age, the balance between bone resorption and bone formation is altered and bone mass decreases. By age 60 years, skeletal mass may be as little as 50% of that at age 30 years.[37]

The incidence of osteoarthritis escalates with age. Normal "wear and tear" begins to affect a substantial number of older adults by age 65 years.

A steady loss of substance along with an increase in the brittleness of bones occurs as a result of the aging process. This loss is far greater in women than in men and is usually not a serious problem among the latter until after age 80 years. In women, however, rapid bone loss occurs after menopause unless preventative therapy is instituted. Estrogen, calcium, vitamin D, and fluoride appear to be helpful for postmenopausal women in this regard.

Bone loss accounts for most of the decrease in height associated with aging. The average man will "shrink" by approximately 3 inches during a normal lifetime and the average woman, approximately 2 inches. The major portion of this loss is from the vertebral column. The reduction of individual vertebral body height, the increased forward curvature of the upper spinal column, and the loss of intervertebral disc space as a result of the gradual degeneration of disc material all account for the decrease in body stature that accompanies natural aging.

Bone fractures dramatically increase within the older adult population. Bones become more brittle, and because vision often is impaired along with the diminution of other sensory neurological input, the frequency of accidental falls multiplies with the resultant increase of long bone fractures. The incidence of hip fractures doubles every 5 years after the age of 60 years, with a 2.5:1 ratio of female morbidity to that of men.

Loss of calcium, inherent in the aging process, contributes to an increased incidence of osteoporosis in older adults. In addition, muscles atrophy and lose symmetry. Coordination and balance are further affected as joint capsules tighten, lose flexibility, and develop contractures. Adipose tissue ultimately replaces lean muscle mass. Abdominal obesity contributes to lordosis of the lumbar spine, with corresponding kyphosis of the thoracic spine. This leads to the common stooped posture so characteristic of older adults.[37,104]

Musculoskeletal changes observed in aging adults include a decrease in muscle mass, a decrease in muscle fiber size, a decrease in the number of myofibrils, and a reduced concentration of mitochondrial enzymes. These changes occur regardless of activity level. Muscle strength diminishes after age 60 years, declining as much as 20% to 30%. Maximal power output (the work rate) decreases by up to 45% after age

50 years. Degenerative joint changes in the weight-bearing joints are evident radiographically in most individuals after age 60 years.

### Neurological

Neurological function substantially decreases with aging. Neurons in the central nervous system undergo a slow, steady decay beginning at approximately 25 years.[37] Yet this decay rarely causes problems as a result of primary aging alone until the seventh or eighth decade of life. Short-term memory decreases, motor activity slows down, and the rate of central information processing slows. The peripheral nervous system exhibits a decline in neuronal conduction speed as well as in the number of neuronal junctions.[41,47] These changes further contribute to the decline in strength, balance, fine motor control, and agility. Tremors, a common affliction among older adults, are another manifestation of an age-related neurological dysfunction. In addition, they also experience major difficulties with balance, which may lead to falls and other accidents.

Sensory perception falls off fairly sharply at approximately age 70 years, which leads to a reduction in the perception of pain and proprioceptive sensations along with a loss of coordination, muscle, and sympathetic tones. Normal physiological changes in both the central and peripheral nervous systems that occur with aging also include a reduction in vibratory sense (60% by age 75 years) in the lower extremities, with a corresponding 20% decrease in reaction time.[48,52]

Herpes zoster affects 10% of patients older than 80 years (who have decreased cell-mediated immunity). Herpes zoster ophthalmicus may produce uveitis or central nervous system manifestations (including ophthalmoplegia) in addition to the telltale vesicular dermatomal skin eruption. Postherpetic neuralgia occurs in up to 10% to 15% of afflicted patients. Prudent administration of antiviral agents such as acyclovir or famciclovir may reduce the severity of, or arrest the development of, postherpetic neuralgia.[95] There have also been anecdotal accounts of stellate ganglion blocks being effective in diminishing the occurrence and degree of postherpetic neuralgia.

The incidence of dementia increases with age. Approximately 10% of those older than 65 years have some degree of cognitive debility. Measured intelligence scores seem to peak between the ages of 18 and 25 years and apparently slowly decrease thereafter. Only rarely does this apparent drop in cognitive ability become a handicap before age 70 years. Even then, for the most part, intellectual functioning remains at a satisfactory level, with the only inconvenience being that the processing and resolution of information by the central nervous system begins to take a little longer. Therefore practitioners need to allow more time with older adults to allow them to respond and provide information they deem necessary. Short-term memory and the ability to recall recent events drop off noticeably for many older persons after age 60 years. The main problem again appears to be the speed of information processing and retrieving, which justifies the exercise of patience when dealing with older individuals.

Neuropsychological problems are more numerous with the older cohort. The incidence of depression and alcohol abuse is significant, along with a marked increase in suicide and suicide attempts. Psychological and social aspects of aging are addressed later in this chapter because of the importance and implications of these potential problems.

### Metabolic Disease

Clinicians should be aware of an increased incidence of metabolic and nutritional derangements in older adults. The prevalence of anemia from vitamin $B_{12}$ deficiency increases with age. In patients with low to normal serum $B_{12}$ levels, increased serum and urinary methylmalonic acid and homocysteine may assist with the diagnosis. In addition, 30% of patients with early vitamin $B_{12}$ deficiency have anemia, but 59% may have reversible memory deficits. For the eye care professional, patients with vitamin $B_{12}$ deficiency may have painless, bilateral, progressive visual loss; a central or cecocentral scotoma on visual field testing; and optic atrophy showing a temporal pallor. Concomitant alcohol and tobacco use should be discontinued.[12]

### Sleep Disorders

Sleep disturbances among aging populations are often multifactorial in nature. They may be caused by such things as physical illness (chronic pain or discomfort, gastroesophageal reflux, cardiac dysfunction with associated orthopnea, or paroxysmal nocturnal dyspnea that may lead to frequent awakenings during the night), medications, and social factors such as retirement or change in daily activity patterns, bereavement, or changes in circadian rhythm.[66] Although some changes in sleep pattern may be seen as part of the normal aging process, they may also be associated with an existing disease.[67] In addition to affecting quality of life, sleep disorders such as apnea have been implicated with an excess mortality rate.[90,122] Sleep apnea and periodic limb movement disorder are the two most common sleep disturbances observed in older adults. In addition to daytime hypersomnolence, sleep apnea may result in hypertension, arrhythmias, or even sudden cardiac death.[61]

**Vision, Balance, and Locomotion**

On the average, changes in the refractive status have been found to occur throughout the human life span.[74,117] Moreover, the prevalence of eye disease increases from a low of approximately 1% in the general population during preschool ages to a high of approximately 85% for those aged 65 and older.[127] Numerous references can be found that discuss diagnostic and therapeutic options for anterior and posterior ocular segment morbidity.[15,34,58]

Visual acuity levels may show marked changes through a person's life. By the seventh decade a progressive loss in the time required for dark adaptation is experienced. Older readers can profit by increased levels of illumination, particularly when supplied in the longer wavelengths. Threshold levels of illumination must be doubled every 13 years for the normal dark-adapted eye to simply discern an object.[142] The presence of an uncorrected refractive error has been found to increase by 1.8 times for every decade of life after age 40 years. For most, the average refractive status of the eye becomes more hyperopic, the pace of change being most rapid during one's fifties, and then subsequently slowing. The horizontal meridian of the cornea most often becomes steeper, accounting in large measure for the against-the-rule minus cylinder astigmatism commonly encountered in older patients.[13,23] Several authors have reviewed the changes that can be anticipated to the eye and adnexa in association with the aging process.[101,118,157]

Dysfunctional visual abilities have been recorded by older adults as being a predominant cause in their loss of mobility, freedom, as well as independence and deterioration of lifestyle.[128] The American Optometric Association recommends a complete eye and vision examination every 2 years for adults between the ages of 18 and 60 years. Annual examinations are strongly suggested thereafter, or as recommended by the patient's vision care provider, particularly if there exists a family history of eye disease such as glaucoma, macular degeneration, or diabetes.[7]

Although applicable to all segments of the population, older adults within minority groups are particularly susceptible to ocular dysfunction.[129,155] One survey found that retinal pathosis, trauma, diabetes, and glaucoma were the major causes of visual loss in a predominantly nonwhite outpatient ophthalmological clinic population.[11]

Impaired vision can lead to isolation, dependence, depression, and sometimes disorientation and confusion for an older person.[164] Moreover, difficulties in ambulation, injuries resulting from falls and motor vehicle accidents, and diminished productivity can all result from dysfunctional vision. A report to the U.S. Secretary of Health and Human Services noted that approximately 13% of Americans aged 65 years and older have some form of visual impairment. Eight percent of this cohort has severe visual debility, such as bilateral blindness or the inability to read a newspaper even when wearing an optimal ophthalmic prescription.

Visual stimuli are major factors in helping to maintain balance. Yet for too many older adults vision is degraded, hence providing inadequate or improper feedback to the vestibular system. The ability to detect and process spatial information visually is commonly reduced in older adults.[29,158] Greater contrast is required for the older eye to detect details, and stereopsis, along with peripheral vision sensitivity, is often reduced for older adults.[142]

In this regard, a number of variables can contribute to falls among older adults, including being male, demonstrating an impaired gait, being frail, and having environmental hazards in the home. Daleiden and Lewis[46] describe and list a number of potential hazards often present in an older person's home. Frequent falls can play a role in accelerating the health decline in older adults. Among this population, "accidents are as important a cause of death as are pneumonia and diabetes."[130]

Visual fields become constricted with advancing age.[8,89] When of sufficient magnitude, the loss in visual field sensitivity can be associated with a decline in mobility performance. Walking speed decreases, and the number of bumps into obstacles increases.[178] Using a Goldman Perimeter one investigator found an inverse relation with age, concluding that a person of 60 years will have a central visual field that is only 52% of that expected for a 20-year-old.[187] In addition, patients with aphakia, whether wearing either an implant or contact lenses after cataract extraction, generally show visual fields that are more constricted than do age-matched phakic control subjects.[109] Age-related diseases that limit acuity and scope of vision, such as macular degeneration, glaucoma, and cataracts, or neural damage to the vision system resulting from stroke, can be causes of accidents.[78] Patients who have had a stroke may have visual field losses, which in turn create mobility and orientation problems for the afflicted individual.[96]

The aging adult should be alerted to his or her personal safety needs. Experts state that a "decline in visual function is one of the most significant normal physiological changes that place the older person at risk for falling."[175] One of the numerous age-related visual debilities that occur is a retardation in the rate of dark adaptation. This results in an increase in the time needed for an older eye to adjust to dim illumination. Glare intolerance increases, along with a loss of depth perception. Stepping from a bright outside environment to a more dim inside environment thus may be difficult, especially if stairs must be climbed or descended in the process. In addition, crystalline lens opacities and brunescence may induce color insensitivities, causing older adults to have trouble discriminating between medicine bottles and among various capsules and tablets of similar size and shape. Inadvertent overdoses or untoward drug interactions can cause confusion and neurological disorientation. One survey found that 25% of older adults may have visual impairments of sufficient magnitude to interfere with taking medicines and complying with therapeutic directions.[169] Thus, as has been noted, "a fall can be a sign of inappropriate medication administration."[56]

Hip fractures (femoral neck fractures) are an important and serious injury associated with high rates of mortality and morbidity among older adults. In the United States alone, the incidence of hip fractures exceeds 250,000 per year, at an estimated cost of $8.7 billion. Hip fractures most commonly occur after falls, or avulsion of the femur may precipitate a fall.[88]

The incidence and severity of falls increase with advancing age. Fall-related expenses approached $13.8 billion in 1995. Eighty-five percent of all injuries sustained by those aged 65 or older result from accidental falls. Of these, 25% have been ascribed to faulty vision.[183] Two thirds of all accidental deaths—the fifth-leading cause of death in older adults—are from falls. Three fourths of these fall-related deaths occur in individuals older than 65 years. More than one third of older patients living in the community will fall, and 5% of these falls result in a bone fracture or hospitalization.[159] Eye trauma can result from falls, further complicating the health status of older adults.[54]

Falls are the single largest cause of restricted activity in older adults. Moreover, falls are the leading cause of injury-related deaths, which total about 4000 each year.[131] Falls are the most common cause of nonfatal injuries and hospital admissions for trauma among older adults.[56] When not the direct cause of death, a fall is often the event that leads to hospitalization for the older patient, and because of secondary complications that result from the injury, only half of those patients then are still alive 1 year after the original episode.[56,175]

In addition to serious injury or death, falls have a significant psychosocial impact on patients, including such conditions as aggravated fear of falling; postfall anxiety; depression; social isolation; and the loss of mobility, self-confidence, independence, and function. Factors that increase the risk of falls are related to those that increase the probability of falls and that decrease the individual's ability to withstand the trauma. Poor physical conditioning, poor nutrition, impaired vision, balance, and neurological dysfunction, as well as slower reflexes and response times, all increase the risk of falls. White women are at a higher risk than other groups for hip fracture because of the increased prevalence of osteoporosis in this subpopulation.

One author cites figures that report that 85% of all injuries sustained by those aged 65 years and older result from accidental falls.[183] Coleman et al[40] found a direct correlation between the loss of visual acuity and the frequency of falls among older women. These findings "suggest that elderly people with impaired acuity and/or declining acuity should be prioritized for intervention to evaluate and correct vision to minimize risk for future falls."[40] When low-vision aids are prescribed, patients need to be carefully supervised in their use and application.[51]

Vision specialists should carefully heed the design and placement of bifocal and trifocal segments. Sudden head flexures can cause vertebrobasilar symptoms of vertigo and ataxia, visual hallucinations, diplopia, and momentary field losses. Reaching up to a shelf can produce the symptoms mentioned when the head is suddenly tilted backward while the patient makes an adjustment to see through the lens segment. Therefore patients should minimize the need for head flexion by storing items that are commonly needed at eye level, such as clothing, medications, personal items, and utensils.[175]

Multidisciplinary consultation is the most desirable approach for prevention of falls among older adults. A few well-directed questions can identify individuals who are at high risk for falls during the next year. Chronic illnesses, such as arthritis and Parkinson's disease, are significant predictors. Tests of neuromuscular coordination, such as the ability to regain a standing position after being seated in a chair and the capability to perform a tandem walk, also are informative.

In addition to detection and correction of vision-related disorders, identifying and communicating with individuals, caregivers, and family who can implement preventive measures in the home or dwelling are essential. Modifications such as the removal of obstacles, slippery surfaces, loose rugs, and electrical cords as well as the use of high-contrast colors and improved lighting in the home environment can help reduce the risk of accidental falls.[55] In addition, hand rails, well-fitting footwear, and other assistive mobility devices may reduce the morbidity and mortality rates associated with falls among older adults.

## AGE-RELATED PHYSIOLOGICAL AND PATHOLOGICAL CHANGES TO THE EYE AND PERIORBITAL TISSUES

Changes to the eye and adnexal structures occur over time, albeit with marked variability among individuals. Included among natural and expected processes are atrophy to the skin and soft tissues of the eyelids and periorbita, laxity of the orbital septum, prolapse of orbital fat, dermatochalasis, levator dehiscence resulting in blepharoptosis, entropion, and ectropion. Dry eye syndromes can occur among aging populations as a result of lacrimal gland dysfunction and decreased production from the accessory tear glands. Meibomian gland and goblet cell dysfunction may also contribute to dry eye symptoms.[68,105] Atrophic changes to the conjunctiva, along with subsequent decrease in goblet cell density, are documented age-related changes and further contribute to dry eye symptoms. Tear film dysfunction may contribute to the reduction in corneal sensitivity observed in older adults.[3] Additional aging changes to the eye include progressively miotic pupils, which become less reactive to light. The risk and incidence of presbyopia, cataract, glaucoma, age-related macular degeneration, and diabetic retinopathy increase with advances in age. In addition, refractive error is present in more than 90% of patients and, when uncompensated, remains a significant cause of visual disability in the nursing home population.

The four leading causes of visual impairment in older adults are age-related macular degeneration, glaucoma, cataract, and diabetic retinopathy. The incidence of primary open-angle glaucoma increases with advancing age, and screening is recommended for patients older than 50 years.[4] The Medicare program now provides for yearly glaucoma screening in high-risk populations. More than 2.25 million Americans older than 40 years have primary open-angle glaucoma, and perhaps half as many have the disease but are unaware of that fact.[31,35] Open-angle glaucoma is an incurable anomaly, but it can be controlled when diagnosis and management are instituted at the earliest possible time. The primary eye care provider again represents a first-line of defense for older adults against this debilitating ocular dysfunction. (See Chapters 5 and 6 for a more complete discussion of anterior and posterior segment eye diseases.)

Cataract surgery continues to be the most common surgical procedure performed among older adults. More than 1.4 million cataract surgeries are performed in the United States each year. Some 300,000 to 400,000 new visually significant cataracts are diagnosed annually in this country alone.[123]

Before attempting to evaluate the unusual, however, the vision care provider must understand what is expected to occur in the relatively normal course of events during the aging process. Mancil and Owsley[118] review the changes that can be anticipated to the eye and adnexa as a person gradually ages. (See Chapter 2 for a more complete discussion of normal age-related vision changes.)

Knowing what is considered within normal limits regarding age-related changes,[29,97] the primary care vision specialist is thus equipped to formulate a differential diagnosis when something unusual is observed. Various texts discuss diagnostic and therapeutic options for anterior and posterior ocular segment morbidity.[15,34,58] Older adults are subject to numerous visual dysfunctions, not the least of which is a natural decrease over time in the intensity of light that reaches the retina. A 60-year-old eye receives approximately one third the amount of light on its retina as does one aged 20 years. This is caused principally by an age-related brunescence that develops in the crystalline lens, selected wavelength absorption by the yellowing of the lens stroma, and senile miosis. Lower levels of visual perception for the older adult are thereby induced, in addition to a decrement in visual acuity. In this regard, at least 25% of older adults may have visual impairments of sufficient magnitude to interfere with taking medicines and complying with therapeutic directions.[169] Recognizing this, the Food and Drug Administration plans to introduce regulations requiring that labels on over-the-counter drug containers be printed in larger type and with greater spacing between characters.[99]

Another common annoyance experienced by those in the seventh decade of life is a progressive loss in the time required for dark adaptation. Older readers can profit by increasing the levels of illumination they use for close work, particularly when these sources supply longer spectral wavelengths.

As mentioned, limitation in light sensitivity stems in part from senile miosis, a situation that results in light rays being concentrated along the visual axis and through the central, thickest part of the yellowing lens. This encourages scattering of the shorter wavelengths and creates an effect of veiling glare that further reduces retinal illumination and contrast sensitivity values. Senile miosis can also shift retinal functioning into the mesopic zone during central field testing when a 1- or 2-meter black tangent screen is used, with the result being the creation of an artificially reduced field plot.[32]

Pathological complications aside, visual acuity levels show marked changes throughout a life span. Care must be exercised in reporting such changes because the methods of measuring visual acuities differ and techniques have not been standardized. In terms of Snellen equivalents, however, distance acuities have been found to range from approximately 20/1200 to 20/150 at birth, with improvement being reached to approximately 20/800 to 20/300 by age 1 month, depending on the test procedure used.[144] Six-month acuity levels by electrophysiological methods may be expected to reach from 20/40 to 20/20, all of which suggest that the uncompromised human eye can display standard-distance Snellen acuity abilities within the first year of life.[56a] Retinal cells continue to mature and motor coordination improves as the child grows, during which time the visual cortex continues to mature and refine its sensory decoding skills. On the average, maximal visual efficiency is reached by age 30 years and remains at peak capacity for the next 20 years. A slow decline begins after age 50 years and continues thereafter. This decrement may be exacerbated by age-related health problems, cataract formation, miosis, changes in the ocular media, cellular losses in the central nervous system, and the falling off of contrast sensitivity responses in combination with decreases in retinal illumination.[141]

The ability to maintain central foveal fixation seems to be unaffected by aging, remaining stable, whereas other visual functions may deteriorate through time.[103] Meanwhile, on average, the refractive status of the eye tends to become more hyperopic, the pace of change being most rapid during one's fifties and then slowing during the sixties and thereafter. As mentioned, the horizontal meridian of the cornea becomes steeper relative to the vertical, accounting in large measure for the against-the-rule minus cylinder astigmatism commonly encountered in older patients.[13,126] For the most part, the issue of changes in ocular motor control as a result of aging is as of yet unresolved. Saccadic accuracy and related functions do not appear to change significantly as a consequence of aging.[36] The authors noted, however, that "increasing age may interact with changes to alter saccadic task performance." In particular, high levels of generalized anxiety may affect some aspects of saccadic eye movements.[160]

## PSYCHOLOGICAL ISSUES

### Overview

The deterioration of mental capabilities that is sometimes observed in association with aging can create serious psychological and emotional problems for the older patient, as well as cause intense stress for the family members involved. It is estimated that currently 1.5 million Americans of all ages have some type of severe, chronic dementia, and an equal number have a more mild form of ongoing and progressive intellectual or cognitive impairment. As the population both increases in number and gradually becomes older, predictions have been made that 7.4 million Americans will be incapacitated by a form of dementia by 2040. In current financial terms this translates into an annual national health care expense of $40 billion for long-term care alone.[17]

Dementia is a general term referring to a broad scope of psychological maladies. It is a collection of multiple, chronic, and acquired neurocognitive deficits that would include such conditions as memory impairment, loss of the ability to perform simple calculations, lack of orientation, language inconsistencies, failure to demonstrate purposeful activity, inability to plan ahead, and loss of behavior control. Acute confusion, focal deficits such as aphasia, and congenital defects (as in the case of mental retardation) should be excluded before a diagnosis of dementia is finalized.

When occurring in older adults, loss of intellectual functioning is often associated with senile changes of the central nervous system.[139] The speed and complexity of cognitive functioning are commonly assumed to decrease during the aging process. No generalization regarding all older adults can be made in this regard, however. Although individual differences may be found within an older cohort, aging alone cannot be said to lead to a decline in all intellectual functions.[162]

The most familiar causes of dementia in older adults are Alzheimer's disease, multi-infarct vascular disease, depression (known also as pseudodementia), and frontal lobe disease. Alzheimer's disease rarely occurs before the age of 50 years but becomes quite common later in life. It is the most frequent cause of dementia in older adults. Less than 15% of dementias are caused by reversible circumstances. Such possibilities should be ruled out, however, and include nutritional deficiency, substance abuse, normal pressure hydrocephalus, drug toxicity, thyroid disease, syphilis, seizures, meningitis, encephalitis, and tumors of the central nervous system.[20]

Although older persons seem to process information more deliberately and are less inclined to make hasty decisions or snap judgments, actual decrements in cognitive abilities do not appear to be indigenous to the aging experience. Only when an individual is close to the end of life may significant losses from past performance levels in such areas as verbal information processing, psychomotor response times, and computational abilities be demonstrated. This decline in mental agility, known as "terminal drop," is a phenomenon recognized by gerontologists, but the etiology is obscure.[23]

Most older persons do not lose their ability to reason so much as they demonstrate a less-rapid response time to stimuli of all descriptions. This slowing of psychomotor and cognitive reactions probably is the most prominent characteristic documented in gerontological research. Each individual has a unique psychological profile and social life history. Psychological deterioration is not ubiquitous. In the absence of disease, growth of character and the ability to learn continue throughout life.

Human response times to all modalities have generally been found to decrease as age increases, even when no other health complications are present. All physical and intellectual abilities do not necessarily decline with age, though. Decreased function in the areas of vision and hearing, along with a slowing of cognitive and physical response times and increased problems with memory, is not uncommon. Yet although certain sensory functions experience desensitization in conjunction with age, many are retained. Changes in physical, emotional, or intellectual capabilities may reflect underlying organic or psychological disease. Too often this natural process of variation is misinterpreted as being a form of senility by insensitive observers as well as unsophisticated health care practitioners. Age-related changes of structure within the central nervous system, including loss of neurons, a decrease in the number of neural synapses, and the gradual accumulation of waste products from cellular metabolism probably contribute to this overall loss of mental efficiency.[53]

Of course, true psychological dysfunctions exist among members of the older generation. Loneliness and despondency are not unknown emotions for those older than 65 years, along with feelings of rejection, worthlessness, and loss of identity. Older individuals who are married have expressed concerns about family and interpersonal relations as·well as sexual impotency. Sensory impairments such as hearing loss have been identified as causes of depression and isolation. These debilities and perceived shortcomings prey on the older person's feelings of self-esteem and can lead to defensive and outright combative behaviors. Regardless of these problems most older adults retain a strong desire to remain independent and be responsible for their own lives, with a minimum of interference being imposed by well-intended relatives, friends, or others.[64,179]

Although older age groups are at higher risk for certain kinds of psychological damage than are younger persons, for the most part few older adults seem interested in or willing to seek the services of mental health specialists. Primary health care practitioners have been urged to be alert for the older patient who shows aberrant or otherwise unexplainable behavioral changes,[27] including the demonstration of an abnormal, irregular, or unsteady gait.[181] Appropriate referrals could be helpful.

The older patient usually is not reluctant to talk about his or her health problems with the sympathetic listener and typically can be led to full disclosure if the interviewer takes the time to inquire. Where inconsistencies, lapses, or uncertainties appear in the dialogue, family members or other providers probably can complete the details regarding specific names, dosages, and schedules of prescribed medications being taken as well as the identities of past and current practitioners who might need to be contacted. Moreover, as debilities are documented, older adults can be reassured and comforted with the knowledge that others have experienced similar problems and have been helped by caring specialists.[143]

Depression and lack of energy are the two most common complaints brought to geriatric counselors by their clients.[65] Depression may occur at any age, but older adults particularly seem to be more susceptible. This condition often develops as a result of prolonged and debilitating illness, loss of function, and the restrictive influences of failing sensory and neurological abilities. In turn, depression can cause eating disorders and loss of appetite, worsen an already sedentary lifestyle, further deteriorate muscle tone and circulatory insufficiencies, and seriously affect the patient's capability and willingness to interact with others.[170]

## Alzheimer's Disease

One of the most devastating maladies that can afflict the aged is senile dementia, also known as *Alzheimer's disease*. In the 1980s more than 2.5 million Americans had this age-related disintegration of the central nervous system. Approximately 150,000 deaths annually were then attributed to Alzheimer's disease or medical complications resulting from the dementia. Sadly, morbidity from Alzheimer's disease has increased dramatically over the past 2 decades. According to recent U.S. government figures, 4.5 million persons had Alzheimer's disease in the United States in 2000. This number is expected to triple by 2050, reaching a count of 13.2 million cases.[81] Such demographic realities stem from the rapid growth of the oldest age groups, who are the most profoundly affected by Alzheimer's disease. The number of U.S. citizens who are aged 85 years and older will more than quadruple in the first half of the twenty-first century. During this same period, individuals who are 75 to 84 years old collectively will reach 4.8 million. Authors generally agree that the number of persons with Alzheimer's disease in the U.S. population will continue to increase unless new discoveries facilitate prevention of the disease.[107]

The course of the ailment is progressive and irreversible. At the onset, one of the inevitable consequences of Alzheimer's disease is a shortening of the patient's otherwise expected life span.[191] No cure is currently available, and the ravages of Alzheimer's disease are the fourth leading cause of death after heart disease, cancer, and stroke among Americans older than 65 years.[112] The exact cause is obscure, although some evidence shows genetic predisposition with a defective gene on the twenty-first chromosome being suspect. Diet has been suggested, with the lack of certain trace elements being blamed along with certain toxins such as aluminum. A slow-acting or latent virus has also been postulated.[43] Recent research suggests defects at the cellular level may play a role in Alzheimer's disease, as well as in stroke, diabetes, heart disease, and other age-related illnesses.[166]

The individual with Alzheimer's disease passes through four general phases, each being marked by increasingly inefficient levels of cognitive ability and regressive social behavior. The first clues of impending disaster are found when friends and family members notice that the stricken individual complains of forgetting the names of well-known acquaintances or not remembering where objects were placed. The patient may experience a mild state of frustration during this phase of the disease but no serious handicap results, and denial of any problem is the usual apology, often with forced attempt at humor. Conditions gradually worsen, however, which leads to the second stage of the malady. Short-term memory losses now become common, whereby the patient is unable to recall events that recently occurred, cannot remember the names of persons to whom they have just been introduced, and start to have difficulty handling money. Certain long-term memory defects also begin to manifest, which can cause work-related errors or result in the patient's becoming lost and disoriented in otherwise familiar environments. The individual may begin to have mild anxiety attacks as he or she recognizes behavioral mishaps that become increasingly embarrassing.

The third stage is one of partial dependency, when the patient must rely on others for basic survival needs such as hygiene, dressing, and eating. Names and addresses can no longer be remembered, and the patient may occasionally lose touch with reality. The disease then progresses into the fourth stage in which the patient is unable to recognize familiar settings and is unaware of present events or those around them. Delusions and paranoia are common complications, emotional mood swings are frequent, obsessive behavior is seen, and the patient is completely unable to care for himself or herself. Secondary infections complicate the picture as the patient becomes susceptible to disease mechanisms as a result of deteriorating lifestyle and related physiological deficiencies. Full-time individual care now is mandatory, leading to the decision by many desperate, heartbroken, and exhausted families to institutionalize the patient.[2,83]

Secondary psychological complications of aging associated with organic dysfunctions are discouraging because so often the primary illnesses are insidious and incurable. Where no progressive physiological complications occur, however, intellectual activity may be as important as physical exercise in reaching and maintaining a healthy state of old age. Those who do nothing more than play cards and board games, keep up with current events, pursue hobbies, and interact actively with alert fellow adults and other individuals seem to retain a high level of cognitive ability and are physically more healthy than those who simply repeat the same routines over again as a daily drudge.[165] The benefits of regular exercise as one grows older, now matter how limited in scope, are well known.[57]

Too often older people increasingly experience feelings of isolation. Loss of sensory facilities in particular decreases their contact with the environment and may induce feelings of loneliness and despondency. Enforced quiescence because of frailty also tends to cut off older adults from the rest of the world. Frustration, anger, and self-pity tend to compound the increasingly narrow world enforced on too many older adults and infirm individuals by the aging process.[33]

Primary vision care is capable of making a significant contribution by helping the older person maintain meaningful sensory (visual) contact with his or her environment. By establishing for the patient an optimal level of visual efficiency, the examiner contributes to the older patient's ability to function as efficiently as possible. In turn that person's capability to achieve meaningful cognitive processing and psychological well-being is enhanced during later years.[156]

The hallmark of serious memory impairment associated with Alzheimer's disease is interference with the ability to function. Although persons older than 60 years typically take longer to learn new information and recall past events, only approximately one of every 100 individuals has debilitating memory loss. Annoying trends of forgetfulness can be countered, however. Prominent among current recommendations is that older persons proactively treat high blood pressure, with ideal values being no greater than 120/80 mm Hg. Moreover, a balanced diet, including abundant supplies of omega-3 fatty acids, is beneficial for optimal mental performance.

As mentioned, a regular exercise program will enhance physical fitness, which translates into better cognitive functioning. Alcohol consumption should be moderate, with recommended limits being no more than approximately 4 oz of wine, 1 oz of spirits, or 10 oz of beer daily. The possible effects of adverse drug interactions should be monitored, especially when taking a number of medications regularly for such commonly encountered age-related ailments as ulcers, chronic pain, depression, anxiety, hypertension, Parkinson's disease, and thyroid conditions.

Sleep deprivation can create stress, which in turn can lead to memory loss and reduced levels of concentration. Good sleep habits, therefore, are a vital part of maintaining mental alertness. In addition, seeking new and stimulating mental challenges seems to encourage the establishment of neuronal synapses within the brain. Reading, learning new games and hobby skills, and developing latent or current musical abilities all work to keep the mind healthy and alert.[182] The implied imperative for quality vision care would seem to be self-evident.

Research suggests that a healthy diet and an increased intake of vitamins C and E may lower the risk of Alzheimer's disease.[182] Moreover, protection from falls and subsequent head injuries becomes increasingly important in the later years of life. Studies have shown that people who have had severe head trauma are more likely to develop Alzheimer's disease and other forms of dementia.[145]

## Depression

Depression is the most common treatable psychiatric disorder among older adults. It also is a key factor in many suicides. As a cohort, older adults have the highest suicide rate in the United States, and almost 20% of those who take their own lives are aged 65 years or older.[10,69]

Most older patients who commit suicide have communicated suicidal ideation to someone. No evidence shows that questions about suicide increase the likelihood of suicide attempts, however. For reasons that are unclear, suicide rates, in conjunction with clinical depression in men older than 65 years, are higher than in older women and are five times greater than those of the general population.[11,69,77]

Approximately 3.1% of the older population show signs of clinical depression, including dysthymia and bipolar disease.[134,148] Many cases go unrecognized, and symptoms that do not meet the criteria for clinical depression per se (termed subsyndromal depression) may occur in up to 15% of the older adult population.[77] Up to 60% of Americans believe that depression is a normal aspect of aging.

Symptoms commonly experienced by older persons with depression include chronic, general fatigue; loss of interest in hobbies; social withdrawal; querulous attitudes and agitation; sleeping disorders; loss of appetite; early morning awakening; unexplained feelings of sadness and personal worthlessness; weight loss; lack of concentration and apparent retardation; loss of self-confidence; difficulty with concentration; and recurrent thoughts of suicide. If a person chronically has five or more of these symptoms and has not been functioning normally for most days during a 2-week period, the individual is likely depressed.[120,134] The signs and symptoms of depression among older adults are similar to those noted in younger age groups, although older persons may place greater emphasis on physical complaints.[11]

Patients may be reluctant to admit to any of these signs, particularly men because they tend to be embarrassed by their symptoms. Older depressed individuals are more likely to manifest somatic or hypochondriacal complaints and minimize their symptoms of depression. Complaints tend to emphasize the individual as not feeling well, feeling different than usual, or feeling that something about his or her life is vaguely wrong. A regular and frequent presentation of subclinical depression can include new medical complaints, increased fatigue, poor concentration, exacerbation of existing symptoms and medical problems, preoccupation with health status, and diminished interest in pleasurable activities. A common disposition among older adults is a recent illness such as a stroke or heart attack. For older patients who are depressed, a precipitating event such as a physical ailment or bereavement can usually be identified. The presence of a malignancy can trigger depression for the older adult, as can less-serious ailments such as a diagnosis of arthritis, multiple sclerosis, or Parkinson's disease. Women may have depression as a result of menopause. Stopping or withdrawing from some drugs can cause symptoms such as anxiety, psychosis, delirium, agitation, or depression.[190] The prolonged use of antiinflammatory drugs such as steroids can induce states of depression. Life-changing events, such as retirement; the loss of loved ones and close friends; or the erosion of personal freedom, independence, and mobility can trigger bouts of depression during a person's later years. Genetic influences cannot be overlooked because a family history of depression increases the individual risk.

A basic component of the ophthalmic examination is a determination of the patient's mood and affect. As a result of frequent visits, if the practitioner observes a cluster of the symptoms described, reasonable cause exists to suspect the presence of depression. Appropriate referrals can be made, along with a record of the telltale signs that have been noted.

## EDUCATIONAL ISSUES

Changes in the delivery of health care are placing professional schools and colleges under accelerating urgency for innovation. Claims have been expressed that the education and training of health care professionals are out of step with the evolving needs of Americans.[110] One survey found that incoming medical students have minimal knowledge about aging, only moderately positive attitudes toward older adults, and a low interest in geriatric medicine. The authors concluded that enhanced training in geriatric medicine is needed, particularly in light of the patient mix that most physicians will see in their future practices.[60] In response to one of these concerns, medicine has taken steps to increase geriatric expertise in surgical and medical subspecialties.[111]

Of added interest regarding the subject of education is Freeman's observation that in the future an increasing number of older adults will return to school, start second or even third careers, and enjoy more leisure time activities, all of which will require specific visual skills.[63] At this point health improvement and maintenance for older persons begins to assume community importance because productive older workers can make significant contributions to local and national economies.

As an academic subject the study of gerontology largely is a post–World War II development.[49] Curriculum models for the inclusion of gerontology into the mainstream of optometric education have existed since at least 1985.[149] But aside from the physiological and psychological aspects of aging, the primary care vision specialist should also be aware of ways by which the lives of older adults can be made less taxing and more enjoyable. Knowledge of this genre can be valuable when the primary care practitioner is counseling the patient and educating older adults concerning both the limitations imposed by the aging process and the means by which such restrictions can be overcome.

In addition to providing vision services, primary care practitioners and allied health providers are obligated to educate their patients continually regarding health maintenance and lifestyles. An issue often confronting the health care provider is how best to educate the older adult regarding beneficial services and regimens. Morris and Ballard[127] found that older adults are most receptive to new information when it is presented in a form that could be used independently, such as newsletters or brochures. Materials printed in Courier, Times

New Roman, and Arial fonts in sizes from 10 to 14 were most desirable. Computers and other electronic media generally received low ratings as sources of information.

Clinicians have numerous innovations available to them that can be beneficial to older patients who have sensory or mobility debilities. Such items as communication enhancement devices, cooking aids, recreation materials, and special clothing for the disabled can be obtained and recommended. Many visually impaired older adults are not aware of the existence of such resources. Furthermore, instruments and equipment are available for professional offices that can amplify voice communications between the doctor and a hearing-disabled patient as well as enhance television and video sound for in-office instructional and educational purposes. A wealth of optical aids on the market can be used by the visually impaired person to enlarge television screens and computer display terminals along with other devices for magnifying print and various reading materials.[116,124]

For decades the professional literature has emphasized the need for preventive as well as remedial measures to be applied during the practice of optometry. Students are taught that preventive health care is designed to enable individuals to live productively and be free of disabilities that could result from disease, injury, or maladaptation. To this end a principal objective of primary medical and optometric preventive health care is to prevent the onset of vision conditions so they will not be detrimental to the full development of the individual's potential and to ensure that visual performance is raised and enhanced to optimal levels. Vision care professionals should also strive to prevent or reverse ongoing vision deterioration so that any interference with the individual's potential would be reversed and visual performance raised above minimal norms and expectations.

Debilities of various kinds are the consorts of advancing age. All sensory functions are affected to a greater or lesser extent, with quality of life being influenced most adversely by losses in the areas of vision.[184] Fewer than 50% of Americans younger than 40 years wear ophthalmic prescriptions, but nearly 9 of 10 who are in their fifth decade or beyond need some form of lens correction, if for no other reason than to counteract the inevitable onset of presbyopia.[84]

In survey findings published in 1989, at least 50 million Americans, or approximately one fifth of the population, did not avail themselves of adequate eye and vision care.[16] Most were either indifferent, taking the visual process somewhat for granted, or simply failed to recognize a problem when it existed. Many also were poorly informed about age-related changes within the vision system, in that one third did not know the symptoms of presbyopia despite recognizing the term. A third also failed to understand the function of a bifocal lens. The fact that bifocal contact lenses are available again was unknown to many, and 29% believed that medical or surgical procedures could relieve a presbyopic status.

When supplying ophthalmic services, vision care professionals are actually treating the whole person, and nowhere is this axiom more apparent or applicable than when dealing with the geriatric patient. The case history is an excellent vehicle by which the practitioner can identify health concerns and communicate with patients about such matters, particularly older adults.[39] Questions concerning specific health conditions such as blood pressure, diabetic family and individual histories, cardiovascular complications, ocular pathological conditions, medication regimens, and psychosocial conditions can be explored and serve as educational overtures for the clinician.

The impetus on higher education institutions to produce health care professionals able to satisfy the particular needs of older patients is not limited to the area of vision services. For example, across America shortages have developed in such critical specialty areas as nephrology and geriatric medicine. The number of physicians now training to become cardiac surgeons is too low to replace those who will retire by the year 2010. In this regard, researchers at the University of California expect the demand for heart surgery to jump 18% by the end of the decade.[86]

As a related issue, the federal government has predicted that the United States will require three times the current number of long-term care providers for the aging baby boomers by the year 2050. Approximately 5.7 million— 6.5 million nurses, nursing aides, and home health and personal care workers—will be required by then as well, compared with the 1.9 million that were needed in 2000.[174]

## SOCIAL ISSUES

Estimations vary regarding the extent of economic resources controlled by older citizens, but the single most important source of income for most older individuals remains their Social Security benefits. Before 1935 there were never fewer than 10 working-age adults for every American older than 65 years. At the start of World War II, nine adults were working for every older adult, and today the differential is approximately 4.5 employed persons for every one who is retired. By the year 2030 this supporting ratio is predicted to be barely two working adults for every one older American.[42]

A larger proportion of today's workers are female and of minority races. With the drop in a younger aged labor pool, older workers are being retained longer by necessity, with retirement options delayed so that business can use the skills and experience of the mature employee. Although older workers accounted for 20% of the work force in 1980, they comprised nearly 33% of all industrial employees at the turn of the century. Changes in work-related benefits have accordingly materialized in the business world, including choices for flex-time working hours and health insurance packages that have altered the insurance and hence the payment scales and the delivery of health care by providers.[24,45]

At present eligibility is gained for Social Security benefits at age 62 years, and a certain number of older adults are ready to forsake the routine and enjoy the fruits of their labors as a retiree.[50] Should a number of retired, older citizens descend on a community because of attractive living conditions, the area's entire social structure can be altered.[82] But not all who qualify for retirement elect the option. McGoldrick[125] summarizes the current research on retirement and its effect on the health and longevity of those who leave the work force as a consequence of age. One survey found that 32% of those who stayed on the job past the time of minimum retirement age did so not for the paycheck, but because they liked to work.[19,72] Industry has found the older employee to be reliable, often to have greater company loyalty than his or her younger counterpart, and to record fewer absentee days.[192] This growing appreciation of the older worker has helped erode many of the stereotypes Americans have held regarding older adults. The fear, distrust, and prejudice that have been directed toward more mature adults are slowly melting as older adults continue to make economic and leadership contributions to society for longer times. Currently approximately 59% of those between the ages of 65 and 69 years receive regular wages.

When dependent on federal supplemental funding alone, many older citizens end up at or near the poverty line.[164] Most older and retired persons have other sources of income, however, which may include pension funds, income from rental properties, and returns from investments. Despite this ancillary support, nearly all older adults are eligible for some additional form of government assistance. How to provide for the health and welfare of older Americans through entitlement programs is a major topic of debate, both at state and national levels.[172]

The general health of one individual apparently influences the health status of his or her spouse. Older adults in poor health often have a partner who also has a poor health status. Couples in which both spouses are in poor health may face higher ratios of long-term care, which is costly for both families and the public.[189]

Economic status is somewhat of a predictor of longevity. One investigation found that "at age 65 the difference in life expectancy between the wealthiest and the poorest quintiles was 6.3 years for men and 2.8 years for women. Moreover, differences in disability-free life expectancy were 14.3 years for men and 7.6 years for women."[16] And it should come as no surprise to recognize that "poor health, low income, and lack of social interaction lead to lower morale, lower contentment, and lower expressed satisfaction, which in turn make individuals more vulnerable to other negative life situations, such as disease."[168]

Successful aging depends on many variables, some of which the primary health care provider can influence by active intervention and counseling. To illustrate, Guralink and Kaplan[75] found that persons who avoided hypertensive complications, did not have arthritis or back pain, were nonsmokers, maintained an appropriate ratio between body weight and height, and consumed only moderate amounts of alcoholic beverages could expect longer life spans than those who did not meet these conditions.

As a corollary, health care providers should be prepared to debunk the current pseudoscientific claims made by producers of antiaging cosmetics and other products on the market. The peddling of such items misleads the gullible public and tends to undermine political and financial support for legitimate biogerontological research into the fundamental aspects of aging.[18]

## ECONOMIC CONSIDERATIONS

Although the supply of health professionals has expanded of late,[167] the costs of providing health care have increased each year for the past several decades. The Kaiser Family Foundation reports that "expenditures in the United States on health care were nearly $1.9 trillion in 2004, more than two and a half times the $717 billion spent in 1990, and more than seven times the $225 billion spent in 1980."[92] In addition, the Foundation states that the outlay in 2004 represented 16% of the national gross domestic product (GDP), which was three times the amount recorded in 1960. About half of this increase occurred from 1980 to 1993, when health as a share of the GDP rose from 9.1% to 13.8%. Concurrently, the average annual growth in private per capita health spending was 3.7%, from 1960 to 2004.

The growing tax burden on state and federal agencies to fund health services has not been fully grasped by many. But as life expectancies increase, "sooner or later Americans will have to work longer and retire later. It will become economically, politically, and morally intolerable for government (aka taxpayers) to support people for a third or even half of their adult lives."[153] Regardless of employment or other sources of income, nearly all older adults are eligible for some additional form of government assistance. Revamping of entitlement programs is a politically sensitive topic, but the issue must be faced in the near future.

An increasing number of employees past the age of 65 years are choosing to stay on the job. Although older workers accounted for 20% of the work force in 1980, by 1985 approximately 25% of men aged 65 to 69 were in the labor force. In 2004 that number was 32.6%. Among

women, the comparable figures were 13.5% and 23.3%.[153]

But the economic picture also has its shadows. In 1984 older Americans consumed more than one third of all the funds spent nationally on personal health care, even though this segment constituted only roughly 12% of the total population. Early in the twenty-first century a growing concern was expressed that too many of our older adults were increasingly unable to assume their copayment obligations to remain eligible for medical subsidies. These older persons were at risk of becoming "health care poor." Too often these aging adults were not able to afford access to modern health care technology and still be able to pay for rent, housing utilities, and basic needs such as food and transportation.

Of concern to providers, Medicare reimbursements to home health care agencies dropped 40% between 1997 and 1999, which represented a reduction of funds from $17.4 billion to $9.3 billion.[9] Concurrently, the incidence of certain age-specific debilities such as Alzheimer's disease are increasing. At present annual direct and indirect costs to a family providing care for a patient with Alzheimer's disease vary from $3700 to $21,000. Indicators suggest these expenses will rise given likely demographic shifts.[21]

## ELDER CARE

The number of older adults who depend on their children for support has steadily increased over the past several years. Government figures project that between 1985 and 2030 the number of those aged 69 to 79 years who rely on younger family members for care and the necessities of life will increase to nearly 26% of that age bracket.[158] This growing dependency will likely lead to greater incidences of elder abuse.

Older adults are starting to have a significant impact on the American economic scene. One positive contribution they make is by remaining in the labor force. But as dependents they are altering lifestyles of those who must care for them, and thus are creating hardships for younger members of society. Because longevity is becoming the rule, 95% of all 40-year-olds now have at least one living parent, as do 80% of all 50-year-olds. Nearly 25% of the total number of older adult workers in business and industry must provide care, either personal or financial, to an aging parent. Three quarters of the individual or hands-on care given to older adults is done by women. Elder care has created high stress levels. One study found that 51% of all caregivers have been forced to take time off from a job to fulfill their obligations to aging parents. Fifty-six percent of those surveyed reported reduced productivity regarding their work, and 29% admitted to increased absenteeism from their jobs.[154]

Too often the women who must provide this care are within the age ranges of 30 to 45 years, have children of their own at home, have ongoing personal and family concerns, and may be involved in a personal career either on a full-time or part-time basis. These women represent a new dilemma in the American social order, that of a grown child with outside adult interests and ambitions being forced to care for homebound aging parents. Caught between their own family needs and the requirements of a caregiver, the "sandwich generation" is itself at risk. All middle-aged adults of both sexes who have elderly parents are vulnerable.[98] Moreover, similar social and economic disruptions to personal family relationships are experienced throughout and across ethnic populations in America.[44]

## ELDER ABUSE

The vision care practitioner may be the first or only physician to see an older patient who has been maltreated. The signs of elder abuse (a form of domestic violence) may be subtle, and early recognition is critical. The national prevalence of elder maltreatment is 4% to 10% and may affect 1.5 to 2 million older adults per year.[5,6] The actual numbers are probably significantly higher because of underreporting. External stress, such as marital, financial, and legal issues; dependent relationships, where the abuser may be beholden to an older patient for finances or housing; existing psychopathology, including mental illness and substance abuse; social isolation; and misinformation, including ignorance about normal aging changes or about the patient's medical or nutritional needs, are the major risk factors leading to elder maltreatment. This mistreatment may take the form of abuse or neglect.[38]

In spite of renewed interests by business and older adults themselves in continued employment, not all older citizens can remain economically productive and independent. Frailty and cognitive debilities may require the older person to withdraw and require care, either on a part-time or full-time basis. As the number of older adults increases, so do the social needs for their housing and life support services. Although most caregivers provide dedicated and loving attention, an increasing number of disturbing reports concerning elder abuse and neglect have been reported. One problem area involves guardianship and the rights that may be forfeited by an older person when placed under the control of a court-appointed custodian. No uniform jurisdictions exist, and each state has its own laws governing how and when an older adult may be declared legally incompetent. Restrictions may vary, but older adults often lose their right to travel, handle money, or buy or sell property once placed under a guardianship decree.

Physical abuse may be defined as an act of violence that causes pain, injury, impairment, or disease, including striking, pushing, force-feeding, and improper use of physical restrains or medications. Psychological or emotional abuse is conduct that causes mental anguish. Financial abuse is misuse of an older person's money or assets for personal gain. Neglect is the failure of a caretaker to provide for a patient's basic needs. Physical neglect includes withholding food or water, medical care, medication, or hygiene. Neglect may be intentional or unintentional and may be fostered by financial constraints or other lack of resources such as transportation and supervision.[5]

Elder maltreatment also includes mental abuse or exploitation and deprivation of basic rights such as privacy and decision-making regarding provisions of care. The vision care practitioner should suspect elder maltreatment (red flags) in circumstances shown in Box 1-1.

Abuse of older adults, whether by an official guardian or family members, unfortunately is not rare in American society.[150] Elder abuse can assume many forms, including psychological abuse, sexual abuse, and the violation of personal and constitutional rights. Cases of negligence, neglect, and financial impoverishment have been recorded. Victims often are aged 75 years or older and tend to be female. When perpetrated by family members, the abuser most likely will be the victim's son, followed by the daughter. While the mistreatment is occurring, the family member is usually experiencing personal stresses in addition to having to care for the older adult. These problems can include alcoholism, substance addiction, marital problems, or employment difficulties. Interestingly, abusers were often abused themselves as a child by the parent, according to one government study.[150] A relatively new perspective to this problem is the abuse of grandparents by their grandchildren or the physical abuse of parents by teenage children. Again, mothers most often are the victims with sons commonly the instigators of violent acts. The aggressors can range in age from 10 to 35 years, with the parents being from 35 to 70 years. At particular risk are aged and frail adults who have teenage children at home or who have taken on the social responsibility of being foster parents for mentally or physically handicapped relatives or state dependents.[76]

An ominous development has emerged concerning elder abuse and is occurring with increasing regularity, particularly in poor, rural communities and at larger urban hospitals. Older and debilitated patients are being brought to hospital emergency departments and virtually abandoned by families who no longer can afford to cope with the aged person. This previously unrecognized issue has not as yet been addressed by governmental agencies but promises to become a matter of intense social concern within the next few years.[79]

Any suspected case of neglect or abuse should prompt a complete written report. Documentation of any suspicious injury is mandatory, including type, size, location, color, and stage of healing. Mandatory reporting of elder abuse varies from state to state, and many localities have abuse hotlines for reporting maltreatment. The professional health care provider should be aware of local services for adult protection, community social service, and law enforcement agencies.[38,91,100,106]

## HEALTH CARE PROVIDERS NEEDED

Although one fourth of Americans live in rural communities, only 12% of all practicing medical physicians reside and practice in small towns. A disturbing maldistribution of traditional health care providers exists throughout the United States, a situation that has placed more than 2000 small communities in jeopardy regarding conventional access to the health care delivery system. During the 1980s, for example, 698 community hospitals closed, either because of a lack of professional staffing or for financial reasons, with half being located in rural and farming communities. This trend has continued; in 1989, 44 of the 80 hospitals that ceased operations were in nonurban locations.[147]

The U.S. Public Health Service claims that 12.5 million residents of small towns have no community-based primary medical health care practitioner available to them. Specialists are in equally short supply, with 52% of all counties in the United States having no office-based obstetrician in residence. Ancillary and support personnel also are lacking because of a nationwide shortage of more than 150,000 registered nurses, with the scarcity being most critical in rural areas. As the population ages, indigent, poor, and older adults are increasingly threatened with having to forego primary health care services unless other providers can be found.[147] Considering their availability and more general distribution throughout the country, their level of training, and the obvious need for services, the rationale for optometrists to practice primary health care seems self-evident. The training of medical primary health care providers with special interest in older adults may not be keeping pace with the burgeoning older population. Conflicting evidence regarding this issue has been documented. For example, during a hearing in Washington, DC, the Congressional Subcommittee on Aging was told that at the start of 2001 only 9000 certified medical geriatricians were practicing in the United States. This figure is less than half of the 20,000 practitioners estimated to be needed to care for the health needs of older adults. At that time testimony described that only three of the 125 medical schools in the country had formal departments of geriatrics. A mere 14 of these medical institutions included geriatrics as a required course, and one third of the schools and colleges did not even offer geriatrics as a separate elective course. The subjects of eye and vision care for the older adult were neither specifically mentioned nor addressed, despite the fact that instances of ocular disease and ophthalmic conditions needing professional attention are known to increase in direct ratio with a population's chronological age.[80]

On the other hand, in March 2001 a survey was conducted among the 144 allopathic and osteopathic medical schools in the United States. A total of 121 program directors responded, representing 84% of those contacted. Of these, 87% reported that their institution did include an identifiable geriatric program, with the majority of these departments having been established after 1984.

The survey authors found that faculty and staff assigned to the various geriatric programs spent a large proportion of their time (40%) in clinical practice. Residency and fellowship education required 10% each of faculty effort, whereas medical student education took only 7.8% of the faculty's time. Stubborn obstacles to achieving the goals of an academic geriatric medicine program have been noted, such as a lack of research faculty, postgraduate fellows in geriatric health care, and poor clinical reimbursement.[185]

Another group of authors conducted a review of medical textbooks and was critical regarding the lack of helpful information given to students regarding terminal patients and end-of-life experiences.[146]

## HEALTH INSURANCE PORTABILITY AND ACCOUNTABILITY ACT

Starting in April 2003, the first federal law to protect medical privacy was mandated. The Health Insurance Portability and Accountability Act (HIPAA) applies to every health provider's office, every hospital, every pharmacy, and to all teaching clinics in which individual records may be circulated or discussed and information about patients shared among practitioners. Registration desks must be situated so that no one can overhear conversations between the receptionist and the patient. Moreover, computer screens must be shielded to prevent anyone in the waiting area from reading the data being entered.

Patients may examine their medical files and have the privilege of copying or amending any part of the record. No other party, aside from the health care practitioner, may have access to a patient's records without that individual's written permission. This includes students, public health workers, employers, marketing agencies, and others who have no immediate responsibility for providing for that person's primary care.

Health care practitioners must notify patients of their privacy rights. This is done most efficiently by stating that such rights exist and then supplying the patient with a written summary of what the law provides. In certain instances, individual patients may not be able to read a page containing a synopsis of the HIPAA regulations. But as long as a good faith effort to inform patients of their rights to privacy has been made, the spirit and intent of the law will have been met (Box 1-2).

At present, compliance with HIPAA is being monitored by the Office for Civil Rights. The

---

**BOX 1-2**

### Patient Rights

- To see, copy, and request corrections of medical (optometric) records
- To know how health care providers intend to use and to disclose personal information
- To prohibit employers and marketing companies from obtaining medical (optometric) records without that person's written authorization
- To request medical (optometric) information be sent to an address other than the one officially listed
- To tell providers and health care facilities not to release any information about a condition—or even reveal the fact that the individual is a resident within a hospital or clinic—to relatives or the public

U.S. Department of Health and Human Services is the chief administrative agency. Violation of the act constitutes a felony, and provisions have been made for federal prosecution of deliberate offenders. More complete details can be found at *www.healthprivacy.org*. Patients may file a grievance with the U.S. Department for Health and Human Services Office for Civil Rights by calling 800-368-1019 or by following links at *www.hhs.gov/ocr/hipaa*. Providers must recognize that the federal government is becoming more aggressive in investigating and prosecuting health care fraud and malfeasance. Although it would likely not be experienced by the conscientious practitioner, agents can appear unannounced at any office for the purpose of serving search warrants for alleged violations of federal law, particularly when a complaint—be it imaginary or substantial—has been filed by a disgruntled former employee or a noisome patient. To obtain a search warrant, authorities do not need actual proof of wrongdoing. Credible allegations may be enough.[108] Disruptions caused by such intrusions can be potentially devastating to a practice.

Prudence dictates that health care providers take steps to avoid entanglements with federal policies. Numerous articles in the current literature carry the theme that, in the extreme, if HIPAA-proposed security rules are enacted in anything like their proposed form, a security officer would be mandatory for every professional health care office and clinic. New software will be required, and office routines will need to be modified. Practitioners should prepare themselves and their staff for reconciliation with the pending HIPAA regulations.

## REFERENCES

1. Altergott K, Vaughn CE: Themes and variations: social aspects of aging. In Rosenbloom AA Jr, Morgan MW, editors: *Vision and aging: general and clinical perspectives*, New York, 1986, Professional Press Books, p 19.
2. *Alzheimer's disease: Report of the Secretary's Task Force on Alzheimer's disease*, Washington, DC, 1984, United States Government Printing Office, p 30.
3. American Academy of Ophthalmology: *Basic and clinical science course. Section 8: external disease and cornea*, San Francisco, 1990, American Academy of Ophthalmology.
4. American Academy of Ophthalmology: *Basic and clinical science course. Section 10: glaucoma*, San Francisco, 1996, American Academy of Ophthalmology.
5. American College of Emergency Physicians: Management of elder abuse and neglect. Policy statement, *Ann Emerg Med* 31:149-50, 1998.
6. American Medical Association: *Diagnostic treatment guidelines on elder abuse and neglect*, Chicago, 1992, American Medical Association, pp 4-37.
7. American Optometric Association: *Recommended examination frequency for the adult patient*. Available at at: http://www.aoa.org/x1929.xml. Accessed March 2006.
8. Anderson DR: *Testing the field of vision*, London, 1982, CV Mosby, p 150.
9. Angelelli J, Fennell M, Hyatt RR, et al: Linkages in the rural community: the balanced budget act and beyond, *Gerontologist* 43:151-7, 2003.
10. Angst J, Angst F, Stassen HH: Suicide risk in patients with major depressive disorder, *J Clin Psychiatry* 60(suppl 2):57-62, 1999.
11. Apter A, Horesh N, Gothelf D, et al: Relationship between self-disclosure and serious suicidal behavior, *Comp Psychiatry* 42:70-5, 2001.
12. Balducci L: Epidemiology of anemia in the elderly—information on diagnostic evaluation, *J Am Geriatr Soc* 51(suppl): 52-9, 2003.
13. Baldwin, WR, Mills D: A longitudinal study of corneal astigmatism and total astigmatism, *Am J Optom Physiol Opt* 58:206-11, 1981.
14. Barrow GM: *Aging: the individual and society*, ed 3, New York, 1986, West.
15. Bell FC, Stenstrom WJ: *Atlas of the peripheral retina*, W.B. Saunders, 1983, Philadelphia.
16. Bertz K: Harris poll: Americans neglect eye care, *Opt Management* 25:4, 1990.
17. Billig N, Fox JH, Reisberg B: Diagnostic dilemma: is it dementia? *Patient Care* 23: 192-220, 1989.
18. Binstock RH: The war on "anti-aging" medicine, *Gerontologist* 4:4-14, 2003.
19. Bird C: The jobs you do, *Modern Maturity* Dec-Jan:40-6, 1989.
20. Blair BD: Frequently missed diagnosis in geriatric psychiatry, *Psychiatr Clin North Am* 21:941-71, 1998.
21. Bloom BS, de Pouvourville N, Straus W: Cost of illness of Alzheimer's disease: how useful are current estimates? *Gerontologist* 43:158-64, 2003.
22. Borska L: Can anyone solve the black vision crisis? *Review of Optometry* 128:50-4, 1991.
23. Botwinick J: *Aging and behavior*, New York, 1978, Springer, pp 25-9.

24. Bowker M: Retires for hire, *Kiwanis Magazine* March:25-7, 53, 1989.

25. Brenner BM, Rector FC Jr, editors: *The kidney,* ed 6, Boston, 1999, W.B. Saunders.

26. Brown BM, Hawkins W: A descriptive study examining primary-level prevention activities of Oregon optometrists, *J Am Optom Assoc* 62:296-303, 1991.

27. Bruce ML, Leaf PJ: Psychiatric disorders and 15-month mortality in a community sampling of older adults, *Am J Public Health* 79:727-30, 1989.

28. Butler RN, Fossel M, Harman SM, et al: Is there an antiaging medicine? *J Gerontol A Biol Sci Med Sci* 57A:B333-8, 2002.

29. Caird FI, Williamson J: *The eye and its disorders in the elderly,* Bristol, England, 1986, John Wright and Sons, pp 30-3.

30. Campanelli LC: Theories of aging. In Lewis CB, editor: *Aging: the health care challenge,* Philadelphia, 1990, FA Davis, pp 7-21.

31. Cantor L: Glaucoma. In *Basic and clinical science course,* Section 10, San Francisco, 1996-1997, American Academy of Ophthalmology.

32. Carter J: *Predictable visual responses to increasing age, J Am Optom Assoc* 53:31-6, 1982.

33. Cason A, Thompson V: Working with the old and dying, *Inst J Psychology* 1:58-69, 1980.

34. Catania L: *Primary care of the anterior segment,* Norwalk, CT, 1988, Appleton and Lange.

35. Chadhry I, Wong S: Recognizing glaucoma: a guide for the primary care physician, *Postgrad Med* 99:247-9, 1996.

36. Ciuffreda KJ, Tannen B: *Eye movement basics for the clinician,* St. Louis, 1995, Mosby, p 52.

37. Clark GS, Siebens HC: Geriatric rehabilitation. In Delisa JA, editor: *Rehabilitation medicine: principles in practice,* ed 3, Philadelphia, 1998, Lippincott-Raven, pp 963-95.

38. Clarke ME, Pierson W: Management of elder abuse in the emergency department, *Emerg Med Clin North Am* 17:631-44, 1999.

39. Cole K, McConnaha DL: Understanding and interacting with older patients, *J Am Optom Assoc* 57:920-5, 1986.

40. Coleman AL, Stone K, Ewing SK, et al: Higher risk of multiple falls among elderly women who lose visual acuity, *Ophthalmology* 111:857-62, 2004.

41. Consortium for Spinal Cord Medicine: *Neurogenic bowel management in adults with spinal cord injury. Clinical practice guidelines 1998,* Washington, DC, 1998, Paralyzed Veterans of America, p 12.

42. Cowan E: Background and history: the crisis in public finance and social security. In Boskin MJ, editor: *The crisis in Social Security,* San Francisco, 1977, Institute for Contemporary Studies.

43. Cowley G, Hager M: Medical mystery tour: what causes Alzheimer's disease? *Newsweek* Dec 18, 1989.

44. Cox C, Monk A: Strain among caregivers: comparing the experiences of African-Americans and Hispanic caregivers of Alzheimer's relatives, *Int J Aging Hum Dev* 43:93-105, 1996.

45. Crooks L: Older Americans in a changing society, *Vital Speeches* 60:556-8, 1989.

46. Daleiden S, Lewis CB: Clinical implications of the neurological changes in the aging process. In Lewis CB, editor: *Aging: the health care challenge,* ed 2, Philadelphia, 1990, FA Davis, pp 171-5.

47. Davidoff G, Werner R, Waring W: Compressive mononeuropathies of the upper extremity in chronic paraplegia, *Paraplegia* 29:17-24, 1991.

48. Dearolf WW 3d, Betz RR, Vogel LC, et al: Scoliosis in pediatric spinal cord-injured patients, *J Pediatr Orthop* 10:214-8, 1990.

49. Decker DL: *Social gerontology,* Boston, 1980, Little, Brown, pp 5-6.

50. Denzer S: Do the elderly want to work? *U.S. News and World Report* May 14, 1990, pp 48-50.

51. DeSylvia DA: Low vision and aging, *Optom Vision Sci* 67:319-22, 1990.

52. Deutsch EM, Sawyer H: *A guide to rehabilitation,* White Plains, NY, 2000, Ahab Press, pp 318-27.

53. Devereaux M, Andrus LH, Scott CD, editors: *Eldercare,* New York, 1981, Green & Stratton, p 51.

54. Eagling EM, Roper-Hall MJ: *Eye injuries: an illustrated guide,* Philadelphia, 1986, J.B. Lippincott.

55. Edmondson JM: *Home safety: it's no accident,* Kalamazoo, MI, 1983, Upjohn Healthcare Services.

56. Eisenberg JS: Your role in fall prevention, *Rev Opt* 15:46-9, 2004.

56a. Eskridge JB, Amos, JF, Bartlett. *Clinical procedures in optometry,* Philadelphia, 1991, Lippincott William & Wilkins, p 521.

57. Ettinger WH, Evans WJ, Weindruch R, et al: Exercise for the elderly, *Patient Care* 23:165-91, 1989.

58. Fedukowicz HB, Stenson S: *External infections of the eye,* ed 3, Norwalk, CT, 1985, Appleton-Century-Crofts.

59. Field M: *Depth and extent of the geriatric problem,* Springfield, IL, 1970, Charles C. Thomas, pp 13-5.

60. Fitzgerald JT, Wray LA, Halter JB, et al: Relating medical students' knowledge, attitudes, and experience in geriatric medicine, *Gerontologist* 43:849-55, 2003.

61. Fleetham JA: Is sleep disordered breathing associated with increased mortality? *Thorax* 53:627-8, 1998.

62. Fowles DG: *A Profile of older Americans,* Publication #PF 3049, Dept D-996, Washington, DC, 1985, American Association of Retired Persons.

63. Freeman PB: Ageless issues. Editor's perspective, *Optometry* 75:737-8, 2004.

64. Gartz CM, Scott J: Analysis of letters to "Dear Abby" concerning old age, *Gerontologist* 15:47-50, 1975.

65. Geba B: *Vitality training for older adults,* New York, 1974, Random House, p 20.

66. Gentili A, Weiner DK, Kuchibhatil M: Factors that disturb sleep in nursing home residents, *Aging (Milano)* 9:207-13, 1997.

67. Gentili A, Edinger JD: Sleep disorders in older people, *Aging (Milano)* 11:137-41, 1999.

68. Gilbard JP: Dry eye disorders. In Albert DM, Jakobiec FA, editors: *Principles and practice of ophthalmology, vol 2,* Philadelphia, 2000, WB Saunders, pp 982-1000.

69. Gliatto MF, Rai AK: Evaluation and treatment of patients with suicidal ideation, *Am Fam Physician* 59:1500-6, 1999.

70. Goldberg AP, Hagberg JM: Physical exercise in the elderly. In Schneider EL, Rowe JW, editors: *Handbook of the biology of aging, ed 3,* Boston, 1990, Academic Press, pp 407-28.

71. Good GW, Augsburger AR: Role of optometrists in combating high blood pressure, *J Am Optom Assoc* 60:352-5, 1989.

72. Grad S: *Income of the population 55 and over: 1984,* Washington, DC, 1985, United States Government Printing Office, p 2.

73. The Graying of Nations. Hearing before the Special Committee on Aging, U.S. Senate, 99th Congress, July 12, 1985. Washington, DC, 1986, U.S. Government Printing Office, pp 4-8.

74. Grosvenor T: *Primary care optometry, ed 3,* Boston, 1996, Butterworth-Heinemann, pp 39-60.

75. Guralink JM, Kaplan GA: Predictors of healthy aging: prospective evidence from the Alameda County study, *Am J Public Health* 79:703-8, 1989.

76. Harben HT: Violence against parents, *Medical Aspects of Human Sexuality* 17:20-44, 1983.

77. Harwitz D, Ravizza L: Suicide and depression, *Emerg Med Clin North Am* 18:263-71, 2000.

78. Hassan SE, Lovie-Kitchin JE, Woods RL: Vision and mobility performance of subjects with age-related macular degeneration, *Optom Vision Sci* 79:697-707, 2002.

79. Hasson J: Families abandoning elderly in hospital emergency rooms, *Muskogee Phoenix* April 15, 1991, Sec. A-6.

80. Hearing Before the Subcommittee on Aging of the Committee on Health, Education, Labor, and Pensions. United States Senate, 107th Congress, First session on examining the effect of the national shortage of geriatric-trained health professionals may have on the growing senior population, June 19, 2001. Washington DC, 2002, U.S. Government Printing Office, p 5.

81. Hebert LE, Scherr PA, Bienias JL et al: Alzheimer's disease in the U.S. population: prevalence and estimates using the 2000 census, *Arch Neurol* 60:1119-22, 2003.

82. Heckheimer EF: Health promotion of the elderly in the community, Philadelphia, 1989, W.B. Saunders.

83. Henig RM: *The myth of senility,* Glenwood, IL, 1985, Scott Forsman, pp 112, 127.

84. Herrin S: The surprising '90s, *Review of Optometry* 127:32, 1990.

85. Hodkinson HM: *An outline of geriatrics, ed 2,* London, 1981, Academic Press.

86. Howell RE: Medical schools must meet demands of aging boomers: opinion, *Tulsa World* 100:G4, 2005.

87. Hyman CL: Tuberculosis: a survey and review of the current literature, *Curr Opin Pulm Med* 1:234-42, 1995.

88. Isaacs B: *The challenge of geriatric medicine,* Oxford, England, 1992, Oxford University Press, p 77.

89. Jaffe GJ, Alvarado JA, Juster RP: Age-related changes in the normal visual field, *Arch Ophthalmol* 104:1021-5, 1986.

90. Jean-Louis G, Kripke DF, Ancoli-Israel S: Sleep duration, illumination, and activity patterns in a population sample—effects of gender and ethnicity, *Biol Psychiatry* 47:921-7, 2000.

91. Jones JS, Veenstra TR, Seamon JP, et al: Elder mistreatment—national survey of emergency physicians, *Am Emerg Med* 30:473-9, 1997.

92. Kaiser Family Foundation: *Trends and indicators in the changing health care marketplace: national health expenditures and their share of gross domestic product, 1960-2004.* Available at http://www.kff.org/insurance/7301/print-sec1.cfm. Accessed March 2006.

93. Kane RL, Solomon DH, Beck JC, et al: *Geriatrics in the United States,* Lexington, MA, 1981, DC Heath, pp 9-11.

94. Kannan CR: *Essential endocrinology,* New York, 1986, Plenum Medical, p 138.

95. Karbassi M, Raizman MB, Schuman JS: Herpes zoster ophthalmicus, *Surv Ophthalmol* 36:395-410, 1992.

96. Kart CS, Metress EK, Metress SP: *Aging, health, and society,* Boston, 1988, Jones and Bartlett, p 218.

97. Keeney VT, Keeney AH: Emotional aspects of visual impairment in the population over sixty

years of age. In Kwitko ML, Weinstock FJ, editors: *Geriatric ophthalmology,* Orlando, FL, 1985, Grune & Stratton.

98. Keith PM, Walker R: Change in thinking about old age among male guardians, *J Aging Studies* 12:255-70, 1998.

99. *The Kiplinger Washington Letter,* 69:6, 1992.

100. Kleinschmidt KC: Elder abuse—a review, *Ann Emerg Med* 30:463-72, 1997.

101. Klopfer J, Rosenberg R, Verma SB: Geriatric and rehabilitative optometry. In Newcomb RD, Marshall EC: *Public health and community optometry,* ed 2, Boston, 1990, Butterworth, pp 341-6.

102. Kogan MD, Kotelchuck M, Alexander GR et al: *Quality of health care. National Healthcare Disparities Report, 2003,* Rockville, MD, 2003, U.S. Government Printing Office.

103. Kosnik W, Fikre J, Sekulor R: Visual fixation stability in older adults, *Invest Ophthalmol Vis Sci* 27:1720-5, 1986.

104. Koval KJ, Zuckerman JD: Hip fractures: I. Overview and evaluation and treatment of femoral-neck fractures, *J Am Acad Orthop Surg* 2:141-9, 1994.

105. Krachmer JH, Mannis MJ, Holland EJ, editors: *Cornea, vol 1,* ed 2, Philadelphia, 2005, Mosby, p 251-40.

106. Kruger RM, Moon CH: Can you spot the signs of elder mistreatment? *Postgrad Med* 106:169-73, 183, 1999.

107. Lanska DJ, editor: *Recognition and initial assessment of Alzheimer's disease and related dementias.* Clinical practice guidelines #19, US Dept of Health and Human Services, Public Health Services, AHCPR Pub No 97-0702-E, Rockville, MD, 1996, chapter 2.

108. Lawler W, Eiland G: Your rights if the feds come knocking, *Med Econ* 80:59, 2003.

109. Lazarus L, Williams DT: Visual field area in phakic, aphakic, and pseudophakic individuals, *Am J Optom Physiol Opt* 65:593-7, 1988.

110. Lee AG: The new competencies and their impact on resident training in ophthalmology, *Surv Ophthalmol* 48:651-62, 2003.

111. Lee AG, Liesegang T: Increasing geriatric expertise in ophthalmology. Guest editorial, *Ophthalmology* 109:635-6, 2002.

112. Leroux C: *Coping and caring: living with Alzheimer's disease,* Washington, DC, 1986, American Association of Retired Persons, p 2.

113. Little JN, Triest RK, editors: *Seismic shifts: the economic impact of demographic change.* Federal Reserve Bank Conference, Boston, June 2000.

114. Longino CF, Bradley DE: A first look at retirement migration trends in 2000, *Gerontolotist* 43:904-7, 2003.

115. LoVecchio F, Oster N, Sturmann K, et al: The use of analgesics in patients with acute abdominal pain, *J Emerg Med* 15:775-9, 1997.

116. Lunzer, FZ: Small gadgets that can change lives, *U.S. News and World Report* March 6, 1989, pp 58-60.

117. Lyle WM: Changes in corneal astigmatism with age, *Am J Optom Arch Am Acad Optom* 48:467-78, 1971.

118. Mancil GL, Owsley C: "Vision through my aging eyes" revisited, *J Am Optom Assoc* 59: 288-94, 1988.

119. Marciniuk DD, McNab BD, Martin WT: Detection of pulmonary tuberculosis in patients with a normal chest radiograph, *Chest* 115: 445-52, 1999.

120. Margolis S, editor: Depression: it's more than just the blues, *Johns Hopkins Med Lett* 15:4, 2003.

121. Mark DB, Naylor CD, Hlatky MA: Use of medical resources and quality of life after acute myocardial infarction in Canada and the United States, *N Engl J Med* 331:1130-5, 1994.

122. Marsh GR: Sleep problems in the elderly, *Consultation—Liaison Psychiatry and Behavioral Medicine* 2:1-14, 1993.

123. Martinez GS, Campbell AJ, Reinken J, et al: Prevalence of ocular disease in a population study of subjects 65 years old and older, *Am J Ophthalmol* 94:181-9, 1982.

124. *MAXIAIDS:* Catalog 2005, ed 2, 2005, Farmingdale, NY: Maxi-Aids.

125. McGoldrick AE: Stress, early retirement, and health. In Markroles KS, Cooper CL, editors: *Aging, stress, and health,* New York, 1989, John Wiley and Sons.

126. Michaels DD: *Visual optics and refraction: a clinical approach,* ed 3, St. Louis, 1985, C.V. Mosby, p 417.

127. Morris ML, Ballard SM: Instructional techniques and environmental considerations in family life education. Programming for midlife and older adults, *Fam Relat* 52:167-73, 2003.

128. Morse AR, Friedman DB: Vision rehabilitation and aging, *Journal of Visual Impairment and Blindness* 80:803-4, 1986.

129. Morse AR, Silberman R, Trief E: Aging and visual impairment, *Journal of Visual Impairment and Blindness* 81:308-12, 1987.

130. Mummah HR, Smith EM: *The geriatric assistant,* New York, 1981, McGraw-Hill, p 151.

131. Newman BY: Health notes: preventing falls, *J Am Optom Assoc* 61:803-4, 1990.

132. Notestein FW, editor: *On population: three essays,* New York, 1960, Mentor Books, pp 13-59.

133. O'Keefe JJ Jr, Lavie CJ Jr, McCallister BD: Insights into the pathogenesis and prevention

of coronary artery disease, *Mayo Clin Proc* 70: 69-79, 1995.

134. Oquendo MA, Malone KM, Mann JJ: Suicide—risk factors and prevention in refractory major depression, *Depress Anxiety* 5: 202-11, 1997.

135. Oscherwitz T, Tulsky JP, Roger S: Detention of persistently nonadherent patients with tuberculosis, *JAMA* 278:843-6, 1997.

136. Owens A: 1995: who will be your patients? *Med Econ* 63:35-53, 1986.

137. Pace S, Burke TF: Intravenous morphine for early pain relief in patients with acute abdominal pain, *Acad Emerg Med* 15:1086-92, 1996.

138. Parker LJ, Vukov LF, Wollan PC: Emergency department evaluation of geriatric patients with acute cholecystitis, *Acad Emerg Med* 4:51-5, 1997.

139. Patten J: *Neurological differential diagnosis,* New York, 1977, Springer-Verlag, pp 105-6.

140. Peplinski LS: Ocular involvement in Behçet's disease, *J Am Optom Assoc* 60:854-57, 1989.

141. Pitts DG: Dark adaptation and aging, *J Am Optom Assoc* 53:37-41, 1982.

142. Pitts DG: The effects of aging on selected visual acuity functions: dark adaptation, visual acuity, stereopsis, and brightness contrast. In: Sekuler R, Klein D, Dismukes K, editors: *Aging and human visual functions,* New York, 1982, Alan Liss, pp 131-59.

143. Poe WD: *The old person in your home,* New York, 1989, Charles Scribner and Sons, p 16.

144. Press LJ, Moore BD: *Clinical pediatric optometry,* Boston, 1993, Butterworth-Heineman, p 38.

145. Rabins PV: Eight simple steps to an agile mind, *Johns Hopkins Med Lett Health after 50* XV:6, 2003.

146. Rabow MW, Hardie GE, Gair JM, et al: End-of-life care content in 50 textbooks from multiple specialties, *JAMA* 283:771-8, 2000.

147. Rakstis TJ: Wanted: small-town health care, *Kiwanis Magazine* 76:30-3, 1991.

148. Rives W: Emergency department assessment of suicidal patients, *Psychiatr Clin North Am* 22:779-87, 1999.

149. Rosenbloom AA: A proposed curriculum model for geriatric optometry, *J Optom Educ* 11:22-4, 1985.

150. Roybal ER: *Elder abuse: a national disgrace,* Washington, DC, 1985, United States Government Printing Office, pp 1-21.

151. Rumsey KE: Implications of biological aging to the optometric patient, *J Am Optom Assoc* 59:295-300, 1988.

152. Sacks FM, Svetkey LP, Vollmer WM, et al: Effects on blood pressure of reduced dietary sodium and the dietary approaches to stop hypertension (DASH) diet. DASH-Sodium Collaborative Research Group, *N Engl J Med* 344:3-10, 2001.

153. Samuelson R: Many US seniors could work longer, *Tulsa World* 2005; Sec. G, p 5.

154. Scharlach AE: Caregiving and employment: completing or complementary roles? *Gerontologist* 34:378-85, 1994.

155. Scheie HG, Albert DM: *Textbook of ophthalmology,* Philadelphia, 1977, W.B. Saunders, pp 462-9.

156. Schmitt EP: Sensory deprivation and remediation among the elderly, Oklahoma City, 1990, Oklahoma Geriatric Education Center, p 3.

157. Sekuler R, Kline D, Dismukes K, editors: *Aging and human visual function. Modern aging research, VII,* New York, 1982, Alan Liss.

158. Sekuler R, Owsley C: The spatial vision of older humans. In Sekuler R, Kline D, Dismukes K, editors: *Aging and human visual function. Modern Aging Research, VII,* New York, 1982, Alan Liss, pp 185-201.

159. *Senate Report #108-395. Keeping seniors safe from falls,* 108th Congress, 2d session, Calendar 785; 2004 Oct 8: Section I.

160. Shafiq-Antonacci R, Maruff P, Whyte S, et al: The effects of age and mood on saccadic function in older individuals, *J Gerontol P Psychol Sci Soc Sci* 54:361-8, 1999.

161. Shephard RJ: *Aging, physical activity, and health,* Toronto, Canada, 1997, University of Toronto.

162. Shock NW: *Aging: some social and biological aspects,* Washington, DC, 1960, American Association for the Advancement of Science, p 252.

163. Shute RH: *Psychology in vision care,* Boston, 1991, Butterworth-Heinemann, pp 114-5.

164. Siegel JA, Davidson M: *Demographic and socioeconomic aspects of aging in the United States,* Washington, DC, 1984, United States Government Printing Office, p 108.

165. Skay RM: *Gerontology: an optometric approach to aging,* Santa Ana, CA, 1984, Optometric Extension Program Foundation, pp 37-41.

166. Sohn E: Energy crisis—failing 'power plants' inside cells give rise to debilitating diseases, *U.S. News and World Report* Nov 3, 2003, pp 52-4.

167. Soroka M, Werner DL: Optometry and ophthalmology—renewed professional rivalry, *J Am Optom Assoc* 62:283-7, 1991.

168. Spirduso WW: *Physical dimensions of aging,* Champaign, IL, 1995, Human Kinetics, p 321.

169. Stephens RC, Haney CA, Underwood S: *Drug taking among the elderly. Treatment and research report,* Washington, DC, 1982, United States Government Printing Office, p 21.

170. Stern EM: Ross M: *You and your aging parents,* New York, 1965, Harper and Row, p 194.

171. Swanson MW: The elderly. In Benjamin WJ, editor: *Borish's clinical refraction,* Philadelphia, 1998, W.B. Saunders, p 1197.

172. Swisher K, editor: *The elderly: opposing viewpoints,* San Diego, CA, 1990, Greenhaven Press.

173. Taeuber CM: *America in transition—an aging society,* Washington, DC, 1983, U.S. Government Printing Office, p 3.

174. Thompson T: Future shortages in long-term care, *Public Health Rep* 118:480, 2003.

175. Tideiksaar R, Kay AD: What causes falls: a logical diagnostic procedure, *Geriatrics* 42:32-50, 1986.

176. Tonner PH, Kampen J, Scholz J: Pathophysiological changes in the elderly, *Best Pract Res Clin Anaesthesiol* 17:163-77, 2003.

177. Trilling JS, Froom J: The urgent need to improve hypertension care, *Arch Fam Med* 9:794-801, 2000.

178. Turano KA, Broman AT, Bandeen-Roche K, et al: Association of visual field loss and mobility performance in older adults: Salisbury eye evaluation study, *Optom Vis Sci* 81:298-307, 2004.

179. Uhlmann RF, Larson EB, Rees TS, et al: Relationship of hearing impairment on dementia and cognitive dysfunction in older adults, *JAMA* 261:1916-9, 1989.

180. U.S. Census Bureau: *National data book 2000, statistical abstract of the United States,* ed 122, Washington, DC, 2000, U.S. Government Printing Office, p 54.

181. Verghese J, Lipton RB, Hall CB, et al: Abnormality of gait as a predictor of non-Alzheimer dementia, *N Engl J Med* 347:1761-8, 2002.

182. Verghese J, Lipton RB, Katz MJ, et al: Leisure activities and the risk of dementia in the elderly, *N Eng J Med* 348:2508-16, 2003.

183. Verma SB: Geriatric optometry—today and tomorrow, *J Optom Educ* 7:9-11, 1982.

184. Verma SB: Vision care for the elderly: problems and directions, *J Am Optom Assoc* 60:296-9, 1989.

185. Warshaw GA, Bragg EJ, Shaull RW, et al: Academic geriatric programs in US allopathic and osteopathic medical schools, *JAMA* 288:2313-9, 2002.

186. Weale RA: *A biography of the eye: development, growth, age,* London 1982, H. K. Lewis, p 13-8.

187. Williams DT: Aging and central visual field area, *Am J Optom Physiol Opt* 60:888-91, 1983.

188. Wilson RJ, Hoffman DJ: Optometry in the multidisciplinary health care setting, *Optom Vis Sci* 66:859-63, 1989.

189. Wilson SE: Socioeconomic status and the prevalence of health problems among married couples in late life, *Am J Public Health* 91:131-5, 2001.

190. Wolfe SM, editor: *Drug induced psychiatric symptoms (part 1 and 2), worst pills, best pills.* Washington, DC, 2002, Public Citizen Health Research Group, pp 73-5, 81-5.

191. Wolfson C, Wolfson DB, Asgharian M, et al: A reevaluation of the duration of survival after the onset of dementia, *N Engl J Med* 344:1111-6, 2001.

192. Wright J: Days Inn policy proves value of senior workers, *Tulsa World* March 17, 1991, Sec. D-3.

## SUGGESTED READINGS

Bressler NM, Bressler SB, West SK, et al: The grading and prevalence of macular degeneration in Chesapeake Bay watermen, *Arch Ophthalmol* 107:847-52, 1989.

Broyles, G: Guardianship puts elderly at mercy of unscrupulous, *Tulsa World* Sept 20, 1987, Sec. A-1.

Carney J: Can a car driver be too old? *Time* Jan 16, 1989, p 28.

Garnett WR, Barr WH, *Geriatric pharmacokinetics,* Kalamazoo, MI, 1984, Upjohn, p 14.

Goroll A, May L, Mullen A: *Primary care medicine,* ed 2, Philadelphia, 1987, Lippincott, pp 449-51.

Gramm S, Barker A: Sensory deprivation training for your office staff, *J Am Optom Assoc* 53:53-4, 1982.

Klein SD, Klein RE: Delivering bad news: the most challenging task in patient education, *J Am Optom Assoc* 58:660-3, 1987.

Kornzweiz AL: The eye in old age. In Rossman I, editor: *Clinical geriatrics,* ed 2, Philadelphia, 1979, J.B. Lippincott.

Kovar MG, Hendershot G, Mathis E: Older people in the United States who receive help with basic activities of daily living, *Am J Public Health* 79:778-9, 1989.

Krieger N, Ketcher G Fulk G: Physiological variables affecting intraocular pressure in a population study, *Am J Optom Physiol Opt* 65:739-44, 1988.

Penisten D: Optometry's 100-year wars, *Review of Optometry* 128:40-3, 1991.

Pirozzolo FJ, Maletta GJ, editors: *The aging nervous system, vol I,* New York, 1980, Praeger, p 50.

Pitts DG: Visual acuity as a function of age, *J Am Optom Assoc* 53:117-24, 1982.

Reisner R: Two professions: two perceptions, *Optometric Management* 26:19-26, 1990.

Ressler LE: Improving elderly recall with bimodal presentation, *Gerontologist* 31:364-70, 1991.

Sheras V: *The 'sandwich generation' cares for aging parents,* Little Rock, AK, 1990, Arkansas Aging Foundation, p 2.

Soroka M: A comparison of charges by optometrists and ophthalmologists under the Medicare program, *J Am Optom Assoc* 62:372-6, 1991.

Stelmack TR: Management of open-angle glaucoma, *J Am Optom Assoc* 58:716-21, 1987.

Vingerling JR, Klaver CC, Hofman A, et al: Epidemiology of age-related maculopathy, *Epidemiol Rev* 17:347-60, 1995.

# CHAPTER 2

# Normal Age-Related Vision Changes

## GUNILLA HAEGERSTROM-PORTNOY and MEREDITH W. MORGAN

This chapter is limited to changes in visual function in the normal, healthy, aging eye that is free from obvious structural or pathological anomalies. This restriction may raise some practical as well as philosophical problems because few eyes that have survived 65 or more years are free from at least some slight sign of deterioration, degeneration, or past or present disease that can escape a scientific, sophisticated search. This chapter uses the concept of "normal" in much the same way the average clinician states that an amblyopic eye is normal—in that it has no immediately apparent structural or pathological defect that could account for reduced acuity. Such an eye is obviously not normal because it has less than normal acuity. In an amblyopic eye, no apparent cause for the reduced acuity is readily found. Conditions that apply to most aged eyes, such as miosis and the absence of accommodation, are considered normal rather than abnormal or pathological.

This approach is used for two main reasons: (1) pathological and degenerative conditions affecting the aging eye are discussed in other chapters, and (2) departure from normal function is a clue that a more detailed and critical examination and search need to be made. This requires that the examiner know what normal function is. Unfortunately, most clinical optometric norms have been established with data from subjects without presbyopia.

The major thrust of the discussion is about the aspects of vision of chief concern to clinicians and ordinarily measured by them. Some attention, however, is given to phenomena that today are primarily of interest to visual scientists but that will someday also be of concern to optometrists. Most of the significant changes in visual function of the aging eye, except for the loss of focusing ability and the increase in variability of measured functions, are not quantified by clinicians in the usual vision examination. Currently nearly all ophthalmologists, as well as most optometrists, assume that aging patients without significant motor imbalance and with good corrected visual acuity at distance and near must have satisfactory or normal visually controlled behavior and therefore need no therapy other than corrective lenses. Some visual scientists, as well as some optometrists, suggest a more sophisticated and comprehensive view of vision is possible.[67]

The increase in variability or dispersion of measured function with increasing age applies to nearly all visual functions. This makes it extremely difficult to identify performance that is clearly subnormal. Some older persons do function as well as younger ones, but the number with "best performance" usually declines with age. For example, Weymouth,[121] using data supplied by Hirsch, reported that in the age bracket of 40 to 44 years 93.5% of patients had a corrected visual acuity of 20/20 or better; in the age bracket from 70 to 74 years, however, only 41.9% had a corrected visual acuity of 20/20 or better, and 56.1% had a corrected visual acuity of 20/40 or better. Most of this decrease in the percentage of individuals with maximum acuity and the greater variability in best-corrected acuity is caused by the effects of degeneration or disease conditions. Some of the decrease, however, cannot be accounted for on that basis. In the 70- to 74-year-old age group, 14.5% of the patients with corrected visual acuity of less than 20/25 had no clinically reportable degenerative or disease conditions; the eyes were clinically normal but visual acuity was not.

Many of the apparent physiological or psychological changes in visual function have a physical cause. Consequently, this chapter first discusses changes in the structure of the eye that could result in a change in visual function and that are detected by clinicians in routine vision examinations. Most of the biometric data discussed are cross-sectional in nature; that is, the data were collected from different subjects, usually without regard to size or sex, at different times and frequently by different examiners using different techniques. Therefore differences in measurements between individuals attributed primarily to age can be only tentatively accepted. Most biometric data concerning the eye, such as length of the eyeball, depth of the anterior chamber, and radius of curvature of the cornea, are smaller for women than for men; smaller adults have smaller eyes. For each decade during the past several decades, human beings have become somewhat larger. Thus changes that indicate that the eyes of older persons are smaller in any dimension may be caused by the fact that older adults are, on average, smaller than younger adults.

## CHANGES IN THE CORNEA WITH AGE

Corneal sensitivity to touch decreases with age. According to Millodot,[80] the threshold for touch almost doubles between the ages of 10 and 80 years, increasing rapidly after the age of 40 years. The cause for this decrease is not known. It is both an advantage and a disadvantage in fitting contact lenses; older patients adapt more readily to contact lenses, but corneal lesions may occur without creating significant subjective symptoms of pain. Millodot and Owens[82] also demonstrated that as corneal sensitivity decreases, the corneal fragility increases in a mirror-image pattern. They found that considerably less pressure is required to damage the corneal epithelium in adults older than 60 years than in younger adults. This combination of reduced sensitivity and increased fragility increases the risk for contact lens wearers. The practitioner, particularly with older patients, should not depend on the presence of symptoms to suggest that the integrity of the cornea needs to be carefully examined at regular intervals.

Reports of the increase in against-the-rule astigmatism in older people have been published since before von Helmholtz. Most cross-sectional studies of refractive error and age confirm this trend. Does this change in the meridian of greatest refractive power of the eye from the 90-degree meridian in youth to the 180-degree meridian in old age signify that the curvature of the cornea changes with age? In 1924, von Helmholtz believed that the natural form of the cornea was such that the meridian of greatest curvature was horizontal, but that the cornea was deformed in youth by the pressure of the lids so that the greatest curvature was vertical in youth. As the lid tension decreases and the ocular tissues harden with age, the cornea goes back to its natural form.[113]

The concept that the corneal curvature changes with age seems to be confirmed by the studies of Kratz and Walton[65] and Phillips.[89] Kratz and Walton reported from a study of clinical records that the best estimate for the correction of astigmatism based on keratometric findings was achieved when the allowance for physiological astigmatism in Javal's formula remained at 0.50 D for all ages. They argued that because the total astigmatism increases against-the-rule throughout life, the cause of the increase must be a change in corneal astigmatism. Their actual data, originally presented in graphic form, are summarized in Table 2-1. The data seem to support the concept that the number of patients having with-the-rule astigmatism decreases with age. Phillips' data from a clinical practice in Great Britain are shown in Table 2-2.

The data from Kratz and Walton and Phillips are unfortunately in relative terms, showing the difference in power of the two principal meridians. Vertical power, and hence the curvature, cannot be categorically stated to have decreased or that horizontal power, and hence the curvature, increased.

**TABLE 2-1**

## Corneal Astigmatism in Kratz and Walton Study

| | Against-the-Rule | With-the-Rule | |
| Decade | Corneal Astigmatism (%) | Corneal Astigmatism (%) | No Corneal Astigmatism (%) |
|---|---|---|---|
| 2 | 18 | 80 | 2 |
| 5 | 11 | 78 | 11 |
| 8 | 30 | 20 | 50 |
| 9 | 75 | 25 | 0 |

Adapted from Kratz JD, Walton WG: A modification of Javal's rule for the correction of astigmatism, *Am J Optom Arch Am. Acad Optom* 26:302, 1942, Copyright 1949 American Academy of Optometry.
Number of patients at each decade is unknown.

In a longitudinal study of 46 patients over a period of 0.5 to 20 years, Exford[31] reported that corneal power in both the horizontal and vertical meridians increased at a rate slightly less than 0.25 D per decade and that no trend was observed that either meridian changed more rapidly than the other.

Mason[75] reported on 475 eyes of people aged 12 to 39 years and 475 eyes of people aged 45 to 79 years. All eyes had at least a 0.25 D with-the-rule corneal astigmatism as measured with a keratometer. Of the younger group, 22% required against-the-rule corrections, whereas 41% of the older group required such corrections. Mason's data, originally presented in graphic form, are restated in Table 2-3.

The data of Mason indicate that some portion of the increase in against-the-rule astigmatism with age must be accounted for on some other basis than changes in corneal curvature because even with matched corneal astigmatisms, more people in the older group had against-the-rule astigmatism than did those in the younger group.

More recent data, however, indicate that the power of the cornea does increase with age, particularly in the horizontal meridian. Baldwin and Mills[3] found, from a retrospective study of longitudinal data from private optometric practice, that the horizontal meridian of the corneas of the same individuals became somewhat steeper over time. Their data are shown in Table 2-4. Anstice[1] reported somewhat similar data (Table 2-5).

Reporting only on the radius of a single meridian, Fledelius[35] reported that the cornea steepens. Unfortunately he did not give both meridians, but he did report separately on men and women. His data are given in Table 2-6.

More recent studies using corneal topography on 734 observers ranging in age from the 20s to the 80s report a linear increase in corneal curvature in the horizontal meridian with age.[47] The vertical meridian also steepened with age but with a much shallower slope. Between the ages of 60 and 70 years, the average cornea was reported to be spherical; after age 70 years, against-the-rule astigmatism became the rule.

Thus with age it appears that the horizontal meridian of the cornea becomes steeper while the vertical changes less. Consequently, the prevalence of against-the-rule astigmatism significantly increases with increasing age. For example, in a random sample of 569 community-living older adults, nearly 50% of those aged

**TABLE 2-2**

## Corneal Astigmatism According to Phillips

| | Against-the-Rule | With-the-Rule | | |
| Age (yr) | Astigmatism (%) | Astigmatism (%) | No Astigmatism (%) | No. Patients |
|---|---|---|---|---|
| 10-20 | 6.8 | 75.5 | 12.7 | 164 |
| 20-30 | 8.2 | 72.3 | 19.5 | 268 |
| 30-40 | 17.7 | 64.1 | 18.2 | 204 |
| 40-50 | 25.6 | 46.9 | 27.5 | 320 |
| 50-60 | 31.7 | 40.5 | 27.8 | 356 |
| 60-70 | 33.9 | 37.7 | 28.4 | 239 |
| 70-80 | 35.0 | 37.2 | 27.8 | 140 |

Adapted from Phillips RA: Changes in corneal astigmatism, *Am J Optom Arch Am Acad. Optom.* 29:379, 1952. Copyright 1952 American Academy of Optometry.

**TABLE 2-3**

## Comparison of Corneal and Ametropic Astigmatism

| With-the-Rule Corneal Astigmatism (D) | Ametropic Astigmatism | | | |
|---|---|---|---|---|
| | Age 12-39 Years | | Ages 45-75 Years | |
| | Against (%) | With (%) | Against (%) | With (%) |
| 0.25 | 40 | 22 | 50 | 10 |
| 0.50 | 21 | 41 | 41 | 30 |
| 0.75 | 15 | 52 | 20 | 45 |
| 1.00 | 9 | 67 | 10 | 55 |
| 1.25 | 5 | 70 | 9 | 65 |
| 1.50 | 2 | 87 | 1 | 66 |
| 1.75 | 1 | 90 | 1 | 67 |
| 2.00 | 1 | 99 | 1 | 88 |

Adapted from Mason FL: *Principles of optometry,* San Francisco, 1940, Carlisle, pp 400-1.
The percentage of those with 0.00 D cylindrical correction for astigmatism has been omitted.

85 years and older had 1.00 D or greater against-the rule astigmatism, whereas as many as 20% in the same age group showed 2.00 D or greater against-the-rule astigmatism.[44] Other recent population studies have demonstrated the same effect.[40]

## CHANGES IN THE ANTERIOR CHAMBER WITH AGE

Weale,[116] quoting Johansen and Raeder, stated that the depth of the anterior chamber decreases from an average of 3.6 mm in the age range of 15 to 20 years to an average of 3.0 mm by 70 years because of growth of the lens. A decrease in the depth of the anterior chamber could make the angle of the anterior chamber at the root of the iris more acute, thus increasing the possibility of interference with aqueous outflow. Likewise, if all other factors remain constant, a decrease in the anterior chamber depth slightly increases the refractive power of the eye, making the eye relatively more myopic. The chemical composition and refractive index of the aqueous appear to be independent of age.

## CHANGES IN THE IRIS WITH AGE

One of the most significant changes in the older eye is senile miosis.[6,117] In addition, the difference in diameter of the pupil in the light- and dark-adapted states becomes less and less. The cause of the miosis is not known but is thought to be the atrophy of the dilator muscle fibers, an increased rigidity of the iris blood vessels, or both. In any event, the pupil becomes smaller at all levels of illumination. The linear loss with age varies from 0.43 mm per decade for low photopic light levels to 0.15 mm per decade for high photopic light levels.[122] These authors also found that pupil size was independent of sex and refractive error. A small increase in the latency of pupillary responses has been found with advancing age.[32,88]

This miosis reduces retinal illuminance and the diameter of retinal blur circles when the eye is out of focus. Consequently, at high levels of illumination, uncorrected visual acuity may appear to improve rather than decrease with age. Likewise, the range of clear vision at near through any addition appears to increase with age, giving the appearance of accommodative change. This miosis makes it difficult to examine the fundus or other structures of the eye

**TABLE 2-4**

## The Longitudinal Change in the Corneal and Refractive Astigmatism over an Approximately 13-Year Period

| Factor | Average Age: 52 Years | | Average Age: 65 Years | |
|---|---|---|---|---|
| | Vertical | Horizontal | Vertical | Horizontal |
| Refraction | +1.09 D | +0.85 D | +1.91 D | +1.15 D |
| Change: 13 years | | | +0.82 D | +0.30 D |
| Cornea | 43.86 D | 43.48 D | 43.93 D | 43.86 D |
| Change: power | | +0.07 D | +0.33 D | |
| Change: radius | | −0.01 mm | −0.07 mm | |
| Refractive astigmatism | −0.24 DC ax 90 | | −0.75 DC ax 90 | |
| Corneal astigmatism | −0.38 DC ax 180 | | −0.07 DC ax 180 | |

Adapted from Baldwin W, Mills D: A longitudinal study of corneal astigmatism and total astigmatism, *Am J Optom Physiol Opt* 58:206-11, 1981.

**TABLE 2-5**

### Cross-Sectional Data of the Differences in Corneal and Refractive Astigmatism of Patients Between the Ages of 25 and 39 Years and Patients Between the Ages of 70 and 74 Years

|  | Mean Astigmatism | |
| --- | --- | --- |
|  | Ages 25-39 Years | Ages 70-74 Years |
| Corneal | −0.75 DC ax 180 | −0.15 DC ax 180 |
| Refractive | −0.30 DC ax 180 | −0.40 DC ax 90 |
| Change, corneal |  | −0.55 DC ax 90 |
| Change, refractive |  | −0.70 DC ax 90 |

Adapted from Anstice J: Astigmatism—its components and their changes with age, *Am J Optom Arch Am Acad Optom* 48:1001-6, 1971.

**TABLE 2-6**

### Cross-Sectional Data of the Mean Corneal Curvature of Patients Between the Ages of 36 and 40 Years and Patients Approximately Age 77 Years

|  | Ages 36-40 Years | Age Approximately 77 Years |
| --- | --- | --- |
| Radius of curvature, M | 7.99 ± 0.29 mm | 7.85 ± 0.27 mm |
| Radius of curvature, F | 7.83 ± 0.20 mm | 7.77 ± 0.27 mm |
| Change, curvature, M |  | −0.14 mm |
| Change, curvature, F |  | −0.06 mm |

Adapted from Fledelius H: Refraction and eye size in the elderly, *Arch Ophthalmol* 66:241-8, 1988.

through the undilated pupil. Subjective refraction becomes more difficult because changes in lens power do not change the diameter of retinal blur circles as much as a similar change in eyes with larger pupils. This means that the optometrist must be prepared to use a 0.50 or 0.75 D instead of the usual 0.37 D crossed cylinder to determine the magnitude and axis of any astigmatism. In other words, the older patient may be less sensitive to lens changes than the younger person because of optical reasons rather than because of any decrease in observational abilities caused by supposed senility.

## CHANGES IN THE LENS WITH AGE

The lens of the eye continues to grow throughout life. Weale,[116] quoting Johansen and Raeder, states that the axial thickness of the lens increases linearly by approximately 28% by age 70 years over that which existed at age 15 to 20 years. This means that if the lens is assumed to be 3.6 mm thick at age 15 to 20 years (the Gullstrand standard), then by age 70 years it will be approximately 4.6 mm thick. The nuclear thickness remains constant while the cortical thicknesses increase. On average, the anterior cortex increases by 0.6 mm and the posterior by 0.4 mm. By using distortion-corrected Scheimpflug photography, Dubbelman et al[26] reported a 4.6-mm axial thickness at age 70 years and 3.4-mm axial thickness at age 20 years.

The transverse or equatorial diameter of the lens appears to increase at a somewhat slower rate than the axial thickness.[8,76,116] In the past, most authorities had assumed that if the lens becomes larger overall from the continuous laying down of new fibers just under the capsule posteriorly and just under the epithelium anteriorly, then it must also become flatter. To quote Duke-Elder,[27] "In this way the lens becomes continuously flatter with age."

Measurements of the curvature of the lens surfaces with slit-lamp techniques indicate that the radius of the central portion of the anterior lens surface decreases by approximately 1 mm per decade between the ages of 40 and 70 years and that the radius of the central portion of the posterior surface remains almost constant (Fig. 2-1).[8,73] Recent results from Dubbelman et al,[26] using distortion-corrected Scheimpflug photography found less of a change in the anterior lens radius and confirmed the nearly constant posterior lens radius. In this study, the radius of the 3-mm zone of the anterior lens surface decreased linearly at the rate of 0.57 mm per decade while the radius of the 3-mm zone of the posterior lens surface decreased linearly at the rate of 0.12 mm per decade. Subjects (n = 102) ranged in age from 16 to 65 years. Their results resembled the results of other studies that used phakometry to assess the curvature of the lens, and the values are similar to the Gullstrand nonaccommodated schematic eye.[48]

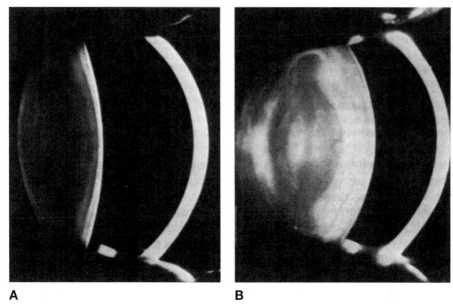

**A**                                          **B**

**Fig. 2-1** Biomicroscopic images of the eye of a 10-year-old boy (**A**) and an 82-year-old man (**B**) to the same scale. These photographs clearly indicate the increase in lens thickness, the decrease in the depth of the anterior chamber, and the apparent increase in the curvature of the lens with increasing age. (From Brown N: The change in lens curvature with age, *Exp Eye Res* 19:175-83, 1974.)

Such an increase in curvature of the anterior lens surface is compatible with the observation that the axial thickness increases faster than the equatorial. However, these comparisons of the physical parameters of the crystalline lens are based on cross-sectional data without regard to the physical size of the subjects.

The lens substance is yellow, not crystal clear; thus, as the lens thickens, it absorbs more and more light selectively.[16,77,98,118] This increase in absorption is caused to a large extent by the increased thickness, but pigment deposition in the nucleus is also increased while the concentration in the cortex does not change but the path length increases.[77] As the lens grows, it accumulates two fluorogens, one of which is activated by light of wavelength 345 nm and emits light of wavelength 420 nm.[69,100] In addition, the mass of some protein molecules of high molecular weight increases toward the nucleus of the lens. In some cases, the index of refraction of these high-mass molecules is greater than the index of their environment, and they can, under some conditions, act as scatter points for light.[111]

The miosis and the growth of the lens do alter visual performance. According to Weale[115-117] and Cullinin,[17] the amount of light reaching the retina in a normal 60-year-old is only roughly one third that reaching the retina of a 20-year-old. This means that an older person must use significantly more light to achieve the same level of retinal illumination as that achieved by a younger person. Mesopia and scotopia occur at higher levels of ambient luminance. In addition, the useful light reaching the retina may be attenuated by fluorescence and scatter. Both fluorescence and scatter tend to reduce contrast. The visual performance of an older person is usually impaired at twilight.

The yellow pigment of the lens absorbs the short wavelengths more than the long. Thus older adults have a decreased sensitivity at the violet end of the spectrum. White objects may appear yellow, and the distinction between blues and greens is decreased. For example, the distinction between a light green wall and a blue-green carpet become less marked with age. Also, the color differences between dark grey and dark brown are less. Because older individuals of the same age show great variation, stating that any given 70-year-old will have significant difficulty with color perception is not accurate. However, color vision of those older than 55 years should be checked at regular intervals.

Contrary to the assumption of many clinicians, not much direct evidence shows that the index of refraction of the lens substance changes with age in the normal eye.[36,86,90,91] However, several authors have calculated the refractive index as a function of age on an individual basis by using biometric data from each subject. Dubbelman and Van der Heijde[25] reported a significant linear decrease in equivalent refractive index with age, and Koretz and Cook[62] stated that according to their calculations, the lens refractive power decreases by approximately 2.00 D during a 50-year period between ages 20 and 70 years because of lens index changes.

The common clinical concept that the lens substance becomes significantly harder and less pliable with age is supported by the fact that the amplitude of accommodation decreases with age and ultimately becomes essentially 0 by the sixth decade of life. However, little direct research data support this concept. Fisher[34] has stated that the reason the lens becomes more difficult to deform with increasing age is not because of lenticular sclerosis, but rather because the capsule loses its elastic force and the lens fibers become more compacted.

Likewise, little or no evidence exists for atrophy or sclerosis of the ciliary muscle.[116,117] In fact, the evidence seems to indicate hypertrophy of the ciliary muscle. Depending somewhat on the supporting pressure exerted by the vitreous, the mechanical aspects of the suspension of the crystalline lens in relation to the ciliary muscle must change as the lens increases in size with age. However, a change great enough to reduce the amplitude of accommodation to practically 0 should increase the static power of the eye as well as reaction time.

## CHANGES IN THE VITREOUS WITH AGE

Millodot[79] found that the magnitude of the chromatic aberration of the eye decreases with age in both the phakic and aphakic eye. Millodot and Leary[81] found that the discrepancy between the magnitude of the ametropia determined by skiametry and subjective methods changes from plus to minus with increasing age. Both observations can be explained if the index of refraction of the vitreous is assumed to increase with age. This would also help explain the loss of reflectance of the fundus observed with an ophthalmoscope and the increase in hyperopia that occurs in the "normal" aging eye. Goodside[37] presented evidence that supports this hypothesis.

If the index of the vitreous increased enough to introduce a concave surface into the refractive system of the eye, to account for the decrease in chromatic aberration the refractive power of the eye would become markedly reduced, and the increase in hypermetropia would be much greater than that reported for the aging eye. This decrease in power could be compensated for in the presence of a corresponding increase in the refractive power of the cornea and lens, as the data seem to indicate. These changes must be investigated more fully before Millodot's hypothesis can be assumed correct.

In addition to a possible change in the refractive index, the vitreous appears to be subject to liquefaction and syneresis with age, which results in an increase in the speed and amplitude of the movements of vitreous floaters and a decreased support for the posterior lens surface. Ordinarily, muscae volitantes have no effect on vision except to give older people something to watch in an otherwise empty field or when bored. Sometimes, however, they can be very distracting during reading.

## RETINAL AND NEURAL CONNECTION CHANGES WITH AGE

The changes in the retina and the neural connections that can accompany the normal aging process are largely inferential rather than directly observable in the normal eye. Consequently, this section emphasizes the changes in visual function rather than observed changes in the retina or neural connections. However, some recent data on cone/rod density and nerve fiber layer density changes with age deserve mention.

Curcio et al[18] measured cone density in human retinas from donors ranging in age from 27 to 90 years and found no consistent change in cone density with age. The number of foveal cones was also stable with age. Thus the loss of acuity found with age in the absence of disease is not caused by a loss of photoreceptors. They did find a significant loss of rod density (as much as 30%) in the central retina but the remaining rods increased in size, maintaining stable rod coverage. Thus losses in scotopic function with age are either optical or postreceptoral. Lovasik et al[72] reported an approximately 20% to 30% thinning of the retinal nerve fiber layer in healthy older subjects (75 to 88 years), particularly in the superior quadrant, with concomitant loss of pattern evoked potential in the same area. The functional impact of these anatomical changes in daily life is unknown.[72]

Clinicians usually assess the integrity of the retina and the visual system by direct observation (ophthalmoscopy and biomicroscopy); the determination of corrected visual acuity; the size and shape of the visual fields using various methods, including the Amsler grid; and contrast sensitivity. On occasion stereoacuity may be determined, and even less frequently, performance on one of the color vision screening and glare sensitivity tests may be determined.

In the absence of a pathological condition, most decline in static corrected visual acuity with age up to approximately age 70 years is accounted for by miosis and the increased density of the lens.[92] In general, however, the number of individuals achieving 20/10 to 20/25 visual acuity declines with age. According to the Framingham study, 95.4% of individuals in the age group from 52 to 64 years have corrected acuity between 20/10 and 20/25.[57] In the age group from 65 to 74 years, this figure declines to 91.9%, and in the age group from 75 to 85 years, it becomes 69.1%. The major causes of this decline for the 75 to 85 years age group are cataract (46%), macular degeneration (28%), glaucoma (7.2%), and general retinal disease (7%). However, an apparent cause for the failure to achieve at least 20/25 acuity cannot be determined for approximately 10% of the patients between ages 75 and 85 years. As age increases, the number of patients apparently free from ocular disease who achieve normal corrected acuity decreases.

Elliott et al[29] compiled visual acuity data by using log MAR charts from several of their previous studies in people with normal ocular health who were tested with best correction. The mean high-contrast visual acuity for those aged 75 years and older (n = 20) was –0.02 or 20/20 +1, an acuity value considerably higher than that reported by Pitts[93] and Weale[119] in their reviews. Elliott et al suggest that strict exclusion criteria and nontruncated charts contributed to their much better results. Unfortunately, they also used acuity to eliminate subjects. Rubin et al[97] reported median high-contrast acuity with best correction in a large random sample (that included observers with ocular disease). The median visual acuity, which worsened linearly with age, became worse than 20/20 at approximately age 75 years. Median values are usually better than means, but no means were reported for direct comparison with other studies.

The size of the visual field as measured under standard conditions decreases with age. That is, the 1/1000 isopter for the average normal 60-year-old will be inside that of an average normal 20-year-old, even when the pupil is controlled.[10,12,19,23] This does not necessarily mean that neural function is diminished because the density of the lens will reduce retinal illuminance even when pupil size is controlled. The retinal illuminance will be reduced even more by light scatter within the eye. Consequently, a slightly reduced field cannot be taken as positive evidence that neural function is reduced. With multiple target presentations and short exposure times, as frequently used in automated perimetry, a more significant loss of field with age than with kinetic perimetry seems to occur. Johnson and Marshal[56] found a linear loss of sensitivity with age in normal observers ranging in age from 20 to 83 years. Standard white-on-white automated perimetry produced a loss of 0.7 dB per decade, and shortwavelength automated perimetry resulted in a much more significant loss of 1.6 dB per decade even after correction for lens density, suggesting additional neural loss in the S cone pathway. Johnson et al[55] had previously shown that even if stimulus conditions are altered to minimize pupil and lens effects, a loss of visual field sensitivity with age of approximately 0.8 dB per decade still occurs in normal observers free of ocular disease. Thus much of the loss of visual field sensitivity with age must be ascribed to neural changes.

The presence of scotomas, or areas of reduced sensitivity, as well as sudden changes in the visual field, is more important than a slightly reduced field. The clinician must make comparisons between recent fields. This means that the visual field should be determined and recorded at regular intervals in the aging patient.

Although individuals with excellent stereopsis do not necessarily have a good ability to judge distance, they do have good binocular motor and sensory integration. Thus the determination of stereoacuity can aid the optometrist in judging whether a patient's visual neural system is functioning properly. Likewise, the integrity of the monocular visual neural system can be judged from a determination of vernier acuity. Vernier acuity can be determined more easily in eyes with a poor optical system (with corneal or lenticular opacities) than visual acuity can; hence it should prove useful in cataractous eyes.

Hofstetter and Bertsch[53] reported that stereoacuity does not decline with age (up to age 42 years, at least) in individuals with good visual acuity. Pitts[92] suspected that stereopsis would decrease with age after 50 years in a randomly selected sample of the population. Zaroff et al[123] tested random dot stereoacuity for brief (100 ms) presentations in 160 normal observers with acuity of 20/30 or better in each eye. The subjects ranged in age from 15 to 79 years. The mean stereo threshold for observers from 15 to 59 years was 37 arc sec. More than 90% of observers younger than 60 years were classified as stereonormal (within ±2 SD or better than 109 arc sec), but fewer than 40% of subjects between ages 60 and 69 years and fewer than 30% of subjects aged 70 to 79 years could be classified as stereonormal. This loss of fine stereoacuity for random dot targets without monocular cues is likely to be of cortical origin.

Vernier alignment thresholds, on the other hand, are fairly robust with normal aging.[30] They are also highly resistant to image degradation, as noted, and can be used to assess neural function in eyes with cataract.

As previously discussed, older adults experience changes in the ability to discriminate colors The spectrum shortens on the violet end, the ability to discriminate blues from blue-greens is lessened, and white objects appear yellow so that the older individuals may have difficulty discriminating between white and unsaturated yellow, between pastel violets and yellow-greens, and between dark browns and grays. These changes occur in the absence of disease and degeneration. Because subtle changes in color vision may be the first sign of disease, the color vision of aging patients should be determined at regular intervals and comparisons made between the eyes of the same individual as well as with a standard. Recently, updated age norms for observers without ocular disease have been published for the Farnsworth-Munsell 100 Hue test, a test of chromatic discrimination often used in the clinic.[59]

The fact that mesopia and scotopia occur at higher levels of ambient illumination in older individuals means that the difficulty with color discrimination that occurs after sunset occurs earlier in the evening for older persons.

All the usual tests of sensory neural integrity may show small but definite decrements in the absence of disease or degeneration.

In clinical testing, such as the determination of visual acuity (spatial resolution), illumination, contrast, and time are optimal rather than near threshold. Also, extraneous stimuli such as competing peripheral objects in the visual field are kept to a minimum. Usually the only significant competing objects in the field of view are optotypes adjacent to the one being resolved. In the real world, however, discrimination, identification, and resolution must frequently be made under low levels of illumination and poor contrast, in the presence of glare, and with competing stimuli located nearby or peripherally to the object of regard and with some stimuli being presented on a variable time scale. As an example, Haegerstrom-Portnoy et al[43] measured acuity under different conditions of contrast, illumination, and glare by using habitual correction in a random population of 900 older observers ranging in age from 58 to 102 years. For those older than 80 years, median standard high-contrast acuity was 20/33. Reducing the contrast from more than 90% to approximately 15% changed the median acuity to 20/66. Reducing the background illumination by a factor of 10 (and keeping contrast at approximately 15%) caused the median acuity to drop to 20/152 while adding glare to a low-contrast acuity chart resulted in a median acuity of

20/214. Performance under adverse conditions could not be predicted on an individual basis from the standard measures of high-contrast acuity, emphasizing the importance of making the measurements on an individual basis.[45]

Different stimuli have a masking effect on each other when adjacent in both space and time. Frequently this masking effect becomes exaggerated or increased when there is deterioration in the visual system some way. Perhaps the best-known example of the effect is the significant improvement in the visual acuity of amblyopic eyes when optotypes are presented one at a time in a restricted field rather than a line or whole chart at a time.

The marked reduction in retinal illuminance with increasing age resulting from miosis, lens absorption, and light scatter already has been discussed briefly, but little has been said concerning contrast, spatial, and temporal interaction.

## CHANGES IN DARK ADAPTATION WITH AGE

Most investigators report that the absolute level of adaptation reached by older adults is less than that reached by younger individuals. Older studies were unclear whether a difference in the rate of adaptation exists.[7,22] However, a recent study testing adults free from ocular disease and correcting for pupil size and lens density differences on an individual basis found a significant delay in rod-mediated dark adaptation in addition to elevated final thresholds.[54] The time required to reach prebleach sensitivity for those in their 70s was more than 10 minutes longer than for those in their 20s. The authors suggest a neural basis for the delay: a slowing of the rhodopsin regeneration. The rate of foveal cone–mediated dark adaptation also slows with age.[15] Mesopia and scotopia occur at higher levels of ambient illumination in older adults than in the young.[12]

## CHANGES IN RECOVERY FROM GLARE WITH AGE

Paulson and Sjöstrand[87] and Reading,[95] among others, have reported that older adults are more sensitive to glare than are younger patients. This is indicated by an increase in reaction and redetection time in the presence of a glare source.

Severin et al,[105,106] among others, advocated a "photostress" test measuring the time required for functional recovery to a specified visual acuity after exposure to a measured flash of light. Elliott and Whitaker[28] have shown a steady increase in glare recovery time with age in normal adults even when differences in lens density and pupil size were taken into account. An exponential function fit their data well; the average glare recovery time for those in their 20s was approximately 10 seconds, whereas those in their 80s required 25 seconds to recover to an acuity target one line larger than that read before glare exposure. This measure thus reflects neural changes in the ability of the retina to recover.

## CONTRAST SENSITIVITY CHANGES WITH AGE

Even in the absence of a glare source, Sekuler[101] and Sekuler and Hutmann[103] have reported that older individuals are only one third as sensitive to low spatial frequencies (below 4 cycles/degree) as younger people are. This loss of contrast sensitivity at low frequencies has not been borne out by a more carefully controlled investigation.[104] If care is used to be certain that the subjects have the proper optical correction and are free from disease and degenerative conditions, it becomes apparent that older people exhibit sensitivity losses predominantly at intermediate and high frequencies. This also reduces peak sensitivity and shifts it to lower frequencies. Most, but not all, of this loss is caused by the decreased retinal illuminance found in older subjects. Burton et al[11] bypassed the eye's optics by imaging laser interference fringes on the retina in older adults with good eye health. A small loss in sensitivity (0.1 to 0.2 log units) was found, but this loss accounted for less than half of the contrast sensitivity loss found by standard viewing methods. These results confirm that most of the loss of contrast sensitivity in the older eye is caused by the preretinal media and pupil changes.

In addition, these same investigators report that older subjects had difficulty in detecting and differentiating between relatively large complex targets, such as faces, at low contrast. Lott et al[71] recently reported a dramatic linear loss of face recognition ability with age even when the acuity was restricted to those with

20/40 or better. Those older than 85 years needed to be at an equivalent distance of 1 m to identify the face and its expression accurately, whereas young observers could perform this task at an equivalent distance of 6 m.[71]

The investigation of the variations of the relation between spatial frequency and contrast sensitivity and its meaning in visual perception is important and can be used to detect visual changes before a loss of visual acuity occurs. It brings to mind the pioneering work of Luckiesh and Moss[74] and Guth.[41,42] They developed a number of methods of determining the relations among luminance, contrast, and target size.[74]

## ATTENTION FACTORS

Older individuals appear to have a decreased resistance to distraction and a decreased ability to attend to one source of information selectively in the presence of competing messages. They exhibit a decreased flexibility in observing all aspects of reversible figures.[46,60] Older observers also exhibit processing deficits for a number of visual perceptual functions.[110]

## TEMPORAL INTERACTION

Kline and Orme-Rogers[61] have presented evidence that indicates that the ability to separate visual events that happen serially declines with age. Events that appear as separate to younger individuals may be reported as joined together by older observers. The loss of flicker fusion sensitivity with age is well known. This decrease in sensitivity persists even when the usual decrease in retinal illuminance is taken into account.[66] Temporal modulation sensitivity decreases more for higher temporal frequencies and more for peripherally placed stimuli.[13] Both forward and backward masking effects increase with increasing age, and "some major slowing in selective attention with pattern recognition processes" appears.[114]

## SPATIAL INTERACTION

The interaction of different objects in the field of vision on the perception of each one separately or all as a complete picture is complex. The interaction may be as simple as that found by the interaction of adjacent optotypes (contour interaction) on each other, as found in the determination of visual acuity, or as complex as locating and recognizing a house number in a cluttered visual space while driving down a street.

Older adults show little decline in localizing suprathreshold peripheral objects in an uncluttered field, but performance declines somewhat when a central visual task is added. If, in addition to the central visual task, the peripheral field is cluttered, the decline in performance becomes significant. With age, the size of the "useful" or "functional" field of view decreases.[4,5,102] This decline in peripheral localization ability occurs in the absence of any significant changes in the clinically determined visual field and appears to be related to attending to both a central task and attempting to localize another target in a complex field at the same time. The only significant correlation of this loss of functional field reported by Ball et al[4,5] is with answers by patients to questions concerning visual search and speed of processing, such as "Do you have to take more time now than you did in the past and be more careful doing things that depend on your vision, such as driving, walking down stairs, and so forth?" More recently, significant correlations have been found between the useful field of view and crash history in older drivers.[85]

Sekuler and Ball[98] have found that peripheral localization in a cluttered field on the testing device can be improved with training. Whether this training actually results in improved performance in the real situation is not known, however, but training undoubtedly makes the older observer more aware of the problem and may result in real improved performance.

## DYNAMIC VISUAL ACUITY CHANGES WITH AGE

Visual acuity for moving targets is less than for stationary targets, and the more rapidly a target moves, the greater is the decrease in dynamic visual acuity. Both Burg[9] and Reading[96] have reported that this decline in acuity with target velocity increases with age. The cause for this decline is not known, but Goodson and Morrison[38] have shown that dynamic acuity can be improved by training. The decline may be related to the decrease in the rate of smooth following movements, and the improvement with training may be caused by the improvement in these movements after visual training. Adjusting for decreased retinal illuminance in older observers essentially eliminated differences in dynamic visual acuity between younger (mean, 19.6 years) and older (mean, 67.6 years) observers for targets presented at a range of velocities (30 to 120 degrees per second) suggesting that eye movement changes may not be required to explain the age-related loss.[70]

One of the consequences of aging is the failure of the organism to completely replace functional cells that have been injured, such as by disease and trauma. This appears to be especially true of the nervous system. For example, studies have shown that the number of nerve fibers in the optic nerve decreases with age.[2,21] This same decrease also takes place in the visual cortex, where nearly half of the neurons drop out by age 70 years.[20] In view of the loss of neural function, it is more surprising that the aged human visual system performs as well as it does rather than be surprised by some loss of acuity, adaptation, color vision, spatial and temporal resolution, or useful field beyond that explained by physical changes in the iris and lens.

## REFRACTIVE ERROR

As has already been reported, the horizontal meridian of the cornea becomes steeper with age and, as a consequence, against-the-rule astigmatism also increases. The changes reported by Hirsch,[49] Anstice,[1] and Baldwin and Mills[3] are between 0.02 D and 0.04 D per year (longitudinal data) after age 40 years.

Along with this change in astigmatism comes an increase in relative hyperopia in the absence of visible lenticular opacities. According to Hirsch,[50] the rate of increase is between 0.03 D and 0.04 D per year after age 47 years. A recent study showed a median increase in hyperopia of 1.25 D from age 60 to 90 years (or 0.04 D per year).[44] The cause for this increase in hyperopia is obscure. As Table 2-7 indicates, most of the apparent changes in the physical characteristics of the eye, determined from cross-sectional data, suggest a relative increase in myopia.

If the indexes of refraction of the Gullstrand Simplified Eye (aqueous = vitreous = 1.336 and lens = 1.416) are assumed, the 40-year-old eye should be a little more than 5.50 D hyperopic

**TABLE 2-7**

### Recent Biometric Data of the Physical Parameters of the Eye

| Parameter | Source | Age 40 Years | Age 60 Years |
|---|---|---|---|
| Cornea, r | Fledelius[35] | 7.91 mm | 7.81 mm |
| Lens, $r_1$ | Brown[8] | 13.4 mm | 10.0 mm |
| Lens, $r_2$ | Brown[8] | −7.8 mm | −7.5 mm |
| Anterior chamber | Weale[120] | 3.2 mm | 2.8 mm |
| Lens thickness | Hockwin[52] | 4.3 mm | 5.0 mm |
| Axial length | Fledelius[35] | 23.5 mm | 23.45 mm |
| Refraction | Calculated | +5.57 D | +3.05 D |

The refractive error was calculated by using assumed indexes of refraction.

and the 70-year-old eye should be almost exactly 3.00 D hyperopic—a 2.50 D increase in relative myopia. The only really significant hyperopia-inducing change is the decrease in axial length. Sorsby, according to Grosvenor,[39] has reported much greater changes than those reported by Fledelius, but the Sorsby "older" grouping was from age 40 years and older (data not included in Table 2-7).

Changes in the index of refraction, particularly a decrease in the index of the nucleus of the lens or an increase in the index of the vitreous, also could account for the real increase in hyperopia. Recent reports agree that changes in the gradient of the refractive index in the older lens contribute to the increase in hyperopia.[25,62] Another possible contributing factor is that cross-sectional data of physical parameters over time are not reliable when making comparisons or determining growth. Adults born in 1920 are, on average, smaller in most dimensions than adults born in 1950. Consequently, smaller dimensions or sharper curvatures are suspect; on the other hand, larger dimensions or longer curvatures may be understated.

The cause of the increase in hyperopia must be definitively determined by future research, taking advantage of the ever-increasing population who have had intraocular lenses for 10 or more years. If the increase in hyperopia continues in these patients, the crystalline lens may lose its current status as the chief contributor to the refractive change.

## MOTOR SYSTEMS CHANGES WITH AGE

Accurate, steady fixation by either eye and by both eyes together is essential for normal binocular vision. Dannheim and Drance[19] reported that under scotopic conditions, aging patients had difficulty with fixation. In contrast, the evidence derived from the maintenance of relatively good static visual acuity and good stereoacuity, as well as the clinical evidence that aging patients usually have normal binocular vision, indicates that under photopic conditions aging individuals maintain good, steady fixation. This has been confirmed by Kosnik et al.[63,64]

### Version Eye Movements

Sharpe and Sylvester[107] compared the monocular pursuit eye movements of 15 patients between the ages of 19 and 32 years with those of 10 patients between the ages of 65 and 77 years. Even at relatively slow target movements, the older patients showed a decreased gain (increased lag) and consequently an increased number of saccades to maintain fixation.

Leigh[68] claims that with advancing age the range of voluntary eye movements becomes limited. If the individual follows a moving target, the restrictions are less marked. Vertical version movements seem to be restricted more than movements in other directions.[14]

In the authors' clinical experience, however, most healthy, vigorous aging patients do not exhibit marked restrictions of version movements, whether voluntary or following. In those instances in which the movements have appeared somewhat restricted, clinically acceptable version movements were restored by home vision training. In instances in which the voluntary and following movements were markedly restricted, the patient either had or was discovered to have neurological disturbances.

### Vergences

#### Tonic Vergence: Distance Heterophoria

Tonic vergence appears to increase somewhat with age, as evidenced by increasing esophoria for distance fixation. The increase is approximately $0.03^{\Delta}$ per year after age 30 years. Hirsch et al[51] found the mean heterophoria to be just over a $0.5^{\Delta}$ exophoria at age 30 years and nearly $0.4^{\Delta}$ esophoria by age 50 years. This variation has no clinical significance and is less than the error of measurement used in clinical testing.

#### Fusional (Disparity) Vergence

According to Sheedy and Saladin,[108] positive fusional vergence decreases with age, but negative fusional vergence does not. The decrease in positive fusional vergence is far greater than the increase in the near exophoria and thus appears to be a real loss in amplitude. In the authors' clinical experience, however, positive fusional vergence in older adults responds well to training; thus the decrease in positive fusional vergence with age does not necessarily represent a permanent or serious loss.

#### Total Vergence

The total vergence as determined from the far point to the near point of convergence does not appear to change significantly with age,[24,78] but some reduction is to be expected.

### Accommodative Convergence and Proximal Convergence

The loss of accommodation with age is generally accepted to be the result of changes in the lens substance, ciliary body, or both. As previously mentioned, Weale[116,117] states that the ciliary muscle undergoes hypertrophy rather than atrophy with age. Shirachi et al[109] believe that the loss of accommodation is caused by the continued growth and hence the decreasing curvature of the lens itself and with a corresponding decrease in mechanical advantage of the ciliary muscle.

The loss of accommodation appears to be caused by changes in the lens or ciliary body rather than by changes in the underlying neural mechanisms. Some blur appreciation may be lost, optically induced as opposed to retinal appreciation, because of miosis and perhaps some neural loss; however, these are minimal at the age at which accommodative ability first matches the depth of focus of the static eye. The fact that convergence is less effective in producing accommodation as age increases may be explained by a reduction in the output of the effector mechanism, the lens, and capsule.[33,58,84] Thus the critical age at which accommodation reaches a minimum, approximately 55 years, affects neither the sensory output from the retina nor the motor neural input to the ciliary muscle.

In reality, a discussion of accommodation and accomodative convergence is not germane to a discussion of the visual functions of the aging eye because presbyopia, in reality, is an affliction of middle age and not old age. By the time a person has become older, that individual has become fully adapted to a static eye with an accommodative amplitude equivalent to the depth of focus. Clinically, the near correction must be made more convex in some patients even after accommodation becomes minimal, but with older adults this increase in the addition is not to replace lost accommodation but rather to replace decreased contrast and resolution by increasing magnification.

Most older adults, on fixating a near object through their reading correction, present a near phoria, indicating more convergence than that of their tonic position. Most of this convergence is stimulated by the proximity of the target, but some of it may be caused by accomodative convergence even though the lens is not changed by the motor impulses to accommodate.

Some direct evidence supplied by impedance cyclography has shown that neural impulses reach the ciliary muscle of patients with presbyopia who have little or no accommodative response.[99,112] In other words, patients with presbyopia attempt to accommodate even when no direct feedback is given in the form of clearer retinal images. Whether the origin of these impulses is reflex in nature because of blurring, nearness, or convergence, or whether it is voluntary is not known.

Indirect evidence has also shown that the accommodative mechanism is probably activated in presbyopic individuals even though little or no gain in clearness of the retinal image occurs. Sheedy and Saladin[108] found that the mean near phoria of a group of young patients was 2.8 $^\Delta$ exophoria, whereas that for a group of patients with presbyopia using a +2.50 addition was 8.7 $^\Delta$ exophoria, or only approximately 6 $^\Delta$ greater than that for younger patients. If this increase in near exophoria were caused entirely by the loss of accommodation, the difference should be nearly 10 to 12.8 $^\Delta$ exophoria because the average AC/A ratio is approximately 4 $^\Delta$/1.00 D. These authors also reported that the near fixation disparity for the younger patients increased from 0.17 minutes of arc of exodisparity to 6.62 minutes of arc through a + 2.50 D addition. The older patients exhibited only 1.48 minutes of arc of exofixation disparity through the same addition. In other words, patients with presbyopia exhibit greater proximal convergence in both the disassociated and associated conditions than do patients without presbyopia under similar conditions. This increased proximal convergence could be conditioned gradually as accommodative convergence is lost with age, or it could be caused, at least in part, by convergence stimuli derived from attempted accommodation.

## VARIABILITY

The variability in visual performance between individuals appears to increase with age for virtually all tasks.[94] This alone tends to make assessment more difficult of whether a below-normal performance on a visual task should be attributed to an optical or neural defect of an aging visual system or just a normal decrease. As previously mentioned, a decrease in dark adaptation, a shift in color perception at the violet end of the spectrum, and a report of increased sensitivity to glare may be mostly attributed to miosis and growth of the lens rather than to a neural defect. However, these changes, although not indicative of degenerative conditions or disease, are nevertheless real and do represent actual decreases in function that may not be apparent from a routine visual examination. Consequently, older patients, in the absence of a pathological condition, may report some decreased visual function that goes undetected by the clinician in routine examination.

Usual clinical procedures do not reveal such conditions as a reduction of temporal resolution or a shrinkage of the functional field; however, these losses usually result in subjective symptoms and complaints that, although real, may be vague and poorly described by the older patient and consequently overlooked by the optometrist, ophthalmologist, or internist. The older person may know that something is wrong, and it is not helpful to be informed by an optometrist or physician that everything is normal and nothing requires attention. For this reason alone a good, simple, clinical measurement of spatial and temporal interaction and a method for the clinical determination of the size of the functional field is needed. In the meantime, however, more attention needs to be paid to the case history and to the older patient's report of visual problems.[83]

All these changes in visual function become much more critical under reduced visual conditions such as driving at night or in fog, when a further decrease in intermediate and high spatial frequency information is especially troublesome; when the rapid interpretation of successive visual stimuli are important, such as in reading road signs or detecting the shape of the sign in an unfamiliar location; or when reading poor-contrast printing or crowded printing under less-than-optimal levels of illumination.

Many of these conditions that result in decreased or more difficult visual performance cannot be avoided or corrected, but they can be explained to the older patient. Most older astute patients already know before they seek optometric care that they perceive more "slowly" and with less certainty than they did when younger. They seek vision care to eliminate or improve their visual performance or to seek assurance that nothing critical is wrong. The optometrist should be certain that patients understand the cause of their symptoms, and they should be advised about ways and means of improving their visual performance by using more light, substituting incandescent for fluorescent light, reducing driving speeds, avoiding looking directly into the headlights of oncoming cars at night, and closing one eye in the presence of momentary glare. With age, the best optical correction becomes increasingly important, as does home visual therapy, when appropriate, to keep ocular movements free and full. Perhaps most important is an understanding and sympathetic optometrist who will someday be an aging viewer of the world and its wonders.

## REFERENCES

1. Anstice J: Astigmatism: its components and their changes with age, *Am J Optom Arch Am Acad Optom* 48:1001-6, 1971.
2. Balazsi A, Rootman J, Drance S, et al: The effect of age on the nerve fiber population of the human optic nerve, *Am J Ophthalmol* 97:760-6, 1984.
3. Baldwin W, Mills D: A longitudinal study of corneal astigmatism and total astigmatism, *Am J Opt Physiol Opt* 58:206-11, 1981.
4. Ball K, Beard B, Roenker R, et al: Age and visual search: expanding the useful field of view, *J Opt Soc Am* 5:2210-9, 1988.
5. Ball K, Owsley C, Beard B: Clinical visual perimetry underestimates peripheral field problems in older adults, *Clin Vis Sci* 5:113-25, 1990.
6. Birren JE, Casperson RC, Botwineck J: Age changes in pupil size, *J Gerontol* 5:267-71, 1960.
7. Birren JE, Shock NW: Age changes in the rate and level of dark adaptation, *J Appl Psychol* 26:407-11, 1950.
8. Brown N: The change in lens curvature with age, *Exp Eye Res* 19:175-83, 1974.
9. Burg A: Visual acuity as measured by dynamic and static tests: a comprehensive evaluation, *J Appl Psychol* 50:460-6, 1966.
10. Burg A: Lateral visual fields as related to age and sex, *J Appl Psychol* 52:10-5, 1968.
11. Burton KB, Owsley C, Sloane ME: Aging and the neural spatial contrast sensitivity: photopic vision, *Vision Res* 33:939-46, 1993.
12. Carter JH: Predictable visual responses to increasing age, *J Am Optom Assoc* 53:31-6, 1982.
13. Casson EJ, Johnson CA, Nelson-Quigg JM: Temporal modulation perimetry: the effects of aging and eccentricity on sensitivity in normals, *Invest Ophthalmol Vis Sci* 34:3096-102, 1993.
14. Chamberlain W: Restriction in upward gaze with advancing age, *Am J Ophthalmol* 71:341-6, 1971.
15. Coile CD, Bekr HD: Foveal dark adaptation, photopigment regeneration, and aging, *Vis Neurosci* 8:27-9, 1992.
16. Coren S, Gergus JS: Density of human lens pigmentation: in vivo measures over an extended age range, *Vis Res* 12:343-6, 1972.
17. Cullinin T: *Low vision in elderly people: light for low vision. Proceedings from a Symposium.* London, 1978, University College.
18. Curcio CA, Millican CL, Allen KA, et al: Aging of the human photoreceptor mosaic: evidence for selective vulnerability of rods in central retina, *Invest Ophthalmol Vis Sci* 34:3278-96, 1993.
19. Dannheim F, Drance SM: Studies of spatial summation of central retinal areas in normal people of all ages, *Can J Optom* 6:311-9, 1971.
20. Devaney K, Johnson H: Neuron loss in the aging visual cortex of man, *J Gerontol* 15:836-41, 1980.
21. Dolman C, McCormack A, Drance S: Aging of the optic nerve, *Arch Ophthalmol* 98:2053-8, 1980.
22. Domey RG, McFarland RA, Chadwick E: Threshold and rate of dark adaptation as functions of age and time, *Hum Factors* 2:109-19, 1960.
23. Drance SM, Berry V, Hughes A: Studies on the effects of age on the central and peripheral

isopter of the visual field in normal subjects, *Am J Ophthalmol* 63:1667-72, 1967.

24. Duane A: The norms of convergence. In Crisp W, Finnoff WC, editors: *Contributions to ophthalmic science*, Menasha, WI, 1926, George Banta Publishing Co., pp 24-46.

25. Dubbelman M, Van der Heijde GL: The shape of the aging human lens: curvature, equivalent refractive index and the lens paradox, *Vision Res* 41:1867-77, 2001.

26. Dubbelman M, Van der Heijde GL, Weeber HA: The thickness of the aging human lens obtained from corrected Scheimpflug images, *Optom Vis Sci* 78:411-6, 2001.

27. Duke-Elder S: *Systems of ophthalmology, vol IV,* St. Louis, 1961, C.V. Mosby, p 322.

28. Elliott DB, Whitaker D: Changes in macular function throughout adulthood, *Doc Ophthalmol* 76:251-9, 1991.

29. Elliott DB, Yang CH, Whitaker D: Visual acuity changes throughout adulthood in normal, healthy eyes: seeing beyond 6/6, *Optom Vis Sci* 72:186-91, 1995.

30. Enoch JM, Werner JS, Haegerstrom-Portnoy G, et al: Forever young: visual functions not affected or minimally affected by aging: a review, *J Gerontol B* 54A:B336-51, 1999.

31. Exford J: A longitudinal study of refractive trends after age forty, *Am J Optom Arch Am Acad Optom* 42:685-92, 1965.

32. Feinberg R, Podolak E: Latency of pupillary reflex to light stimulation and its relationship to aging. In Welford AT, Birmen JE, editors: *Behavior, aging and the nervous systems,* Springfield, IL, 1965, Charles Thomas.

33. Fincham EF: The proportion of ciliary muscular force required for accommodation, *J Physiol (London)* 128:99-122, 1955.

34. Fisher RJ: The mechanics of accommodation in relation to presbyopia. In Stark L, Obrecht G, editors: *Presbyopia*, New York, 1987, Professional Press-Fairchild Publications.

35. Fledelius H: Refraction and eye size in the elderly, *Arch Ophthalmol* 66:241-8, 1988.

36. Glasser A, Campbell MC: Biometric, optical and physical changes in the isolated human crystalline lens with age in relation to presbyopia, *Vision Res* 39:1991-2015, 1999.

37. Goodside V: The anterior limiting membrane and the retinal light reflexes, *Am J Optom* 41:288-92, 1956.

38. Goodson JE, Morrison TR: Effects of surround stimuli upon dynamic visual acuity. Presented at Tri-Service Aeromedical Research Coordinating Panel, Pensacola, FL, December 1979.

39. Grosvenor T: Reduction in axial length with age: an emmetropizing mechanism for the adult eye? *Am J Optom Physiol Opt* 64:657-63, 1987.

40. Gudmundsdottir E, Jonasson F, Jonsson V, et al: With the rule astigmatism is not the rule in the elderly. Reykjavik Eye Study: a population based study of refraction and visual acuity in citizens of Reykjavik 50 years and older, *Acta Ophthalmol Scand* 78:642-6, 2000.

41. Guth SK: Effects of age on visibility, *Am J Optom Arch Am Acad Optom* 34:463-77, 1957.

42. Guth SK: Prentice memorial lecture: the science of seeing—a search for criteria, *Am J Optom Physiol Opt* 58:870-85, 1981.

43. Haegerstrom-Portnoy G, Schneck ME, Brabyn J: Seeing into old age: vision function beyond acuity, *Optom Vis Sci* 76:141-58, 1999.

44. Haegerstrom-Portnoy G, Schneck ME, Brabyn JA, et al: Development of refractive error into old age, *Optom Vis Sci* 70:643-9, 2002.

45. Haegerstrom-Portnoy G, Schneck ME, et al: The relation between visual acuity and other spatial vision measures, *Optom Vis Sci* 77:653-62, 2000.

46. Hartman LP, Sekuler R: Spatial vision and aging: 2. Criterion effects, *J Gerontol* 35:700-6, 1980.

47. Hayashi K, Hayashi H, Hayashi F: Topographic analysis of the changes in the corneal shape due to aging, *Cornea* 14:527-32, 1995.

48. Hemenger RP, Garner LF, Ooi CS: Change with age of the refractive index gradient of the human ocular lens, *Invest Ophthalmol Vis Sci* 36:703-7, 1995.

49. Hirsch MJ: Changes in astigmatism after the age of forty, *Am J Optom Arch Am Acad Optom* 36:395-405, 1959.

50. Hirsch M: Refractive changes with age. In Hirsch M, Wick R, editors: *Vision and aging*, Philadelphia, 1960, Chilton.

51. Hirsch MJ, Alpern M, Schultz HL: The variation of phoria with age, *Am J Optom Arch Am Acad Optom* 24:535-41, 1948.

52. Hockwin O: Biometry of the anterior eye segment. In Stark L, Obrecht G, editors: *Presbyopia*, New York, 1987, Professional Press-Fairchild Publications.

53. Hofstetter HW, Bertsch JD: Does stereopsis change with age? *Am J Optom Physiol Opt* 53:644-67, 1976.

54. Jackson GR, Owsley C, McGwin G Jr: Aging and dark adaptation, *Vis Res* 39:3975-82, 1999.

55. Johnson CA, Adams AJ, Lewis RA: Evidence for a neural basis of age-related visual field loss in normal observers, *Invest Ophthalmol Vis Sci* 30:2056-64, 1989.

56. Johnson CA, Marshall D Jr: Aging effects for opponent mechanisms in the central visual field, *Optom Vis Sci* 72:75-82, 1995.

57. Kahn HA, Leibowitz HM, Ganley JP, et al: The Framingham Eye Study: 1. Outline on major prevalence findings, *Am J Epidemiol* 106:17-41, 1977.

58. Kent P: Convergent accommodation, *Am J Optom Arch Am Acad Optom* 35:393-406, 1958.

59. Kinnear PR, Sahraie A: New Farnsworth-Munsell 100 hue test norms of normal observers for each year of age 5-22 and for age decades 30-70, *Br J Ophthalmol* 86:1408-11, 2002.

60. Kline D, Birren JE: Age differences in backward dichoptic masking, *Exp Aging Res* 1:17-25, 1975.

61. Kline DW, Orme-Rogers C: Examination of stimulus persistence as the basis for superior visual identification performance among older adults, *J Gerontol* 33:76-81, 1978.

62. Koretz JF, Cook CA: Aging of the optics of the human eye: lens refraction models and principal plane locations, *Optom Vis Sci* 78:396-404, 2001.

63. Kosnik W, Fikre J, Sekuler R: Visual fixation stability in older adults, *Invest Ophthalmol Vis Sci* 27:1720-3, 1986.

64. Kosnik W, Kline D, Fikre J, et al: Ocular fixation control as a function of age and exposure duration, *Psychol Aging* 2:302-5, 1987.

65. Kratz JD, Walton WG: A modification of Javal's rule for the correction of astigmatism, *Am J Optom Arch Am Acad Optom* 26:295-306, 1949.

66. Kuyk T, Wisson M: Aging related foveal flicker sensitivity losses in normal observers, *Optom Vis Sci* 68:786-9, 1991.

67. Leibowitz H, Post R, Ginsburg A: The role of fine detail in visually controlled behavior, *Invest Opthalmol Vis Sci* 19:846-8, 1980.

68. Leigh RJ: The Impoverishment of ocular motility in the elderly, In Sekuler R, Kline D, Dismukes K, editors: *Aging and human visual function*, New York, 1983, Liss, 1983, pp 173-180.

69. Lerman S, Borkman R: Spectroscopic Evaluation and classification of normal, aging and cataractous lens, *Ophthalmic Rev* 8:335-53, 1976.

70. Long GM, Crambert RF: The nature and basis of age-related changes in dynamic visual acuity, *Psychol Aging* 5:138-43, 1990.

71. Lott LA, Haegerstrom-Portnoy G, Schneck ME et al: Face and object recognition in elders, *Invest Opthalmol Vis Sci* 42:S863, 2001.

72. Lovasik JV, Kergoat MJ, Justino L, et al: Neuroretinal basis of visual impairment in the very elderly. *Graefes Arch Clin Exp Ophthalmol* 241:48-55, 2003.

73. Lowe R, Clark B: Radius of curvature of the anterior lens surface, *Br J Ophthalmol* 57:471-4 1973.

74. Luckiesh M, Moss FK: *Seeing*, Baltimore, 1983, Williams and Wilkins.

75. Mason FL: *Principles of optometry*, San Francisco, 1940, Carlisle.

76. Mellerio J: Light absorption and scatter in the human lens, *Vis Res* 11:129-41, 1971.

77. Mellerio J: Yellowing of the human lens: nuclear and cortical contributions, *Vis Res* 27:1581-7, 1987.

78. Mellick A: Convergence: an investigation into the normal standards of age group, *Br J Ophthalmol* 33:755-63, 1949.

79. Millodot M: The influence of age on the chromatic aberration of the eye: 5, *Grafes Archiv fur Klinische und Experimentelle Ophthalmologie* 198:235-43, 1976.

80. Millodot M: The influence of age on the sensitivity of the cornea, *Invest Opthalmol Vis Sci* 16:240-72, 1977.

81. Millodot M, Leary D: The discrepancy between retinoscopic and subjective measurements: effects of age, *Am J Optom Physiol Opt* 55:309-16, 1978.

82. Millodot M, Owens H: The influence of age on the fragility of the cornea, *Acta Ophthalmol (Copenh)* 62:819-24, 1984.

83. Morgan M: Vision through my aging eyes, *J Am Optom Assoc* 59:278-80, 1988.

84. Morgan MW: The ciliary body in accommodation and accommodative convergence, *Am J Optom Arch Am Acad Optom* 31:219-29, 1954.

85. Owsley C, McGwin G, Ball K: Vision impairment, eye disease, and injurious motor vehicle crashes in the elderly, *Ophthalmic Epidemiol* 5:101-13, 1998.

86. Parsons JH: *The pathology of the eye, vol 3*, London, 1906, Hodder and Staughton, p 929.

87. Paulson LE, Sjöstrand J: Contrast sensitivity in the presence of a glare light, *Invest Opthalmol Vis Sci* 19:401-6, 1980.

88. Pfeifer MA, Weinberg CR, Cook D, et al: Differential changes of autonomic nervous system function with age in man, *Am J Med* 75:249-58, 1983.

89. Phillips RA: Changes in corneal astigmatism, *Am J Optom Arch Am Acad Optom* 29:379-80, 1952.

90. Pierscionek BK: Refractive index contours in the human lens, *Exp Eye Res* 64:887-93, 1997.

91. Pierscionek B, Chan D, Emis J, et al: Non-destructive method of constructing three-dimensional gradient index models for the crystalline lens, *Theory and Experiment* 65: 481-91, 1988.

92. Pitts DG: The effects of aging on selected visual functions: dark adaptation, visual acuity, and stereopsis, and brightness contrast. In Sekuler R, Kline D, Dismukes K, editors: *Aging and human visual function*, New York, 1982, pp 131-59.

93. Pitts DG: Visual acuity as a function of age, *J Am Optom Assoc* 53:117-24, 1982.

94. Ratwinick J: *Aging and behavior: a comprehensive investigation of research findings,* New York, 1978, Springer.

95. Reading VM: Disability glare and age, *Vis Res* 8:207-14, 1968.

96. Reading VM: Visual resolution as measured by dynamic and static tests, *Pflugers Archly fur die Gesamte Physiologie* 338:17-26, 1972.

97. Rubin GS, West SK, Munoz B, et al: A comprehensive assessment of visual impairment in a population of older Americans, *Invest Ophthalmol Vis Sci* 38:557-68, 1997.

98. Said FS, Weale RA: Variation with age of the spectral transmissivity of the living human crystalline lens, *Gerontologica* 3:1213-31, 1959.

99. Saladin JJ, Stark L: Presbyopia: New evidence from impedance cyclography supporting the Hess-Gullstrand theory, *Vis Res* 15:537-41, 1975.

100. Satchi K: Fluorescence in human lens, *Exp Eye Res* 16:167-72, 1973.

101. Sekuler R: Human aging and spatial vision, *Science* 209:1255, 1980.

102. Sekuler R, Ball K: Visual localization, age and practice *J Optom Soc Am* A3:864-7, 1986.

103. Sekuler R, Hutman L: Spatial vision and aging: 1. Contrast sensitivity, *J Gerontol* 35:692-9, 1980.

104. Sekuler R, Owsley C, Hutman L Assessing spatial vision of older people, *Am J Optom Physiol Opt* 59:961-8, 1983.

105. Severin SL, Tour RL, Kershaw RH: Macular function and the photo-stress test: 1, *Arch Ophthalmol* 77:2-7, 1967a.

106. Severin SL, Tour RL, Kershaw RH: Macular function and the photo-stress test: 2, *Arch Ophthalmol* 77:163-7, 1967b.

107. Sharpe JA, Sylvester TO: Effect of aging on horizontal smooth pursuit, *Invest Opthalmol Vis Sci* 17:465-8, 1978.

108. Sheedy JE, Saladin JJ: Exophoria at near in presbyopia, *Am J Optom Physiol Opt* 52:474-81, 1975.

109. Shirachi D, Lui J, Lee M, et al: Accommodation dynamics: 1. Range of nonlinearity, *Am J Optom Physiol Opt* 55:631-41, 1978.

110. Spear PD: Neural basis of visual deficits during aging, *Vision Res* 33:2589-609, 1993.

111. Spector A: Aging of the lens and cataract formation. In Sekuler R, Kline D, Dismukes K, editors: *Aging and human visual function*, New York, 1983, Liss, pp 27-43.

112. Swegmark G: Studies with impedance cyclography on human ocular accommodation at different ages, *Acta Ophthalmol* 47:1186-206, 1969.

113. von Helmholtz H: In Southall JPC, editor: *Physiological optics, vol 1*, New York, 1924, Optical Society of America.

114. Walsh D: The development of visual information processes in adulthood and old age, In Sekuler R, Klein D, Dismukes K, editors: *Aging and human visual function*, New York, 1982, Alan Liss, p 222.

115. Weale RA: Retinal illumination and age, *Trans Illuminating Engineering Soc* 26:95-100, 1961.

116. Weale RA: Presbyopia, *Br J Ophthalmol* 46:660-8, 1962.

117. Weale RA: *The aging eye*, London, 1963, Lewis.

118. Weale RA: The effects of the aging lens on vision, *Ciba Foundation Symposium* 19:5-20, 1973.

119. Weale RA: Senile changes in visual acuity, *Trans Ophthalmol Soc UK* 95:36-8, 1975.

120. Weale RA: *Biography of the eye,* London, 1982, H.K. Lewis.

121. Weymouth F: Effect of age on visual acuity. In Hirsch MJ, Wick RE, editors: *Vision of the aging patient*, Philadelphia, 1960, Chilton, pp 37-62.

122. Winn B, Whitaker D, Elliott DB, et al: Factors affecting light-adapted pupil size in normal human subjects, *Invest Ophthalmol Vis Sci* 35:1132-7, 1994.

123. Zaroff CM, Knutelska M, Frumkes TE: Variation in stereoacuity: normative description, fixation disparity, and the roles of aging and gender, *Invest Ophthalmol Vis Sci* 44:891-900, 2003.

# CHAPTER 3

# Age-Related Systemic Diseases

**WALTER I. FRIED**

Older adults are subject to most of the diseases that affect the rest of the population. However, the eye care practitioner soon realizes that certain diseases are quite common and may cause eye-related problems. Many of these conditions have direct bearing on medical and surgical treatment and must be taken into account in the treatment plan. This chapter discusses the most common diseases and syndromes that affect this population and their eye care.

## HYPERTENSION

### Definition and Epidemiology

Hypertension may severely harm affected individuals in many ways. It is defined over a continuum of blood pressure readings in Table 3-1, adapted from the National Institutes of Health (NIH), Seventh report of the Joint National Committee on Prevention, Detection, Evaluation, and Treatment of High Blood Pressure.

Patients with prehypertension are encouraged to reduce their blood pressure with diet and lifestyle changes to prevent progression to frank hypertension. Systolic pressure tends to increase indefinitely, but diastolic pressure tends to stabilize or decrease after age 60 years. Hypertension in older adults is extremely common; high systolic or diastolic pressure is present in more than half of the population older than 65 years. Cardiovascular-related morbidity and mortality rates increase as levels of hypertension rise, although high systolic pressure seems to be more predictive of cardiovascular complications than high diastolic pressure. Systolic pressure greater than 160 mm Hg increases the cardiovascular mortality risk by two to five times, triples the risk of stroke, and doubles overall mortality risk.[10] Hypertension predisposes older adults to vascular end-organ complications, such as heart failure, stroke, renal failure, coronary artery disease, peripheral vascular disease, and ophthalmic vascular occlusion.

Essential (primary) hypertension is the most common condition, affecting at least 90% of patients and resulting from changes in any of the regulatory mechanisms that maintain normal arterial pressure. Secondary hypertension affects the other 10% and may be caused by several conditions, most commonly renal artery stenosis, usually caused by atherosclerosis, but hyperaldosteronism, pheochromocytoma, polycystic kidney disease, aortic coarctation, and Cushing syndrome are other possible causes. Secondary hypertension should be suspected if previously controlled hypertension suddenly becomes difficult to control.

### Risk Factors

Antihypertensive therapy is effective in lowering the risk of these complications. It should start with adjustments to modifiable risk factors, including cigarette smoking, obesity, a sedentary lifestyle, high dietary sodium levels, alcohol consumption, and poor nutrition. The effect of lifestyle modification can be significant. For example, a pack a day cigarette habit can raise

**TABLE 3-1**

## Hypertension Guidelines

| Category | Systolic (mm Hg) | Diastolic (mm Hg) |
| --- | --- | --- |
| Normal | <120 | <80 |
| Prehypertension | 120-139 | 80-89 |
| Hypertension | | |
|     Stage 1 | 140-159 | 90-99 |
|     Stage 2 | ≥160 | ≥100 |

the risk of coronary artery disease 25 times, whereas a reduction of 2 g in the average American's 6 g of daily dietary salt can lower blood pressure by 7 mm Hg. Consumption of more than 1 oz/day of alcohol may elevate blood pressure and make patients more resistant to antihypertensive therapy. [4]

### Signs and Symptoms

Essential hypertension is considered uncomplicated when no target organ damage has occurred. These patients are usually asymptomatic. The most common symptoms usually ascribed to hypertension are headache, epistaxis, and tinnitus, but these symptoms are just as common among persons without hypertension.

The presence of symptoms or signs in patients with essential hypertension suggests target organ damage. Early cardiac involvement may cause easy fatigability, palpitations, and atrial or ectopic ventricular beats. Left ventricular hypertrophy from persistently high blood pressure may cause chest pain even without occlusive coronary artery disease because of increased myocardial oxygen demand. Later cardiac involvement with heart failure may cause exertional dyspnea, orthopnea, peripheral edema, and increased ventricular irritability. Hypertensive complications in the brain result in stroke, with subsequent sensory or motor deficits. Eye involvement may include glaucoma, hypertensive retinopathy, and vein or artery occlusion.

### Pathogenesis

The renin-angiotensin system is the feedback mechanism for maintaining blood pressure. Renin is an enzyme that acts on a circulating substrate, angiotensinogen, cleaving it to produce the decapeptide, angiotensin. The renin-angiotensin system plays an important role in regulating blood volume, arterial pressure, and

cardiac and vascular function. Angiotensin converting enzyme (ACE), which is found in vascular tissue, cleaves off two amino acids to form the octapeptide angiotensin II, which acts on its receptors on the blood vessels to cause constriction. Angiotensin II also works indirectly to increase blood volume by causing the adrenal cortex to release aldosterone, which then acts on the kidneys to increase fluid retention and stimulates thirst centers within the brain. Angiotensin II also stimulates cardiac and vascular hypertrophy.

### Treatment

This pathway is important in the treatment of hypertension. ACE inhibitors and angiotensin II receptor blockers are used to decrease arterial pressure and blood volume. Angiotensin II receptor blockers are more effective in patients with high renin hypertension. However, older adults exhibit higher total peripheral resistance and reduced compliance of the large arteries compared with younger patients. Most older patients with essential hypertension show reductions in intravascular volume as arterial pressure and total peripheral resistance increase. The reduction of plasma renin activity and angiotensin II levels in older adults suggests less correlation between intravascular volume and the renin-angiotensin system than expected. The relative nonresponsiveness of renin to intravascular volume may explain why patients with hypertension respond well to diuretics and calcium channel blockers. As diuretics decrease the intravascular volume, no corresponding renin-induced peripheral constriction raises the blood pressure. Similarly, as calcium channel blockers reduce peripheral resistance, the blood volume is not correspondingly elevated. Interestingly, calcium channel blockers have not been shown to improve cardiovascular morbidity and mortality risk better than other drugs.

Despite low plasma renin and angiotensin II levels, ACE inhibitors in older adults are effective in controlling hypertension. The explanation has been thought to be a tissue-based renin-angiotensin system within the vascular myocyte that contributes to vascular smooth muscle tone and arterial remodeling. Blocking that system would lower peripheral resistance, resulting in lowered blood pressure. Up to 20% of patients on ACE inhibitors develop a dry cough not seen with angiotensin II receptor blockers, so they are a useful as a second-line alternative for those patients who cannot tolerate ACE inhibitors.

Diuretics remain the first-line treatment of hypertension by decreasing plasma volume and cardiac output. Thiazide diuretics affect the kidney distal tubules and accelerate sodium and potassium loss. Loop diuretics inhibit electrolyte resorption in the ascending loop of Henle. Potassium-sparing diuretics are similar in action to the thiazides but are not as effective. They are used in tandem with thiazides to minimize potassium loss.

Catecholamines stimulate beta-adrenergic receptors on vascular, bronchial, and cardiac tissue, resulting in vasoconstriction, bronchodilation, tachycardia, and increased myocardial contraction. Beta-1 receptors are found on vascular and cardiac tissue and beta-2 on bronchial tissue. Beta blockers reverse the effects of the receptors and also decrease the secretion of renin. Nonselective beta blockers work on all receptors, whereas cardioselective blockers work more preferentially on beta-1 receptors. Beta blockers with sympathomimetic activity, when used with other beta blockers, minimize their bradycardiac effect.

Alpha-1 inhibitors block postsynaptic alpha-1 receptors, causing dilation of arteries and veins. Direct vasodilators lower peripheral resistance. Sympatholytics work on the central nervous system vasomotor center, decreasing sympathetic output, which reduces peripheral vascular resistance, cardiac output, and blood pressure.

Treatment should take into account blood pressure level, risk factors, any cardiovascular disease or other target organ damage, and the potential for adverse side effects from treatment.

Treatment modalities adapted from the NIH are listed in Table 3-2.[10]

**TABLE 3-2**

### Hypertension Treatment Modalities

| Class | Drug | Usual dose range (mg/day) | Usual Daily Frequency |
|---|---|---|---|
| Thiazide diuretics | chlorothiazide (Diuril) | 125-500 | 1-2 |
| | chlorthalidone | 12.5-25 | 1 |
| | hydrochlorothiazide (Microzide, HydroDIURIL*) | 12.5-50 | 1 |
| | polythiazide (Renese*) | 2-4 | 1 |
| | indapamide (Lozol*) | 1.25-2.5 | 1 |
| | metolazone (Mykrox) | 0.5-1.0 | 1 |
| | metolazone (Zaroxolyn) | 2.5-5 | 1 |
| Loop diuretics | bumetanide (Bumex*) | 0.5-2 | 2 |
| | furosemide (Lasix) | 20-80 | 2 |
| | torsemide (Demadex*) | 2.5-10 | 1 |
| Potassium-sparing diuretics | amiloride (Midamor*) | 5-10 | 1-2 |
| | triamterene (Dyrenium) | 50-100 | 1-2 |
| Aldosterone receptor blockers | eplerenone (Inspra) | 50-100 | 1 |
| | spironolactone (Aldactone*) | 25-50 | 1 |
| Beta blockers | atenolol (Tenormin*) | 25-100 | 1 |
| | betaxolol (Kerlone*) | 5-20 | 1 |
| | bisoprolol (Zebeta*) | 2.5-10 | 1 |
| | metoprolol (Lopressor*) | 50-100 | 1-2 |
| | metoprolol extended release (Toprol XL) | 50-100 | 1 |
| | nadolol (Corgard*) | 40-120 | 1 |
| | propranolol (Inderal) | 40-160 | 2 |
| | propranolol long acting (Inderal LA*) | 60-180 | 1 |
| | timolol (Blocadren*) | 20-40 | 2 |
| Beta blockers with intrinsic sympathomimetic activity | acebutolol (Sectral*) | 200-800 | 2 |
| | penbutolol (Levatol) pindolol | 10-40 | 1 |
| | | 10-40 | 2 |
| Combined alpha and beta blockers | carvedilol (Coreg) | 12.5-50 | 2 |
| | labetalol (Normodyne, Trandate*) | 200-800 | 2 |

*Continued*

**TABLE 3-2—cont'd**

## Hypertension Treatment Modalities

| Class | Drug | Usual dose range (mg/day) | Usual Daily Frequency |
|---|---|---|---|
| ACE inhibitors | benazepril (Lotensin*) | 10-40 | 1 |
| | captopril (Capoten*) | 25-100 | 2 |
| | enalapril (Vasotec*) | 5-40 | 1-2 |
| | fosinopril (Monopril) | 10-40 | 1 |
| | lisinopril (Prinivil, Zestril*) | 10-40 | 1 |
| | moexipril (Univasc) | 7.5-30 | 1 |
| | perindopril (Aceon) | 4-8 | 1 |
| | quinapril (Accupril) | 10-80 | 1 |
| | ramipril (Altace) | 2.5-20 | 1 |
| | trandolapril (Mavik) | 1-4 | 1 |
| Angiotensin II antagonists | candesartan (Atacand) | 8-32 | 1 |
| | eprosartan (Teveten) | 400-800 | 1-2 |
| | irbesartan (Avapro) | 150-300 | 1 |
| | losartan (Cozaar) | 25-100 | 1-2 |
| | olmesartan (Benicar) | 20-40 | 1 |
| | telmisartan (Micardis) | 20-80 | 1 |
| | valsartan (Diovan) | 80-320 | 1-2 |
| Calcium channel blockers, non-dihydropyridines | diltiazem extended release (Cardizem CD, Dilacor XR, Tiazac*) | 180-420 | 1 |
| | diltiazem long acting (Cardizem LA) | 120-540 | 1 |
| | verapamil immediate release (Calan, Isoptin*) | 80-320 | 2 |
| | verapamil long acting (Calan SR, Isoptin SR*) | 120-480 | 1-2 |
| | verapamil (COER-24, Covera HS, Verelan PM) | 120-360 | 1 |
| Calcium channel blockers, dihydropyridines | amlodipine (Norvasc) | 2.5-10 | 1 |
| | felodipine (Plendil) | 2.5-10 | 1 |
| | isradipine (Dynacirc CR) | 60-120 | 2 |
| | nicardipine sustained release (Cardene SR) | 30-60 | 2 |
| | nifedipine long acting (Adalat CC, Procardia XL) | | |
| | nisoldipine (Sular) | 10-40 | 1 |
| Alpha-1 blockers | doxazosin (Cardura) | 1-16 | 1 |
| | prazosin (Minipress*) | 2-20 | 2-3 |
| | terazosin (Hytrin) | 1-20 | 1-2 |
| Central alpha-2 agonists and other centrally acting drugs | clonidine (Catapres*) | 0.1-0.8 | 2 |
| | clonidine patch (Catapres-TTS) | 0.1-0.3 | 1 weekly |
| | methyldopa (Aldomet*) | 250-1000 | 2 |
| | reserpine | 0.1-0.25 | 1 |
| | guanfacine (Tenex*) | 0.5-2 | 1 |
| Direct vasodilators | hydralazine (Apresoline*) | 25-100 | 2 |
| | minoxidil (Loniten*) | 2.5-80 | 1-2 |

Adapted from the *Physicians' desk reference*, ed 57, Montvale, NJ, 2003, Thomson PDR.
*Available now or soon to become available in generic preparations.
Brand names are in parentheses.

## Adverse Effects

Older patients with hypertension are more likely to have orthostatic hypotension caused by the use of peripherally acting adrenergic inhibitors. Transient hypotension may also occur when ACE inhibitor treatment is initiated. Side effects of centrally acting drugs include depression, forgetfulness, vivid dreams, hallucinations, and sleep problems. Diuretics, peripherally acting adrenergic inhibitors, and beta blockers may cause impotence. Beta blockers are known to cause hallucinations and postural hypotension, aggravate asthma, and reduce the heart rate. Direct vasodilators may cause reflex tachycardia and orthostatic hypotension.

Pseudohypertension may occur in older patients with stiff arteries because the sphygmomanometer cuff cannot completely occlude the sclerotic brachial artery, resulting in a falsely elevated reading.

Control of blood pressure is important before eye surgery. Hypertension may lead to excessive bleeding during orbital and plastic procedures. The risk of choroidal hemorrhage during cataract, glaucoma, and retinal surgery is much greater with uncontrolled hypertension.

## HYPERCOAGULABILITY AND ANTICOAGULATION

Hypercoagulability predisposes older adults to intravascular thrombosis. The most important risk factor is probably atherosclerosis, although the venous system is involved, suggesting a multifactorial cause. The thrombotic syndromes include deep vein thrombosis with subsequent pulmonary embolism and arterial thromboembolism, which can lead to myocardial infarction and stroke.

### Pathogenesis

Three underlying conditions that contribute to intravascular thrombosis are known as Virchow's triad (Box 3-1).

The blood vessel luminal surface must be regular enough to avoid hypercoagulability and have some prothrombotic qualities to allow protective clotting. Atherosclerosis contributes to stimulating unwanted clotting when fibrin deposition leads to plaque growth and subsequent plaque rupture, which then may stimulate abnormal clotting. Atherosclerosis itself has an inflammatory aspect, which also contributes to abnormal clotting by facilitating the release of mediators such as cytokines and chemokines that contribute to thrombosis. Inflammation may cause changes in the vessel intima with platelet adherence activation and resulting fibrin deposition. In older adults the most prominent inflammatory causes of thrombosis are polyarteritis nodosa and giant cell arteritis.

Fibrinogen levels increase in older adults, but whether elevated levels alone without

atherosclerosis increases the risk of clotting is unclear. High blood levels of homocysteine increase the risk for thrombotic episodes. The homozygous state of hyperhomocysteinemia results in severe neurological and developmental abnormalities, but heterozygotic individuals may have a tendency for thrombosis as their only abnormality. Therefore hyperhomocysteinemia may not be diagnosed until these individuals are older. Acquired hyperhomocysteinemia is usually caused by nutritional deficiencies of pyridoxine, vitamin $B_{12}$, and folate, which are cofactors in homocysteine metabolism.

Venous stasis occurs during periods of immobilization, such as after major surgery or serious medical conditions. Cataract surgery with large unsutured incisions, as performed in the early to mid twentieth century, had relatively high morbidity and mortality rates because of the long period of bed rest required. Clots may occur after relatively short periods, such as during long airline flights where patients sit in restricted quarters for an extended period.

In older adults the most common medical indication for anticoagulation therapy is atrial fibrillation or flutter with valvular disease because thrombus formation in the atria and atrial appendages may lead to thromboembolism and stroke. The incidence of thromboembolism after acute myocardial infarction is approximately 20%, so anticoagulant treatment is usually started with heparin and continued with warfarin. The use of heparin after ischemic stroke has been shown to reduce the incidence of venous thrombosis by 50%.

In general intravenous drugs, such as heparin, or fibrinolytic agents are used short term for hospitalized patients, and oral drugs, such as warfarin and antiplatelet drugs, are used long term for outpatients.

### Heparin

Low-molecular-weight heparins are administered subcutaneously and can be used in almost any setting. Unfractionated heparin is the most widely used intravenous anticoagulant. It binds to antithrombin and accelerates the inhibitory interaction between antithrombin and thrombin and factor X. Activated partial thromboplastin time is a test sensitive to this interaction and is used to monitor heparin effectiveness for

---

**BOX 3-1**

### Virchow's Triad

1. Abnormality in the vessel wall
2. Abnormalities within the circulating blood
3. Stasis of blood flow

dosing. The therapeutic level is 1.5 to 2.5 times control. High levels indicate a risk of hemorrhage. Low-molecular-weight heparins are given by intravenous or subcutaneous routes and are used for deep vein thrombosis prophylaxis and treatment and in the treatment of acute coronary syndromes. Heparin and warfarin prevent clotting but have no effect on clots already formed, so thrombolytics are used as initial treatment.

## Warfarin, Fibrinolytic Agents, and Platelet Antagonists

Warfarin is a frequently used anticoagulant in clinical practice, indicated for prophylaxis and treatment of thromboembolism. Its action is reversed by vitamin K, so even the amount of green leafy vegetables in the diet may substantially alter warfarin response. Its activity may be changed by interactions with numerous other medications, so new drugs must be prescribed with caution. The prothrombin time is the method most commonly used for monitoring warfarin therapy because prothrombin time increases in response to depression of three of the four vitamin K–dependent coagulation proteins. Bleeding is the most common complication of long-term warfarin therapy.[2]

The available fibrinolytic agents, tissue plasminogen activator and streptokinase, along with newer generation agents, convert the inactive proenzyme plasminogen to the active enzyme plasmin, which is responsible for dissolution of fibrin.

Acute myocardial infarction, ischemic stroke, and massive pulmonary embolism are helped significantly by fibrinolytic-based reperfusion, although serious hemorrhage is a risk. Fibrinolytic agents are most effective when administered within 3 hours of symptom onset after careful screening to exclude hemorrhagic stroke.

Platelets start the thrombotic process by adhering to an abnormal surface and aggregating to form an initial platelet plug, which stimulates further aggregation and triggers the coagulation cascade.

Aspirin irreversibly acetylates cyclooxygenase, impairing prostaglandin metabolism and thromboxane $A_2$ synthesis, thereby inhibiting platelet aggregation in response to collagen, adenosine diphosphate, and thrombin. The inhibitory effect of aspirin persists for the 7-day life span of the platelet because platelets lack the synthetic capacity to regenerate cyclooxygenase. The antithrombotic effect of aspirin can be achieved with maintenance doses ranging from 80 to 325 mg/day. Low-dose aspirin may be added to the warfarin regimen to help patients with mechanical heart valves if they continue to have problems with thrombosis.

The platelet glycoprotein IIb/IIIa antagonists abciximab, tirofiban, and eptifibatide are indicated in acute coronary syndromes and during high-risk percutaneous coronary procedures because they completely block platelet aggregation.

Ticlopidine inhibits aggregation provoked by adenosine diphosphate, collagen, epinephrine, arachidonic acid, thrombin, and platelet-activating factor, with varying success. It also inhibits the platelet release action and may impair platelet adhesion as well. Clopidogrel is useful for reducing the risk of myocardial infarction in patients with atherosclerosis.

## ATHEROSCLEROSIS

Atherosclerosis is a disorder affecting medium and large arteries. Hyperlipidemia may induce intimal fatty streaks, which are followed first by fibrous plaques and then by atherosclerotic plaques, which are patchy subintimal deposits of lipids and connective tissue that reduce or obstruct blood flow. Atherosclerosis includes the syndromes of coronary artery disease, cerebrovascular disease, and peripheral vascular disease.

The incidence of atherosclerosis increases with age. During the last 30 years, the mortality rate for atherosclerosis has markedly decreased in the United States, most likely because of more attention paid to the control of modifiable risk factors.

### Risk Factors

Nonmodifiable risk factors include age (older than 45 years for men, older than 55 years for women), premature menopause, male sex, and a family history of premature atherosclerosis.

Modifiable risk factors include hypertension, particularly for older adults. For men and women of all ages, the overall risk of atherosclerosis is two to three times higher in persons with moderate to severe hypertension than in those with normal blood pressure. High diastolic blood pressure in older adults is a more important risk factor for men than for women.

Blood lipid levels, including a high level of total or low-density lipoprotein cholesterol and a low level of high-density lipoprotein cholesterol are also risk factors, but the correlation may not be as marked in older adults. High triglyceride levels occur in the independent risk factors of obesity, glucose intolerance, and low high-density lipoprotein levels.

Cigarette smoking increases the risk and complications of atherosclerosis. Smoking can exacerbate ischemia because the carbon monoxide in cigarette smoke reduces the oxygen-carrying capacity of hemoglobin, and nicotine can affect vascular smooth muscle and platelets and lead to thrombosis after the arteries have been damaged by atherosclerosis. Smoking may trigger ventricular arrhythmia, most likely by enhancing sympathetic tone and reducing the threshold for ventricular fibrillation.

Chronic high blood glucose level is another strong risk factor. Obesity, even at an advanced age, is a significant risk factor for atherosclerosis.[5] It leads to increases in other risk factors, including blood pressure and elevations in cholesterol, triglyceride, and blood glucose levels and a decrease in high-density lipoprotein cholesterol level.

Exercise reduces the risk of cardiovascular events by positively affecting all these risk factors.

Blood-related risk factors include a high plasma fibrinogen level, high white blood cell count, a high hematocrit level, and low vital capacity in all men and in women who smoke.

Homocysteine is toxic to vascular endothelium, resulting in the proliferation of vascular smooth muscle cells. High homocysteine levels are thrombogenic and may affect blood coagulation by increasing the atherogenic properties of low-density lipoprotein particles. Folic acid, vitamin $B_6$, and vitamin $B_{12}$ supplements are safe, effective, and inexpensive but have not been shown to reduce mortality and morbidity rates.

Left ventricular hypertrophy detected by electrocardiography or echocardiography is an independent risk factor in older patients who may respond to medical treatment.

### Symptoms and Signs

Onset of symptoms is usually gradual as the arteries narrow, unless a sudden occlusion or vascular failure leads to a catastrophic event. The various symptoms are related to the specific blood vessels that are occluded.

### Diagnosis and Treatment

The diagnosis of atherosclerosis is made on the basis of patient symptoms and physical findings, with confirmation of arterial narrowing by arteriography or Doppler ultrasonography.

Treatment is aimed at treating the underlying risk factors with lifestyle changes and medication. The cholesterol-lowering statins have been shown to be valuable for both lowering total cholesterol and low-density lipoprotein and also having antiinflammatory properties.[7]

## CORONARY ARTERY DISEASE
### Definition and Epidemiology

Coronary artery disease is defined as a disorder in which one or more coronary arteries are narrowed by atherosclerotic plaque or vascular spasm.

Thirty percent of patients older than 65 years have clinical manifestations of coronary artery disease, and 70% of patients older than 70 years have a greater than 50% blockage in at least one major coronary artery. The prevalence is higher in younger men than in women, but by age 75 years the incidence in both sexes is equal. Over the last 30 years the rates and severity of coronary artery disease have been declining, most likely because of reductions in cholesterol level, better treatment of hypertension, and lower smoking rates.

### Risk Factors and Prevention

Risk factors and prevention are similar to those of atherosclerosis.

### Diagnosis

Diagnosis is usually made on the basis of symptoms and signs and is confirmed by coronary angiographic evidence of significant coronary artery obstruction or by evidence of a previous myocardial infarction (MI). Noninvasive procedures such as electrocardiography (ECG), exercise stress testing, and echocardiography are used to detect myocardial ischemia. Complex ventricular arrhythmias or silent myocardial ischemia detected by 24-hour ambulatory ECG monitoring is predictive of future coronary events. The risk is higher in patients with left ventricular hypertrophy or with an abnormal left ventricular ejection fraction detected by echocardiography.

## Syndromes

Angina pectoris is a clinical syndrome caused by myocardial ischemia. It is characterized by dyspnea (shortness of breath), chest discomfort, pressure, or pain. It is usually precipitated by exertion and relieved by rest or sublingual nitroglycerin. Older adults are more likely to have dyspnea on exertion than chest pain.

The chest pain is usually described as tightness or heaviness, or constricting, pressing, squeezing, strangling, or burning discomfort in the substernal or adjacent area of the chest and may extend to one or both shoulders, arms, fingers neck, jaws, teeth, or left shoulder region.

Anginal pain in older adults is less likely to be retrosternal than in younger patients and may be misinterpreted as pain from degenerative joint disease, peptic ulcer disease, or hiatal hernia. Anginal symptoms may be precipitated by physical exertion, emotional stress, heavy meals, or exposure to cold weather. The pain, which lasts 1 to 15 minutes, can usually be relieved within 3 minutes by sublingual nitroglycerin, rest, or resolution of emotional stress.

Attacks of angina may vary in frequency from several per day to occasional attacks weeks or months apart. Acute coronary syndromes are a continuum of unstable angina, non–Q-wave infarction, and Q-wave infarction. The Q wave refers to specific changes on the ECG when necrosis of an area of the wall is total. Unstable angina and non–Q-wave infarction represent a significant increase in the frequency and duration of chest pain caused by ischemia. Although temporary changes in the ECG may occur during these episodes in both conditions, non–Q-wave infarction represents small infarcts or necrosis as detected by changes in cardiac injury markers. Either may progress to Q-wave infarction, which is typically caused by plaque rupture resulting in full-thickness ventricular wall necrosis. Symptoms may actually improve once an area of the cardiac wall undergoes the change from ischemia to necrosis. Circulating chemical markers used in the detection of acute necrosis include heart and skeletal muscle enzymes and troponins, important regulatory elements in cardiac muscle that are not found in healthy individuals.

The usual treatment of underlying risk factors is important. Aspirin 160 to 325 mg daily reduces the incidence of MI, stroke, and cardiovascular death. Nitrates prevent and relieve angina. Nitroglycerin as a sublingual spray or tablet or as a transdermal ointment or skin patch is the drug most commonly used. Long-acting nitrates such as isosorbide mononitrate and dinitrate help prevent recurrent episodes of angina. Complications of nitrates include episodes of hypotension, which may cause symptoms ranging from lightheadedness to syncope.

Beta blockers are effective in preventing myocardial ischemia. Calcium channel blockers such as verapamil should be used in patients who have a normal left ventricular ejection fraction if nitrates and beta blockers are contraindicated, poorly tolerated, or ineffective. Surgical coronary revascularization by percutaneous transluminal coronary angioplasty (PTCA) or coronary artery bypass grafting can be performed for persistent angina that interferes with quality of life or if the patient is at high risk for further complications. PTCA consists of threading a balloon catheter into a narrowed vessel and inflating the balloon to widen the lumen at the site of the stenosis. The chance of the vessel occluding within 6 months can be up to 40%. The insertion of a wire mesh stent during angioplasty improves long-term outcome by up to 50%.

Clinically recognized or unrecognized MI occurs in 35% of older adults. Major symptoms of MI in older adults are chest pain, dyspnea, neurological symptoms, and gastrointestinal symptoms such as epigastric distress, vomiting, nausea, heartburn, and indigestion. Older patients with acute MI tend to delay longer than younger patients in seeking medical assistance and are more likely than younger ones to have complications, including pulmonary edema, heart failure, left ventricular dysfunction, cardiogenic shock, conduction disturbances requiring insertion of a pacemaker, atrial fibrillation or atrial flutter, and death. Rupture of the left ventricular free wall, a papillary muscle, or the interventricular septum may occur without warning, usually 1 to 4 days after an MI. Such rupture is an ominous sign but surgery may be successful, especially in the case of papillary muscle rupture, and with decreased success rates with interventricular rupture or ventricular outer wall rupture. The same medications used for angina are indicated for the treatment of MI, with the addition of morphine sulfate for pain and vascular dilation and diuretics for the treatment of heart failure.

An ACE inhibitor is recommended for patients with acute MI who have stable blood pressure and heart failure, a large anterior MI, or decreased left ventricular ejection fraction to reduce the risk of death, severe heart failure, and severe left ventricular systolic dysfunction.

Reperfusion therapy (thrombolytics or PTCA) during acute MI can reduce the absolute and percent mortality rate more among older patients than among younger patients. PTCA has a higher success rate in acute MI than thrombolytic therapy has if the procedure can start within 90 minutes of the onset of symptoms. As of now, not enough trials have compared the risks and benefits of each to make a definite recommendation regarding preferred immediate therapy. Medical therapy alone is preferred for most older patients who have had an MI, but if revascularization is indicated PTCA is generally preferred to coronary artery bypass grafting. Streptokinase may be preferable to recombinant human tissue plasminogen activator for older adults because it causes fewer episodes of stroke and cerebral hemorrhage and is less expensive.

Long-term management includes the control of risk factors. Long-term drug therapy may include antiplatelet drugs, anticoagulants, beta blockers, nitrates, and ACE inhibitors. Automatic implantable cardioverter-defibrillators and surgical revascularization are options for some patients. Long-term beta-blocker therapy reduces rates of recurrent MI and sudden cardiac death more in older patients than in younger ones.

## CONGESTIVE HEART FAILURE

### Definition

Congestive heart failure (CHF) is a condition in which cardiac output is insufficient to meet physiological demands because of impaired function of one or both cardiac ventricles. Compensated CHF refers to the adequate control of symptoms, decompensated CHF refers to symptomatic CHF, and refractory CHF is the term used when previous attempts to relieve symptoms have failed. Heart failure is common in patients older than 65 years. It is now the most common diagnosis among hospitalized older patients.

The cardinal symptoms and signs of heart failure include dyspnea, fatigue, orthopnea, and edema.

The diagnosis is based on clinical findings. Patients may not report the symptoms and attribute them to old age if they progress slowly. Evaluation of new-onset heart failure should include an imaging test, usually echocardiography, to evaluate left ventricular systolic function and help determine the primary cause of heart failure such as cardiac tamponade, aortic stenosis, or severe valvular regurgitation. The causes of pure right-sided failure include chronic pulmonary disease, pulmonary hypertension, right-sided valve disease, right-sided infarction, or constrictive pericarditis.

Ejection fraction is a measurement of ventricular function and is defined as stroke volume divided by end-diastolic volume. Normal ejection fraction is 50% to 65%. Usual findings in primarily diastolic heart failure include a normal or high ejection fraction, a normal or small left ventricle, thickened ventricular walls with concentric hypertrophy, and no segmental wall motion abnormalities. In contrast, patients with primarily systolic heart failure usually have a significantly reduced left ventricular ejection fraction to less than 40%, a dilated left ventricle, and multiple regional wall motion abnormalities. Patients with mixed heart failure may have combined systolic and diastolic dysfunction with an ejection fraction of 40% to 50%. No reliable measurement for diastolic dysfunction is available because measurements of diastolic filling by echocardiography can be affected by blood pressure, drugs, and aging. Because patients with active myocardial ischemia can present with heart failure, a workup for coronary artery disease is usually indicated.

For 70-year-old patients, the annual mortality rate is 9% for diastolic heart failure and 18% for systolic heart failure. Recent hospitalization for heart failure indicates a poor prognosis whether the heart failure is systolic or diastolic.

## Treatment

Treatment measures include attempts to identify and manage exacerbating factors or disorders, including controlling dietary sodium intake, drug compliance, and blood pressure. Proper management of these factors can often prevent acute episodes. Other measures include attention to the risk factors associated with atherosclerosis, including smoking and alcohol cessation and control of hyperlipidemia and diabetes, and possibly cardiovascular rehabilitation. Pneumococcal and influenza vaccinations are also recommended.

Pharmacological therapy for systolic heart failure with only mild symptoms without significant edema usually begins with an ACE inhibitor. If volume overload and edema are present, treatment starts with a diuretic at the lowest effective dose. Digoxin is added for severe symptoms or if atrial fibrillation develops. Therapy for patients with diastolic heart failure is usually related to control of blood pressure. Digoxin therapy for symptomatic heart failure remains important. It can improve exercise tolerance, alleviate symptoms, and reduce the incidence of acute decompensation.

Antiarrhythmic therapy, including drugs and electrical cardioversion, may be necessary to restore and maintain sinus rhythm in the presence of atrial fibrillation. Atrial contraction may be necessary for adequate ventricular filling in older adults.

High-risk patients include those with a history of sustained ventricular tachycardia, ventricular fibrillation, or resuscitated sudden cardiac death. Amiodarone and automatic implantable defibrillators have been shown to reduce the risk of sudden cardiac death.

Warfarin is indicated for patients with systolic heart failure and atrial fibrillation or prior embolism to prevent emboli, but older adults are at increased risk of adverse effects from anticoagulants.

Surgical treatment includes coronary revascularization in patients with coronary artery disease and myocardial ischemia. Valve replacement surgery is warranted if the cause of heart failure is valvular disease. Even though survival rates after heart transplantation have improved steadily, transplantation is rarely performed in older patients because the availability of donor organs is limited.

## CEREBROVASCULAR DISEASE

Cerebrovascular disease is a heterogeneous group of vascular disorders that result in brain injury. The two main categories are stroke and transient ischemic attack (TIA).

Each year approximately 750,000 Americans have a stroke, and approximately 150,000 of them die. Stroke is the third leading cause of death in the United States and in most other industrialized countries. At any time, there are approximately 2 million stroke survivors in the United States. Stroke incidence and mortality rate increase with age, especially after age 65 years. This age group comprises almost three fourths of all stroke victims and almost 90% of the mortality rate of stroke. Stroke causes loss of motor and cognitive skills, resulting in much greater dependency on the families and other caregivers. The complications of stroke may be more devastating than the stroke itself because strokes activate the body's clotting system, which can lead to potentially devastating complications such as venous thromboembolism and MI.

The extent of neurological recovery depends on the mechanism, location, and size of the lesion, with approximately 90% of neurological recovery usually occurring within 3 months. The remaining 10% occurs more slowly. Recovery after hemorrhagic stroke is slower. Depression is common after a stroke and may impede recovery. Patients with access to rehabilitation, therapists, and home caregivers do best.

Strokes are either ischemic or hemorrhagic, with an 80:20 ratio. Ischemic strokes are caused by insufficient blood flow to a region of the brain. Risk factors include hypertension, heart disease, arrhythmias (most commonly atrial fibrillation), hyperlipidemia, and atherosclerotic vascular changes. Atherosclerosis is a major cause of ischemic stroke. Coronary and peripheral vascular occlusive disease and hyperlipidemia are strongly correlated. Hematological abnormalities such as polycythemia and thrombocytosis are major causes of vascular occlusion, especially with preexisting atherosclerosis. A hypercoagulable state, sometimes seen in cancer and other systemic disorders, may also lead to obstruction of a previously narrowed vessel. TIAs may recur for weeks or months.

TIAs are focal neurological abnormalities of sudden onset and brief duration caused by cerebrovascular disease. They are caused by temporary blockage of blood flow to the brain. Although by definition they last less than 24 hours, more than three fourths last less than 5 minutes. A third of individuals with TIAs eventually have a stroke. Symptoms are identical to those of a stroke but are temporary and do not cause permanent damage. The symptoms give information about the location of the diseased vessels that caused them.

Emboli can arise from the aortic arch, from plaques, from dissections of the large extracranial and intracranial arteries, and from valvular heart disease or myocardial ischemia, especially in the presence of atrial fibrillation.

Neurological symptoms usually begin abruptly, often while the patient is awake and active. When emboli pass distally, the deficit may worsen or improve. Visualization of the emboli by angiography is usually not possible after 2 days have elapsed. Neurological signs are identical to those of large-vessel atherosclerosis.

If the emboli cause a permanent defect, computed tomography and magnetic resonance imaging usually show superficial wedge-shaped infarcts. Many infarcts may be detected in different vascular areas. Ultrasonography, computed tomography, angiography, and magnetic resonance angiography show embolic sources within the proximal extracranial arteries.

ECG may be useful for detecting myocardial ischemia, chamber hypertrophy, or arrhythmias. Echocardiography detects valvular heart disease, regions of decreased contractility, tumors such as myxomas, and chamber hypertrophy. Holter monitoring can detect intermittent arrhythmias.

Temporary disruption of blood flow may result in ischemia without infarction, but when ischemia is prolonged infarction occurs and localized brain function is permanently lost. Brain function is somewhat plastic, so that some lost function may be taken over by nearby areas. A narrowed or occluded artery supplying a local brain region is the usual cause of ischemia.

Specific symptoms and signs relate to the anatomy of the involved artery and the area it supplies. They may be sensory, motor, or both.

Headache is also common and is probably caused by dilation of collateral arterial channels.

Transient decreases in arterial flow in the internal carotid artery in the neck cause attacks of transient monocular blindness (amaurosis fugax) on the side of the lesion. These attacks are usually described as being like a shade falling or a curtain moving across the eye from the side. They usually last from 30 seconds to a few minutes.

Hemispheric ischemia may produce weakness or numbness of the contralateral limbs and the face. Aphasia is common when the left internal carotid artery is involved. Plaque disease and stenosis are most severe at the origin of the internal carotid artery, where it branches from the common carotid artery.

Stenosis in the intracranial internal carotid artery proximal to the ophthalmic artery branch causes symptoms similar to those affecting the internal carotid in the neck, but no neck bruit is present and noninvasive studies of the internal carotid artery find no abnormalities. Stenosis beyond the ophthalmic artery origin shows hemispheric ischemic symptoms such as lateralized weakness, sensory loss, or visual neglect without clinical or radiological evidence of decreased ophthalmic artery flow. Aphasia is a common finding in left hemispheric ischemia, and defective drawing and copying ability and left-sided visual neglect are common in right hemispheric ischemia.

Symptoms of ischemia related to vertebral artery disease in the neck are evanescent dizziness, vertigo, diplopia, and visual loss, especially on neck extension. Occlusion or severe stenosis of an intracranial vertebral artery blocks flow through the posterior inferior cerebellar artery branch and causes ischemia of the lateral medulla and the cerebellum, which can result in staggering gait, ataxia, sensations of disequilibrium, and nausea.

Middle cerebral artery disease usually causes weakness and numbness of the contralateral limbs, trunk, and especially the face. Left-sided damage usually causes aphasia, whereas damage to the right usually causes visuospatial dysfunction and left-sided neglect.

Anterior cerebral artery disease may cause contralateral weakness and numbness with occasional loss of spontaneity or interest in the surroundings.

Posterior cerebral artery atherosclerosis causes symptoms related to the visual fields. Patients may have transient attacks of hemianopia or scotomata. A large lesion that includes parts of the temporal lobe may result in memory loss, alexia, and agitated delirium.

Lacunar infarcts are small, deep infarcts caused by occlusion of penetrating brain arteries. Lacunes are less than 2 cm at their greatest diameter and affect only deeper structures.

TIAs in penetrating arterial disease are less common than in large vessel disease. The most common syndromes are pure motor hemiparesis and pure sensory stroke, which may be subtle enough to be missed by both patients and their families. Multiple lacunes may lead to dementia or parkinsonism. Lacunes may not be visible on computed tomography or magnetic resonance imaging scans and may need to be diagnosed clinically.

Treatment is similar to other atherosclerotic diseases and includes lifestyle changes, control of blood pressure and diabetes, and reduction of blood fibrinogen levels. Treatment of TIAs should include specific medical or surgical treatment for the underlying cardiac disorder. Thrombolytic treatment can be given if the patient is seen soon after the embolic event with evidence of a thromboembolism in an intracranial artery. If the patient is vulnerable to further emboli, long-term anticoagulant therapy may be indicated.

Hemorrhagic stroke is caused by bleeding into brain tissue or meningeal spaces. Intracranial hemorrhage, which is most often caused by aneurysms, vascular malformations, bleeding disorders, hypertension, amyloid angiopathy, and use of illicit drugs, accounts for approximately 20% of strokes. Subarachnoid hemorrhage is bleeding into the subarachnoid space and accounts for approximately 10% of all strokes but a much higher percentage of deaths from stroke. Subarachnoid hemorrhage increases the pressure within the cranium, impairs the drainage of cerebrospinal fluid, and irritates the arteries at the base of the brain. The blood is usually released quickly into the subarachnoid space at arterial pressure and becomes widely dispersed around the brain and spinal cord. Delayed vasoconstriction of the cerebral arteries, beginning more than 48 hours after hemorrhage and possibly continuing for more than a week, is common. Vasoconstriction with delayed brain ischemia is likely when the hemorrhage is large or produces thick, focal collections of blood.

The most common causes of hemorrhagic stroke in older adults are cerebral aneurysms, hematological and anticoagulant overuse bleeding disorders, head trauma, and amyloid angiopathy, which is a degenerative hyalinization of the arteries in the brain and subarachnoid spaces. Head trauma, most often from falls, is often undiagnosed because the patient may be confused or amnesic and cannot clearly describe the event.

Amyloid angiopathy can cause subarachnoid or intracerebral hemorrhage. Patients often have multiple, recurrent bleeding episodes that can result in dementia because of Alzheimer-like changes in the cortex.

Symptoms always start with sudden, severe headache. The pain is usually diffuse but may radiate down the back or down the lower limbs in a sciatic pattern. The sudden increase in intracranial pressure may cause nausea and vomiting. Patients usually cannot perform any activity and often become restless, agitated, and confused.

At presentation, patients are usually not paralyzed and often do not have important focal neurological signs. The most apparent abnormality is usually a change in the level of consciousness, resulting in restlessness, delirium, sleepiness, stupor, or coma. Stiff neck, difficulty concentrating, impaired short-term memory, and impaired extensor plantar reflexes are also common.

Subdural hematoma is an accumulation of blood between the dura mater and the arachnoid, usually from bleeding of the bridging veins. Blunt head trauma causes brain motion within the skull, shearing off the bridging veins between the brain's surface and adjacent dural venous sinuses. The blood leaks and accumulates slowly. Subdural hematomas may be acute (caused by severe head trauma) or chronic (usually caused by minor trauma). Chronic subdural hematomas typically occur in older persons taking anticoagulants or in alcoholics who have some degree of brain atrophy. The most common findings are headache, decreased alertness, and abnormalities of hemispheric function. Neurological abnormalities are usually mild. Seizures, when present, indicate contusion of underlying brain tissue. As the hematoma enlarges, headache worsens and consciousness can deteriorate. An ipsilateral Babinski sign and ipsilateral third-nerve paresis indicate midbrain compression.

## Treatment

Options include surgical and medical treatment. Endarterectomy is the procedure of choice for ischemic problems if an extracranial artery is open but more than 70% stenotic, if the lesion is surgically accessible, and no medical contraindication is present. Angioplasty with or without stenting is used if the patient is not a surgical candidate or the arterial lesion is not surgically accessible. Thrombolysis may be used when a patient presents soon after the onset of symptoms of brain ischemia but before infarction, after the arterial occlusion is identified by diagnostic tests. Thrombolysis is contraindicated in cases of uncontrolled hypertension, bleeding disorders, or large infarcts because of the possibility of hemorrhage.

Heparins may be used when thrombolysis is not indicated. Warfarin should be started 2 to 4 days after initiation of heparin and is usually continued for 1 to 3 months. Longer term warfarin therapy should be used when the vascular lesion is severely stenotic and inaccessible or the patient is not a candidate for or declines surgery.

Antiplatelet drugs such as aspirin are prescribed when the vascular lesion is not severely stenotic. Treatment of elevated plasma homocysteine levels should be instituted, such as in the treatment of atherosclerosis.

In the case of hemorrhagic stroke, aneurysms and vascular malformations must be repaired. If the hemorrhage is a warfarin complication, hypoprothrombinemia must be quickly reversed with vitamin K or fresh frozen plasma. In the case of head trauma, immediate evaluation and treatment of accompanying brain contusions, hematomas, and lacerations are necessary. Corticosteroids help control increased intracranial pressure and brain swelling. When vasoconstriction is present, both nimodipine and hypervolemic therapy should be considered.

## PERIPHERAL ARTERIAL DISEASE

### Definition

Peripheral arterial disease is common in older adults. Atherosclerosis, exacerbated by cigarette smoking and diabetes, is the most common cause. Arteriosclerosis obliterans is the occlusion of blood supply to the extremities by atherosclerotic plaques in the peripheral arteries. It parallels atherosclerosis in the coronary and cerebral arteries, developing slowly and insidiously.

### Risk Factors

Risk factors are similar to those of atherosclerosis. Increased hematocrit levels by any cause increase resistance to blood circulation and consequently raise the risk of intimal injury to the vessel wall. The incidence of limb amputation is 10 times higher in those who continue to smoke after developing arterial occlusion than in those who quit.

### Symptoms and Signs

Almost 70% of a vessel's lumen must be occluded before symptoms develop, so most patients are asymptomatic.

The cardinal and most specific symptom is intermittent claudication, which is pain, tightness, or weakness in an exercising muscle, usually the calf, which recovers during rest. It occurs during walking and is described as squeezing. Claudication may occur at rest when the occlusion reaches 90% and is an ominous portent for the development of gangrene. The pain is paresthetic and burning, most severe distally, and typically worse at night, preventing sleep. Diabetic patients with neuropathy may develop gangrene without pain.

Gangrene first appears as nonblanching cyanosis, followed by blackening and mummification. Cellulitis and deeper infections may soon follow.

### Diagnosis

The absence of peripheral pulses strongly suggests peripheral atherosclerosis. A fasting full lipid profile, including total cholesterol, high-density lipoprotein, low-density lipoprotein, and triglyceride levels, should be obtained. The homocysteine level should be measured, and if high, vitamin $B_{12}$ levels should be measured.

### Treatment

In asymptomatic patients, therapy consists primarily of preventive measures involving foot care, exercise, and control of risk factors.

Patients are advised to avoid positions that may impair circulation, such as crossing the legs while sitting. If clinically present, atherosclerosis should be treated. Patients with intermittent claudication may also need drug therapy with vasodilators. Pentoxifylline decreases blood viscosity and improves red blood cell flexibility; however, it has not been shown to improve endurance enough to be useful. Cilostazol improves walking distance ability comparable to that produced by pentoxifylline, but it is a phosphodiesterase and may cause cardiovascular toxicity, so it should be used with extreme caution. It is contraindicated in patients with heart failure.

The most effective treatments for intermittent claudication—arterial bypass surgery or percutaneous transluminal angioplasty—are usually reserved for patients with severe claudication caused by isolated aortoiliac disease. They are also indicated for severe cutaneous ischemia involving the feet with pain at rest and dependent rubor, especially with tissue loss, to relieve disabling pain and prevent amputation.

## DIABETES MELLITUS

Diabetes mellitus is a syndrome characterized by hyperglycemia caused by a relative or absolute insulin insufficiency. Type 1 diabetes, also known as juvenile diabetes, is characterized by primary destruction of the insulin-producing cells in the pancreas by an autoimmune process. Type 2, also known as maturity-onset diabetes, is caused by insulin resistance, the ineffectiveness of skeletal muscles to use insulin to absorb glucose and of the hepatic cells to limit glucose production. The number of beta cells in the pancreas does not seem to be altered in most cases of type 2 diabetes. The incidence of type 2 diabetes increases with age, resulting in a prevalence of between 10% and 20% in the seven to eighth decade. The incidence is much higher in some ethnic groups, including Native Americans, Hispanics, and black Americans. Most cases are diagnosed during routine medical examinations, although the diagnosis may be made during the workup for complications such as retinopathy or cranial nerve palsies. Chronic pancreatitis may lead to diabetes through the destruction of the insulin and glucagon-secreting islet cells.

### Pathogenesis

Insulin resistance is common as aging progresses and is normally compensated by the increased production of insulin by the body. Genetically determined post insulin receptor defects seem to be present in the skeletal muscle cells, which lead to hyperinsulinemia and insulin resistance syndrome, characterized by visceral abdominal obesity, hypertension, hyperlipidemia, and coronary artery disease. Patients with visceral abdominal obesity who lose weight may see their blood glucose levels return to normal. Diabetic patients may have normal or even higher levels of fasting blood insulin, but the glucose-simulated insulin response is markedly diminished, causing the high blood glucose levels. The hyperglycemia itself may in turn further decrease insulin sensitivity. Newly diagnosed patients who become well controlled often see their need for hypoglycemic medication reduced. Patients with unexplained, frequent, and rapid swings in blood sugar are known as brittle diabetics. They most commonly have low residual insulin secretory capacity or autonomous neuropathy with impaired gastric emptying.

### Symptoms and Signs

Patients with type 2 diabetes may be asymptomatic on diagnosis with blood glucose levels less than 200 mg/dL or may present with symptomatic hyperglycemia, nonketotic hyperglycemic-hyperosmolar coma, or a complication of diabetes. Symptomatic hyperglycemia usually starts with polyuria, followed by polydipsia and weight loss caused by glucosuria and osmotic diuresis, resulting in dehydration. Because the ability of the kidney to reabsorb filtered glucose increases with age, older patients may have significant hyperglycemia without polyuria. Symptoms of hyperglycemia include blurred vision caused by transient induced hyperopia, fatigue, nausea, and sensitivity to bacterial and fungal infections. Women may have perineal itching from vaginal candidiasis. Many patients with type 2 diabetes do not have the classic symptoms, instead presenting with a history that may include reactive hypoglycemia, a history of giving birth to large babies, and systemic hypertension.

## Complications

Hyperglycemia increases the risk of macrovascular disease fivefold, although not as much as hypertension or smoking. Dyslipidemia results in higher concentrations of smaller, denser, more atherogenic low-density lipoprotein particles than in patients without diabetes, leading to higher complication rates of stroke, coronary artery disease, claudication, skin breakdown, and infections. They respond to treatment of concomitant risk factors such as hypertension and hyperlipidemia.

Microvascular complications such as retinopathy, nephropathy, and neuropathy respond to tight glycemic control and usually occur after years of poorly controlled hyperglycemia, although some patients present at diagnosis with these complications. Approximately 85% of patients with diabetes eventually have some form of retinopathy. The incidence of diabetic nephropathy develops in less than a third of type 2 diabetics. It is aggravated by concomitant hyperglycemia and hypertension, leading to end-stage renal disease.[3,9]

Diabetic neuropathy most often presents as a distal, symmetric, predominantly sensory polyneuropathy usually described as a "stocking glove" distribution. Numbness, tingling, and paresthesias in the extremities may be present, with occasional severe, deep-seated pain and hyperesthesias. Acute, painful, self-limited mononeuropathies attributed to nerve infarctions affecting the third, fourth, or sixth cranial nerve occur more often in older patients. They usually improve over weeks to months. Symptoms of autonomic neuropathy include postural hypotension, disordered sweating, impotence, and retrograde ejaculation in men, impaired bladder function, delayed gastric emptying, esophageal dysfunction, constipation or diarrhea, and nocturnal diarrhea. Foot ulcers and joint problems caused by sensory denervation are important causes of morbidity in patients with diabetes because patients will ignore or not be aware of trauma from such common causes as poorly fitting shoes or items in the shoes. Decreased cellular immunity caused by acute hyperglycemia and circulatory deficits caused by chronic hyperglycemia result in infection.

Older patients with diabetes are thought to have similar cognitive function as nondiabetic patients but are twice as likely to exhibit symptoms of depression.

## Diagnosis

Either a repeated random blood glucose level greater than 200 mg/dL or a fasting blood glucose level greater than 125 mg/dL in nonpregnant adults is considered diagnostic for diabetes. An oral glucose tolerance test, 75 g anhydrous glucose dissolved in water, is a helpful test in patients whose fasting blood glucose level is less than 126 mg/dL and who are symptomatic. Test results are positive if blood glucose levels are 200 mg/dL or more at 2 hours.

## Glucose Surveillance

The major advance in glycemic control has been self-monitoring of blood glucose. At-home devices to measure blood glucose—which work by the insertion of a glucose oxidase–impregnated paper strip, onto which a drop of capillary blood has been placed, into an electronic reflectance meter instrument—allow close control of blood glucose levels for patients taking insulin and are now being used by some patients who are taking an oral medication.

Elevated glycosylated hemoglobin (Hb A1c) often indicates existing diabetes. All membrane-bound proteins react with glucose at a rate proportional to the plasma glucose level. Because hemoglobin resides in the red blood cells, which have a life expectancy of 30 to 60 days, the level of glycosylated hemoglobin gives a measure of glucose control over approximately the previous 60 days. A linear relation exists between Hb A1c levels and the rate at which complications develop. A1c should be determined every 3 months to estimate blood glucose control with a goal of less than 7%, which seems to be protective of complications. Fructosamine is formed by a chemical reaction of glucose with plasma protein and reflects glucose control in the previous 1 to 3 weeks. A fructosamine assay may show a change in control before Hb A1c does. Hyperglycemia is responsible for most of the long-term microvascular complications of diabetes.

## Treatment

### Lifestyle Changes

Weight management is important, especially in obese patients with diabetes. Insulin sensitivity increases when obese patients are in negative caloric balance even before much extra weight is lost. Improved hyperglycemia improves glucose toxicity, leading to better metabolic control. Weight maintenance or even weight gain may be indicated for patients who are lean because they are relatively malnourished.

Diet management aims to tightly control the timing, size, and composition of meals to best match the insulin regimen. All insulin-treated patients require detailed diet management. A dietitian can tailor the plan to meet the patient's needs.

Regular exercise increases insulin sensitivity if the exercise is sufficient to lower the resting heart rate. All patients with diabetes should be encouraged to exercise as much as they can, especially walking, swimming, and other aerobic activities, being careful to modify the insulin dosage to account for the increased insulin sensitivity.

### Pharmacotherapy

The mainstay of treatment for type 2 diabetes is oral medication (Table 3-3). Single or combination drug therapy is often successful and is preferred in achieving good metabolic control for many years. These drugs include the antihyperglycemic drugs, which include biguanides, alpha-glucosidase inhibitors, and thiazolidinediones, as well as oral hypoglycemic drugs, sulfonylureas, and meglitinide analogs. The antihyperglycemic drugs should be used for patients who received an early diagnosis of diabetes because they rarely cause hypoglycemia.

Combination therapy is often useful when oral antidiabetic drugs with different mechanisms of action are used together. For example, the combination of metformin and glyburide is likely to decrease Hb A1c levels by approximately 2% more than glyburide can alone. When combined with insulin, metformin and thiazolidinediones allow for decreased insulin dosage while improving metabolic control. Although the incidence of hypoglycemia is low when these drugs are combined with insulin, patients should be instructed to decrease their

**TABLE 3-3**

## Oral Diabetic Drugs

| Classes | Drug | Mechanism of Action | Side Effects |
|---|---|---|---|
| Sulfonureas<br>First-generation<br>Second-generation<br>(requires smaller doses) | chlorpropamide (Diabinese)<br>glipizide (Glucotrol, Glucotrol XL)<br>glyburide (Micronase, Glynase, DiaBeta)<br>glimepiride (Amaryl) | Stimulate pancreas to produce insulin | May interact with alcohol to cause vomiting<br>May cause hypoglycemia |
| Meglitinides | repaglinide (Prandin)<br>nateglinide (Starlix) | Stimulate pancreas to produce insulin | May cause hypoglycemia |
| Biguanides | metformin (Glucophage) | Decrease liver glucose production<br>Make muscle tissue more sensitive to insulin | Diarrhea |
| Alpha-glucosidase inhibitor | acarbose (Precose)<br>meglutol (Glyset) | Blocks intestinal starch breakdown<br>Slows breakdown of some sugars, such as sucrose<br>Results in slow rise of blood sugar after eating | Gas and diarrhea |
| Thiazolidinediones | rosiglitazone (Avandia)<br>troglitazone (Rezulin)<br>pioglitazone (ACTOS) | Increase insulin sensitivity in muscle and fat<br>Reduce liver glucose production | Rare liver toxicity |

Adapted from McCarren M: *Diabetes forecast, resource guide*, Alexandria, VA, 2005, American Diabetes Association, p 58. Brand names are in parentheses.

**TABLE 3-4**

## Insulins Commonly Used in the United States

| Generic Name | Brand Name | Form | Manufacturer |
|---|---|---|---|
| **Rapid acting** | | | |
| Insulin lispro | Humalog* | Analog | Eli Lilly and Company |
| Insulin aspart | NovoLog* | Analog | Novo Nordisk Pharmaceuticals, Inc. |
| **Regular** | | | |
| Regular | Humulin R | Human | Eli Lilly and Company |
| Regular | Novolin R* | Human | Novo Nordisk |
| | ReliOn (Wal-Mart) | | Pharmaceuticals, Inc. |
| **Intermediate acting** | | | |
| NPH | Humulin N* | Human | Eli Lilly and Company |
| NPH | Novolin N* | Human | Novo Nordisk |
| | ReliOn (Wal-Mart) | | Pharmaceuticals, Inc. |
| **Long acting** | | | |
| Insulin glargine | Lantus | Analog | Aventis Pharmaceuticals |
| **Mixtures** | | | |
| 70% NPH/30% regular | Humulin 70/30* | Human | Eli Lilly and Company |
| 70% NPH/30% regular | Novolin 70/30*† | Human | Novo Nordisk |
| 75% lispro protamine/25% lispro | ReliOn (Wal-Mart) | Analog | Pharmaceuticals, Inc. |
| 70% aspart protamine/30% aspart | Humalog Mix 75/25* | Analog | Eli Lilly and Company |
| | NovoLog Mix 70/30*† | | Novo Nordisk Pharmaceuticals, Inc. |

Adapted from McCarren M: *Diabetes forecast, resource guide*, Alexandria, VA, 2005, American Diabetes Association p 58.
*Available in prefilled disposable pens or cartridges for reusable pens.
†Note difference between Novolin 70/30 (70% NPH/30% regular) and NovoLog Mix 70/30 (70% aspart protamine/30% rapid-acting aspart).

daily insulin dosage by 10% to 20% when blood glucose levels decline to between 140 and 200 mg/dL.

Insulin is injected subcutaneously with disposable syringes. Insulin preparations are rapid acting, intermediate acting, or long acting (Table 3-4). Mixtures of insulin preparations with different onsets and durations of action are often given in a single injection by drawing measured doses of two preparations into the same syringe immediately before use. The critical determinant of the onset and duration of action is the rate of insulin absorption from the injection site (Table 3-5). The insulin dose is adjusted to maintain the preprandial blood glucose level between 80 and 150 mg/dL.

Episodes of hypoglycemia may occur because of an incorrect insulin dose, a temporary change in diet or exercise, or without an obvious reason. Patients should be able to recognize symptoms of hypoglycemia, although they may not experience adrenergic symptoms, which may result in rapid onset of coma. All patients with diabetes should carry candy, sugar, or glucose tablets and a card, bracelet, or

**TABLE 3-5**

## Human and Analog Insulin: Time of Action

| Insulin | Onset | Peak (hr) | Duration of action (hr) |
|---|---|---|---|
| Lispro, aspart | <15 min | 1-2 | 3-4 |
| Regular | 0.5-1 hr | 2-3 | 3-6 |
| NPH | 2-4 hr | 4-10 | 10-16 |
| Glargine | 2-4 hr | Peakless | 20-24 |

Adapted from McCarren M: *Diabetes forecast, resource guide*, Alexandria, VA, 2005, American Diabetes Association, p 58.

necklace that identifies them as diabetic in case of an emergency. Family members should be taught how to administer glucagon, which can raise blood glucose in emergency situations.

The common elevation of blood glucose levels in the early morning before breakfast is known as the dawn phenomenon. It is frequently exaggerated in patients with type 1 diabetes and in some patients with type 2 diabetes. Fasting blood glucose levels rise because of an increase in hepatic glucose production, probably related to a midnight spike in growth hormone. The Somogyi phenomenon sometimes seen refers to a marked increase in fasting blood glucose levels with an increase in plasma ketones after nocturnal hypoglycemia.

The healthy, lean adult secretes approximately 33 U insulin per day. Insulin resistance may increase insulin requirements to 200 U/day and is associated with marked increases in the plasma insulin–binding capacity. Patients with diabetes commonly have coexisting illnesses that aggravate hyperglycemia, such as infection or coronary artery disease. Bed rest and a regular diet may also aggravate hyperglycemia. Conversely, if the patient is anorectic or vomits, or if food intake is reduced, continuation of drugs may cause hypoglycemia.

The effects of surgical procedures (including the prior emotional stress, the effects of general anesthesia, and the trauma of the procedure) can markedly increase blood glucose levels in diabetic patients and induce diabetic ketoacidosis in patients with type 1 diabetes. Patients undergoing cataract or retinal surgery with intravenous sedation are told to fast and delay their insulin injection until after surgery, when a reduced dose may be given depending on blood glucose measurement. Patients who undergo cataract surgery with oral midazolam (Versed) and no intravenous sedation are encouraged to eat a light breakfast and take their usual insulin.

## THYROID DISORDERS

### Physiology

The thyroid gland produces thyroxine (T4) and triiodothyronine (T3). Thyroid function is governed by a feedback interaction of hypothalamic, pituitary, and thyroid activity. Thyrotropin-releasing hormone is secreted by the hypothalamus, which causes the anterior pituitary to produce and secrete thyrotropin (thyroid stimulating hormone [TSH]), which stimulates the thyroid to secrete T3 and T4. Diagnosis of thyroid abnormality is made by measuring serum levels of TSH and free T4.

### Hypothyroidism

Hypothyroidism has a prevalence of 2% to 5% in older adults. The prevalence rises with age and is higher in women. The most common causes are chronic immune thyroiditis, also known as Hashimoto's disease, previous treatment for hyperthyroidism, and idiopathic hyperthyroidism. Older patients have few of the classic symptoms of hypothyroidism, such as chilliness, weight gain, muscle cramps, fatigue, weakness, depression, constipation, and coarse, dry skin. They do present with typical geriatric symptoms, confusion, anorexia, weight loss, falling, incontinence, and decreased mobility.

### Hyperthyroidism

Hyperthyroidism, or thyrotoxicosis, is the consequence of excess thyroid hormone. The prevalence in all adult age groups is approximately 1%. It may be caused by nodules of hyperactive thyroid tissue in the thyroid gland or by Graves' disease, an autoimmune disorder in which an antibody to the TSH receptor on thyroid follicular cells is produced with TSH-like activity. An overproduction of T3 is usually present and, to a lesser extent, T4, with the liver converting the excess T4 to T3. The cause in older adults is more often a nodular toxic goiter than Graves' disease.

Symptoms in older adults include tachycardia, weight loss, and fatigue. Ocular signs, including exophthalmos, are usually absent. Anxiety, sweating, and hyperactive reflexes are much less common than in young patients. Symptoms may be restricted to heart failure and angina. Atrial fibrillation is the most common and most potentially fatal presenting complication in older adults. Other important complications are depression, myopathy, and osteoporosis. Thyroid storm is a rare complication that occurs when a stressful illness or iodine-131 therapy leads to massive leakage of thyroid hormones into the bloodstream. Even though serum T3 and T4 levels are not more elevated than in typical hyperthyroidism, fever, extreme tachycardia, nausea, vomiting, and heart failure may occur, leading to death if not treated quickly.[1]

### Treatment

Treatment for Graves' disease or a single nodule is radioactive sodium iodide [131]I. Multinodule toxic goiter does not respond well to [131]I, so the preferred treatment is surgical removal.

Further testing to differentiate the various thyroid syndromes includes radioactive iodine uptake, a 24-hour test of the thyroid's ability to concentrate radioactive iodine that is used to differentiate Graves' disease, nodular goiter, and subacute thyroiditis. Several antibodies are related to thyroid disease. The most common, thyroid microsomal antibody, is found in approximately 95% of patients with Hashimoto's thyroiditis, in 55% of patients with Graves' disease, and in 10% of patients who do not seem to have thyroid disease. Patients with Hashimoto's disease, Graves' disease, or thyroid carcinoma may also have antibodies to thyroglobulin. Graves' disease is characterized by two types of antibodies to TSH receptors: one stimulates these receptors and the other inhibits TSH binding to the receptor and thus does not stimulate thyroid function. Risk factors for ophthalmopathy in Graves' disease include both high levels of thyroid stimulating immunoglobulin and the absence of antithyroperoxidase antibody.

## CHRONIC OBSTRUCTIVE PULMONARY DISEASE

### Definition

Chronic obstructive pulmonary disease (COPD) is a group of diseases including chronic bronchitis and emphysema that are characterized by airway obstruction.

Chronic bronchitis is a clinical diagnosis and is characterized by a productive cough caused by hypertrophied mucous glands in the bronchi. Emphysema is a pathological diagnosis and is characterized by enlarged alveolar spaces of the terminal bronchi and destructive changes in their terminal septae, without obvious fibrosis, that reduce the surface area for gas exchange.

Peripheral airway disease is characterized by fibrosis, inflammation, and tortuosity in the small airways.

Cigarette smoking is believed to contribute to COPD in more than 80% of cases, with most patients having smoked at least a pack a day for more than 20 years before the onset of the common symptoms of cough, sputum, and dyspnea.

### Symptoms and Signs

The most common symptoms of COPD are cough, increased sputum production, dyspnea, and wheezing. A productive cough usually begins several years after a person starts to smoke. Coughing can be severe enough to cause rib fractures in patients with osteoporosis.

Dyspnea usually begins after age 50 years and worsens progressively. Variations in the degree of dyspnea and wheezing are indicative of bronchospasm.

Two stereotypical patients define the variation of the disease. Most patients have features of both stereotypes. The patient with end-stage emphysema is nicknamed a "pink puffer" and is typically thin and barrel chested and exhibits pursed-lip breathing. This patient typically uses extrathoracic muscles to breathe and has reduced diaphragmatic excursions. He or she produces minimal sputum and has relatively constant dyspnea. The patient with end-stage pure, chronic bronchitis, nicknamed a "blue bloater," is typically overweight and has a chronic productive cough because damage to the endothelium has impaired the mucociliary response that clears bacteria and mucus. Inflammation and secretions are the obstructive component of chronic bronchitis, but the pulmonary capillary bed is relatively undamaged. Ventilation is decreased and cardiac output is increased, which results in rapid circulation in the poorly ventilated lung, leading to hypoxemia and polycythemia and, eventually, hypercapnia and respiratory acidosis followed by pulmonary artery vasoconstriction and right-sided heart failure.

### Diagnosis

Spirometry documents the obstructive component of the disease. In early or moderate COPD, prolonged forced expiration (over 4 seconds) is the first clinically measurable change. With emphysema, a determination of lung volume by the helium dilution technique or body plethysmography shows an increased functional reserve capacity, which is the lung volume after normal expiration, and residual capacity, which is the lung volume after forced expiration. With chronic bronchitis, functional reserve capacity and residual capacity may be near normal. The diffusing capacity is low in emphysema but is near normal in chronic bronchitis. An increased dead space is common in patients with emphysema. Carbon monoxide diffusing capacity is decreased in proportion to the severity of emphysema. Arterial blood gases reveal mild-to-moderate hypoxemia without hypercapnia in the early stages but, with progression, hypoxemia becomes more severe and hypercapnia develops. Secondary polycythemia caused by chronic hypoxemia may develop in severe COPD or in those patients who smoke excessively.

### Treatment

Adequate hydration is necessary for liquefaction and expectoration of sputum. Potassium iodine solutions may be helpful. Older adults may become dehydrated because of loss of the thirst sensation, so they must be told to drink adequate amounts of fluids daily. Pursed-lip breathing may reduce dyspnea by allowing more complete emptying of the lungs, which in turn allows the diaphragm to achieve a more efficient length.

Bronchospasm is a temporary narrowing of the airways resulting in wheezing and may be alleviated by bronchodilator use. Higher doses of bronchodilators and oral corticosteroids may also be necessary during acute infections (Table 3-6). Right-sided heart failure and biventricular failure are the two most common forms of cardiac decompensation in older patients with COPD. Right-sided heart failure usually results from alveolar hypoxia-induced pulmonary hypertension. Pulmonary vasodilators may be helpful for some patients with severe pulmonary and systemic hypertension.[8]

Hypercapnia commonly accompanies severe airway obstruction, but it is generally not dangerous when blood pH is near normal. Neurological skills may be impaired by hypoxemia and hypercapnia.

## ANEMIA

Anemia is defined as a decrease in red blood cells or hemoglobin resulting from blood loss or impaired production or destruction of red blood cells.

The most diagnostically useful way to classify anemia is by mean corpuscular volume. This method groups forms of anemia into three categories: microcytic, normocytic, and macrocytic. Symptoms and signs include fatigue, shortness of breath, worsening angina, and peripheral edema, which are signs more common with anemia when older patients also have preexisting atherosclerotic heart disease or heart failure. Mental status changes, including confusion, depression, agitation, apathy, and dizziness, may occur as presenting symptoms of anemia. Pallor of the oral mucosa and conjunctiva can usually be seen.

### Microcytic Anemia

Microcytic anemia is defined as a mean corpuscular volume of less than 80 fL. In older adults, common forms of microcytic anemia include iron-deficiency anemia and thalassemia minor. Because the body stores of iron increase with age, iron-deficiency anemia is rare in patients without malabsorption from blood loss, most often from the gastrointestinal tract. Iron deficiency may lead to central nervous system dysfunction.

Iron-deficiency anemia is characterized by small, pale red blood cells and depleted iron

**TABLE 3-6**

## Medications in COPD

| Drug | Mode of Action | Risk |
|------|----------------|------|
| Theophylline | Bronchodilator, mild respiratory stimulant | |
| Ipratropium bromide | Reverses bronchospasm | Atropine derivative, may precipitate narrow-angle glaucoma or urinary retention in patients with prostatic hypertrophy |
| Inhaled beta-2 sympathomimetics | Airway dilation | |
| Corticosteroids | Reduce inflammatory response in acute exacerbation of bronchospasm | |
| Influenza and pneumococcal vaccination | Prevention of acute comorbid condition | |
| Nifedipine and hydralazine | Pulmonary dilation | |

stores. The peripheral blood smear is populated with microcytic hypochromic cells, and the mean corpuscular volume, the mean corpuscular hemoglobin, and the mean corpuscular hemoglobin concentration are usually reduced. Serum ferritin levels less than 10 µg/L are diagnostic of iron deficiency.

A bone marrow aspirate stain reveals no iron or only trace amounts. For all patients, stools should be screened for occult blood. Additional gastrointestinal tract evaluation with radiology or endoscopy may be performed.

Treatment involves finding and eliminating the source of bleeding and correcting the iron deficiency with oral iron. Parenteral iron may be used for patients who have severe malabsorption, who cannot tolerate oral iron, or when iron losses through bleeding exceed what can be replaced orally.

Thalassemia minor produces a microcytosis with or without mild anemia in persons who are heterozygous for genes that produce few or no beta- or delta-globin chains. Because thalassemia minor is asymptomatic, the microcytosis throughout life may have been overlooked or misdiagnosed as iron deficiency; thus thalassemia minor may not be diagnosed until old age. No treatment is required for thalassemia minor, and iron therapy is contraindicated because it may cause iron overload.

### Normocytic Anemias

Normocytic anemia is defined by a mean corpuscular volume of 80 to 100 fL. Anemia of chronic disease is the most common form of normocytic anemia in older adults, accounting for up to 10% of anemias in this population. The most common and most important causes are chronic infection or inflammation, cancer, renal insufficiency, chronic liver disease, endocrine disorders, and malnutrition.

Acquired hemolytic anemia increases in incidence with age. The causes are idiopathic autoimmune hemolysis, secondary immune hemolysis caused by lymphoproliferative diseases, and drug-induced hemolysis.

All forms of hemolytic anemia require folic acid treatment because this vitamin is depleted with the increased bone marrow production of erythrocytes.

Idiopathic autoimmune hemolysis caused by warm-reacting antibodies of immunoglobulin

G responds to corticosteroid therapy, followed by splenectomy or immunosuppressive drugs.

Idiopathic cold agglutinin disease is caused by pathologic cold-reacting autoantibodies, which occur in a high concentration, resulting in hemolysis. Cold agglutinins react with polysaccharide antigens of the ABO system present on the red blood cells of all human beings. They attach to the red blood cells in the peripheral cooler circulation and dissociate from them as the blood returns to the warmer central circulation. The disease is best treated by avoiding exposure to cold. Corticosteroids and splenectomy are seldom helpful. Secondary immune hemolysis usually improves only with treatment of the underlying illness. Drug-induced hemolysis should be treated by discontinuation of the responsible drug.

Aplastic anemia is a normochromic-normocytic anemia resulting from decreased bone marrow production of red blood cells alone or of all cell lines. Aplastic anemia is not common, but its incidence increases with age. In this disorder the reticulocyte count is low; serum levels of iron, vitamin $B_{12}$, and folate are normal, and the bone marrow is hypoplastic. If thrombocytopenia occurs, bleeding may become a problem. The overall mortality rate is greater than 50%.

Idiopathic aplastic anemia is usually a disease of adolescents and young adults but can occur in old age. Secondary aplastic anemia is more common in older adults and may be caused by chemicals, radiation, or drugs (especially chemotherapeutic drugs), chloramphenicol, gold, and anticonvulsants. Thymoma and chronic lymphocytic leukemia sometimes cause pure red blood cell aplasia.

All potentially causative drugs must be discontinued. The definitive treatment is bone marrow transplantation. However, ongoing supportive treatment with transfusions is required in patients older than 65 years, who usually cannot tolerate bone marrow transplants. Prednisone or cyclophosphamide may be effective.

### Macrocytic Anemias

Macrocytic anemia is defined by a mean corpuscular volume greater than 100 fL. Macrocytic anemia in older adults is often megaloblastic because of vitamin $B_{12}$ or folate deficiency.

Macrocytic anemia may also be caused by hypothyroidism, chronic liver disease, or hemolytic anemia as well as by drugs such as chemotherapeutic drugs and anticonvulsants.

Vitamin $B_{12}$ deficiency anemia accounts for up to 9% of all forms of anemia in older adults, and 3% to 12% of all older persons have low serum vitamin $B_{12}$ levels. Neurological damage and dementia may occur before anemia or any hematological changes are found.

In older adults, the most common cause of low serum vitamin $B_{12}$ is an inability to split vitamin $B_{12}$ from the specific proteins in food to which it is bound, most likely from a deficiency of hydrochloric acid or pancreatic enzymes. Low stomach acidity is present in 15% of older adults and is the major known cause of vitamin $B_{12}$ deficiency.

Vitamin $B_{12}$ deficiency anemia may also result from a lack of intrinsic factor, which prevents vitamin $B_{12}$ absorption (pernicious anemia). In this autoimmune disease, antibodies are produced against parietal cells in which intrinsic factor is synthesized or against intrinsic factor itself. Pernicious anemia occurs in approximately 1% of persons older than 60 years and is often associated with other autoimmune disorders.

Vitamin $B_{12}$ deficiency anemia may be caused by other gastrointestinal abnormalities, including gastrectomy, small-bowel disease or surgery, prolonged antacid use, antibiotic-induced intestinal bacterial overgrowth, *Helicobacter pylori* infection, or even a strict vegan diet.

Vitamin $B_{12}$ deficiency takes years to develop, and its symptoms are subtle. Neurological changes, when they occur, may predate the anemia. Various neuropsychiatric syndromes, including dementia, depression, and mania, may occur even without anemia and often remain after the deficiency is treated. Even though the anemia is usually reversible, the neurological changes may be permanent.

Laboratory findings besides macrocytic anemia include the presence of hypersegmented polymorphonuclear leukocytes on peripheral blood smear and large platelets. The mean corpuscular volume and red blood cell distribution width are typically elevated. Leukopenia and thrombocytopenia may occur. Serum levels of bilirubin, ferritin, and lactic dehydrogenase may be elevated because of ineffective erythropoiesis. Bone marrow shows megaloblastic changes if anemia is present.

Treatment of vitamin $B_{12}$ deficiency in pernicious anemia or hypochlorhydria consists of lifelong vitamin $B_{12}$ administration. Treatment with folic acid alone may improve the hematological disorder; however, it will not prevent or improve the neurological changes associated with vitamin $B_{12}$ deficiency, so the correct diagnosis must be made.

Folate deficiency produces changes in the peripheral blood smear and bone marrow identical to those caused by vitamin $B_{12}$ deficiency. It is probably uncommon in ambulatory older adults who are well nourished, but the actual incidence is unknown.

Normal body stores of folate can be depleted in 3 to 6 months. Rapid folate deficiency can be caused by malabsorption, poor nutrition, alcoholism, and states of increased folate use such as in hemolytic anemia and with neoplasia. Certain drugs such as anticonvulsants, nitrofurantoin, triamterene, and trimethoprim also can cause folate deficiency.

Pure folate deficiency may result in neurological changes virtually indistinguishable from those caused by vitamin $B_{12}$ deficiency. This may be caused, in part, by elevated serum levels of homocysteine in folate, vitamin $B_{12}$, and vitamin $B_6$ deficiencies.

A diagnosis of folate deficiency anemia is confirmed by the presence of macrocytic red blood cells and hypersegmented neutrophils in the peripheral blood smear and a low red blood cell folate level. Serum vitamin $B_{12}$ levels are normal unless a concurrent $B_{12}$ deficiency is present. Serum folate levels fluctuate rapidly and do not necessarily reflect body stores. Red blood cell folate levels are more stable and therefore more reliable. Serum homocysteine level is elevated, but methylmalonic acid levels are normal. Bone marrow is histologically indistinguishable from that seen in vitamin $B_{12}$ deficiency, but bone marrow aspiration or biopsy is rarely needed. Therapy consists of daily folic acid supplements.

## VASCULITIC SYNDROMES

The vasculitic syndromes that most affect older adults are giant cell (temporal) arteritis and polymyalgia rheumatica. Giant cell (temporal) arteritis is a chronic inflammatory process involving the extracranial arteries. Polymyalgia rheumatica is a syndrome characterized by pain and stiffness in muscles of the limb girdles.

These disorders occur almost exclusively in older adults. They may occur separately, but a clinical overlap is found in up to 50% of patients. The annual incidence may be as much as 1 in 200 in older adults and increases strikingly with age in that both syndromes are 10 times more common in patients older than 80 years than in the 50- to 59-year-old age group. They are associated with HLA-DR4, are twice as common in women than in men, and are more common in whites than in blacks.

### Etiology and Pathology

In giant cell arteritis, round cell infiltration of the intima and inner part of the media is characteristic. Histiocytes, lymphocytes, and monocytes predominate, but the presence of multinucleated Langhans giant cells is more diagnostic. The inflammatory process involves stenosis of occlusion of short segments of the artery and is usually circumferential. The superficial temporal artery is most frequently biopsied because it is most accessible, but the vertebral, ophthalmic, and posterior ciliary arteries are often concurrently involved, resulting in severe ophthalmic complications. In polymyalgia rheumatica, skeletal muscle is histologically normal. Synovitis characterized by round cell infiltration and synovial proliferation may often occur. The hips and shoulders are usually affected, although the knees and sternoclavicular joints may also be involved.

### Symptoms, Signs, and Diagnosis

Both disorders are often associated with fatigue, weight loss, and fever. Weight loss or fever is sometimes the only finding. In patients with polymyalgia rheumatica, signs or symptoms of giant cell arteritis must be sought; if such signs and symptoms are present, complications may be sudden and serious and the initial dose of corticosteroids used for treatment is higher.

In giant cell arteritis, the typical presenting feature is a continuous, throbbing, temporal headache. Ischemia of the masseter muscles, tongue, and pharynx, which causes pain during chewing, talking, or swallowing, is referred to as jaw claudication. Stenosis of the ophthalmic artery and its branches can cause ocular or orbital pain, amaurosis fugax, visual field defects, blurring, or sudden, permanent blindness from central retinal artery occlusion. Ischemia of an extraocular muscle may cause diplopia.

The temporal arteries may be tender, red, swollen, and nodular, with diminished pulses. Less commonly, pulses over other head and neck arteries are reduced or absent.

Polymyalgia rheumatica usually presents as severe bilateral pain and stiffness of the shoulders and thighs that is worse in the morning, leading to immobility and other functional losses such as difficulty with washing or dressing. Wrists, knees, and fingers may be swollen and tender.[6]

The most useful laboratory test is the erythrocyte sedimentation rate, which is usually more than 40 mm/hr and is often greater than 100 mm/hr. C-reactive protein and interleukin-6 levels are also usually elevated in both disorders but may be normal. Patients often have normochromic-normocytic anemia.

Temporal artery biopsy is the most specific test for giant cell arteritis and should be performed in all patients with clinical features of this disorder. Treatment with corticosteroids can be started up to 1 week before biopsy without affecting biopsy results so that treatment should not be delayed. A 5-cm section of artery should be excised because a shorter section may miss the affected segment. Round cell and Langhans giant cell infiltration of the media are pathognomonic. A negative biopsy occurs in 5% to 10% of the cases, so a biopsy of the contralateral artery may be justified.

The role of temporal artery biopsy in patients with symptoms of only polymyalgia rheumatica is controversial. In this case, treatment is based on the patient's symptoms and erythrocyte sedimentation rate without a biopsy.

### Treatment

Corticosteroids are the treatment of choice for giant cell arteritis, polymyalgia rheumatica, and polyarteritis nodosa. The drugs produce a dramatic response, so treatment should start when giant cell arteritis is clinically suspected even before the diagnosis is proven by biopsy to prevent ocular complications.

Efficacy is monitored by serial erythrocyte sedimentation rate measurements and clinical response. The corticosteroid dosage should start at 60 mg/day of prednisone and then be gradually reduced to a maintenance dose of as little as 5 mg/day for up to 2 years. The dosage should be the lowest possible that controls symptoms. After corticosteroids are discontinued, the patient should be monitored for at least 6 months with treatment restarted if symptoms return.

Corticosteroid side effects in older adults include fluid retention, increased appetite, acceleration of osteoporosis, confusion, and hyperglycemia in diabetics. Dormant tuberculosis may become active. Stress doses of corticosteroid may be needed for further medical problems.

Cyclophosphamide is the treatment of choice for Wegener's granulomatosis. Other measures include high-dose corticosteroids, immunosuppressants, antihypertensive therapy, careful fluid management, attention to renal impairment, and blood transfusion. Early diagnosis and aggressive treatment are necessary to prevent end-organ damage.

## REFERENCES

1. AACE Thyroid Task Force: American Association of Clinical Endocrinologists medical guidelines for clinical practice for the evaluation and treatment of hyperthyroidism and hypothyroidism, *Endocr Pract* 8:457-69, 2002.
2. Ansell J, Hirsh J, Poller L, et al: The pharmacology and management of the vitamin K antagonists: the Seventh ACCP Conference on Antithrombotic and Thrombolytic Therapy, *Chest* 126(3 suppl):204S-33S, 2004.
3. Arauz-Pacheco C, Parrott MA, Raskin P: American Diabetes Association. Treatment of hypertension in adults with diabetes, *Diabetes Care* 26(suppl 1):S80-2, 2003.
4. Chobanian AV, Bakris GL, Black HR, et al: Seventh report of the Joint National Committee on Prevention, Detection, Evaluation, and Treatment of High Blood Pressure, *Hypertension* 42:1206-53, 2003.
5. Hubert HB, Feinleib M, McNamara PM, et al: Obesity as an independent risk factor for cardiovascular disease: a 26-year follow-up of participants in the Framingham Heart Study, *Circulation* 67:968-77, 1983.
6. Hunder, GG, Arend, WP, Bloch, DA, et al: The American College of Rheumatology 1990 criteria for the classification of vasculitis. Introduction, *Arthritis Rheum* 33:1065, 1990.
7. National Cholesterol Education Program: Third Report of the National Cholesterol Education Program (NCEP) expert panel on detection, evaluation, and treatment of high blood cholesterol in adults (Adult Treatment Panel III) final report, *Circulation* 106:3143-421, 2002.
8. National Collaborating Center for Chronic Conditions: Chronic obstructive pulmonary disease. National clinical guideline on management of chronic obstructive pulmonary disease in adults in primary and secondary care, *Thorax* 59(suppl 1):1-232, 2004.
9. Snow V, Weiss KB, Mottur-Pilson C: The evidence base for tight blood pressure control in the management of type 2 diabetes mellitus, *Ann Intern Med* 138:587-92, 2003.
10. Vasan RS, Larson MG, Leip EP, et al: Assessment of frequency of progression to hypertension in nonhypertensive participants in the Framingham Heart Study: a cohort study, *Lancet* 358:1682-6, 2001.

## SUGGESTED READINGS

Beers MH, Berkow R: *The Merck manual of diagnosis and therapy,* ed 17, http://www.merck.com/mrkshared/mmanual/home.jsp.
Roccella EJ, Kaplan NM: Interpretation and evaluation of clinical guidelines. In Izzo JL Jr, Black HR, editors: *Hypertension primer,* Dallas, 2003, American Heart Association, pp 126-7.

# CHAPTER 4

# Age-Related Neurological Diseases

**JAMES GOODWIN**

This chapter concentrates on conditions that have a special propensity for occurring in older people, although most of the diseases discussed affect younger people as well. This chapter emphasizes the particulars that should be sought in taking a history and the physical findings important to recognize in each of these diseases.

In many of these conditions treatment will not be the primary role of the optometrist, so this review emphasizes how to recognize the diseases and how to monitor the visual and ocular effects of the disease so the optometrist can play an important role in the management of the disease by providing feedback to neurologists, neurosurgeons, and general physicians involved in disease management.

## TEMPORAL ARTERITIS

Temporal arteritis is the quintessential disease of the older adult because it occurs only in persons older than 55 years. Horton et al[23] are usually credited with the first published account of the disease with a pathological description, although a clinical case without disease had been reported as early as 1889 by Hutchinson,[24] describing a patient named Rumbold whose temporal arteries were painful, swollen, and reddened.

The disease is characterized by granulomatous inflammation that is most intense in the inner tunica media and internal elastic lamina of medium to large arteries. Fragmentation of the internal elastic lamina and intimal hyperplasia that narrows or occludes the lumen occur. Characteristically the inflammatory infiltrate includes multinucleated giant cells, but these may be absent from the lesion in some stages of the process.[13,26] The most frequently involved sites are the extracranial portions of the internal and external carotid and vertebral arteries. The aortic arch and the thoracic and abdominal portions of the aorta are frequently involved, which increases the risk of developing an aortic aneurysm.[9,34]

The disease is nearly unheard of in patients younger than 55 years, and the incidence increases dramatically among patients in their 70s and 80s. The incidence in women is more than twice that in men both in Scandinavia and in the northern United States.[1,36]

Headache is the most common presenting symptom and local pain and tenderness may be present along the superficial temporal arteries, but often the pain is diffuse and nonspecific.[15] An important clinical syndrome to identify if present is jaw claudication because this is fairly specific for temporal arteritis. Severe and diffuse stenosis of internal and external carotid arteries is required to deprive the masseter muscles of blood flow sufficient enough to produce ischemic pain, and it is seldom seen as a result of atherosclerotic vascular disease. Patients with jaw claudication describe crescendo pain in the masseter muscles that begins some time after beginning to chew, increases in intensity with continued chewing, and abates fairly rapidly after cessation of chewing. Establishing the time course of the pain is important to distinguish claudication from jaw pain of dental origin, which usually is present in maximal intensity at the onset of chewing. Other findings that may be present include ulceration of the scalp, tongue, palate, or oral mucosa and occasionally lack of palpable pulses in the arms or legs.

Symptoms and signs of systemic illness are frequently but not always present. These include lack of energy, fatigue, listlessness, depression, weight loss, low-grade fever, leukocytosis, and especially elevation of the erythrocyte sedimentation rate and C-reactive protein level. Much reliance has traditionally been placed on finding significant erythrocyte sedimentation rate elevation in the diagnosis of temporal arteritis, but the erythrocyte sedimentation rate may be normal or only slightly elevated in 10% of patients.[44] Elevation of C-reactive protein level greater than 2.45 mg/dL is somewhat more sensitive than erythrocyte sedimentation rate elevation as a diagnostic indicator, but combined elevation of both the C-reactive protein and the erythrocyte sedimentation rate (more than 47 mm/hr) is the most specific supporting evidence for the diagnosis.[17]

Immunoglobulin G anticardiolipin antibody and interleukin-6 (IL-6) titers may be elevated when the disease is active and can be used to monitor for relapses during treatment because the titers rise if the inflammation becomes active again. Weyand et al[50] found IL-6 levels to be a more sensitive indicator of disease activity than either the erythrocyte sedimentation rate or C-reactive protein level.[35]

Temporal artery biopsy has traditionally been the benchmark for definitive diagnosis in temporal arteritis since the original report by Horton describing the disease in temporal artery specimens.[23] The superficial temporal artery is accessible and is frequently involved enough to provide the most common site for biopsy. The inflammatory arterial lesion is, however, segmental, finding a normal biopsy specimen from an artery that is involved in adjacent segments is not uncommon.[28] In response to the presence of "skip areas" along the artery, some have suggested that selective angiography of the external carotid artery could help the surgeon chose a portion of the artery that shows narrowed or irregular lumen to increase the yield of positive biopsy specimens.[12] Magnetic resonance angiography is useful in this regard as well, particularly because the intracranial vessels can be subtracted from the image, leaving the superficial temporal artery view unobstructed by the usual tangle of underlying intracranial vessels.[38]

Polymyalgia rheumatica is a rheumatic condition that is sometimes associated with temporal arteritis. In particular, a person with polymyalgia rheumatica may go on to have temporal arteritis with all its associated ischemic complications. Polymyalgia rheumatica, like temporal arteritis, occurs selectively in persons older than 50 years and is characterized by pain and stiffness in the axial joints, including the shoulder and pelvic girdles. It is characteristic for active movement of involved portions of the extremities (neck, shoulder, and hip joints) to cause more pain than passive movement. This means the examiner can slowly and gently move the affected joint through its full range while the patient may not be able to move it at all because of pain. This finding is consistent with the fact no significant inflammatory involvement of the joints, tendons, or bursae is involved, as has been confirmed on joint or synovial biopsy, which shows only mild and nonspecific inflammatory changes.[14] One hypothesis has been that the pain in polymyalgia rheumatica is referred pain from inflammation in the aortic arch and abdominal aorta.[16] Histological evidence for this was provided by autopsy study of patients with polymyalgia rheumatica.[41] Polymyalgia rheumatica characteristically raises the erythrocyte sedimentation rate even more than temporal arteritis, with values usually 100 or more. Patients with polymyalgia rheumatica also have the same systemic symptoms as those with temporal arteritis, including malaise, weight loss, and poor appetite.

The complications of temporal arteritis are ischemic in nature. The most common occurrence is sudden blindness in one or both eyes caused by either anterior ischemic optic neuropathy or central retinal artery occlusion. The incidence of blindness in temporal arteritis in large series varies a great deal, probably reflecting variation in the use of steroid treatment at different times in the history of this disease and in different countries. It was not until 1950 that treatment with corticosteroids was suggested to prevent ischemic complications in this disease.[46,47] In the Mayo Clinic experience the incidence of total blindness in the presteroid era was 17%, and in later patients treated with corticosteroids it was 9%.[4] Other reports on the incidence of vision impairment in more recent series are much more favorable: 14 (8.4%) of 166 from the Mayo Clinic[7] and 10 (3.8%) of 264 in Denmark.[11]

In temporal arteritis most cases of ischemic blindness are caused by anterior ischemic optic neuropathy. In one early series the prevalence was 64% from anterior ischemic optic neuropathy compared with 7% from central retinal artery occlusion.[49] A long-term (1973 to 1995) prospective series from an eye department indicated the ratio was 81% anterior ischemic optic neuropathy and 14% central retinal artery occlusion.[18] These authors made the important observation that 30% of patients had amaurosis fugax, which offers a prime opportunity to promptly initiate high-dose corticosteroid treatment early enough to prevent permanent blindness.

Corticosteroids have been the mainstay of treatment for temporal arteritis since their use was introduced in 1950.[46,47]

The pain of polymyalgia rheumatica typically responds to low-dose corticosteroids, and patients are typically treated with prednisone 10 to 15 mg/day. Experience has shown that patients with the clinical syndrome of polymyalgia rheumatica have a low risk for ischemic blindness and stroke, so maintenance treatment with just enough prednisone to control pain and stiffness is sufficient. If affected patients have headache, jaw claudication, or any of the other typical symptoms of temporal arteritis, however, the dose of prednisone should be immediately raised to the range of 80 to 100 mg/day because the risk of ischemic blindness and stroke in these patients is the same as in any other patient with temporal arteritis.

The high incidence of side effects when older patients must be treated for long intervals with drugs such as prednisone in doses greater than 60 mg/day led some authors to question whether lower doses would be just as effective with a lesser incidence of side effects.[8,39]

However, the observations on which these authors concluded that treatment with doses less than 40 mg/day was not associated with greater visual or ischemic morbidity hinged on outcomes in only five patients. A study of 35 patients with temporal arteritis alone or associated with symptoms of polymyalgia rheumatica treated with no more than 40 mg/day prednisone found that only two patients had visual complications. Follow-up of this cohort of patients for a median of 60 weeks indicated that only one patient had lost vision permanently in one eye.[30-32] Another study comparing outcomes in 77 patients with temporal arteritis found no differences in the incidence of ischemic complications between groups receiving prednisone at dosages of 40 mg/day or less and groups receiving more than 60 mg/day.[40]

Occasional case reports documenting marked vision recovery after optic nerve or retinal ischemic complications in temporal arteritis have led to recommendations that corticosteroid treatment be initiated with intravenous methylprednisolone in doses of 1 to 2 g/day for several days followed by high-dose oral prednisone.[37] A survey of 114 eyes in 84 patients treated initially with intravenous methylprednisolone showed that only 4% showed significantly improved visual function.[20] Initiating treatment with a high-dose pulse of intravenous methylprednisolone has also been recommended to prevent the occasional occurrence of an ischemic complication during the first few days of treatment with conventional high-dose oral prednisone, which has been documented in individual case reports, although ischemic blindness and stroke can still occur despite the addition of intravenous methylprednisolone pulses.[45]

Adjunctive immunosuppressive agents such as azathioprine, cyclophosphamide, or methotrexate have been reported to be effective in reducing the prednisone dosage required to suppress disease and symptom activity in patients with temporal arteritis who have intolerable steroid side effects and in whom the required prednisone dosage is too high.[2,5,42] The only adjunctive agent that has been submitted to a multicenter, randomized, double-blind, placebo-controlled trial for its steroid-sparing effect in temporal arteritis is methotrexate, and it was not found to be effective.[21]

## ANTERIOR ISCHEMIC OPTIC NEUROPATHY

Anterior ischemic optic neuropathy presents with painless, usually abrupt loss of vision in one eye. The most common visual field defect is inferior altitudinal or lower half (Fig. 4-1), although upper-half defects occur as well as central scotoma and broad inferior or superior arcuate defects. Another variation includes inferior or superior altitudinal paracentral scotoma when a more limited area of optic nerve ischemia is present. The disorder is ischemic infarction of the optic nerve head, presumably from progressive narrowing of one or more of the short posterior ciliary arteries that supply arterial blood to the anastomotic circle of Zinn and Haller, from which small branches supply the choroid and optic nerve head. Because the lesion is so close to the optic disc, there is

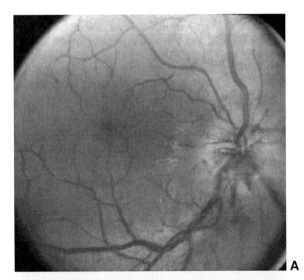

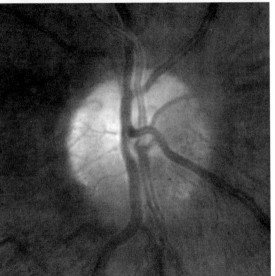

**Fig. 4-2** **A,** Optic disc early in the course of anterior ischemic optic neuropathy, when pronounced edema and relative pallor of the upper half are visible. **B,** Involved optic disc after optic atrophy has ensued, showing relative pallor in the upper half of the disc.

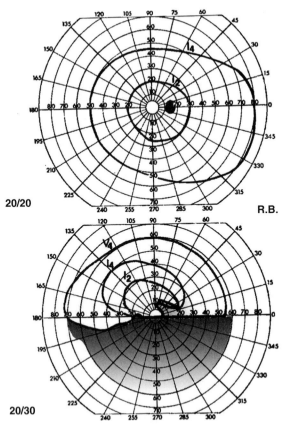

**Fig. 4-1** Goldmann visual field charts. *Top,* Normal right eye visual field. *Bottom,* Left eye inferior altitudinal visual field defect resulting from anterior ischemic optic neuropathy.

almost always marked optic disc edema, which is virtually always present in the acute stages (Fig. 4-2).

Individual case reports have shown that the disc probably swells before vision is lost. This has been observed in patients who had anterior ischemic optic neuropathy involving one eye and had the onset of second-eye involvement during follow-up when a return visit revealed disc edema without vision loss. Most often the vision is lost in the second eye within a matter of days from when the edema was observed.

"Pallid edema" is particularly characteristic of anterior ischemic optic neuropathy; the hyperemia that usually accompanies disc edema is replaced by pallor, presumably because of the impaired vascular flow at the disc, even at the outset when the swelling is still prominent. The degree of edema may initially be greater in the infarcted part of the disc, which would be the upper half when the altitudinal visual field defect is inferior and the lower half when the field defect is superior. Even though the infarction conforms to an altitudinal pattern, a generalized attrition of optic nerve axons is probably present because the visual field isopters are usually contracted concentrically in the remaining field quadrants, indicating a more global loss of visual sensitivity (see Fig. 4-1).

The disc edema always recedes within a few weeks as the infarcted axons lose integrity and undergo atrophy. Figure 4-2 depicts the optic disc early in the course of anterior ischemic optic neuropathy when pronounced edema is present and later after optic atrophy has ensued showing relative pallor in the upper half of the disc.

Most commonly the severe altitudinal visual field defect does not improve. The visual acuity may be reduced a few lines at the outset and then improve over the next several weeks even though the visual field defect does not measurably change. This would seem to involve return of function in a small area of visual field quite close to fixation in the quadrants that are relatively uninvolved, which is difficult to measure by perimetry.[25]

Most cases of anterior ischemic optic neuropathy are not in the setting of temporal arteritis and are presumably caused by arteriosclerosis.[3] The importance of recognizing the minority of cases caused by temporal arteritis is the fact that involvement of the other eye is likely to occur within hours or days of the first eye involvement—a preventable condition if treated immediately with high-dose oral steroids or intravenous methylprednisolone. The lost visual field in anterior ischemic optic neuropathy is likely to be permanent regardless of treatment even in the setting of temporal arteritis, although individual reports have been published of visual improvement with aggressive early treatment with cytotoxic drugs together with prednisone in cases of temporal arteritis with anterior ischemic optic neuropathy.[6] Some evidence has also shown that daily aspirin prophylaxis in patients with nonarteritic anterior ischemic optic neuropathy reduces the incidence of recurrence in the other eye.[29] Recurrence of anterior ischemic optic neuropathy in the same eye is unusual (6.4%, or 53 of 829 eyes in one study) in nonarteritic anterior ischemic optic neuropathy.[19]

## RETINAL ARTERY OCCLUSION

Central and branch retinal artery occlusion leads to painless acute vision loss that is most likely to be permanent regardless of treatment. The vision loss usually involves the entire visual field with central retinal artery occlusion and usually results in an upper or lower half (altitudinal) visual field defect when the occlusion involves the lower or upper main branch, respectively. Occlusion of more distal branches results in various sectoral field defects depending on the location of the resulting retinal infarction. Because of the optical properties of the eye, upper retinal infarcts result in lower-half visual field loss, and lower retinal infarcts result in upper visual field defects.

If the fundus can be observed within a few minutes of first vision loss, the artery may be occluded and all that is visible of the arterial tree is a branching pattern of threadlike "ghost vessels" that represents the collapsed walls of the vessels without blood in the lumen. This is a reminder that when the retinal artery in the fundus is "seen," what is actually visualized is mainly the blood column in the lumen and virtually nothing of the artery wall. The occluding embolus may be visible in the central retinal artery or in a branch, but sometimes the occluding embolus is lodged in a retrobulbar portion of the central retinal artery and is not visible even when the intraocular portion of the retinal artery is without blood flow. At this stage of the process the retina has usually suffered irreversible ischemia, and the biochemical cascade of events leading to infarction have occurred. The retina is nonfunctional and the eye is blind, but the retina itself still appears normal.

After a few minutes the embolus usually breaks up and begins to dislodge and blood once again flows in the retinal artery and its branches, which reestablishes the normal appearance of the blood column. An interval of up to many hours may occur in which smaller embolic particles are seen either stationary in the more distal branches or moving slowly outward in these branches.[10,19]

It takes approximately 12 hours for the infarcted retina to become edematous and white in appearance on fundus examination. Patients usually take at least an hour to arrive at a physician's office or an emergency treatment facility, and by this time the fundus examination reveals normal-appearing central retinal artery and branches (blood in the lumen of the artery) and normal-looking retina because retinal whitening (edema) has not had time to develop: in short, a blind eye with normal fundus examination. This situation may lead to the erroneous conclusion either that the patient is faking the blindness or that the problem is a retrobulbar form of optic neuropathy. The issue of functional visual loss can be ruled out by the presence of a relative afferent papillary defect, which is an obligate finding in central retinal artery occlusion at the time the eye is blind, presuming normal (or at least better) visual function in the other eye. If no relative afferent papillary defect is present in a patient claiming blindness in one eye with normal fundus appearance, functional visual loss is established as the diagnosis. In other words, central retinal artery occlusion with monocular blindness or visual field defect in the case of branch artery occlusion *must* have a concomitant relative afferent papillary defect.

The issue of retrobulbar optic neuropathy is not so easy to settle during this interval between when the retinal arterial blood column has become reestablished and before retinal whitening is expected to occur if the problem is central retinal artery occlusion. In both cases a blind eye with normal-appearing fundus and a relative afferent papillary defect will be present. For these two conditions to be differentiated definitively, the patient must be reexamined, probably 24 hours later.

The retinal edema at the twelfth hour may be just perceptible and may be easily missed, especially if any problem exists with the quality of the fundus view. Also, retinal edema is easier to perceive in branch occlusion because a line of

transition will be present between edematous retina in the involved upper- or lower-half retina and the normal retina adjacent to it. Even subtle whitening can be distinguished by observing the difference across this line of transition (Fig. 4-3). With central retinal artery occlusion no transition is present because the entire retina is involved. In this case the most sensitive finding will be the presence of a relative cherry-red spot at the fovea. Because the fovea is a small round area where most of the inner retinal cellular elements have been displaced laterally to provide the least obstructed path for light rays to the foveal photoreceptors, the retina is extremely thin at this location.

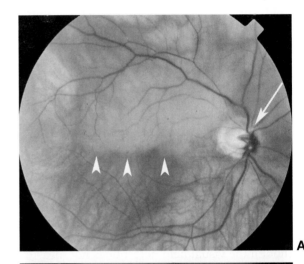

**A**

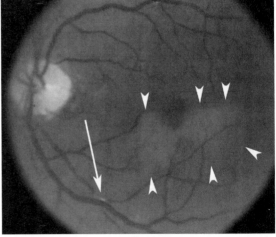

**B**

**Fig. 4-3** Branch retinal artery occlusion. **A,** Upper branch occlusion. **B,** Lower branch occlusion. Line of transition between edematous (whitened) retina and normal retina is indicated (*arrowheads*). White platelet-fibrin emboli are also visible (*arrows*).

Therefore the retinal whitening will be nearly absent at the fovea, and the view of the underlying choroidal blood filtered through the retinal pigment epithelium is unobstructed. This makes the central fovea appear unnaturally bright red against the surrounding whitened retina—hence the relative cherry-red spot. The word "relative" is important because the red of the fovea is not truly exaggerated; it is normal but the surrounding white opacity makes it appear redder than expected. The same scenario underlies the relative cherry-red spot in Tay-Sachs disease and other lipid storage diseases where the retinal opacity surrounding the fovea is produced by lipid stored abnormally in retinal ganglion cells rather than edema.

Paralleling brain edema after ischemic infarction, the retinal edema after central retinal artery occlusion or branch retinal artery occlusion reaches its peak at approximately 72 hours and then subsides gradually over the subsequent 2 to 3 weeks. After this interval the patient again has one blind eye, a relative afferent papillary defect and a relatively normal-looking fundus because the blood column is normal, the retina is no longer whitened, and the optic disc has not had time to develop pallor and involution of capillaries. However, this second normal interval should be relatively short because the area of infarction is relatively close to the nerve head and only a few weeks pass before Wallerian degeneration of retinal ganglion cell axons reach the nerve head and start to produce the appearance of optic atrophy with pallor and reduction in capillary content of the disc head. Thus the final stage of the process after central retinal artery occlusion or branch retinal artery occlusion is a patient with one blind eye, relative afferent papillary defect, and optic disc pallor. This is the permanent residual stage, and if this is the first observation, distinguishing between the final permanent stage after central retinal artery occlusion or after anterior ischemic optic neuropathy is not possible. Both will have a history of acute painless vision loss in one eye, generally at least several weeks previously; a relative afferent papillary defect in the involved eye will be present as well as pallor of the involved optic disc without swelling. Branch retinal artery occlusion probably mimics anterior ischemic optic neuropathy even more than central retinal artery occlusion because pallor will be restricted to the upper- or lower-half disc depending on whether the upper or lower branch was occluded. In the final stage after ischemic optic neuropathy when the disc edema has subsided, half-disc pallor corresponding to the altitudinal visual field loss is most often present.

Patients having recurrent emboli into the retinal vasculature from the internal carotid artery or from the heart or proximal aorta may present with transient episodes of vision loss in one eye—a syndrome called amaurosis fugax. Platelet-fibrin emboli are usually responsible for transient interruption of blood flow in the retinal artery or its branches, and these appear dull and white on fundus view when present (see Fig. 4-3). Between episodes of amaurosis fugax, when vision is fully normal, bright shiny emboli emanating from ulcerated atheromata in the internal carotid artery may be observed. Hollenhorst[22] described these and characterized them as consisting of cholesterol crystals based on the highly refractile yellow appearance and the fact that their needlelike shape allows them to lodge without interrupting the flow of blood. This is why they are most often seen without ongoing vision defect or retinal whitening (Fig. 4-4).

## CEREBRAL VASCULAR DISORDERS

Strokes can occur at any age, even in newborns and children, but only older adults have them with any frequency. The basis for most strokes in older adults is atherosclerosis or arteriosclerosis. The most potent risk factor for arteriosclerosis is age, but other common ones include systemic hypertension, diabetes mellitus, hyperlipidemia, and hypercholesterolemia.

Manifestations of cerebral vascular disease include ischemic stroke from in situ thrombosis or, more commonly, from embolism originating in the heart or more proximal arteries, cerebral hemorrhage, or ischemic cranial neuropathy.

The neuro-ophthalmological manifestations of stroke are many, but as a practical issue for an office-based practice of optometry or ophthalmology, patients seldom have acute stroke-related symptoms. This is probably due to other neurological signs and symptoms that overshadow the eye-related ones and the fact that the patient most commonly presents primarily

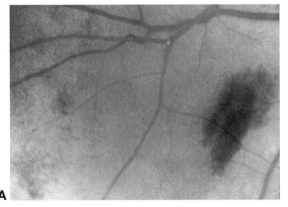

**A**

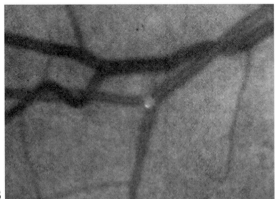

**B**

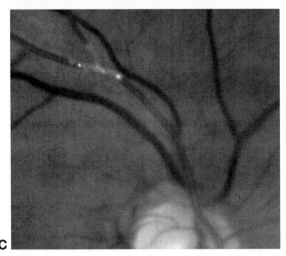

**C**

**Fig. 4-4 A,** Retinal arteriolar cholesterol emboli (Hollenhorst plaques). **B,** Close view of **A. C,** Longer cholesterol embolus that spans an arteriolar bifurcation. No retinal infarction is related to these cholesterol emboli.

to an emergency service, his or her primary physician, or a neurologist. The two most common exceptions are homonymous hemianopsia from calcarine (medial occipital lobe) infarction and diplopia from ischemic neu-

ropathy of the third, fourth, and sixth cranial nerves. In these instances the visual symptoms occur without overshadowing other neurological symptoms and the patient generally sees an eye care professional first.

**Calcarine Cortex Infarction**

Embolism or thrombosis involving the posterior cerebral artery or its calcarine branch presents with sudden onset of homonymous hemianopsia contralateral to the side of the medial occipital infarction involving Brodmann's area 17 and surrounding portions of area 18. A process called diaschisis may cause complete blindness at first and is defined as bilateral loss of cerebral function in the presence of unilateral disease. This generally passes within a few hours, leaving a dense homonymous hemianopsia except for sparing of the central 2 to 5 degrees of field surrounding fixation and possibly sparing of the unpaired or monocular temporal crescent in the most peripheral part of the hemianopic field (Fig. 4-5). In Figure 4-6 magnetic resonance imaging reveals infarction involving the left calcarine cortex and the resulting visual field defect limited to the right upper quadrant. The white arrows in parts *A* and *B* indicate the area of infarction, which appears white. The white arrowhead in part *B* indicates the left calcarine fissure; the infarction is limited to the lower bank of the calcarine fissure. Note also that the infarct does not extend all the way to the occipital pole and that this determines an area of central sparing within the involved right upper quadrant.

Central sparing is based on collateral vascular supply by distal branches of the middle cerebral artery to the occipital pole, where the fixation area of the visual field is represented in the calcarine cortex. Sparing of the unpaired temporal crescent is based on potential collateral supply to the most anterior portion of calcarine cortex, where the most peripheral part of the visual field is represented. Because the involved nasal field of the eye contralateral to the hemianopsia (left eye with right homonymous hemianopsia) extends only to approximately 50 to 55 degrees eccentricity and the involved temporal visual field of the other eye extends to approximately 80 degrees, the spared 20 to 30 degrees of peripheral visual field is only represented in the eye ipsilateral to the hemi-

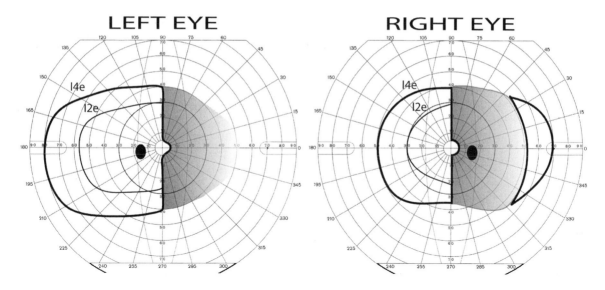

**Fig. 4-5** Goldmann visual field showing right homonymous hemianopsia with central sparing and sparing of the unpaired or monocular temporal crescent. This is a typical visual field defect from a left calcarine cortex (medial occipital lobe) infarction.

anopsia (right eye with right homonymous hemianopsia).

Another important diagnostic feature of visual field defects with lesions of the primary visual cortex is nearly total congruity. Congruity refers to the extent to which the spatial features (size, shape, and location) and the severity or density of the visual field defect is identical in the two eyes. For each point in the visual field the input from the two eyes converges on the same column of visual cortical cells, so whatever the disease process, it affects the visual field of the two eyes in an identical fashion. This is the anatomical basis of the rule that visual field defects from lesions of the primary visual cortex in Brodmann's area 17 are perfectly congruous. In more anterior portions of the visual radiations and in the optic tract in particular, the point-by-point inputs from the two eyes are not constrained anatomically to be in exactly the same place in the either the tract or the radiations; therefore the visual field defect in the two eyes may differ in spatial extent and density. A high degree of incongruity characterizes homonymous hemianopsia from incomplete optic tract lesions, although the tract is such a compact bundle of axons that most tract lesions give rise to total hemianopsia, which is nonspecific as a localizing feature and can occur with retrochiasmal lesions at all loci within the afferent visual system. A degree of incongruity intermediate between what is usually found with incomplete optic tract lesions on one hand and occipital cortical lesions on the other often characterizes homonymous visual field loss from lesions in the geniculocalcarine radiations.

With occipital infarction the visual field may show some improvement over time, but as a general rule the patient is left with permanent dense hemianopsia. The initial involvement may involve only an upper or lower quadrant rather than complete hemianopsia if only sub-branches of the calcarine artery are involved with single or multiple emboli. Multiple bilateral occipital embolic infarctions may present a diagnostically difficult visual field picture with multiple subquadrantic areas of field loss bilaterally, all homonymous and congruous as is the case with any occipital cortical lesion.

### Ischemic Cranial Neuropathy

Acute ischemic lesions of the third (oculomotor), fourth (trochlear), or sixth (abducens) cranial nerves present with sudden onset of diplopia and often pain in and around the eye on the same side. The basis for the associated pain is not clear but it is a regular feature of these lesions and may be quite severe. The pain tends to fade and disappear within 1 to 3 weeks of

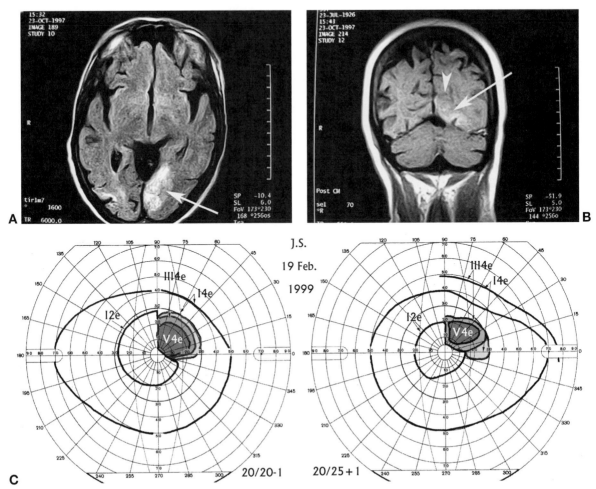

**Fig. 4-6** Left lower bank calcarine infarction. **A,** T1-weighted axial magnetic resonance image showing the area of infarction (*arrow*) in the medial occipital lobe sparing a small part of the occipital pole. **B,** T1-weighted coronal magnetic resonance image showing the infarction (*arrow*), which is limited to the lower bank of the calcarine fissure (*arrowhead*). **C,** Goldmann visual fields in the same patient. The right-hand field chart is the right eye, and the left-hand field chart is the left eye. A dense right upper quadrant homonymous scotoma shows a high degree of congruity between the two eyes. The small area of spared field next to fixation in that quadrant is present because the infarction illustrated in **A** does not extend all the way to the occipital pole. The sparing of visual field beyond the scotoma exists because the infarct does not extend all the way to the most anterior part of the calcarine cortex, which can also be seen in **A**. The scotoma is limited to the upper quadrant because the infarct is limited to the lower bank of the calcarine cortex.

onset, but the cranial nerve palsy generally requires 8 to 12 weeks to recover. Remarkably, they almost always completely recover in that time frame.

## Third Cranial Nerve Palsy

The muscles innervated by the third cranial nerve include the levator palpebrae superioris muscle, which lifts the upper eyelid; the medial rectus muscle, which adducts the eye; the superior rectus muscle, which elevates the eye; the inferior rectus muscle, which depresses the eye; and the inferior oblique muscle, which elevates the globe and the iris sphincter pupillae, which constricts the pupil. Acute third cranial nerve palsy therefore presents with marked, often complete, ptosis, with the globe depressed and abducted ("down and out") on account of remaining tone in the lateral rectus muscle, innervated by the sixth cranial nerve, and in the superior oblique muscle, innervated by the fourth cranial nerve. Involvement of the pupillary sphincter causes the pupil to be dilated and relatively fixed or nonreactive to light and effort to fixate a near point, the two main stimuli for pupillary constriction.

The condition of the pupil is a critical issue in diagnosis of acute third cranial nerve palsy. When the cause is ischemia within the trunk of the third nerve, the pupil is relatively spared, probably because the ischemia involves the interior of the nerve trunk and the pupillary parasympathetic fibers run in the most peripheral or superficial parts of the nerve trunk.

The most important other cause of acute third nerve palsy is a "berry" aneurysm at the posterior communicating artery junction with the internal carotid siphon. The dome of these aneurysms is immediately adjacent to the third cranial nerve in its subarachnoid portion, and enlargement of the aneurysm or blood leakage into the third nerve usually presents with acute third nerve palsy with or without symptoms of generalized subarachnoid hemorrhage (sudden massive headache and stiff neck followed by low back pain as the blood descends along the spinal cord). Because aneurysm enlargement and blood leakage both involve the peripheral portions of the third nerve trunk, prominent pupillary dilation and nonreactivity to light or near stimuli are usually present.

In any older patient with acute third nerve palsy, careful assessment of the state of the pupil must be made. One difficulty is that in ischemic third nerve palsy the pupil may be involved to some degree, but always to a lesser degree than the extraocular muscles. This means that in a patient with nearly complete ptosis and paralysis of the superior and inferior rectus muscles, the medial rectus muscle, and the inferior oblique muscle, the pupil might be a little larger than the other and might be a little more sluggishly reactive than the other and still be compatible with ischemia rather than aneurysm. However, any patient with *partial* or *mild* external ophthalmoplegia should have a completely normal pupil to qualify as ischemic rather than aneurysmal.[33,48] Even with a normal pupil, patients with partial external involvement should be watched carefully for increasing pupillary involvement because this has been shown to be delayed for up to 7 days after onset of third nerve palsy in some cases caused by aneurysm.[27]

### Fourth Cranial Nerve Palsy

The fourth cranial nerve, or trochlear nerve, innervates a single extraocular muscle on each side—the superior oblique muscle. This muscle is the primary depressor of the globe when in adduction and has a secondary action to intort or incyclodeviate the globe—that is, to rotate the eye about an anteroposterior axis, moving the 12 o'clock meridian of the iris toward the nose or midline. The torsional action of the superior oblique muscle is greatest and the depressive action is weakest with the globe in abduction. In each horizontal position of gaze, the action of the superior oblique muscle is a mixture of depression and intorsion, and in primary gaze the two actions are fairly equal.

These mixed actions of the superior oblique muscle determine that in primary gaze the patient with fourth nerve palsy will have vertical diplopia from hyperdeviation of the involved eye (relatively elevated compared with the other eye) and tilting of the deviated image on account of excyclodeviation (extorsion) caused by relative weakness of the intorsion function and unbalanced tone in the muscle that maintains excyclodeviation, the inferior oblique, innervated by the third cranial nerve.

The patient with fourth cranial nerve palsy is likely to soon have a compensatory head posture defined by head tilt away from the side of the lesion to artificially intort the globe, head turn away from the side of the lesion to move the involved eye out of adduction and into abduction where the vertical deviation is less, and chin-down position to move the eye into a more elevated position where less of the deficient depressive function is needed.

### Sixth Cranial Nerve Palsy

The sixth cranial nerve, or abducens nerve, also innervates a single extraocular muscle on either side, the abducens muscle, which has the single function of abducting the eye. Patients with sixth nerve palsy have horizontal diplopia with esotropia or deviation of the eye inward toward the nose.

## Anterior Circulation (Carotid Artery Distribution) Ischemic Stroke

As previously mentioned, many patients with stroke involving the cerebral hemispheres have homonymous hemianopsia as part of the symptom complex, but optometry professionals are not often called on to demonstrate this or quantify it with perimetry because the patient is often hemiplegic or mentally obtunded as well (at least in the acute stages of the illness) and they are not able to cooperate with visual sensory testing. Many of these patients remain mentally compromised or aphasic (specific loss of language capability), remain severely weak on one side, and are not able to cooperate with quantitative perimetry.

When eye care professionals are consulted for bedside examination while the patient is still in the hospital, it is often for fairly limited examination to determine the patient's gross level of visual function or to develop a set of eye movement findings to determine the patient's localizing value.

## Bedside Vision Testing in Neurologically Impaired Patients

### Visual Acuity

Visual acuity must be checked with a near card, but getting decent light onto the card with the patient lying down or propped up in bed can be a challenge in many hospital rooms. Optometry clinicians should carry a good hand light such as a Finoff head on the ophthalmoscope handle. This gives a uniform, bright illumination that can be directed on the card where the patient should read. Most penlights project a halo of light with a dark center that can confound attempts to use them for reading illumination or pupil testing. Many patients arrive at the hospital under emergency conditions and do not have their glasses with them. Often the most that can be done at the bedside is to get the best corrected acuity with the patient viewing through a pinhole, which should be carried in a kit for bedside examination. Under battlefield conditions, a hole can be punched in an index card with a safety pin for this purpose.

### Visual Fields: Confrontation Testing

The best way to test visual field at the bedside is with "confrontation" techniques, so named because the examiner faces the patient, usually from a distance of approximately 1 m. This usually requires the patient to be propped up somewhat in the bed, but it can be done with the patient completely supine.

Finger counting is the usual starting point and the most sensitive screening test for confrontation visual field testing. Mental obtundation and aphasia are big hurdles, but testing can be done on some patients with these afflictions. Many obtunded patients can be roused by loud calls or gentle shaking, even only for short intervals, but the arousal may have to be repeated to test each quadrant of each eye. The patient's eyes should be occluded one at a time for monocular testing; with some luck the patient may be able to hold a hand over one eye. This may not be possible with hemiplegia and other problems, so an occluder that can be strapped on the patient's head should be carried in the bedside kit. A suggested method is for the optometrist to close one eye and look at the patient's eye being tested to align the respective hemianopic midlines. The clinician then presents the fingers of his or her hand individually in the four quadrants with either one or two presentations per quadrant. This should take no more than 10 to 15 seconds per eye but could take longer depending on what must be done to maintain the patient's attention. Presenting one, two, or all fingers is most practical because it provides enough alternatives to determine if the patient can count fingers.

Some degree of quantitation can be obtained with confrontation visual field testing, depending on the patient's mental status. If, for instance, the patient cannot count fingers in a particular quadrant, then grosser stimuli can be presented to see how dense the defect is.

The hierarchy of usual stimuli from more challenging (requiring higher visual sensitivity) to less challenging (requiring less visual sensitivity) next to finger counting is hand motion and light perception, with and without "projection" (the ability to locate the source of the light). Hand motion is fairly straightforward—just wiggle the fingers or make a to-and-fro waving motion with the hand in each of the quadrants. Light perception testing is a little trickier. When shining a hand light into the patient's eye it reflects widely within the eye; even if the light circle of a direct ophthalmoscope is selectively focused on hemianopic portions of the retina, light scatter would stimulate nonhemianopic retina and the patient may detect light without actually seeing the point source. This problem of light scatter can be minimized by working in the brightest possible ambient illumination, which may be difficult in the usual hospital room. Ask the patient to say "now" or another word immediately if he or she sees the *source of the light*, the actual point of light that is the hand light's bulb. If the response is positive, that quadrant can be listed as having *light perception with projection*. Bare light perception without projection is not useful as a test of visual field because that perception cannot be localized to any particular quadrant or even half visual field.

A sensitive parameter to measure visual field by confrontation is subjective perception of a bright red object with a shift toward a duller or less saturated color in areas of defective visual field. This may well be abnormal in a mildly affected quadrant of visual field when the ability to count fingers is preserved. Therefore, if the patient counts fingers accurately in all quadrants, presenting a small bright red object to each quadrant is recommended for the patient's subjective response. Unfortunately, this requires uniform decent illumination, which is not allowed in any inpatient facility. A single red object can be moved back and forth between the right and left sides of the visual field, first in the upper quadrants and then in the lower quadrants; then ask the patient if the red changes to "less red" in any location. The patient finds it easier to make that judgment if two equally red objects, one in the right quadrant and the second in the left, are provided for simultaneous comparison of color saturation. In the defective field the color shift may be either toward a bleached-out orange or yellow or in the direction of darkening toward amber, but in either case the stimulus appears "less red" in the area of involved visual field. Whether the field defect changes to normal across the vertical hemianopic midline—which is highly characteristic of neurological visual field defects and is the defining feature of neurological hemianopsia—can even be determined with reasonable accuracy. The clinician should move the red object in the defective quadrant toward the midline and keep tabs on his or her own hemianopic midline while fixating the patient's

open eye while the patient is fixating your open eye. This method reliably assesses whether the patient indicates change in the red toward normal exactly as the clinician brings the stimulus across that mutual hemianopic midline.

So, with these limited sets of hierarchical stimuli from most sensitive (hardest to detect) to least sensitive (easiest to detect), it can be determined, whether, for instance, the patient has a homonymous hemianopsia that is worse in the upper quadrant or in the lower quadrant. Upper quadrant predominance of the defect is characteristic of temporal lobe lesions involving the geniculocalcarine radiations coursing toward the lower bank of the calcarine cortex. Lower quadrant predominance indicates a lesion in the parietal lobe involving the geniculocalcarine pathways en route to the upper bank of the calcarine cortex. (See Chapter 18 for further discussion of vision care in nontraditional settings.)

### Eye Movement Disorders with Anterior Circulation Strokes: Disorders of Conjugate Gaze

The cerebral hemispheres are the site of elaborate neuronal control circuitry for eye movements. This subject is beyond the scope of this chapter, but some simple eye movement findings can be characteristic of focal cerebral lesions such as cerebral infarction. The overriding principle behind cerebral eye movement abnormalities is that the two eyes remain relatively parallel with respect to one another and continue to move together, as is the case for normal conjugate gaze. The dynamics of the eye movements characterize the alterations caused by cerebral strokes.

In the acute stage of any sizeable cerebral infarction or hemorrhage, regardless of exact location, the eyes may be deviated away from the side of the stroke because of the unbalanced tone of the motor control circuits in the normal hemisphere, which cannot be shut down immediately. Each hemisphere in general exerts a tone that tends to deviate the eyes contralateral to the hemisphere in question. This torsional bias can be strong and can involve postural muscles in addition to eye muscles, such that the patient's eyes are in the extreme of lateral gaze away from the damaged hemisphere and his or her head and neck are strongly turned in the same direction. The patient is likely to have homonymous hemianopsia contralateral to the lesion as well. For instance, a patient with an acute right hemisphere infarct may lie for the first few days with the head turned all the way to the left with the eyes in an extreme left gaze as well. Visitors are usually advised to sit on the side opposite a homonymous hemianopsia so the patient can see them, but when the gaze and head are so strongly turned to the left, the only place the patient may still be able to see visitors is, paradoxically, on the left side of the bed.

After that initial period of extreme deviation, the patient usually regains the capacity over the course of several days to keep eyes more toward midline and eventually look all the way to the right and left. This then leads to the more subtle abnormalities of conjugate gaze that may be different with frontal lobe–versus parietal lobe–predominant lesions.

The two main conjugate eye movement systems that are organized at the level of the cerebral hemispheres are the saccade system and the ocular pursuit system. These two systems can be conceptualized in fairly intuitive ways. Being foveate animals, human beings can only see with high resolution and find detail in a fairly small area of central field a few degrees around the fixation point. So, to take in the visual scene, human beings must constantly refixate the gaze at different points around the visual environment and construct out of that dynamic input scenario a conscious perception of a stationary visual scene. The saccade system underlies these refixational eye movements to "palpate" the visual environment. The term *saccade* comes from a Greek word that refers to the flicking of a sail in the wind. Saccades are rapid conjugate eye movements that dart from one stationary object to another in the visual scene. Saccades become abnormal predominately in the presence of frontal lobe lesions, and in general that abnormality is that they become *hypometric,* or smaller than intended. Most human beings can make a 15-degree conjugate refixation in one large saccade and perhaps a tiny second saccade in the same direction to correct a small degree of hypometria. A patient who has recovered from the initial eye deviation after, for example, a right frontal infarction, may persist in having hypometric saccades when making refixations to his or her left. This can easily be tested for at the

bedside with a confrontation method that is similar to the visual field testing previously outlined, except the output is the clinician's observation of the patient's eye movements when asked to look first at the nose and then sequentially to the clinician's uplifted right and left hands on either side. Again considering a patient with right frontal stroke, refixations to the right from midline (the clinician's nose) are done in one or two saccades as normal, but leftward refixations (contraversive to the involved hemisphere), first back to the clinician's nose and then to the right hand in his left peripheral visual field, may require 8 to 10 small saccades in succession. This succession of hypometric saccades has a distinctive "ratchety" look because the neuronal machinery that generates saccades requires an approximately 200-msec lag before each saccade is generated. This patient could be described as having hypometric saccades to the left, which is consistent with a component of selective right frontal lobe dysfunction.

The other major cerebral conjugate gaze dynamic control system is that for ocular pursuit. The act of looking at an object usually involves acquiring the image of the object on the fovea of both eyes by a saccade or refixation. If that object happens to be moving relative to the viewer's position, he or she must produce a conjugate following eye movement that is matched in direction and velocity to that of the object. This is the business of the pursuit system, which becomes abnormal primarily after parietal lobe lesions. Unlike the saccade system, which is contraversive, the pursuit system is ipsiversive, with each hemisphere controlling pursuit in the same direction as the side of the hemisphere. For example, a right hemisphere parietal lobe lesion gives abnormal pursuit of objects moving to the right and not the left.

The abnormality that is caused by lesions involving the pursuit mechanism is pursuit that is too slow and does not match the velocity of the object being pursued. Because of this the eyes fall progressively behind the object, and eventually the brain ascertains, by monitoring visual data coming in from the afferent visual system, that the eye is no longer looking directly at the moving object. If voluntary commands are issued to the eye movement systems to look at a particular thing, which at some point is not being looked at, a saccade is generated to reacquire the image of that object onto the fovea of our eyes. A saccade is, of course, a rapid darting eye movement. In this case it will be in the same direction as the pursuit movement because the eye was behind or to the left of the object moving rightward. Things have not improved for the pursuit mechanism, and in a fraction of a second the eyes have again fallen behind and another forward saccade is generated. This cycle continues endlessly, all while the eye continues to pursue in the defective direction.

This succession of forward saccades has that same ratchety look as the succession of hypometric saccades with frontal lobe lesions previously discussed. But the mechanism of that succession of ratchety movements is completely different. The saccades were all too small in the case of frontal disease; with parietal lobe disease, the saccades are normal but the pursuit is defective. Remember that the task the patient is asked to perform is different for saccade testing ("Look back and forth between my nose and my hands"; nothing is moving in the environment) and pursuit testing ("Watch my hand as I move it right and left in front of you"). This is how pursuit can be tested in the same confrontation setting used for saccade testing. For pursuit, move the hand, with or without some other object for the patient to follow, at moderate speed from the extreme of the patient's right gaze to the extreme of his or her left gaze. The best speed for this kind of testing is 3 to 4 seconds to go across one time.

### *Posterior Circulation (Basilar-Vertebral Artery) Ischemic Stroke*

Strictly speaking, occipital or calcarine artery territory infarction is a manifestation of disease in the posterior or basilar-vertebral artery territory. This section mainly discusses the characteristic eye movement abnormalities that can result from brainstem infarction. The same findings can occur with brainstem hemorrhage, but these are much less common than infarction in this territory.

### Eye Movement Disorders with Posterior Circulation Strokes

#### *Cranial Nerve Involvement*

Brainstem infarction can involve the intraparenchymal portions of the trunks of the third, fourth, and sixth cranial nerves and produces the same clinical features as the primarily

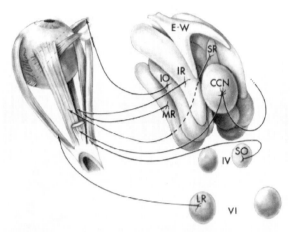

**Fig. 4-7** Third cranial (oculomotor) nerve nucleus and the extraocular muscles innervated by the various subnuclei. Also shown are the nuclei for the fourth and sixth cranial nerves. The superior rectus muscle receives crossed innervation from the contralateral subnucleus, as does the superior oblique muscle from the contralateral fourth nerve nucleus. The levator palpebrae muscle on either side receives both ipsilateral and contralateral innervation from the caudal central nucleus. *E-W*, Edinger-Westphal parasympathetic subnucleus innervating the pupillary sphincter muscle; *IR*, inferior rectus; *IO*, inferior oblique; *MR*, medial rectus; *CCN*, caudal central nucleus innervating both levator palpebrae muscles; *SO*, superior oblique (fourth cranial or trochlear nerve); *LR*, lateral rectus (abducens nucleus and sixth cranial nerve). (Reprinted from Glaser JS: *Neuro-ophthalmology*, ed 3, New York, 1999, Lippincott Williams & Wilkins.)

ischemic lesions in the more distal portions of these cranial nerves, as outlined above. Two exceptions are nuclear involvement of the third nerve and the sixth nerve, both relatively rare occurrences.

The nucleus of the third cranial nerve consists of a series of cell columns in pairs on either side of midline in the dorsal rostral midbrain (Fig. 4-7). Most of the muscles innervated by the third nerve receive only uncrossed input from the ipsilateral subnucleus, but the levator palpebrae superioris muscle receives bilateral input and the superior rectus muscle receives contralateral input. These two features lead to the distinguishing features of nuclear third nerve palsy, namely, bilateral ptosis and bilateral elevation palsy. The contralateral elevation palsy results from direct involvement of the superior rectus subnucleus, and its crossed output, and the ipsilateral elevation palsy result from damage of the fibers that have crossed from the opposite superior rectus subnucleus as they pass through the damaged ipsilateral nucleus.

### Disorders of Conjugate Gaze

Horizontal conjugate gaze is mediated by the sixth cranial nerve, or abducens nucleus (Figs. 4-8 and 4-9), which receives supranuclear input from the hemisphere conjugate gaze pathways. These include the outputs from the contralateral frontal saccade system and from the ipsilateral parietal pursuit system by way of intermediary connections in the pontine paramedian reticular formation, which is a diffuse array of cells in the reticular formation immediately surrounding the abducens nucleus on either side. The supranuclear pathway from the contraversive frontal saccade system (see Fig. 4-8) probably decussates (crosses midline) just caudal to the fourth nerve nucleus. Whether the ipsiversive parietal pursuit system output never decussates or decussates twice in its course to the pontine paramedian reticular formation is not clear. The special feature of the abducens nucleus is that it has a dual cell population—large cells that give rise to ipsilateral output by the sixth cranial nerve to the lateral rectus muscle on the same

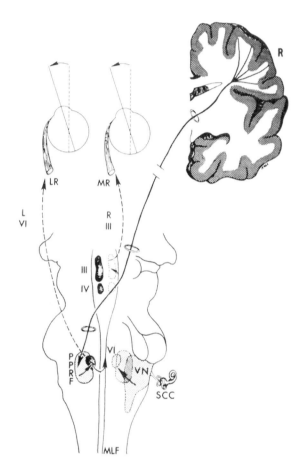

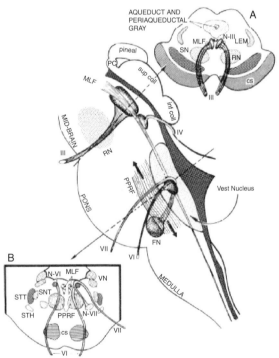

**Fig. 4-8** Brainstem pathways for conjugate horizontal gaze as viewed from above. The supranuclear input for saccades to the left *(L)* pontine paramedian reticular formation *(PPRF)* from the right *(R)* frontal lobe is shown. The ipsilateral input to the left PPRF from the parietal lobe for pursuit movements is not shown. The MLF carries, among other fibers, the output from the small cell population of the left abducens nucleus that has crossed to the right MLF to innervate the right medial rectus *(MR)* subnucleus of the third cranial nerve nucleus and from there activates the right medial MR muscle. *III, IV, VI,* Nuclei for the third, fourth, and sixth cranial nerves, respectively; *L VI,* course of the left sixth cranial nerve to the lateral rectus muscle *(LR)* of the left eye. (Reprinted from Glaser JS: *Neuro-ophthalmology,* ed 3, New York, 1999, Lippincott Williams & Wilkins.)

**Fig. 4-9** Sagittal diagrammatic view of the brainstem and cross sections through the brainstem at the level of the midbrain and the low pons, showing the third and sixth cranial nerve nuclei, the path of the fascicles of the third and sixth cranial nerves, and the pontine paramedian reticular formation. (Reprinted from Glaser: JS: *Neuro-ophthalmology,* ed 3, New York, 1999, Lippincott Williams & Wilkins.)

side and small cells that send axons up the contralateral medial longitudinal fascicules to the opposite medial rectus subnucleus of the third nerve complex, and thus to the medial rectus of the other eye. The combined activation of the ipsilateral lateral rectus and the contralateral medial rectus gives rise to conjugate ocular deviation. Put another way, each abducens nucleus is ipsiversive: the right abducens nucleus leads to abduction of the right eye (rightward movement) and adduction of the left eye (rightward movement).

### Internuclear Ophthalmoplegia (Syndrome of the Medial Longitudinal Fasciculus)

Internuclear ophthalmoplegia (INO) is a distinctive ocular motility syndrome that results from a lesion anywhere along the course of the medial longitudinal fasciculus (MLF) between the abducens nucleus in the caudal pons and the third cranial nerve nucleus in the midbrain (hence, "internuclear"). Because the input of the horizontal conjugate gaze system to the medial rectus subnucleus has been interrupted ipsilateral to the involved MLF, failure of adduction of that eye occurs. The conjugate gaze pathways to the contralateral lateral rectus muscle from the large cell population of the abducens nucleus on that side is not interrupted, so no interference with abduction of the contralateral eye occurs. Figure 4-8 shows leftward conjugate gaze by activation of the left paramedian pontine reticular formation and abducens nucleus. Imagine a lesion (not shown) along the right MLF rostral to the abducens nuclei. This blocks innervation coming from the small cell population of the left abducens nucleus en route to the right medial rectus nucleus and muscle. Therefore the right eye would fail to adduct (move left). The outflow from the left abducens to the left lateral rectus muscle (large cell population of the abducens nucleus) is not involved, so the left eye abducts fully.

The most distinctive feature of MLF syndrome or INO is that often, but not always, the abducting eye exhibits jerk nystagmus with fast phase in the direction of abduction. Why this instability occurs is not known. INO is distinguished from third cranial nerve palsy by the isolated involvement of adduction in the absence of pupillary mydriasis, ptosis, or vertical motility limitation.

INO is most frequently encountered in younger persons as a manifestation of multiple sclerosis. It can be caused by small lacunar infarcts in the brainstem in older adults but is not common, probably because the MLF is in the dorsal part of the brainstem where collateral blood supply from the long circumferential branches of the basilar artery supplements the flow from the paramedian branches that supply the dorsal medial brainstem and MLF.

### Intracranial Hemorrhage

Intracranial hemorrhage may lead to elevated intracranial pressure, causing papilledema. Papilledema is defined as bilateral optic nerve head swelling caused by elevated intracranial pressure specifically. The earliest stages of papilledema may be difficult to discern from normal and consist of slight thickening of the nerve, especially on the nasal side where the optic disc is naturally thicker than the temporal side. Stasis of axoplasmic flow causes accumulation of water in the axons of the retinal nerve fiber layer, and the resulting whitish opacity of the nerve fiber layer obscures from view the underlying disc margin. The margins of the choroid and retinal pigment epithelium, inside of which is the fenestrated bare white sclera of the cribriform plate, account for the white appearance of the "disc." Of course, the whiteness of the normal disc is modified by hemoglobin in capillaries within the tissue of the nerve fiber layer, which imparts the normal pink hue to the optic disc. As the nerve fiber layer swells, vascular congestion often increases the redness of the swollen disc, making it appear hyperemic. Because the retinal arterioles and veins dip in and out of the normal nerve fiber layer as they cross the disc margin, the opacity of the swollen layer obscures sections of these vessels as well as the underlying disc margin.

Visual function is usually normal in papilledema until a late stage when degeneration of the swollen axons may lead to devastating vision loss. This early normal visual function distinguishes papilledema from other forms of disc swelling in which disease directly affects the nerve head— most commonly either optic neuritis (inflammation) or anterior ischemic optic neuropathy (ischemia). The loss of vision that accompanies incipient postpapilledema optic atrophy is stereotyped for reasons that are not entirely clear. The first change from normal vision is loss of the inferior nasal part of the peripheral visual field, followed by concentric contraction of the peripheral field in all quadrants. Only after peripheral visual field has been extensively lost will central visual functions be lost, including visual acuity and color vision.

The following two syndromes related to posterior fossa hemorrhage have distinctive neuro-ophthalmological manifestations.

## Thalamic Hemorrhage

Hemorrhage into the thalamus on one side gives rise to characteristic ocular motility and pupillary phenomena. Vertical gaze palsy is common, especially upgaze palsy leading to downward deviation of both eyes. In addition horizontal conjugate deviation of the eyes toward the side of the lesion or, less commonly, away from the side of the lesion ("wrong-way eyes") can also occur. The pupils are often asymmetrically miotic, smaller on the side of the lesion, and fixed to light.

Other neurological findings include dense contralateral hemisensory defect and some degree of contralateral hemiparesis.

## Pontine Hemorrhage

The pons in the brainstem is a site of predilection for hypertensive intracerebral hemorrhage. Primary hemorrhage in the cerebellum, typically centered on the dentate nucleus, can secondarily break into the pons and cause a similar set of eye findings.

The patient with primary or secondary pontine hemorrhage typically hash sudden coma from involvement of the reticular activating system on both sides. Quadriplegia from involvement of the pyramidal tracts ventrally commonly occurs. The pupils are pinpoint but reactive, probably reflecting bilateral disruption of the sympathetic pathways through the dorsolateral parts of the pons. Complete horizontal gaze palsy leaves only vertical movements of the eyes and characteristic repetitive conjugate downward jerks followed by slower return to primary position—called "ocular bobbing" because of the similarity in movement to a bobber in water when a fish nibbles at a fishing line. Bobbing is the most characteristic

pattern for repetitive eye movements in pontine lesions, although a variant with slow conjugate downward movement followed by rapid upward return to primary gaze is called "ocular dipping"—perhaps referring to dipping a ladle in soup or water (although ladling soup with a rapid upward jerk sounds messy). Converse bobbing or reverse dipping has been used to describe rapid upward conjugate deviation followed by slower downward return to primary gaze that can also be seen with pontine lesions.[43]

## REFERENCES

1. Baldursson O, Steinsson K, Bjornsson J, et al: Giant cell arteritis in Iceland. An epidemiologic and histopathologic analysis, *Arthritis Rheum* 37:1007-12, 1994.
2. Barilla-LaBarca ML, Lenschow DJ, Brasington RD Jr: Polymyalgia rheumatica/temporal arteritis: recent advances, *Curr Rheumatol Rep* 4:39-46, 2002.
3. Beri M, Klugman MR, Kohler JA, et al: Anterior ischemic optic neuropathy. VII. Incidence of bilaterality and various influencing factors, *Ophthalmology* 94:1020-28, 1987.
4. Birkhead NC, Wagener HP, Shick RM: Treatment of temporal arteritis with adrenal corticosteroids: results in fifty-five cases in which lesion was proved at biopsy, *JAMA* 163:821-7, 1957.
5. Buttner T, Heye N, Przuntek H: Temporal arteritis with cerebral complications: report of four cases, *Eur Neurol* 34:162-7, 1994.
6. Calguneri M, Cobankara V, Ozatli D, et al: Is visual loss due to giant cell arteritis reversible? *Yonsei Med J* 44:155-8, 2003.
7. Caselli RJ, Hunder GG, Whisnant JP: Neurologic disease in biopsy-proven giant cell (temporal) arteritis, *Neurology* 38:352-9, 1988.
8. Delecoeuillerie G, Joly P, Cohen dL, et al: Polymyalgia rheumatica and temporal arteritis: a retrospective analysis of prognostic features and different corticosteroid regimens (11 year survey of 210 patients), *Ann Rheum Dis* 47:733-739, 1988.
9. Evans JM, O'Fallon WM, Hunder GG: Increased incidence of aortic aneurysm and dissection in giant cell (temporal) arteritis. A population-based study, *Ann Intern Med* 122:502-7, 1995.
10. Fisher CM: Observations of the fundus oculi in transient monocular blindness, *Neurology* 9:333-47, 1959.
11. Fledelius HC, Nissen KR: Giant cell arteritis and visual loss. A 3-year retrospective hospital investigation in a Danish county, *Acta Ophthalmol (Copenh)* 70:801-5, 1992.

12. Gillanders LA: Temporal arteriography, *Clin Radiol* 20:149-56, 1969.

13. Gilmour JR: Giant-cell chronic arteritis, *J Pathol* 53:263-77, 1941.

14. Gordon I: Polymyalgia rheumatica. A clinical study of 21 cases, *Q J Med* 29:473-88, 1960.

15. Hamilton CRS, Shelley WM, Tumulty PA: Giant cell arteritis. Including temporal arteritis and polymyalgia rheumatica, *Medicine (Baltimore)* 50:1-27, 1971.

16. Hamrin B: Polymyalgia arteritica with morphological changes in the large arteries, *Acta Med Scand Suppl* 533:4-164, 1972.

17. Hayreh SS, Podhajsky PA, Raman R, et al: Giant cell arteritis: validity and reliability of various diagnostic criteria, *Am J Ophthalmol* 123:285-96, 1997.

18. Hayreh SS, Podhajsky PA, Zimmerman B: Ocular manifestations of giant cell arteritis, *Am J Ophthalmol* 125:509-20, 1998.

19. Hayreh SS, Podhajsky PA, Zimmerman B: Ipsilateral recurrence of nonarteritic anterior ischemic optic neuropathy, *Am J Ophthalmol* 132:734-42, 2001.

20. Hayreh SS, Zimmerman B, Kardon RH: Visual improvement with corticosteroid therapy in giant cell arteritis. Report of a large study and review of literature, *Acta Ophthalmol Scand* 80:355-67, 2002.

21. Hoffman GS, Cid MC, Hellmann DB, et al: A multicenter, randomized, double-blind, placebo-controlled trial of adjuvant methotrexate treatment for giant cell arteritis, *Arthritis Rheum* 46:1309-18, 2002.

22. Hollenhorst RW: Significance of bright plaques in the retinal arterioles, *JAMA* 178:23-29, 1961.

23. Horton BT, Magath TB, Brown GE: An undescribed form of arteritis of the temporal vessels, *Proc Mayo Clin* 7:700-701, 1932.

24. Hutchinson J: Disease of the arteries, *Arch Surg* 1:323-9, 1889.

25. Ischemic Optic Neuropathy Study Group: Characteristics of patients with nonarteritic anterior ischemic optic neuropathy eligible for the Ischemic Optic Neuropathy Decompression Trial, *Arch Ophthalmol* 114:1366-74, 1996.

26. Kimmelstiel P, Gilmour MT, Hodges HH: Degeneration of elastic fibers in granulomatous giant cell arteritis (temporal arteritis), *Arch Pathol* 54:157-68, 1952.

27. Kissel JT, Burde RM, Klingele TG, et al: Pupil-sparing oculomotor palsies with internal carotid-posterior communicating artery aneurysms, *Ann Neurol* 13:149-54, 1983.

28. Klein RG, Campbell RJ, Hunder GG, et al: Skip lesions in temporal arteritis, *Proc Mayo Clin* 51:504-10, 1976.

29. Kupersmith MJ, Frohman L, Sanderson M, et al: Aspirin reduces the incidence of second eye NAION: a retrospective study, *J Neuroophthalmol* 17:250-3, 1997.

30. Kyle V, Hazleman BL: Treatment of polymyalgia rheumatica and giant cell arteritis. I. Steroid regimens in the first two months, *Ann Rheum Dis* 48:658-61, 1989a.

31. Kyle V, Hazleman BL: Treatment of polymyalgia rheumatica and giant cell arteritis. II. Relation between steroid dose and steroid associated side effects, *Ann Rheum Dis* 48:662-6, 1989b.

32. Kyle V, Hazleman BL: The clinical and laboratory course of polymyalgia rheumatica/giant cell arteritis after the first two months of treatment, *Ann Rheum Dis* 52:847-50, 1993.

33. Lee SH, Lee SS, Park KY, et al: Isolated oculomotor nerve palsy: diagnostic approach using the degree of external and internal dysfunction, *Clin Neurol Neurosurg* 104:136-41, 2002.

34. Lie JT: Aortic and extracranial large vessel giant cell arteritis: a review of 72 cases with histopathologic documentation, *Semin Arthritis Rheum* 24:422-31, 1995.

35. Liozon F, Jauberteau-Marchan MO, Boutros-Toni F, et al: Anticardiolipin antibodies and Horton disease [in French], *Ann Med Interne (Paris)* 146:541-7, 1995.

36. Machado E, Michet C, Ballard D, et al: Trends in incidence and clinical presentation of temporal arteritis in Olmsted County, Minnesota, 1950-1985, *Arthritis Rheum* 31:745-9, 1988.

37. Matzkin DC, Slamovits TL, Sachs R, et al: Visual recovery in two patients after intravenous methylprednisolone treatment of central retinal artery occlusion secondary to giant-cell arteritis, *Ophthalmology* 99:68-71, 1992.

38. Mitomo T, Funyu T, Takahashi Y, et al: Giant cell arteritis and magnetic resonance angiography, *Arthritis Rheum* 41:1702, 1998.

39. Myles AB, Perera T, Ridley MG: Prevention of blindness in giant cell arteritis by corticosteroid treatment, *Br J Rheumatol* 31:103-5, 1992.

40. Nesher G, Rubinow A, Sonnenblick M: Efficacy and adverse effects of different corticosteroid dose regimens in temporal arteritis: a retrospective study, *Clin Exp Rheumatol* 15:303-6, 1997.

41. Ostberg G: On arteritis with special reference to polymyalgia arteritica, *Acta Path Microbiol Scand* 237:1-59, 1973.

42. Roblot P: Immunosuppressive agents in Horton's disease. Which drug for which indication? [in French]. *Ann Med Interne (Paris)* 149:441-7, 1998.

43. Rosenberg ML: Spontaneous vertical eye movements in coma, *Ann Neurol* 20: 635-7, 1986.

44. Salvarani C, Hunder GG: Giant cell arteritis with low erythrocyte sedimentation rate: frequency of occurrence in a population-based study, *Arthritis Rheum* 45:140-5, 2001.

45. Schmidt D, Vaith P, Hetzel A: Prevention of serious ophthalmic and cerebral complications in temporal arteritis? *Clin Exp Rheumatol* 18(4 suppl 20):S61-3, 2000.

46. Shick RM, Baggenstoss AH, Paulley HF: Effects of cortisone and ACTH on periarteritis nodosa and cranial arteritis, *Proc Mayo Clin* 25:492-4, 1950a.

47. Shick RM, Baggenstoss AH, Paulley HF: Effects of cortisone and ACTH on periarteritis nodosa and cranial arteritis, *Proc Mayo Clin* 25:135, 1950b.

48. Trobe JD: Isolated pupil-sparing third nerve palsy, *Ophthalmology* 92:58-61, 1985.

49. Wagener HP, Hollenhorst RW: The ocular lesions of temporal arteritis, *Am J Ophthalmol* 45:617-30, 1958.

50. Weyand CM, Fulbright JW, Hunder GG, et al: Treatment of giant cell arteritis: interleukin-6 as a biologic marker of disease activity, *Arthritis Rheum* 43:1041-8, 2000.

# CHAPTER 5

# Anterior Segment Diseases in the Older Adult

## MICHAEL J. GIESE and SHELLEY M. WU

This chapter addresses the common clinical findings associated with aging. Also reviewed are changes induced by exposure to environmental elements. This chapter is organized in anatomical sequence from anterior to posterior, specifically from the periorbital dermis to the lens.

## EYELIDS

The most visible aging changes occur in the eyelids and the surrounding skin. Patients with lid disorders may report pain, red eyes, itching, dryness, and swelling.

As aging occurs, eyelids tend to become dry, wrinkled, less elastic, and thinner. A reduction in the secretions from eccrine sweat glands and atrophy of apocrine structures (e.g., glands of Moll) cause these changes. Desquamation of skin slows with age, leading to a wrinkled appearance. However, keratinization of the lid margin increases with age, imparting a thick, leathery character. Thinning is primarily associated with changes in the subepithelial compartments. Basal epithelial cell replication decreases, causing a reduction in the efficacy of its healing mechanisms. Langerhans cells (antigen presenting cells) and melanocytes also decrease. These physiological changes elevate the risk of neoplasia from ultraviolet (UV) A and B radiation exposure. Numerous sources have supported the causative relation between sun exposure and neoplasms.

Other sun-related skin damage commonly observed in older adults is pigment changes ("sun spots") and erythema ("liver spots"). They are the result of altered focal melanin synthesis rates. The frequently observed coarse wrinkles along facial musculature are a result of elastotic collagen loss. UV exposure is also associated with an increase in inflammatory cells, namely, mast cells and fibroblasts. Consequently, a decreased immunity to viral, fungal, bacterial, and neoplastic diseases occurs with greater frequency in aged eyelids.

Unrelated to UV exposure, eyelid connective tissue also undergoes age-related pathological changes. These changes reduce tensile strength, leading to increased laxity. The commonly observed lid malpositions in older adults include senile ptosis, increased laxity, ectropion, and entropion.

The most common form of pathological change is involutional blepharoptosis. Typically bilateral, this is the result of the decreased ability to elevate the upper lid. The condition appears to worsen during superior gaze. Histological evidence suggests changes in the integrity of levator aponeurosis and its attachments to the tarsal plate as a possible cause. A decreased lower lid position is seen in 85% of individuals between the ages of 71 and 89 years.[30] Affected individuals have an inferior lid resting position lowered by 1 to 2 mm compared with individuals who are age 30 years and younger. The upper lid resting position was also found to change by 0.4 mm per decade after age 30 years. Lid laxity is easily evaluated by performing the "pinch test," in which the ability of the lid to return to its normal resting position is evaluated. The palpebral fissure width is shortened to 25 mm at age 50 years from 27.1 mm for individuals aged 49 years and younger.[14]

Physiological changes, altered lower lid position, shortened horizontal palpebral fissure widths, and reduced lid retractor function cause the inferior lid and punctum to roll outward. This displacement is called an ectropion, and it can lead to tarsal conjunctival dryness and inflammation from exposure to the external environment (Fig. 5-1). Chronic ectropion causes thickening of the lid margins, epiphora, excoriation of the skin, and exposure keratitis. The opposite of ectropion is referred to as entropion (eyelid turned out), which can also occur when lid laxity, combined with relatively normal orbicular muscle tension, causes inversion of the lid margin (Fig. 5-2).

Lid closure problems are often associated with tear film instability. This instability does not allow the tears to protect the eyes and prevent drying, especially during sleep. Treatment includes artificial tears, bland ointments, shields, and possibly tarsorrhaphy.

## Other Common Lid Disorders in Older Persons

### Acquired Lesions of the Lids

Blepharitis, or infection of the lid margin, is common in older adults (Fig. 5-3). The lid margins are red, thickened, and may have a scalloped appearance. This condition can be associated with seborrhea of the eyebrows, skin

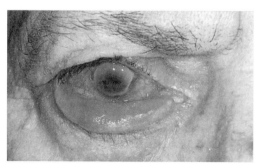

**Fig. 5-1** Ectropion. (From Parrish RK II, editor: *The University of Miami Bascom Palmer Eye Institute atlas of ophthalmology*, Philadelphia, 2000, Butterworth-Heinemann.)

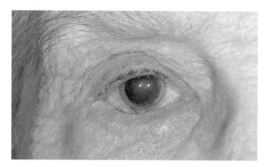

**Fig. 5-2** Entropion. (From Parrish RK II, editor: *The University of Miami Bascom Palmer Eye Institute atlas of ophthalmology*, Philadelphia, 2000, Butterworth-Heinemann.)

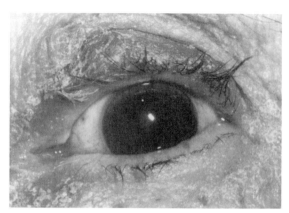

**Fig. 5-3** Staphylococcal blepharitis. (From Roberts DK, Terry JE: *Ocular disease: diagnosis & treatment*, ed 2, Boston, 1996, Butterworth-Heinemann.)

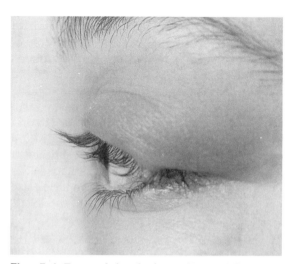

**Fig. 5-4** External hordeolum. (From Silbert JA: *Anterior segment complications of contact lens wear*, ed 2, Boston, 2000, Butterworth-Heinemann.)

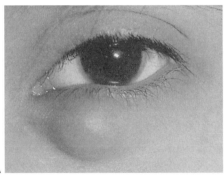
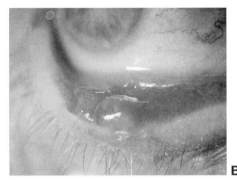

A                                                                                        B

**Fig. 5-5** Chalazion. **A,** external; **B,** internal. (From Kanski JJ, Bolton A: *Illustrated tutorials in clinical ophthalmology,* Boston, 2001, Butterworth-Heinemann.)

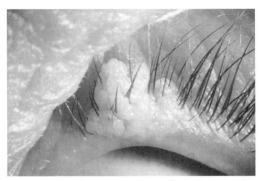

**Fig. 5-6** Squamous papilloma. (From Parrish RK II, editor: *The University of Miami Bascom Palmer Eye Institute atlas of ophthalmology,* Philadelphia, 2000, Butterworth-Heinemann.)

of the nose, cheeks, and scalp. This disease is chronic and sometimes disabling but can be managed with proper lid hygiene and antibiotics if necessary.

Meibomian gland dysfunction increases in frequency with age. Both changes in the gland orifice and alterations in blinking mechanisms appear to contribute to the condition. Various other lid lesions can result from meibomian gland disorders. An acute purulent inflammation of either the glands of Zeis or Moll or the sebaceous glands produces an external hordeolum (Fig. 5-4). If the inflammation is in the meibomian gland, it is called an internal hordeolum. Meibomian glands are often infected with *Staphylococcus* organisms that can lead to numerous and frequent infections. Another commonly seen lid lesion is the chalazion. Chalazae are granulomas that develop around

inflamed meibomian glands (Fig. 5-5). The clinical presentation includes a round, firm, and often painless lesion at the tarsal plate. Individuals with acne rosacea and seborrheic dermatitis have increased risk of having chalazae.

Various cysts are also commonly seen on the lids and lid margins. A cyst of Moll clinically presents as a small, round, translucent, fluid-filled lesion with no associated pain. A cyst of Zeis has a similar presentation but has a less-translucent appearance.

### Benign Lesions of the Lids

Squamous papilloma is a widely used term used to describe numerous lesions. They are the most common benign eyelid lesions and appear in middle-aged and older individuals. Clinically they present as multiple, flesh-colored lesions attached to the lid margin by either a pedicle or a broad base (Fig. 5-6). Histologically, squamous papillomas consist of vascularized connective tissue covered by acanthotic epithelium. These lesions are different from wartlike lesions, which consist of inflammatory hypertrophy with viral inclusions. Only surgical excision is necessary for removal of squamous papillomatous lesions.

Seborrheic keratosis, also known as basal cell papilloma or other names, is mostly found in the aging population (Fig. 5-7). It presents in a wide variety of clinical appearances and sizes. They are often well-circumscribed, greasy, and frequently hyperpigmented single or multiple lesions.

Keratoacanthomas are elevated, dome-shaped lesions found in sun-exposed areas of the skin (Fig. 5-8). They are rapidly growing and can

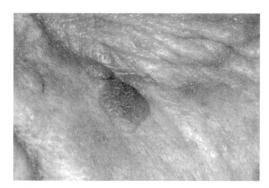

**Fig. 5-7** Seborrheic keratosis. (From Parrish RK II, editor: *The University of Miami Bascom Palmer Eye Institute atlas of ophthalmology*, Philadelphia, 2000, Butterworth-Heinemann.)

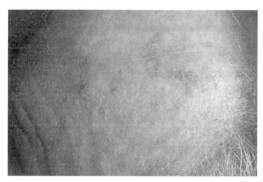

**Fig. 5-9** Actinic keratosis. (From Parrish RK II, editor: *The University of Miami Bascom Palmer Eye Institute atlas of ophthalmology*, Philadelphia, 2000, Butterworth-Heinemann.)

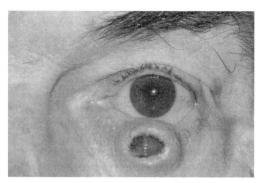

**Fig. 5-8** Keratoacanthoma. (From Parrish RK II, editor: *The University of Miami Bascom Palmer Eye Institute atlas of ophthalmology*, Philadelphia, 2000, Butterworth-Heinemann.)

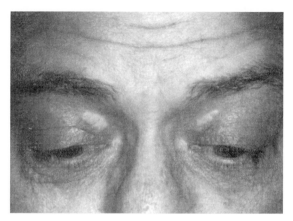

**Fig. 5-10** Xanthelasma. (From Roberts DK, Terry JE: *Ocular disease: diagnosis & treatment*, ed 2, Boston, 1996, Butterworth-Heinemann.)

develop in weeks. They may undergo involutional changes, leaving a scar and possibly tissue damage if they occur at the eyelid margin. These lesions tend to have a craterlike appearance with telangiectatic vessels. They may be the result of inflammation or be associated with a viral element. These lesions are commonly misdiagnosed as squamous cell or basal cell carcinoma and therefore must be closely watched. Treatment of these lesions is conservative.

Actinic keratosis (aka solar keratosis) often affects the fair-skinned older population and is the most common precancerous cutaneous lesion in middle-aged individuals (Fig. 5-9). As the common name suggests, these lesions are the result of UV damage to the epidermis. They typically present as multiple yellow or erythematous lesions, oval in shape and with a nodular horny or wartlike configuration. They are rough and scaly in appearance. Approximately 13% of untreated lesions can transform into squamous cell carcinoma.[5,27]

Xanthelasma are elevated, yellowish plaquelike lesions usually located on the eyelids in the inner canthal area (Fig. 5-10). They are most commonly seen in women. These lesions are composed of histiocytes filled with lipid material in the superficial dermis. One third of these lesions may be associated with elevated cholesterol or triglycerides.[1] Treatment usually consists of excision or carbon dioxide laser treatment.

Cutaneous horns are filiform lesions on the surface of the skin that consist of an overproduction of keratin (Fig. 5-11). Squamous cell carcinoma should be ruled out prior to removal of these lesions.

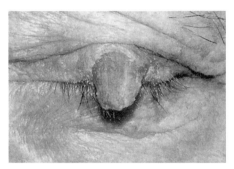

**Fig. 5-11** Cutaneous horn. (From Kanski JJ, Bolton A: *Illustrated tutorials in clinical ophthalmology,* Boston, 2001, Butterworth-Heinemann.)

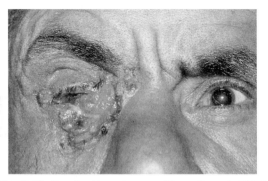

**Fig. 5-12** Basal cell carcinoma. (From Parrish RK II, editor: *The University of Miami Bascom Palmer Eye Institute atlas of ophthalmology,* Philadelphia, 2000, Butterworth-Heinemann.)

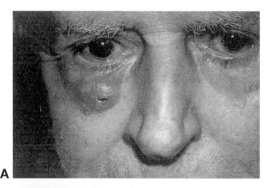

**A**

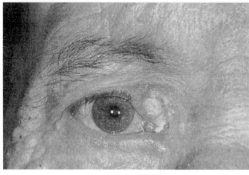

**B**

**Fig. 5-13 A** and **B,** Squamous cell carcinoma. (From Parrish RK II, editor: *The University of Miami Bascom Palmer Eye Institute atlas of ophthalmology,* Philadelphia, 2000, Butterworth-Heinemann.)

### Malignant Lid Lesions

Basal cell carcinoma is the most common malignant lid tumor (90% of all lid malignancies).[29] The tumor is slow growing, focally invasive, but not metastatic. The typical basal cell occurs in the lower lid or inner canthus (Fig. 5-12). Three types have been characterized: nodular, ulcerative, and sclerosing. Clinical presentation is widely variable, as their names suggest. The nodular type usually manifests as pearly or waxy nodules with telangiectatic vessels. A central ulceration may develop as a result of the growth of the tumor outpacing the blood supply. Unlike squamous cell carcinoma, a surface crust is typically not found in basal cell carcinoma.

Squamous cell carcinoma (Fig. 5-13) is possibly the second most common lid malignancy (9% of all periocular cutaneous tumors).[29] However, it is more aggressive than basal cell carcinoma, and, unlike basal cell carcinoma, it can metastasize to regional lymph nodes. The lesions can develop from premalignant lesions such as actinic keratosis. Clinical presentation typically begins with a hard nodule with rough crust on the surface. Eventually ulceration develops in this area. Early detection is crucial because of its metastatic potential; an oncology evaluation must be considered.

Sebaceous gland carcinoma is less common than basal and squamous cell carcinoma (Fig. 5-14). This lesion has the potential to metastasize to regional lymph nodes and orbit and has an associated mortality rate. It most commonly arises from meibomian glands and occasionally from the glands of Zeis. Early clinical presentation may be subtle and mimic recurrent chalazion or chronic conjunctivitis. Older women have a higher risk than older men. Two types of sebaceous gland carcinomas with different clinical presentations have been characterized: nodular and spreading. A nodular carcinoma is a firm, yellow, and slow growing lesion that can mimic a chronic chalazia. Spreading sebaceous

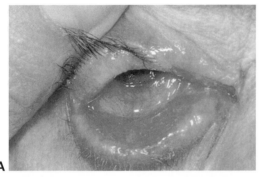

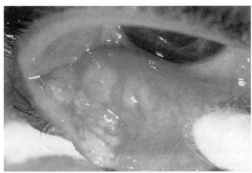

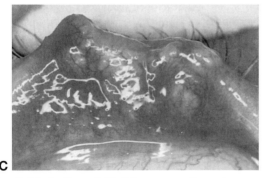

**Fig. 5-14 A, B,** and **C,** Sebaceous cell carcinoma. (From Parrish RK II, editor: *The University of Miami Bascom Palmer Eye Institute atlas of ophthalmology,* Philadelphia, 2000, Butterworth-Heinemann.)

gland carcinoma has a subtle clinical presentation. The tumor spreads into the dermis and presents as a diffuse area of thickening and inflammation along the lid margin, which can mimic chronic, nonresponsive blepharitis. Spread can occur in the palpebral, fornical, or bulbar conjunctiva. The last can involve corneal neovascularization and conjunctival injection similar to conjunctivitis or superior limbic keratoconjunctivitis. If diagnosed early, surgery can be performed; however, if advanced spread to numerous areas is detected, a complete exenteration may be required.

## LACRIMAL GLAND AND TEAR DRAINAGE SYSTEM

The incidence of dry eyes is substantial in the general population and significant in older adults. Reduction in tear quantity and quality in aging eyes has been noted and supported by histopathological evidence. The force and completeness of blinking are also reduced.

Dry eye syndromes are frequently complicated by lid-cornea incongruities (ectropion, trichiasis, pterygium, lid margin hypertrophy) or orbicularis weakness. Corneal sensitivity may also be decreased. The problem therefore is not only that the patient has a dry eye, but also that he or she does not blink normally in response to the dryness. This results in dry spots (dellen), which may progress to erosion and ulceration. Symptoms include irritation, foreign body sensation, intolerance to dust and smoke and, occasionally, excessive tearing. Biomicroscopy reveals an irregular tear meniscus containing mucous debris, corneal filaments, punctate staining in the lower half of the cornea, a rapid tear breakup time (less than 10 seconds) and a positive Schirmer test result. In some cases the clinical picture resembles papillary conjunctivitis.[21] Atrophy and fibrosis of acinar elements and periductal fibrosis have been reported. These changes tend to be seen more in women than in men and lead to a 50% decrease in basal tear secretion observed for 50-year-old individuals compared with younger eyes.[20] Changes are also found in the cellular components of the lacrimal gland. Lymphocyte infiltration may lead to changes in other immunological elements such as immunoglobulin A, chemotactic factors, and other proteins. This might support the increase in dacryoadenitis in aging patients. Basal tear production clearly decreases with age, and thus the increase of epiphora also seen in older adults may imply alterations in the nasal lacrimal outflow system. However, no consistent findings have been reported to support age-related changes in the drainage system.

## CONJUNCTIVA

The conjunctiva can be involved in allergic reactions; infections; and toxic, mechanical, traumatic, degenerative, and vascular changes. Patients may report hyperemia, exudates, itchy or burning sensations, tearing, and chemosis.

## Palpebral

Certain elements change with age and others do not. Epithelium and goblet cells remain stable with age. However, immunological cells such as mast cells remain unchanged, whereas a reduction in Langerhans cells is observed. Enlarged vascular luminal changes are noted, which may contribute to increased conjunctiva injection seen in older adults. Other vascular changes include a decrease in capillary numbers, which may contribute to ischemia in the orbicular muscle and the muscle of Riolan in the lids. Many other histological changes occur, and all affect the eyelids of older adults.

## Bulbar Conjunctiva

The epithelium of the bulbar conjunctiva thickens with age. In contrast, subepithelial layers thin, whereas elastin degenerates. Consequently the subepithelial layers become mobile and fragile.

Aging effects on the bulbar conjunctiva are most visible in the interpalpebral areas because of the exposure to environmental elements. Pingueculae are found in 97% of individuals older than 50 years and in only 7% of individuals younger than 20 years.[25] The onset can occur earlier in the population with more UV exposure; however, almost every 80-year-old will have them even without sun exposure. Thus both aging and UV factors contribute to the occurrence of these lesions, which are composed of degenerated basophilic subepithelial tissues and fibers.

The causative relation between pingueculae and pterygia is debatable, and less evidence exists to support the idea that the latter entity is age related.

## Conjunctival Melanoma

Conjunctival melanoma (Fig. 15-15) usually arises in the older population (mean age, 62 years).[29] It most commonly arises from primary acquired melanosis and rarely from preexisting nevi. The mortality rate is related to the origin of the tumor, with those arising from primary acquired melanosis having the greatest rate. These lesion show great variability; can reoccur; and can metastasize to the brain, lung, or liver.

## CORNEA

Cornea size remains stable at 11.7 mm.[17] The diameter may slightly decrease by 0.4 mm after the age of 40 years, possibly because of expansion of the corneoscleral junction. Corneal thickness also appears to remain stable with aging. Corneal curvature, on the contrary, appears to change with age—from steep to flat at puberty to steep again in adults. The aspherical character of the cornea changes from with-the-rule in 92.8% of youth to against-the-rule in 85.7% in older adults.[3,13,15,28] This change also coincides with the change in lid laxity, but currently no direct relation has been substantiated.

## Corneal Sensitivity

A decrease of corneal sensitivity beginning at age 40 years occurs.[22] It continues to decline with age. Surprisingly, no evidence suggests age-related changes in the corneal nerves themselves.

## Tear Film

The prevalence of bacterial infection increases in older adults. This can be explained by the increase in adherence of bacterial organisms to

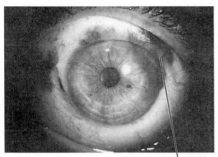
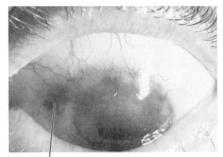

Malignant melanoma

**Fig. 5-15** Conjunctival melanoma. (From Kaiser PK, Friedman NJ: *The Massachusetts Eye & Ear Infirmary illustrated manual of ophthalmology*, Philadelphia, 2004, Saunders.)

the mucin component of tears. The decrease in tear production and quality has been previously discussed.

### Epithelium

Several clinical observations of epithelial changes caused by aging are worth mentioning. Spontaneous changes in the corneal-limbal surface in the form of shallow dimples measuring 1.5 to 2 mm in diameter can occur in aging eyes. They are known as Fuch's dimples and can last up to 48 hours and resolve spontaneously. Histopathological evidence shows thinning in the epithelium, Bowman's membrane, and anterior stroma. Descemet's membrane increases in thickness with age. Stromal edema progresses, and endothelial cells flatten with age. Possible causes of Fuch's dimples include local atherosclerotic changes, changes in neurotrophic factors, and desiccation.

Other pathological changes common in aging epithelium include epithelial basement membrane dystrophy (aka map-dot-fingerprint dystrophy [Fig. 5-16]), which is typically a bilateral change in the epithelial attachment to the basement membrane. It is found in 75% of individuals older than 50 years.[35] However, genetic patterns have been observed in some families. Histological evidence suggests active reduplication of basal lamina into epithelial cells at the strata.

A Hudson-Stähli line is a deposition of iron in the cytoplasm of epithelial cells that occurs in 75% of individuals older than 50 years.[11] The source of iron comes from tears, which typically pool at the junction of lid closure, where the Hudson-Stähli line is commonly found.

### Bowman's Layer

In Bowman's layer collagen fibers insert obliquely into the corneal stroma. The tension of insertion weakens as the fibers change in structure with age. This change can be observed clinically as the anterior crocodile shagreen (aka mosaic shagreen of Vogt). The findings are common in those aged 50 years and older. However, hereditary and traumatic variables have also been noted.

Limbal girdle of Vogt, found in 60% of individuals older than 40 years, is another commonly observed age-related change in Bowman's layer.[6] It appears as a linear, yellow-white deposit at the corneal limbus. It is most commonly seen nasally more than temporally and between the 3 and 9 o'clock positions. Histopathological data suggest it is caused by degeneration of Bowman's layer and the anterior stroma, with deposition of calcium and hyalinization of the peripheral cornea. The epithelium overlying this area also undergoes hypertrophy.

### Stroma

Aged corneas appear to be more hazy than younger corneas. This is mostly caused by the increase in density of the stroma, resulting in increased light scatter. Recent studies have suggested that stromal collagen increases in diameter over time. In addition, the transparency of stroma is intimately affected by the integrity of the endothelium.

Arcus senilis is lipid deposition in the peripheral stroma usually occurring bilaterally (Fig. 5-17). This change is seen in 60% of individuals between the ages of 40 and 60 years, 80% of individuals between the ages of 60 and 70 years, and 100% of individuals older than 80 years.[8] In men younger than 50 years arcus senilis may be related to the development of coronary artery disease.[4] It is also associated with increased cholesterol and low-density lipoproteins in patients older than 50 years.[24] When seen in young individuals, this finding may be associated with systemic lipid disorders. Histopathological observations suggest a deposition of cholesterol, cholesterol esters, neutral fats, and phospholipids in the extracellular

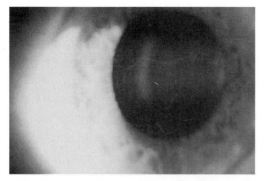

**Fig. 5-16** Epithelial basement membrane dystrophy. (From Parrish RK II, editor: *The University of Miami Bascom Palmer Eye Institute atlas of ophthalmology,* Philadelphia, 2000, Butterworth-Heinemann.)

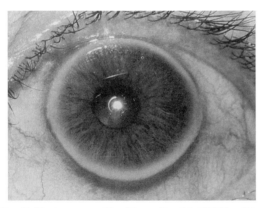

**Fig. 5-17** Arcus senilis. (From Parrish RK II, editor: *The University of Miami Bascom Palmer Eye Institute atlas of ophthalmology,* Philadelphia, 2000, Butterworth-Heinemann.)

space of the stroma. The source of material leakage is suspected to come from perilimbal vasculature. Hereditary and systemic factors also play a role.

Senile marginal atrophy (aka furrow degeneration) is a noninflammatory peripheral corneal thinning commonly associated with arcus senilis. It is a focal depression caused by collagen fragmentation with intact overlying epithelium.

Posterior crocodile shagreen has a similar clinical appearance to the anterior form except it occurs in the posterior stroma. It can be seen both centrally and peripherally.

### Endothelium and Descemet's Membrane

Descemet's membrane continues to reproduce posteriorly throughout life, and its thickness doubles every 40 years. The thickness increases from 2 μm at age 10 years to 10 μm at age 80 years.[2,18] The thickness remains even across the membrane until age 30 years, when excess nodular tissue begins to form in the peripheral cornea. The findings were noted by Hassle in 1846, and Henle in 1866, thus the name Hassle-Henle bodies. These protrusions of excess basement membrane material increase in number and size and eventually present in the central cornea as they become a pathological state known as corneal guttata. The exact cause is not known; however, alteration in the homeostasis of endothelial cells may be contributory.

Corneal endothelial cells are key to corneal dehydration and clarity. These cells do not regenerate after birth. Therefore if cells are lost, adjacent cells migrate into the space. The density of endothelial cells declines with age from 3000 cells/mm² at birth to as low as 900 cells/mm² at age 80 years.[16] However, age-related cell density numbers are highly variable.

### IRIS

Age-related iris changes are often visible. Iris thinning and flattening are easily appreciated on slit lamp examination. Thinning at the pupillary margin allows the sphincter muscle to become visible. Depigmentation in the posterior iris epithelium, particularly at the pupillary margins, occurs in 90% of 60-year-olds and 100% of 80-year-olds.[9] The released pigment cells can be seen with slit lamp examination in or on the anterior chamber, trabecular meshwork, corneal endothelium, and lens.

Histopathological changes include a decrease in fibroblasts and stromal melanocytes but an associated increase in myofibroblasts. The most prominent histopathological change is blood vessel sclerosis, hyalinization of the media and adventitia, which may be consistent with the clinical observations of increased basal levels of aqueous flare in the anterior chamber from leaky iris vessels.

Another visible age-related iris change is senile miosis. Additionally, the pupillary responses to both light and near are reduced. Many hypotheses explaining these findings have been proposed but none have been confirmed. The decrease in pupil size does not appear to have a significant effect on vision.

### Uveitis

Uveitis tends to be seen primarily in the younger population. Even with a declining immune system, the incidence of uveitis declines in older adults. Infectious causes of uveitis are more often seen. Ruling out masquerade syndromes is more important when diagnosing uveitis in the older patient.

### Iris Melanoma

Iris melanomas tend to be diagnosed 10 to 20 years earlier than choroidal melanomas (typically diagnosed in the 60s). Being vigilant and watching for malignant changes of iris lesions in older adults is still important.

## CILIARY BODY

The effect of age on the ciliary body primarily concerns its structure and function. The entire ciliary body becomes larger and shorter by middle age, shifting most of its tissue anteriorly. This anterior movement continues throughout the aging process. The ciliary body shortens longitudinally from approximately 4 mm at 30 years to half of that by age 70 years.[23, 31] The changes reduce the space between the ciliary body and the lens and displace the iris root anteriorly, further narrowing the anterior chamber angle.

The muscular components atrophy with age and are replaced by dense connective tissue within and between muscle layers. Hence muscle mobility is reduced and elasticity declines. These ciliary body alteration and lenticular changes partly contribute to presbyopia.

Similar to the vessels in the iris, the vessels in the stroma of ciliary bodies undergo arteriosclerotic changes and become smaller in caliber. The epithelial basement membrane thickens, hyalinizes, and calcifies, which affects aqueous humor production.

Another age-related change is the development of cysts in the pars plana. Cysts are found in as many as 34% of people older than 70 years.[26]

The aging changes in the ciliary body may have some effects on the production and chemical makeup of the aqueous humor. Aqueous reportedly decreases in production by 2.5% each decade after the age of 30 years.[7] Older individuals also have increased aqueous humor protein levels. The significance of these changes is not clear.

## TRABECULAR MESHWORK

The trabecular meshwork changes in size with age. A 40% increase in the width of the trabecular beams occurs between birth and age 70 years.[32,33]

Endothelial cells lining the trabecular meshwork also change with age. The quantity of endothelial cells changes; most studies suggest a decrease, but this finding is controversial. The remaining cells appear to migrate to cover the unoccupied areas, similar to corneal endothelial cells. However, migration is incomplete, leading to the speculation that the aqueous channel opening is compromised. It can be further compromised by the deposition of extracellular materials found around the trabecular beams. The deposition and trabecular meshwork enlargement are particularly prominent near Schlemm's canal.

Schlemm's canal undergoes aging changes as well. The endothelial cells lining Schlemm's canal degenerate at the rate of 430 cells per year after age 40 years.[12] In addition, the vacuoles in these cells, thought to be responsible for transferring aqueous to the canalicular system, decrease with age.

Aging changes in the trabecular meshwork are particular important because of the role the meshwork may play in glaucoma. Histopathological findings suggest that aqueous outflow facility decreases at the trabecular meshwork in older adults. The cause of glaucoma is unquestionably complex and multifactorial. As the outflow decreases with aging, any external assault to the complex dynamic can offset the delicate balance and cause glaucomatous damage.

## LENS AND ZONULES

Clinicians and patients alike often consider cataracts a normal aging change. As stressed at the beginning of this chapter, aging changes and pathological changes occurring in aging eyes are often difficult to differentiate. Cataract is in fact considered a "pathological acceleration of different biochemical processes occurring during the normal aging process."[27a]

Structural changes include increasing lens thickness in the anterior posterior direction. The curvature of the anterior aspect flattens faster than the posterior curvature with age. The weight and volume continue to change as the lens grows. Such growth contributes to the shallowing of the anterior chamber from 2.9 mm at 20 years to 2.45 mm at 60 years.[10,19,34] This change perhaps further increases the risk of narrow-angle glaucoma.

Lenses grow by adding new cells and fibers generated from epithelial cells on top of previous cells. The growth rate slows as maturation continues, and variation in the growth rates creates different optical appearances when viewing the lens with a slit lamp. Aged epithelial cells become shorter in shape, and vacuoles begin to accumulate in the cells.

Many other structural changes occur and include anterior capsule thickening and growth that may play a role in the loss of accommodation in older adults. Lens rigidity increases with age because of alterations to lipid composition, which are important to maintain lens fiber cell membranes. Marked elevations in cholesterol and suppressed levels of phosphatidylethanolamine, phosphatidylserine, and fatty acids are found in individuals older than 60 years. Little is known about aging changes in the zonules. Limited studies have shown few aging changes in biochemical, structural, or physiological properties. The only change found has been an anterior shift in the zonular fibers and lens insertion sites. No studies have confirmed whether this change contributes to the loss of accommodation.

In addition to the structural changes discussed, numerous biochemical changes also occur, specifically in proteins, lipids, water, and ions. In the young lens, the structural proteins consist of various molecular weights. In the aging lens, the higher molecular weight insoluble proteins become the majority. This shift in the protein composition is caused by protein glycosylation and aggregation. Protein composition is maintained in young eyes by active processes that remove these abnormal proteins. Increased inhibitors to trypsin, a proteolytic enzyme partially responsible for removing the abnormal proteins, are found at elevated levels in aged lenses. Inhibitors to several glycosidases, sodium, potassium, and adenosine triphosphatase have also been found. Glycosylation also contributes to other age-related changes in the lens, such as opacity formation, and a decrease in metabolic activity.

The mechanisms that protect the lens from oxidative damage and free radicals also become compromised with age. Glutathione, a scavenger for oxygen free radicals, decreases dramatically in the nucleus but remains stable in the epithelium. Additional proteolytic antioxidants are also reduced.

Water and ion composition is also altered in the aged lens. Ion-specific channels transport more ions across membranes, passively drawing more water into the lens.

The optical quality of the lens is also affected by age. Aged lenses increasingly absorb more of the light spectrum. Most absorption occurs at the nucleus and is minimal at the cortex. The absorption of blue light can alter a person's color perception and reduce the transmission of this wavelength onto the retina. Lens scattering increases significantly after age of 50 years because of the alterations in lens nuclear fibers. The primary region for scattering is the lens nucleus and anterior cortex.

The knowledge of normal aging changes is important for an eye care professional to diagnose and treat non–age-related pathological conditions properly. However, separating one from another is often difficult. With the advancement of diagnostic technologies, more knowledge will be gained on this topic, and the better clinicians will be able to help patients grow older in a healthy manner.

## REFERENCES

1. Allander E, Bjornsson OJ, Kolbeinsson A, et al: Incidence of xanthelasma in the general population, *Int J Epidemiol* 1:211, 1972.
2. Alvarado J, Murphy C: Histological determination of the normal human corneal dimensions as a function of age [abstract], *Invest Ophthalmol Vis Sci* 22(suppl 32):37, 1982.
3. Anstice J: Astigmatism—its components and their changes with age, *Am J Optom Arch Am Acad Optom* 48:1001-5, 1971.
4. Chambless LE, Fuchs FD, Linn S, et al: The association of corneal arcus with coronary heart disease and cardiovascular disease mortality in the Lipid Research Clinics Mortality Follow-up Study, *Am J Public Health* 80:1200-4, 1990.
5. Chew CKS, Hykin PG, Jansweijer C, et al: The casual level of meibomian lipids in humans, *Curr Eye Res* 12:255-9, 1993.
6. Collier M: Incidence in France of Vogt's white-belt shaped limbic degeneration as a function of age and sex. Respective incidence of types I and II and their localization, *Arch Ophthalmol* 20:588-93, 1960.
7. Diestelhorst M, Krieglstein GK: Physiologic aging in aqueous humor minute volume of the human eye, *Ophthalmology* 91:575-7, 1994.
8. Duke-Elder S: Corneal degenerations, dystrophies, and pigmentations—age changes. In Duke-Elder S, Leigh AG, editors: *System of ophthalmology, vol VIII, diseases of the outer eye*, St. Louis, 1965, C.V. Mosby, pp 867-80.
9. Duke-Elder S: Senile changes in the iris. In Duke-Elder S, Perkins ES, editors: *System of ophthalmology, vol IX, diseases of the uveal tract*, St. Louis, 1966, C.V. Mosby, pp 665-76.
10. Duke-Elder S, Wybar K: The dimensions of the lens. In Duke-Elder S, editor: *System of ophthal-*

*mology. The anatomy of the visual system, vol II,* St. Louis, 1961, C.V. Mosby, pp 312-3.

11. Gass JDM: The iron lines of the superficial cornea. Hudson-Stähli line, Stocker's line, and Fleischer's ring, *Arch Ophthalmol* 71:348-58, 1964.

12. Grierson I, Howes RC, Wang Q: Age-related changes in the canal of Schlemm, *Exp Eye Res* 39:505-12, 1984.

13. Hayashi K, Hayashi H. Hayashi F: Topographic analysis of the changes in corneal shape due to aging, *Cornea* 14:527-32, 1995.

14. Hill JC: Analysis of senile changes in the palpebral fissure, *Trans Ophthalmol Soc UK* 95: 49-53, 1975.

15. Hirsch MJ: Changes in astigmatism after the age of forty, *Am J Optom Arch Am Acad Optom* 36:395, 1959.

16. Hoffer KJ, Kraff MC: Normal endothelial cell count range, *Ophthalmology* 87:861-8, 1980.

17. Hymes C: The postnatal growth of the cornea and palpebral fissure and the protection of the eyeball in early life, *J Comp Neurol* 48:415-8, 1929.

18. Johnson DH, Bourne WM, Campbell RJ: The ultrastructure of Descemet's membrane. I. Changes with age in normal corneas, *Arch Ophthalmol* 100:1942-7, 1982.

19. Kashima K, Trus BL, Unser M, et al: Aging studies on normal lens using the Scheimpflug slit-lamp camera, *Invest Ophthalmol Vis Sci* 34: 263-9, 1993.

20. Marquardt R, Wenz FH: Studies relating to tear film stability [In German], *Klin Monatsbl Augenheilkd* 176:879-4, 1980.

21. Michaels DD: Ocular disease in the elderly. In Rosenbloom A, Morgan M, editors: *Vision and aging,* ed 2, Stoneham, MA, 1993, Butterworth-Heinemann.

22. Millodot M: The influence of age on the sensitivity of the cornea, *Invest Ophthalmol Vis Sci* 16: 240-3, 1977.

23. Nishida A, Mizutani S: Quantitative and morphometric studies of age-related changes in human ciliary muscle, *Jpn J Ophthalmol* 36:380-7, 1992.

24. Nishimoto JH, Townsend JC, Selvin GJ, et al: Corneal arcus as an indicator of hypercholesterolemia, *J Am Optom Assoc* 61:44-9, 1990.

25. Obata H, Yamamoto 5, Horiuchi H, et al: Histopathologic study of human lacrimal gland. A statistical analysis with special reference to aging, *Ophthalmology* 102:678-86, 1995.

26. Okun E: Gross and microscopic pathology in autopsy eyes. IV. Pars plana cysts, *Am J Ophthalmol* 51:1221-9, 1961.

27. Pascucci SE. Lemp MA, Cavavagh HD, et al: An analysis of age related morphologic changes of human meibomian glands, *Invest Ophthalmol Vis Sci* 29(suppl):213, 1988.

27a. Pereira PC, Ramalho JS, Faro CJ, et al. Age-related changes in normal and cataractous human lens crystallins, separated by fast-performance liquid chromatography, *Ophthalmic Res* 26:149-57, 1994.

28. Phillips RA: Changes in corneal astigmatism, *Am J Optom Arch Am Acad Optom* 29:379-82, 1952.

29. Shields CL, Shields JA, Gunduz K, et al: Conjunctival melanoma: risk factors for recurrence, exenteration, metastasis and death in 150 consecutive patients, *Arch Ophthalmol* 118:1497-507, 2000.

30. Shore JW: Changes in lower eyelid resting position, movement, and tone with age, *Am J Ophthalmol* 99:415-23, 1985.

31. Tamm S, Tamm E, Rohen JW: Age related changes of the human ciliary muscle. A quantitative morphometric study, *Mech Ageing Dev* 62:209-21, 1992.

32. Tripathi RC, Tripathi BJ: Functional anatomy of the anterior chamber angle. In Jakobiec FA, editor: *Ocular anatomy, embryology, and teratology,* Philadelphia, 1982, Harper & Row, pp 197-284.

33. Valu L, Feher J: Altersveranderungen des Trabekel-Systems, *Albrecht Von Graefes Arch Klin Exp Ophthalmol* 175:322-36, 1968.

34. Weekers R, Delmarcelle Y, Luyckx-Bacus J, et al: Morphological changes of the lens with age and cataract, *Ciba Found Symp* 19:25-40, 1973.

35. Werblin TP, Hirst LW, Stark WJ, et al: Prevalence of map-dot-fingerprint changes in the cornea, *Br J Ophthalmol* 65:401-9, 1981

# CHAPTER 6

# Posterior Segment Diseases in the Older Adult

SOHAIL J. HASAN and JACK A. COHEN

It has been said that the eyes are the "window to the soul." This may be true, but the posterior segment of the eye is also a window to the body. Indeed, the innermost region of the eye provides a glimpse at many ocular and systemic diseases of the aging body.

Accordingly, this chapter addresses the posterior segment of the eye in the older adult. A short discussion on anatomical changes of the posterior segment is followed by some guidelines for clinical evaluation. The posterior segment manifestations of ocular disease and manifestations of systemic disease are then explored.

## ANATOMICAL CHANGES OF THE POSTERIOR SEGMENT

A number of posterior segment changes are associated with aging. Age changes of the vitreous consist of liquefaction, cavitation, shrinkage, and detachments. Fibrillar aggregates may cast a shadow on the retina if the pupil is small and become visible as muscae volitantes. Contraction of the vitreous gel with a separation of solid and liquid components is called syneresis. This may occur 10 to 20 years earlier in myopic eyes.

The choroid is the vascular and pigmented tunic of the eye. Blood vessels reach it from both anterior and posterior vessels and nourish the outer half of the retina and all of the fovea. The thickness of the choroid gradually diminishes with age because of arteriolar sclerosis, even in the absence of systemic vascular disease.

Atrophic changes are particularly prominent around the optic disc (senile peripapillary atrophy). Diffuse attenuation of pigment occurs regularly with age and gives the senescent fundus its tessellated appearance.

The retina is the central nervous system outpost of the brain. Because it cannot regenerate, retinal disorders are always sight threatening. The aging retina becomes thinner from the loss of neural cells. In the periphery actual spaces appear, which may coalesce to form vacuoles (peripheral cystic degeneration). Lipofuscin, the degradation product of photoreceptor discs, accumulates in pigment epithelial cells and displaces melanin. The glistening ophthalmoscopic reflexes of the youthful fundus disappear, and the foveal reflex is lost. Degenerative changes in the optic nerve include corpora amylacea and arenacea. These basophilic staining bodies are visible only on histological specimens and have no clinical significance.

This list of changes peculiar to the posterior segment may suggest that the older eye does not see because nothing is as it used to be. In fact, visual function remains remarkably efficient in the absence of disease. Acuity declines very little, visual fields remain full, and night vision is only slightly impaired. Of course, annoyances develop, fortunately mostly minor. Older adults must learn to put up with color deficiencies under reduced illumination and fluorescent lights and spots and dots in the visual field.

## CLINICAL EVALUATION OF THE POSTERIOR SEGMENT

Examination of the posterior segment in the aged eye does not differ in essentials from any other eye, except it takes more time, more tact, and more patience. It takes more time because older people frequently have many nonspecific complaints that are poorly expressed and sequentially muddled. Some symptoms may go unreported because of memory loss, fear, or indifference. It takes more tact because, in the nature of things, some senescent diseases are not only chronic, but are irreparable. Clinicians must suppress their own feelings of impotence and stress the positive aspects. It takes more patience because the aged eye often suffers multiple defects that must be sorted out. For example, a person with reduced acuity may have some corneal endothelial changes, some lens vacuoles, some macular pigment dispersion, some amblyopia, and some misplaced spectacles. These causes must be partitioned because each can contribute to the decreased vision, which may not even be the chief complaint.

Older patients should never be treated condescendingly, called by their first names, or addressed by fatuous words of endearment. "It gives me great pleasure to converse with the aged," wrote Plato. "They have been over the road that all of us must travel, and know where it is rough and difficult, and where it is level and easy."*

To define an illness, goes the proverb, don't ask the doctor; ask the patient. Expert diagnosticians consistently emphasize listening to patients because they are telling you the diagnosis. But listening must be analytical to develop the sequence of the disease process, and it must be informed to group the findings into recognizable syndromes. Psychogenic symptoms are not unusual and often represent attempts to gain attention, affection, or respect. The office visit can be a major event in the life of older adults, and the clinician should seize this opportunity to bolster their confidence and dignity.

Much information can be obtained by simple observation, indeed, as soon as the patient walks into the room. Skin color and texture, posture and gait, cranial and facial features, ptosis and ectropion, head tilt and strabismus all have diagnostic meaning to the alert examiner. A shrewd guess of the life course can be made by comparing the apparent and stated age of the patient. Old photographs are sometimes helpful to separate acute from chronic afflictions.

Of all the criteria of visual performance, acuity is the simplest, the most widely used, and the most clinically rewarding. The Snellen chart is poorly standardized and poorly calibrated, and the test is sometimes poorly administered. But it is surprisingly accurate, and it has maintained that reputation after a century of practical use. The responses of patients with scotomas, hemianopia, amblyopia, latent nystagmus, ptosis, myopia, and presbyopia—although not diagnostic—are highly suggestive. The decreased acuity of macular edema may be accompanied by metamorphopsia and that of corneal edema by halos and coronas. Of course, all this information will be missed if the acuity examination is delegated to an assistant.

The absence of light perception is a serious diagnosis and carries with it many therapeutic limitations. Patients tend to confabulate invisible targets because hope springs eternal, and surgical procedures to restore function will be disappointing for all concerned if light perception is absent. The diagnosis should therefore be made on the basis of subjective responses as well as objective evidence of an amaurotic pupil.

Contrast sensitivity is a further method of evaluating acuity. Unlike high-contrast optotypes, gratings can be adjusted spatially and temporally to analyze high- and low-frequency loss. But the tests take more time and are not easily understood by older patients. Clinical correlations with disease also have not been established. Contrast sensitivity, like standard acuity, is influenced by refractive errors. Moreover, no optical aids are available to correct low-frequency loss.

Vision takes time, a factor usually ignored in practice not because it is irrelevant, but because no convenient clinical tests are available to measure it. Dynamic visual acuity, flicker fusion

---

*Modified from Michaels D: Ocular disease in the elderly. In Rosenbloom AA Jr, Morgan MW, *Vision and aging*, ed 2, Stoneham, MA, 1993, Butterworth-Heinemann, p. 116.

frequency, perceptual span, reaction time, light adaptation, and masking are examples of theoretically important but clinically unexplored functions. Exceptions are the time delay in optic nerve conduction manifest as the Marcus Gunn pupil or the analogous Pulfrich phenomenon, the time delay of glare recovery in macular disease, and the focusing inertia patients report in early presbyopia.

In contrast to central acuity, perimetry measures the peripheral field of vision. Perimetry is indicated in any older patient who has headache as a primary complaint; who reports flashes, floaters, or curtains in the field of vision; who has episodes of transient visual loss or transient refractive changes; who exhibits personality and cognitive changes, diplopia, or other neuro-ophthalmic signs and symptoms; whose visual deficit cannot be explained by external or ophthalmoscopic findings; and whose intraocular tensions are outside the normal range. Although different parts of the visual field interact to function as a whole, separating the central and more peripheral fields is useful. Each can be studied independently by tangent screen and perimeter. Central fields should be done with optical correction and peripheral fields without spectacles. Larger-than-average targets may be needed for older patients; stimulus size should also be commensurate with available vision. Central fields have the greatest utility in detecting early glaucomatous damage, and peripheral fields are useful in detecting neuro-ophthalmic disorders. Central fields are usually unrewarding in the very old adults, those with poor vision, and those with aphakia. In unreliable or bedridden patients, a good confrontation field will identify any significant hemianopia or quadrantic defect. The double-finger counting technique provides rapid information with minimal effort. Senescent changes in isopter dimensions are common and mostly artifacts caused by poor or unsteady fixation, slow reaction time, limited attention span, a large nose, an overhanging brow, sagging lids, or thick spectacle frames. Another common error in glaucoma follow-up is to attribute progressive field loss to poor pressure control when increasing lens opacities are actually responsible. To guard against this, fields should be periodically repeated with the pupil dilated. Computerized perimetry is a continuously evolving refinement. Data storage allows comparison of successive fields in the same patient and simultaneous comparison to normals.

The pupil is of significant importance in neuro-ophthalmic diseases and the evaluation of any eye with media opacities. If the fundus cannot be seen, an estimate of retinal integrity can still be formulated by noting whether the consensual reflex is present in the other eye.

Pupillary reflexes (direct and consensual) should be obtained with a good light. The best near reflex target is the patient's own finger. Responses are graded from 1+ to 4+. Anisocoria can be detected only if the eyes are inspected in both dim and bright light. A spurious anisocoria results from a bound-down pupil after an old injury or uveitis. In Horner's syndrome, the abnormal pupil is miotic; in Adie's syndrome, the abnormal pupil is mydriatic. A blind eye still exhibits a near and consensual reflex. Light-near dissociation is not always luetic; more common causes are pituitary lesions, myotonic dystrophy, Adie's syndrome, and aberrant regeneration of the third nerve. The afferent pupillary defect (Marcus Gunn pupil) is best elicited with the swinging flashlight test. When a light is shined from one eye to the other, the clinician sees a pupil dilation instead of constriction: an apparent paradoxical reaction. The significance of the Marcus Gunn pupil is that it almost always means a conduction defect in the optic nerve. Macular disease, media opacities, and amblyopia do not cause afferent pupil defects. A fixed, dilated pupil is usually caused by drugs, third nerve palsy, or compression. Myopathies never involve the pupil.

Intraocular tension readings should be obtained in every older patient at every routine examination. Applanation tonometry is preferred over Schiøtz' tonometer because it is not influenced by ocular rigidity. At any ocular pressure level, however, the risks of glaucomatous damage increase with age. The debate whether ophthalmoscopy or perimetry detects the earliest glaucoma changes ignores the fact that the two methods are complementary, not exclusive. Selective perimetry may save time by concentrating on paracentral scotomas and nasal steps.

Biomicroscopy is a unique method of ophthalmic examination not duplicated by any other technique. It affords visibility of anatomical details both magnified, in depth, and stereoscopic. It serves as a guide in diagnosis, prognosis, and treatment. For example, vitreous prolapse and adhesions may follow lens dislocation or cataract extraction. Iris atrophy, discoloration, adhesions, ruptures, nodules, new vessels, and tumors are readily seen.

Fundus details can also be analyzed with direct and indirect ophthalmoscopy. Both methods are based on illuminating the patient's fundus and observing this area with an appropriate optical system. The direct method uses the optics of the patient's eye to obtain a real image; in the indirect method, the reflected rays are focused by the condensing lens to produce an inverted aerial image. Magnification is inversely proportional to the power of the condensing lens. The usual magnification obtained by the direct method is approximately 15× and with the indirect, approximately 3× (depending on the condensing lens). The field of view is thus approximately 2 disc diameters with the direct technique and 8 disc diameters with the indirect. The direct method can be compared with the high power and the indirect to the low power of the microscope. The indirect method is indispensable for observation of peripheral degenerative changes common in older adults. A third method of examination is fundus biomicroscopy with a preset Hruby or contact lens. This technique combines the optical advantage of the slit beam with the magnification of the biomicroscope and could be compared with the oil-immersion power of the microscope. The Hruby lens needs no topical anesthetic; contact lenses require both topical anesthesia and gonioscopic solution. Several wide-angle contact lenses (e.g., panfunduscope) are now available that give an excellent overall view of the fundus almost up to the ora serrata without mirrors or scleral depression. Subtle vitreous changes can be observed, including cells, cavities, and detachments. Fundus areas of elevation and depression are seen in optic sections, and hemorrhages, exudates, and pigments can be localized in depth. Optic disc imaging with electronic optical instruments and laser scanning are recent advances in diagnostic techniques.

Fundus features of the aged eye that deserve special emphasis are those related to diseases common in later life, namely, the optic disc changes of glaucoma and ischemic neuropathies, the vascular changes of hypertension and arteriosclerosis, diabetic retinopathy in all its variations, macular degeneration, peripheral retinal degenerations, retinal detachment, and the normal aging changes of the choroid and retina previously described.

The integrity of macular function is frequently compromised in older adults, and the diagnosis may not be obvious from ophthalmoscopic inspection, even under high magnification. A few simple tests are available, however, that can help localize disease to this area. The Amsler grid is a self-administered tangent screen test confined to the central 20 degrees. A reasonably intelligent patient can be instructed to report any distortions in the grid. The test is especially applicable in serous macular detachments and also can be used to follow the progress of the disorder by giving the patient some graph paper for home use. The photostress test is a measure of macular glare recovery. The time each eye takes to recover the maximal acuity of which it is capable after exposure to a strong light is compared. In macular disease, recovery time is significantly prolonged, presumably because photopigment regeneration is delayed. Neutral-density filters can differentiate between organic and functional amblyopia. The filter reduces acuity more severely in macular and optic nerve disease than in functional amblyopia.

In contrast to macular disease, optic neuritis causes a decrease in vision characterized by a central scotoma, sometimes a generalized field reduction, defective color vision, and a normal photostress test result. In comparing brightness, the patient may report that it appears reduced on the side of the neuritis. This is the subjective analogue of the Marcus Gunn pupil. The swinging flashlight test is, of course, positive in neuritis and normal in macular disease. Red-free ophthalmoscopy may also reveal nerve fiber dropout, atrophy of the disc, and fewer disc capillaries. If the retina is also involved (neuroretinitis), papillitis and perifoveal exudates may be present.

Gonioscopy is indicated in the initial workup of every patient with glaucoma. It differentiates open- from closed-angle mechanisms, which require fundamentally different treatment. The most popular technique uses the biomicroscope and a mirrored Goldmann contact lens applied to the topically anesthetized eye. This lens produces an inverted image of the opposite angle. The mirror makes an angle of 64 degrees so that the lower chamber angle, for example, is seen when the mirror is placed above. Slit lamp magnification of 16× to 20× is most suitable, and both broad and narrow beams help define the configuration of the angle. The goniolens is then rotated to study the angle circumferentially. Other indirect contact lenses include the Zeiss, Posner, Sussman, Thorpe, and Ritch lenses. The angle can also be viewed by using a direct contact lens. Examples include the Koeppe, Layden, Swan-Jacobs, and Hoskins-Barkan lenses. These lenses provide a direct panoramic view of the angle. The patient is usually examined in the supine position with a binocular microscope. The angle can be classified by a number of different grading systems. Some examples include the Scheie, Shaffer, and Spaeth grading systems. Peripheral anterior synechiae may also block aqueous outflow and can result from uveitis, trauma, previous angle closure, and intraocular surgery. Thus a combined mechanism may result from a flat chamber after a procedure for open-angle glaucoma. New vessels, blood, pigment, tumor cells, and foreign bodies can be observed. Congenital adhesions are present in iridocorneal dysgenesis syndromes.

Unlike pathology textbooks, patients seldom know the names of their diseases. Diagnosis proceeds from signs and symptoms, not the other way around. Moreover, textbook descriptions tend to emphasize advanced, or at least typical, features of disease, whereas in practice minimal signs are often present. Classic patterns of disease are also altered in older adults because of greater response variability and concurrent illnesses. Older patients may forget or confuse therapeutic admonitions and instructions. Finally, compliance in diagnostic tests is seldom perfect; hence cross-checks should be incorporated in the examination to confirm validity.

## POSTERIOR SEGMENT MANIFESTATIONS OF OCULAR DISEASE

One advantage of aging is that it need not be repeated. But this is not true for diseases. For example, clinical manifestations of retinitis pig-

mentosa, migraine, diabetes, and multiple sclerosis may recur and progress in later life. Older adults are prone to diseases of old age and also to the aggregate effects of illnesses whose onset is earlier and that may even be congenital. This pathological background must always be remembered in the differential diagnosis. In all instances, moreover, vision-threatening conditions get priority. Obviously identifying disorders for which effective treatment is available is most important. Thus papilledema is a critical diagnosis; recognition of optic atrophy can be placed on the back burner. Fortunately medical and surgical therapy is constantly evolving; many diseases for which no treatment was available only a few years ago can now be controlled or even cured.

### Diseases of the Uveal Tract

Although uveitis is common, its prevalence decreases with age. It is classified as anterior or posterior. The division into granulomatous and nongranulomatous may be confusing because the two forms are not the result of different causes and can, in fact, appear sequentially. Uveitis in older adults can be associated with surgical trauma, hypersensitivity to drugs or crystalline lens material, reactions to degeneration products in chronically sick eyes, intraocular tumors, systemic infections, severe ischemia, *Herpes zoster ophthalmicus,* and intraocular foreign bodies. This discussion is limited to posterior uveitis.

The signs and symptoms of posterior uveitis are characteristic. Vitreous opacities are inflammatory cells, red blood cells, tissue cells, and debris, best seen with fundus biomicroscopy and retroillumination. Vitreous exudate produces a positive Tyndall phenomenon. If the vitreous is detached, a flare still appears in the retrovitreal space. Vitreous detachment is caused by liquefaction and shrinkage. With vitreous collapse a ring floater may be visible to the patient, representing previous attachment to the optic disc. Retinal edema is common in posterior uveitis and, if the macula is involved, causes reduced vision. Prolonged macular edema leads to cystic changes and permanent loss of central vision. Disc edema is usually transitory and is the result of irritation, particularly when the inflammatory process is nearby (e.g., Jensen's juxtapapillary choroiditis). Active chorioretinal lesions appear gray or white and vary in size, shape, depth, and outline. Poorly defined edges indicate infiltration. Deeper lesions are obscured by overlying tissue, and associated vitreous haze is less marked. Satellite lesions may appear in the vicinity of older, healed areas. Retinal detachment follows serious exudation, but holes are generally absent. Perivasculitis may occur from cellular infiltration or by retrograde inflammation into the perivascular spaces. Exudates, bleeding, and occlusion are secondary complications. Visual disturbances are often associated with photopsia, metamorphopsia, and scotomas.

Serous choroidal detachment can be a complication of intraocular and retinal detachment surgery. The combination of trauma and hypotony causes an abnormal aqueous flow into the space between the ciliochoroid and sclera. The result is a dramatic ophthalmoscopic picture of a large, dark bulge protruding into the vitreous, which may be mistaken for a tumor or retinal detachment. Central vision is usually unaffected unless the posterior fundus is involved, but some pain is common. The effusion tends to subside after 1 or 2 weeks. The most serious complication is a flat anterior chamber that, if an intraocular implant is present, becomes a surgical emergency.

Choroidal melanomas are the most important malignant intraocular tumors of older adults. Approximately half of all uveal melanomas occur in the fifth and sixth decades of life. The chief symptom is a change in visual acuity that depends on tumor size and position and associated retinal detachment. Scotomas may

be interpreted as blurred vision. Macular edema can cause metamorphopsia. Pain and redness are uncommon. The chief sign is the discovery of a mass in the fundus. Appearance can vary from a small, flat lesion resembling a nevus to a large, protuberant mass that invades the retina and vitreous. Retinal detachment invariably occurs, which may make visualization of the underlying solid tumor difficult. Pigmentation can vary greatly and may be absent. The differential diagnosis includes nevi, melanocytomas, metastatic neoplasms, hemangiomas, and disciform degeneration. Because so much depends on a proper diagnosis, patients exhibiting a suspected mass in the fundus must be referred to an ophthalmologist who has experience with gradations of appearance and malignancy and who can promptly initiate ancillary diagnostic tests (Fig. 6-1).

**Diseases of the Retina**

Retinal disease is a dominant cause of visual disability in older adults. It is also a topic of extraordinary interest for several reasons. First, visual impairment can usually be related to the ophthalmoscopic picture. Second, the histological substrate can often be deduced from fundus appearance. Third, advances such as fluorescein angiography, ocular coherence tomography, and electrophysiologic tests have clarified the basis for both pathological and clinical findings. Fourth, new advances in therapeutic techniques such as photodynamic therapy, intravitreal medications, vitrectomy, and retinal microsurgery have brought about exciting changes in prognosis.

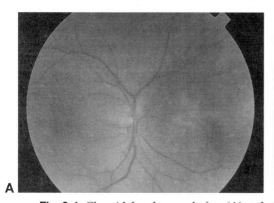
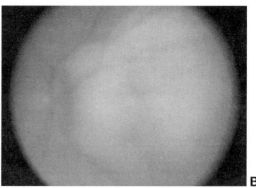

A    B

**Fig. 6-1** Choroidal melanoma before (**A**) and after (**B**) transpupillary therapy. Transpupillary thermal therapy is a relatively new form of uveal melanoma treatment. (Reprinted from Parrish RK, editor: *Atlas of ophthalmology,* Boston, 2000, Butterworth-Heinemann.)

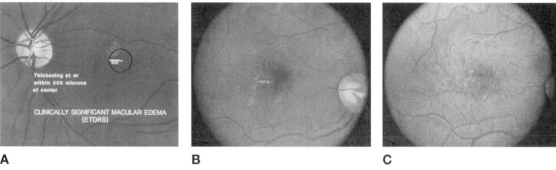

**A**        **B**        **C**

**Fig. 6-2** Clinically significant diabetic macular edema. Shown are a schematic representation of thickening within 500 μm of the center (**A**) and a patient meeting the criteria before (**B**) and after (**C**) treatment. (Reprinted from Parrish RK, editor: *Atlas of ophthalmology*, Boston, 2000, Butterworth-Heinemann.)

Despite its histological and functional complexity, most diseases produce rather stereotyped retinal changes. These include edema, infarcts, exudates, hemorrhages, pigment dispersion, vascular changes, atrophy, deposits of foreign cells or material, cysts, holes, breaks, schisis, and detachments. In interpreting retinal lesions size, shape, location, color, border, depth, effect on adjacent tissue, translucency, and elevation should be noted.

Retinal edema may be localized or general, chronic or evanescent. The retina appears boggy, pale red or white, and more or less thickened. Color changes are most evident when compared with a normal area. The cherry-red macular spot of central retinal artery occlusion is a classic example. Macular edema is suggested by a loss of transparency, thickening of Henle's layer, and distortion of the narrow beam of the slit lamp on fundus biomicroscopy (Fig. 6-2). The patient may report metamorphopsia.

Infarcts, or "cotton wool spots," are sometimes called soft exudates. They are white, fluffy, located mostly in the posterior pole, and invariably superficial (i.e., they often cover retinal vessels) and do not stain with fluorescein (Fig. 6-3). Histopathologically, infarcts represent focal swelling of nerve fibers (cytoid bodies).

Exudates (also called hard exudates) are yellow to white lesions with sharp margins that are most abundant in the posterior poles. Occasionally they are arranged in a circinate or star-shaped pattern. They occur in the middle retinal layers and consist of fatty material. Hard exudates should be differentiated from drusen of Bruch's membrane. The latter are not asso-

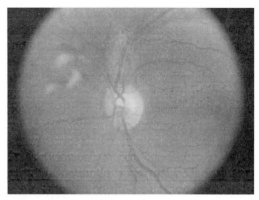

**Fig. 6-3** Cotton wool spots indicating ischemia in radiation retinopathy. (Reprinted from Parrish RK, editor: *Atlas of ophthalmology*, Boston, 2000, Butterworth-Heinemann.)

ciated with retinopathy and may stain with fluorescein, whereas exudates obscure background choroidal fluorescence. Hemorrhages may be subretinal, intraretinal, or preretinal. Subretinal blood has a gray-green color. Intraretinal hemorrhages are punctate or rounded when in the deeper layers and flame shaped when in the nerve fiber layer. Preretinal blood tends to form large masses and may have a fluid level. Extensive retinal hemorrhages are usually the result of venous congestion. Hemorrhages with a white center (Roth spots) can occur in leukemia, anemia, and endocarditis, for example. Vitreous hemorrhage may result from breaks in proliferating new vessels or from a retinal tear and detachment. Even vitreous hemorrhage should be assumed to hide a retinal detachment in older patients until proven otherwise.

Pigment dispersion is a reaction to injury and may represent pigment epithelium cell migration or loss or phagocytosis. Although nonspecific, the pigment distribution sometimes presents as a diagnostic pattern, as in retinitis pigmentosa. Vascular changes consist of alterations in the pattern, reflexes, diameters, and crossings of retinal arteries and veins. Narrowing, tortuosity, congestion, sheathing, obstruction, vascular shunts, and new vessels are adaptations to pressure changes, ischemia, and infection. Atrophy refers to loss of cells or diminution of cell size. Repair may be complete or incomplete, resulting in holes, cysts, or glial proliferation. If pigment epithelium and choroid are absent, the white sclera is visible. Areas of atrophy are frequently surrounded by pigmented margins, which distinguish them from colobomatas.

Foreign cells are illustrated by metastatic tumors; foreign material is usually endogenous and can include cholesterol, hemosiderin, melanin, and lipoids. Bright, scintillating spots overlying an artery are atheromatous emboli. Breaks in Bruch's membrane are illustrated by angioid streaks, lacquer cracks, and traumatic ruptures. Schisis represents splitting within the retina, usually from merging of cystic areas. Detachments represent a splitting between the neural and pigment epithelial layers. Fluid or vessels may cause the pigment epithelium to detach from Bruch's membrane.

In evaluating a retinal lesion shadowing, parallax, ophthalmoscope focus, red-free light, and observation of what structures overlie or are in turn obscured by the lesion can be used. The depth of the lesion may also be evident from limitations imposed by surrounding tissue, as in flame-shaped hemorrhages and macular star exudates. The slit beam of fundus biomicroscopy confirms elevations or depressions.

Fluorescein angiography has greatly aided the interpretation of fundus disease and made purely descriptive discussions in older textbooks obsolete. Intravenous injection of fluorescein allows observation of ocular circulation and adequacy of blood-aqueous barriers. A permanent record is obtained by sequential photography. Normally fluorescein does not stain the retina because retinal vessels and pigment epithelium have tight junctions that act as barriers. Fluorescein does escape from normal choriocapillaries (background fluorescence). Detachment of the pigment epithelium allows dye to pool in the involved area. Areas where pigment is lost act as windows to the underlying choroidal fluorescence (window defects). Blood and exudates in the retina obscure background fluorescence. Damaged retinal vessels leak dye into the retina itself. Fluorescein angiography may be indicated in diabetes, macular edema, nonrhegmatogenous detachments, disciform degeneration, vascular occlusion syndromes, sickle cell disease, presumed histoplasmosis, and suspected neovascularization.

Macular degeneration is by far the most important retinal disease in older adults. Age-related macular degeneration is the leading cause of blindness in older patients around the world. The average age of onset is 65 years, and the second eye is generally involved within 4 years. Loss of central vision results from exudative detachment of pigment epithelium, choroidal neovascularization and hemorrhage, or geographic atrophy of the pigment epithelium. Although the disease is primarily an aging phenomenon, a hereditary dystrophy may also be implicated. There is also progressive loss of choroidal capillaries with age. In the nonexudative or "dry" form of macular degeneration, secondary changes develop in Bruch's membrane characterized by drusen and irregular pigment changes (Fig. 6-4).

Drusen usually increase in size and number and may cause minor visual loss. This may be followed by direct progression to geographic atrophy, or intermediate stages of serous detachment may occur. Recently the Age Related Eye Disease Study, a trial funded by the National Institutes of Health, has shown that certain patients with this disease can reduce their risk of progressing to more advanced stages of macular degeneration by taking nutritional supplementation consisting of high doses of vitamin A, vitamin E, vitamin C, zinc, and copper. The appropriate study doses of these elements have been integrated into many over-the-counter vitamin preparations. Another form of this disease is characterized by an ingrowth of fibrovascular tissue from the choroid through breaks in Bruch's membrane. This form of choroidal neovascularization is also known as exudative, or "wet," macular degeneration.

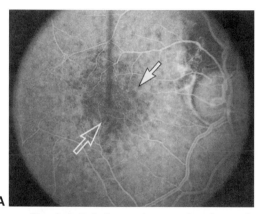
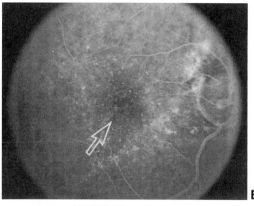

A

B

**Fig. 6-4** Soft drusen in age-related macular degeneration (AMD). Drusen are common; more than 50% to 95% of patients older than 43 years have at least one drusen in the macula. Drusen are accepted as the earliest sign of AMD, but only a small percentage of patients with bilateral drusen actually develop changes of atrophic or exudative AMD that significantly affect their vision. Small, hard drusen (usually <63 μm) appear as flat discrete yellow deposits at the level of Bruch's membrane and do not usually cause significant vision loss or progress to the formation of choroidal neovascularization. Hard drusen are easily seen on the fluorescein angiogram; they stain early and may fade during the recirculation phase. Large, soft drusen (usually >63 μm) are larger than hard drusen and are slightly raised and have less distinct margins than hard drusen. They are also more commonly associated with vision loss in AMD. Early in the angiogram, soft drusen may appear hypofluorescent; later in the angiogram, they may be hyperfluorescent or remain hypofluorescent. The patient shown has 20/20 vision. The hypofluorescent area superior to the disc is secondary to laser treatment for a peripapillary choroidal neovascular membrane. On the earlier frame (**A**) of the fluorescein angiogram the small, hard drusen (*small arrow*) are becoming visible, but the large, soft drusen are hypofluorescent (*open arrow*). Only in the late views (**B**) do some of the soft drusen become fluorescent (*open arrow*); others remain fluorescent even in the late views. Pooling of fluorescein in and around soft drusen is thought to indicate an increased risk for development of exudative disease. (Reprinted from Parrish RK, editor: *Atlas of ophthalmology,* Boston, 2000, Butterworth-Heinemann.)

The presence of new vessels is suggested by clinical observation of a yellow to gray circular patch, subretinal pigment, and a ring of hemorrhage or exudates. Rupture and bleeding of these new vessels may cause sudden, total loss of central vision. Repair may be followed by a disciform atrophic scar that varies in color from white to brown or even black. Further hemorrhages may occur at the margins of the disciform lesion. The treatment of choroidal neovascularization is variable. Verteporfin (Visudyne) has been approved for the treatment of some forms of neovascular growth. This photodynamic agent is selectively taken up by neovascular tissues and then activated by a laser light to induce vascular thrombosis with a visual stabilizing effect. Many other therapeutic options are being developed and evaluated for exuda-

tive macular degeneration. Some examples include laser photocoagulation, intravitreal injection of angiogenic inhibitors, subfoveal surgery, and various other pharmacological agents.

A number of other conditions may be associated with neovascularization in older adults. In degenerative myopia, hemorrhage with pigmentary and atrophic scarring results in a Fuch's spot. Drusen of the optic nerve may be associated with macular edema. Angioid streaks represent breaks in Bruch's membrane through which choroidal vessels can gain access to the retina.

Occlusive disease of the retinal circulation may involve either arteries or veins. Central artery occlusion is the most dramatic, the most sudden, and the most catastrophic of all ocular

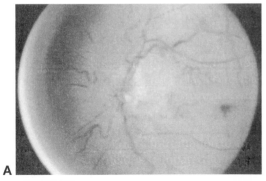

A

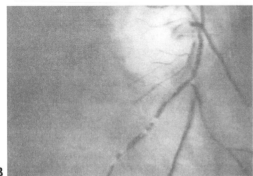

B

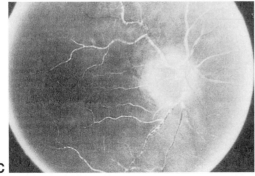

C

**Fig. 6-5 A,** Central retinal artery occlusion with retinal opacification caused by edema, particularly in the posterior pole, where the nerve fiber and ganglion cell layers are thickest. A cherry-red spot occurs in the foveola because the retina in the foveal region is thin. This permits visibility of the underlying intact choroidal vasculature, which stands out in relation to the surrounding opaque and edematous retina. Central retinal artery occlusion with segmentation ("boxcarring") of blood flow. **B,** Most common fluorescein angiographic sign with central retinal artery occlusion is a delay in arteriovenous transit time. **C,** The late-phase angiogram may show staining of the optic disc, but staining of the retinal vessels is rare. (Reprinted from Parrish RK, editor: *Atlas of ophthalmology,* Boston, 2000, Butterworth-Heinemann.)

diseases (Fig. 6-5). A history of previous transient ischemic attacks may be revealed in some patients. The cause can be thrombotic or embolic. Most, but not all, patients have accompanying systemic vascular disorders (carotid atheromas, giant cell arteritis, valvular heart disease, hypertension, or diabetes). Branch retinal artery occlusion usually involves the temporal vessels, and visual loss depends on macular involvement.

Central retinal vein occlusion is also a disease of older people, with a peak incidence in the sixth decade (Fig. 6-6). The pathogenesis remains unknown, but concomitant arterial disease and local thrombotic factors are implicated. Inflammatory causes are unusual. The clinical picture in central retinal vein obstruction is a sudden, painless decrease of vision, but

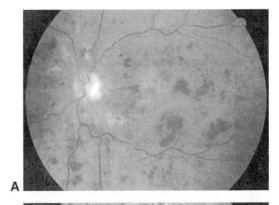

A

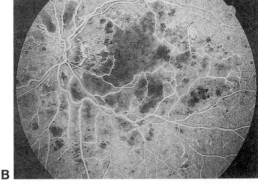

B

**Fig. 6-6** Central retinal vein occlusion associated with dilated retinal veins, retinal hemorrhages, and macular edema. **A,** Clinical appearance. **B,** Angiographic appearance. Patients with central retinal vein occlusion have retinal hemorrhages in all four quadrants, dilated and tortuous veins, and cotton wool spots. A swollen optic disc and retinal edema may be present. (Reprinted from Parrish RK, editor: *Atlas of ophthalmology,* Boston, 2000, Butterworth-Heinemann.)

not as profound as that with arterial occlusion. The ophthalmoscopic picture of massive hemorrhages with dilated vessels is characteristic. Pathological changes are caused by hemorrhagic infarction with destruction of neural elements. The most dreaded complication is neovascular glaucoma, which begins approximately 3 months later. The relation between preexisting glaucoma and vein obstruction dictates a careful workup in the opposite eye. Branch vein obstruction is much more common than central vein obstruction and usually involves the superior temporal vessel (two thirds of cases) or the inferior temporal vessel (one third of cases). The patient may describe acuity loss or distorted vision. If the macula is not involved, no symptoms may be present. The ophthalmoscopic picture is a segmental area of hemorrhages and exudates.

Flashes and floaters are common complaints of older adults. They may represent only innocuous vitreous syneresis but can also be precursors of serious vitreoretinal disease. Floaters are usually vitreous opacities or aggregates; the closer they are to the retina, the more obvious the shadow they cast. When the pupil is small, as when reading outdoors, the opacity is more likely to block the light and become visible. Movement depends on the fluidity of the vitreous. Traction on the retina or bumping of detached vitreous against the retina causes flashes, often compared to lightning streaks. They differ from the scintillating scotomas of migraine, which are bilateral, colorful, and uninfluenced by eye movements. The incidence of retinal complications in patients reporting flashes and floaters is 10% to 15%. Separating the innocuous from the pathological requires meticulous examination with the indirect ophthalmoscope, fundus biomicroscope, and perimeter.

Retinal detachment is a serious and complex disease that may occur with (rhegmatogenous) or without retinal breaks. (Fig. 6-7) Most rhegmatogenous forms begin in the peripheral retina. Predisposing peripheral degenerations that may lead to holes include lattice degeneration, zonular traction tufts, and degenerative retinoschisis. The retinal break connects the vitreous cavity to the subretinal space. Symptoms include blurred vision, flashes, floaters, and a curtain of visual loss corresponding to the

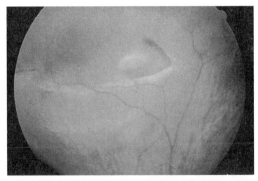

**Fig. 6-7** Appearance of rhegmatogenous retinal detachment. Certain clinical features distinguish the detachments from tractional or exudative detachments, including association with acute posterior vitreous detachment, the presence of a full-thickness break, subretinal fluid, and retinal elevation extending posteriorly from the peripheral breaks near the ora serrata, pigment dusting in the vitreous cavity, irregular folds along the surface lines (rather than smooth, domelike configuration), and absence of shifting fluid (the surface retina may undulate with eye movement). (Reprinted from Parrish RK, editor: *Atlas of ophthalmology,* Boston, 2000, Butterworth-Heinemann.)

detached area. Ophthalmoscopy reveals the typical gray membrane with folds or bulla when highly elevated. Aphakia and myopia predispose to retinal detachment, probably on the basis of vitreous detachment and traction. Identification and localization of all retinal breaks are important because these are surgically treatable lesions. An adhesive chorioretinitis surrounding the break can be created by cryotherapy or photocoagulation to reduce the risk of fluid undermining the retina.

In general, untreated rhegmatogenous detachments are progressive and spread from the ora to the disc. They usually have regular convex borders with pigment (demarcation) lines at stationary edges. In contrast, nonrhegmatogenous detachments tend to be confined to either the peripheral or central fundus, with irregular, sometimes concave borders and no pigment lines. Peripheral cystoid degeneration has a characteristic stippled appearance and does not progress. Retinoschisis tends to be circular, without folds, and does not undulate with movement. Areas of retinal edema are shallow and nonprogressive, with irregular borders that gradually regress. Exudative detachments from

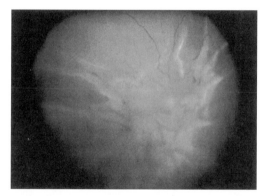

**Fig. 6-8** Complex retinal detachment caused by proliferative vitreoretinopathy. In some cases of rhegmatogenous detachment, certain physiological changes occur in the vitreous cavity and on the retinal surface (e.g., proliferative vitreoretinopathy) to contribute a tractional component to the retinal detachment. Retinal pigment epithelium passing through the retinal break and leukocytes infiltrating the vitreous cavity can migrate onto the retinal surface, proliferate, and form a fibrotic membrane. Ultimately this membrane can contract and thereby apply traction against the retinal surface. Proliferative vitreoretinopathy complicates approximately 5% to 7% of all cases of rhegmatogenous retinal detachment, often causing recurrent detachment, hypotony caused by detachment of the ciliary body, or visually significant macular pucker 6 to 12 weeks after initial successful reattachment. Biological and clinical factors (giant retinal tears, vitreous hemorrhage, ocular inflammation, large choroidal detachment) can identify eyes at particularly high risk. (Reprinted from Parrish RK, editor: *Atlas of ophthalmology*, Boston, 2000, Butterworth-Heinemann.)

tumors and inflammation show gravitation of fluid, fluid shifts, and a bullous configuration. Tractional detachments occur in proliferative diabetic retinopathy, lattice degeneration, chorioretinitis, trauma, aphakia, and after the use of strong miotics. The combination of rhegmatogenous and traction detachments may result in massive vitreous retraction with a crumpled retina and star folds. Complications of surgical repair of retinal detachment include uveitis, glaucoma, cataracts, hazy media, proliferative vitreoretinopathy (preretinal membranes), and refractive changes (Fig. 6-8).

Preretinal macular gliosis is a disorder of older eyes characterized by a membrane on the surface of the retina. Preexisting retinal disease may be present, or the condition may be primary. The ophthalmoscope reveals traction lines, vascular tortuosity, and a cellophane appearance. Posterior vitreous detachment is common. The pathology is migration of glial cells through breaks in the internal limiting membrane. The usual predisposing causes of preretinal membranes are retinal detachment, diabetic retinopathy, retinal vein obstruction, inflammation, and photocoagulation.

## Diseases of the Optic Nerve

Diseases of the optic nerve may be inflammatory, compressive, vascular, infiltrative, degenerative, toxic, or traumatic.

Inflammation of the optic nerve, characterized by hyperemia, edema, and cells in the vitreous, may accompany any inflammatory process of the retina. When inflammation affects the nerve head, the term papillitis expresses the ophthalmoscopic appearance. If the retro-ocular portion of the nerve is involved, the disc appears normal and diagnosis depends on acuity, fields, pupil signs, and color or brightness comparison. The differential diagnosis of papillitis includes edema, high refractive errors, drusen, tilted-disc syndrome, myelinated nerve fibers, and preretinal gliosis. Although demyelinating diseases rarely start in later life, the residua of previous episodes may be visible as optic atrophy.

Disc edema, in contrast to papilledema, is the result of local ocular disease (Fig. 6-9). Progressive visual loss, an afferent pupillary sign, color defects, and field changes occur if

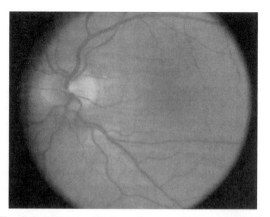

**Fig. 6-9** Patient with disc edema and choroidal folds. (Reprinted from Parrish RK, editor: *Atlas of ophthalmology*, Boston, 2000, Butterworth-Heinemann.)

conduction is compromised. Disc edema can be unilateral, whereas edema from raised intracranial pressure is always bilateral, although it may be asymmetric (e.g., if prior optic atrophy is present on one side). Unilateral disc edema may be found in orbital disease, optic nerve tumors, uveitis, periphlebitis, intraocular tumors, papillitis, occlusive disease of retinal veins, hypotension after intraocular surgery, drusen, ischemic neuropathies, and accelerated hypertension. The pathophysiology of unilateral disc edema may involve neural elements (axon transport block), neurological elements (e.g., drusen), and vascular components (e.g., central retinal vein obstruction or ischemic neuropathies). Fluorescein angiography and ultrasonography can be helpful in the differential diagnosis. Papilledema is discussed under neuro-ophthalmic disorders.

Low-tension glaucoma refers to a disorder characterized by normal intraocular pressures, normal diurnal pressure curves, and normal tonography yet is complicated by progressive glaucomatous-type field loss and disc cupping. The mechanism may involve an imbalance in ocular pulse volume and systemic blood pressure. The disease is difficult to treat and may involve central fixation much earlier than ordinary open-angle glaucoma. A more common disorder of the optic nerve—characterized by pathological cupping and sector field defects but which is not progressive—is shock optic neuropathy. The mechanism is a hemodynamic crisis such as cardiac failure or acute blood loss in an older patient. Overcontrol of hypertension may result in decreased perfusion pressure and nerve damage (Figs. 6-10 and 6-11).

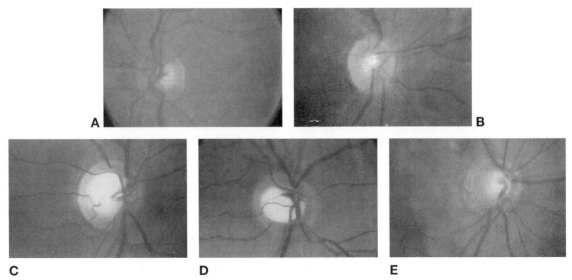

**Fig. 6-10** Normal variants of the optic nerve. The normal optic nerve has a round physiological cup surrounded by the neuroretinal rim. The neuroretinal rim is formed by the edges of the neural retina, retinal pigment epithelium, choroid, and sclera at the disc margin. The inferior neuroretinal rim is usually the thicker quadrant. Normal or abnormal optic nerves can be surrounded by crescents. These crescents may represent defects on the retinal pigment epithelium (either atrophic or hypertrophic) and possibly a misalignment of the retinal-choroidal layer. These peripapillary crescents can be pigmented, choroidal, or scleral. **A,** Normal cupping with healthy neuroretinal rim. **B,** A small cup in a smaller optic nerve, again with healthy neuroretinal rim. **C,** A big nerve with a large cup in a patient without glaucoma. **D,** The horizontal cup is larger than the vertical cup in this normal rim. The larger vertical cupping is more typical of glaucomatous damage. **E,** An optic nerve of a patient without glaucoma with a distinct peripapillary crescent, probably representing a misalignment of the retinal choroidal layers. (Reprinted from Parrish RK, editor: *Atlas of ophthalmology*, Boston, 2000, Butterworth-Heinemann.)

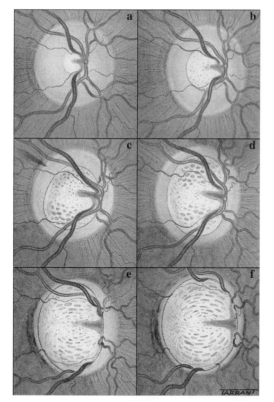

**Fig. 6-11** Progression of glaucomatous cupping. **A,** Normal (c:d ratio, 0.2). **B,** Concentric enlargement (c:d ratio, 0.5). **C,** Inferior expansion with retinal nerve fiber loss. **D,** Superior expansion with retinal nerve fiber loss. **E,** Advanced cupping with nasal displacement of vessels. **F,** Total cupping with loss of all retinal nerve fibers. (Reprinted from Kanski JJ, Bolton A: *Illustrated tutorials in clinical ophthalmology,* Oxford, 2001, Butterworth-Heinemann.)

Ischemic optic neuropathy is primarily a disease of older adults, with a peak incidence in the sixth decade. A sudden loss of vision in one eye occurs, with practically no visual recovery. The ophthalmoscope reveals pallid (often sectoral) disc edema. Perimetry shows a typical altitudinal defect, although isolated central scotomas are also found. The nerve gradually becomes atrophic. A recurrent attack in the same eye is very rare, but months to years later a similar, often symmetrical attack occurs in the opposite eye. The second eye may be involved in one third of cases, and in one half of these within 6 months. Disc edema in the second eye, coupled with atrophy in the other, may be con-

fused with Foster-Kennedy syndrome. Foster-Kennedy syndrome results from simultaneous raised intracranial pressure and optic nerve compression secondary to a tumor (classically, a meningioma of the olfactory groove or, more commonly, from a meningioma of the sphenoid wing).

Ischemic optic neuropathy involves an infarction of the prelaminar portion of the optic nerve. Associated diseases commonly found in these patients include hypertension, diabetes, arteriosclerotic heart disease, and cerebrovascular disease, but the relation, if any, remains unclear. No satisfactory treatment exists for this disorder. The differential diagnosis mainly includes two other entities: hypertensive optic neuropathy and temporal arteritis, both of which are treatable. These are discussed under systemic disorders.

Toxic optic neuropathies present as a painless, bilateral, progressive loss of visual acuity. Visual fields may show a central or caecocentral scotoma with sloping margins. Among the causes implicated are malnutrition, pernicious anemia, tobacco or alcohol toxicity, heavy metals, chemicals such as methanol and benzene, and assorted drugs (ethambutol, isoniazid, streptomycin, chloramphenicol, quinine, penicillamine, disulfiram, vitamin A excess, steroids, and cancer chemotherapy). The importance of recognizing these disorders is that the damage is potentially reversible if nutritional deficiencies are replaced or toxins removed.

Optic atrophy in older adults entails a difficult differential diagnosis. Care must be taken not to call every pale disc atrophic unless confirmatory acuity and visual field evidence are present. The most common cause is glaucoma, followed by vascular, demyelinating, compressive, and traumatic disorders. Drusen of the disc may give it a pale appearance.

Injuries to the optic nerve may occur at any age and can be direct or indirect. Direct injuries are caused by sharp instruments and missiles. Indirect avulsions and fractures are generally the result of head trauma. Visual loss is immediate and often complete. Pupillary signs are positive. Radiographic evidence is often nonconclusive. The mechanism of indirect injury is probably on a concussion basis, with contusion and edema of the nerve tissue, interruption of its vascular supply, or an actual tear.

## Glaucoma

Glaucoma is a leading cause of blindness throughout the world. Because the incidence of elevated intraocular pressure and the susceptibility of optic nerve damage increase with age, early recognition is a fundamental responsibility in the care of older adults.

Glaucoma refers to a group of diseases characterized by optic nerve damage with or without visual field changes that may be related to elevated intraocular pressure. Two broad categories are recognized on the basis of whether the anterior chamber angle is open or narrow. In addition, glaucoma may be classified as primary or secondary. Primary glaucomas are probably genetically influenced, although the exact cause is unknown. Secondary glaucomas are the result of some prior or concurrent ocular abnormality or trauma. Secondary glaucomas may have open angles (as in steroid-induced pressure rise) or closed angles (for example, those induced by a swollen cataractous lens). Space precludes discussion of these many entities, which encompass a vast and detailed literature. This section is limited to primary open-angle glaucoma and, specifically, to its early recognition.

Patients with primary open-angle glaucoma have no symptoms, and the condition is almost invariably discovered by checking intraocular tensions on routine examination. Three groups are typically identified at the initial office visit: normal patients, patients with suspected glaucoma, and patients with definite glaucomatous disease. The first group has normal discs, normal fields, and an intraocular tension less than 21 mm Hg. The second group has a tension greater than 21 mm Hg and therefore require further investigation. The third group has a tension that is obviously abnormal (e.g., greater than 30 mm Hg) or in whom the diagnosis is already established. The third group also includes those who have ophthalmoscopic or visual field changes consistent with glaucoma even though intraocular pressure appears to be within normal limits. This section emphasizes the second group.

At what pressure level is suspicion warranted? Although no absolute value exists, 21 mm Hg applanation is widely accepted. After the sixth decade, 23 mm Hg might be considered the upper limit of normal. Care must be taken to avoid tonometric artifacts such as incomplete patient relaxation, incorrect instrument calibration, corneal edema, and postural effects.

What factors increase the risks of glaucoma? Several conditions are recognized as predisposing eyes to optic nerve damage: a family history of glaucoma, advanced age, myopia, previous retinal vein occlusion, pressure rise induced by steroids, diabetes, pseudoexfoliation of the lens capsule, evidence of prior uveitis, albinism, postoperative complications such as vitreous loss, and vascular crises such as changes in blood pressure or blood volume.

How are the earliest features of glaucomatous damage detected? The two primary techniques are ophthalmoscopy of the optic disc and perimetry. Although optic disc cupping is highly correlated with field changes, the relation is by no means absolute. Older patients tend to demonstrate field loss before disc changes; hence the two techniques complement each other. Moreover, field changes are unequivocal, whereas disc anomalies are more open to interpretation. Finally, ophthalmoscopy is objective, whereas perimetry is a psychophysical measurement.

What are the earliest optic disc changes in glaucoma? The best way to detect early disc changes is with fundus biomicroscopy. The next best way is with the narrow beam of the direct ophthalmoscope. In evaluating appearance with respect to glaucoma, the most important factor is the size of the optic cup compared with the size of the entire nerve head (cup/disc ratio). This comparison is usually made in the horizontal meridian, although it can be made in any direction. An asymmetric cup/disc ratio found by comparing one eye to the other is also highly suspicious. Although the size of the cup can be defined by color change, the configuration is more important. These estimates should be made (and recorded) on every patient to gain familiarity with normal variations. The cup is usually centrally located; extension to the disc margin—especially above, below, and temporally—is highly suspicious. The depth of the excavation determines how much blood vessels are pushed aside (bayonet appearance) as they climb up the cup. Patients with such symptoms are likely to have advanced rather than early field defects. Small, flame-shaped hemorrhages may be found near or crossing the disc margin. Other patterns of abnormal cupping such as ovalization, saucerization, temporal unfolding, polar notching, and increased translucency of the neural rim have also been described. Glaucomatous changes must always be interpreted in light of many normal disc variations. A drawing or photograph is of great help in documenting progression.

What are the earliest field changes in glaucoma? The most important is the nerve fiber bundle defect, although it is not pathognomonic; ischemic neuropathies, branch vessel occlusion, neuritis, drusen, and even chiasmal lesions can produce them. In the early stages nerve fiber damage can cause small paracentral and arcuate scotomas and later, nasal steps and sector-shaped defects. These are best demonstrated by tangent screen examination with emphasis on the innermost 30 degrees. In advanced glaucoma, the perimeter can record progressive, overall, concentric contraction, which eventually results in a temporal island of vision and culminates in total blindness. Automated instruments can be programmed to search for early features of glaucoma, but they require an alert and cooperative patient. These desirable characteristics are not always available in the older population.

Eyes that have suspicious pressures but no field or disc defect always present a challenge. Potential visual damage months or years down the line must be balanced with the inconvenience, side effects, and expense of lifelong treatment. Obviously, the higher the pressure, the greater the risk of eventual damage. And in the context of this text, the older the patient, the greater the risk.

## POSTERIOR SEGMENT MANIFESTATIONS OF SYSTEMIC DISEASE

As previously suggested, the eyes are the windows of the soul, but to the physician—whatever the specialty—the eyes provide a glimpse into the state of general health or disease. When the eye care professional refers a patient to a medical colleague, the latter naturally assumes that purely ocular disease has been ruled out. Thus the neurologist, asked to evaluate a patient with suspected optic neuropathy, is likely to proceed on the basis that visual loss is not caused by amblyopia, refractive error, or macular disease.

### Arteriosclerosis

Normal retinal vessels are actually invisible; what is seen ophthalmoscopically are blood columns. When the walls become opacified, usually by arteriolosclerosis, color changes occur and stripelike densities may appear along the vessel surface. Colors have been compared to copper or, in more advanced stages, silver wire. These changes do not imply vascular obstruction, which is more closely related to the width of the light reflex along the surface of the blood column. In contrast, yellowish stripes along the sides of a vessel, called perivascular sheathing, are caused by exudation into the surrounding spaces. Perivascular sheathing is characteristically seen along veins in papilledema and along arteries in hypertension. Sclerosis may also result in generalized narrowing, so the normal 2:3 ratio of arteries to veins is altered (Figs. 6-12 and 6-13).

The retinal arteries lie mainly in the nerve fiber and ganglion cell layer. At its entrance within the nerve, the central artery has several layers of smooth muscle; this decreases to two or three at the equator. An anatomical peculiarity is that arteries and veins share a common adventitial coat; hence one can be compressed by the other (arteriovenous nicking). Branch retinal vein obstruction is most commonly caused by this mechanism, and it increases in frequency with age. More rarely occlusion is the result of stagnation and primary thrombus formation or intrinsic venous disease. In the acute stage, the ophthalmoscopic picture has been described as if the involved retinal area had been brushed with red paint because of the massive hemorrhages. In the chronic stage retinal edema, serous detachment, vessel collaterals, exudates, microaneurysms, and neovascularization can be seen. Visual loss is caused by macular edema and vitreous hemorrhage. Central retinal vein occlusion has the same pathogenesis, but the entire retina is involved because of compression at the lamina cribrosa. Macular edema always occurs. The most serious complications are vitreous hemorrhage and neovascular glaucoma.

Branch retinal artery occlusion is usually the result of embolization. Cotton wool spots

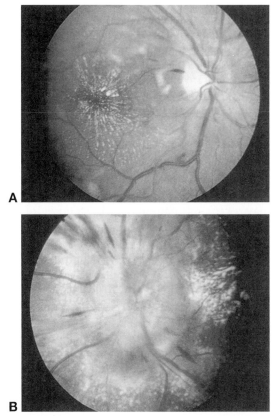

**Fig. 6-12** Grade 3 (**A**) and grade 4 (**B**) hypertensive retinopathy. Prolonged elevated blood pressure or an acute, severe increase in blood pressure may be associated with a breakdown of the inner blood-retina barrier and subsequent extravasation of plasma and erythrocytes. This is accompanied by retinal hemorrhages (dot-blot if present in the deep, vertically oriented retinal layers and flame-shaped if located in the more horizontally oriented nerve fiber layer) and hard exudates, predominantly in the macular region. In severe cases a macular star configuration intraretinal lipid may be present (**B**). Cotton wool spots, nonspecific features of inner retinal ischemia, result from interruption of axonal orthograde and retrograde organelle transport in the ganglion cell axons, with accumulation of mitochondria and lamellar dense nerve fibers. (Reprinted from Parrish RK, editor: *Atlas of ophthalmology*, Boston, 2000, Butterworth-Heinemann.)

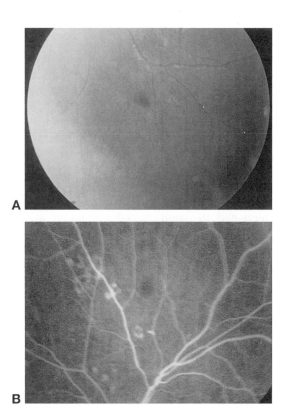

**Fig. 6-13** Healed Elschnig spots. Hypertensive choroidopathy typically occurs in young patients with acute hypertension. Fibrinoid necrosis of choroidal vessels may lead to patchy nonperfused areas of the choriocapillaris, most easily seen on fluorescein angiography. Patches of retinal pigment epithelium overlying occluded choriocapillaris appear yellow and leak fluorescein (acute Elschnig spots). As these lesions heal, the overlying retinal pigment epithelium may be hyperpigmented with a surrounding halo of hypopigmentation (**A**). These healed Elschnig spots no longer leak fluorescein, although fluorescein is transmitted through the hypopigmented halo (**B**). Siegrist streaks refer to linear configuration of hyperpigmentation over choroidal arteries in chronic hypertension. On fluorescein angiography these streaks show hypoperfusion in early phases and some degree of leakage in late phases. Localized retinal or retinal pigment epithelial detachments may develop because of a breakdown of the inner blood-retina barrier with retinal endothelial cell decompensation or retinal pigment epithelial decompensation from fibrinoid necrosis of choroidal arteries with choriocapillaris occlusion. (Reprinted from Parrish RK, editor: *Atlas of ophthalmology*, Boston, 2000, Butterworth-Heinemann.)

appear in the region of nonperfusion and may last for days or weeks. In hypertension, occlusion may be caused by focal arteriolar necrosis. The occlusions seen in collagen diseases are probably on a hypertensive basis. Central retinal artery obstruction is usually caused by atheromatous changes but may be caused by emboli or hemorrhages beneath the atheromas. Rarer causes are arteritis and trauma. The clinical picture is a white, edematous retina with a cherry-red macular spot and narrowed arteries. The cherry-red spot differs from lipoidoses, where the macula actually contains material deposited in ganglion cells. A wider area of perfusion may be observed with a patent cilioretinal artery. Central retinal artery occlusion causes total visual loss without recovery. The scotoma of branch artery occlusion is confined to the involved area. Involvement of the opposite eye, fortunately, is rare. Obstruction of small vessels behind the lamina cribrosa may give rise to ischemic optic neuropathy. Arcuate scotomas of vascular occlusion may be centered on the disc rather than on the macula, as they are in neurological disorders.

## Hypertension

The ophthalmic manifestations of hypertension can be classified in various ways, the most popular of which is the Keith, Wagener, Barker classification. It recognizes four stages of progressive severity (Table 6-1). In fact, a qualitative change between the early and later stages probably occurs. Only approximately 1% of patients with hypertension undergo the malignant phase; even with the advent of effective therapy, only half of these survive for more than 5 years.

The diagnosis of hypertension is made with a blood pressure cuff, not an ophthalmoscope. Nevertheless, fundus changes provide clues to

**TABLE 6-1**

**Keith-Wagener Classification of Hypertension**

| Grade 1 | Mild narrowing or sclerosis of retinal vessels |
|---------|-----------------------------------------------|
| Grade 2 | Focal constrictions, arteriovenous nicking |
| Grade 3 | Cotton wool spots, hemorrhages, retinal edema |
| Grade 4 | Papilledema |

severity and progression, particularly when the disease enters the accelerated stage. These include linear or flame-shaped hemorrhages, cotton wool spots, hard exudates, and blot hemorrhages. Of course, exudates and hemorrhages are found in diseases other than hypertension; hence the association between these and general medical features (e.g., high blood pressure, dyspnea, proteinuria, and chest and cardiac findings) is crucial. Unusual but known mechanisms of hypertension must be ruled out (e.g., pheochromocytoma, Cushing's syndrome, renal disease, aldosteronism, oral contraceptives, and coarctation). Unilateral hypertension fundus changes may occur in patients with stenosis of the carotid system, which maintains lower pressures on that side.

The pathophysiology of vascular changes in hypertension can be studied in experimental hypertension followed by fluorescein angiography. Recall that the retinal circulation is controlled by autoregulation, which permits a nearly constant blood flow over a wide range of perfusion pressures (i.e., mean arterial pressure minus intraocular pressure). A rapid rise in arterial pressure causes vasoconstriction; the precapillary arterioles become occluded and eventually necrose. The vessel loses its ability to remain constricted, and dilation and plasma leakage follow. Fluorescein demonstrates this breakdown of the blood-retinal barrier. Further leakage into the vessel wall causes capillary occlusion, retinal edema, cotton wool spots, and hemorrhages. The presence of arteriosclerosis modifies the response of retinal arterioles to pressure changes. This is probably the reason for focal constriction.

The malignant phase of hypertension is characterized by retinal and disc edema in addition to exudates and hemorrhages. The disorder is fibrinoid necrosis of the arterioles. The patient may report headaches, shortness of breath, and blurred vision, and signs and symptoms of renal failure may be present. Papilledema is caused by accumulated cotton wool spots at the disc rather than hypertensive encephalopathy, although axoplasmic transport block may occur in both. Prolonged disc edema may result in atrophy. Hypertensive optic neuropathy must be distinguished from ischemic neuropathy and neuropathy associated with temporal arteritis.

## Diabetes

Ophthalmic complications of diabetes are partly metabolic (crystalline lens swelling and cataracts) but mostly vascular (diabetic retinopathy). Although the vascular changes are mainly evident in the fundus, they also may involve conjunctiva, iris, choroid, ciliary body, and nerves (diabetic neuropathy). Diabetic fundus changes may be classified into nonproliferative retinopathy (in which the disease is essentially within the retina) and proliferative retinopathy (in which the changes extend over the retinal surface and into the vitreous).

Probably the earliest change in diabetic retinopathy is increased capillary permeability. This has been demonstrated by an elegant technique that measures small amounts of fluorescein in the vitreous. Leakage can be demonstrated within 6 months after onset, even in those without clinically recognizable retinopathy.

Although fundus changes in diabetes are not characteristic, they are generally so typical that the diagnosis can be suspected without difficulty. Mild background retinopathy is characterized by microaneurysms and punctate hemorrhages in the posterior pole, particularly in the region temporal to the macula. The arrangement is haphazard, but occasionally they border an area of soft exudate. Cotton wool spots gradually become more numerous but are less white and less opaque than those seen in hypertension. Microaneurysms are much more numerous than suspected from ophthalmoscopic observation. This has been repeatedly demonstrated by fluorescein angiography. Microaneurysms are round, range in size from 15 μm to 50 μm, and vary in color from venous to arterial blood. Histopathologically they are seen chiefly on the venous side of the capillary and represent bulges caused by a selective loss of mural pericytes. Some aneurysms become hyalinized, and their lumens are lined with degenerated endothelial cells. The cause remains unclear; weakness of the wall, traction, and abortive new vessel formation have all been postulated. Aneurysms differ from blot hemorrhages in that the latter are absorbed and disappear. Capillary closure with areas of nonperfusion persists after the associated cotton wool spot is absorbed. Shunt vessels, connecting arterioles to venules, appear. Damaged vessel walls take up fluorescein.

Venous changes include dilation, tortuosity, beading, and sheathing, and arteriosclerotic changes are accelerated. Hard exudates appear as yellow to white lesions that may coalesce or form a circinate or star pattern around the macula. The visual prognosis is poor if a ring is formed around the macula or hard exudates encroach on the fovea. Hard exudates may improve with time. The most common cause of poor vision, however, is macular edema. It tends to be symmetric, progressive, and surrounded by an area of nonperfusion larger than normal. Edema is the result of abnormal vascular permeability. If the site of leakage can be identified, and it is some distance from the fovea, photocoagulation may help. Longstanding edema, macular hemorrhage, holes, or membranes may benefit from intravitreal steroid injection or vitrectomy.

Proliferative diabetic retinopathy is characterized by the formation of new vessels, which may develop either on the disc or in the periphery. New disc vessels have a poorer prognosis because they tend to bleed into the vitreous. The pathophysiology of new vessel formation is unknown, but ischemia and anoxia are undoubtedly major factors. The vessels are accompanied by a thin film of fibrous tissue that runs across the retinal surface and through the internal limiting membrane. Hemorrhage and retinal detachment may result from vitreous contracture. This form of vitreous collapse differs from the normal aging process by being more gradual and incomplete. Traction and epiretinal membranes may respond to vitrectomy and retinal microsurgery, in which epiretinal membranes are actually peeled off the surface with specially designed instruments (Figs 6-14 through 6-16).

New iris vessels may involve the angle and produce neovascular glaucoma (Fig. 6-17). The mechanism (presumably anoxia) is unknown and the prognosis is poor. Other causes of neovascular glaucoma must be kept in mind: retinal vein occlusion, central retinal artery occlusion, malignant melanoma, and retinal detachment. Recurrent anterior chamber hemorrhages progressively compromise aqueous outflow. These eyes respond poorly to miotics and carbonic anhydrase inhibitors. Laser photocoagulation with or without vitrectomy holds some promise for controlling this serious disease.

Diabetic neuropathy may affect any part of the nervous system. It presents most commonly as a peripheral neuropathy. Symptoms are palsies, paresthesias, numbness, and pain.

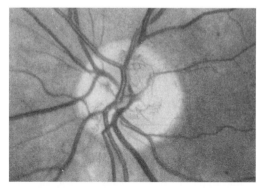

**Fig. 6-14** Proliferative diabetic retinopathy (PDR). This image is the standard photograph from the Diabetic Retinopathy Study and is one definition of high-risk PDR, which portends a high rate of severe visual loss. The Diabetic Retinopathy Study defined high risk PDR as three or four of the following retinopathy risk factors: (1) any neovascularization, (2) location of neovascularization on or within a disk diameter of the optic disc, (3) severe degree of neovascularization (more than or equal to the standard photograph for disc neovascularization or more than the standard photograph showing approximately two disc areas of neovascularization elsewhere), and (4) vitreous hemorrhage. (Reprinted from the Diabetic Retinopathy Study Research Group: Four risk factors for severe visual loss in diabetic retinopathy: DRS #3, *Arch Ophthalmol* 97:654-5, 1979.)

Diabetic neuropathy may involve any of the ocular motor nerves (painful ophthalmoplegia); hence diplopia may be the presenting symptom. Pathologically, small-vessel occlusion with local demyelination is present, but recovery within weeks to months is the rule. Aberrant regeneration does not occur, and the pupil is spared. Differential diagnosis includes trauma, tumor, aneurysm, migraine, and increased intracranial pressure. Decompensated strabismus is an unlikely cause.

### Giant Cell Arteritis

Giant cell arteritis (temporal arteritis, cranial arteritis, polymyalgia rheumatica) is an inflammatory disease of arteries in older adults. The cause is unknown, but both humoral and cellular immune reactions to elastic arterial tissue have been postulated. Any large- or medium-sized artery may be involved, and the condition has a predilection for extracranial vessels. The peak incidence is in the 60- to 75-year-old range. Both sexes are affected, with a slight predominance in women. The disease is not rare; approximately 1.7% of 889 postmortem cases demonstrated the condition when temporal artery sections were taken. Familial associations are uncommon, but a geographic preference for northern climates has been noted. The condition is uncommon in the black population.

The importance of recognizing this disease is that it is potentially blinding for both eyes con-

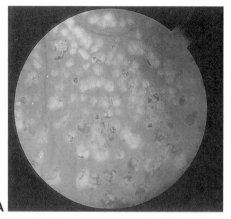

A

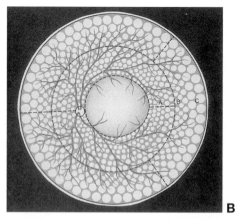

B

**Fig. 6-15** Laser panretinal photocoagulation. **A,** Initial treatment consists of 2000 to 3000 burns. The spot size (200-500 μm) depends on contact lens magnification. Burn duration usually varies from 0.10-0.05 seconds. **B,** Area covered by panretinal photocoagulation. (Reprinted from Kanski JJ, Bolton A: *Illustrated tutorials in clinical ophthalmology*, Oxford, 2001, Butterworth-Heinemann.)

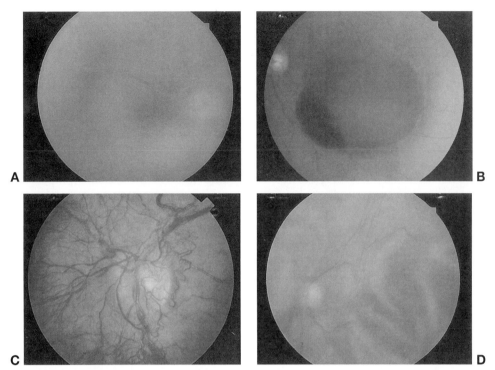

**Fig. 6-16** Indications for vitreoretinal surgery. **A,** Severe persistent vitreous hemorrhage. **B,** Dense, persistent perimacular hemorrhage. **C,** Progressive proliferation despite laser therapy. **D,** Retinal detachment involving macula. (Reprinted from Kanski JJ, Bolton A: *Illustrated tutorials in clinical ophthalmology,* Oxford, 2001, Butterworth-Heinemann.)

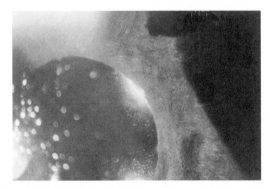

**Fig. 6-17** Rubeosis iridis in a patient with the ocular ischemic syndrome in the left eye. (Reprinted from Parrish RK, editor: *Atlas of ophthalmology,* Boston, 2000, Butterworth-Heinemann.)

secutively, it may be fatal, and treatment is available that may avoid these complications.

Systemic symptoms include headache, malaise, low-grade fever, scalp tenderness, jaw claudication, arthralgias and myalgias, anorexia, weight loss, depression, and tenderness of the course of the temporal arteries, which may feel thickened.

Ophthalmic findings include a sudden, transient loss of vision (amaurosis fugax) that may persist for minutes to hours. This may be followed by unilateral blindness that may be partial or complete. The disorder is an ischemic optic neuropathy. The opposite eye may be involved within a week or months later. If untreated, 65% of patients have bilateral disease, and almost one third of these are totally blind. Ophthalmoplegia with ptosis or other extraocular muscle palsy occurs in 5% of the patients. More rarely, presenting findings are central artery occlusion or anterior segment ischemia with neovascular glaucoma. Ophthalmoscopy shows a pale (not hyperemic), swollen disc. Disc edema may be minimal, but the margins are blurred and a few hemorrhages may be seen. The arterioles of the affected eye are narrowed and often show focal constrictions. The visual deficit is generally out of proportion to the mild disc changes. After about a week, disc edema disappears and the optic nerve gradually becomes pale. The narrowed arteries persist, and no improvement in vision is expected.

One of the most significant laboratory findings in giant cell arteritis is an elevated erythrocyte sedimentation rate (ESR). The Westergren method is most reliable. A guideline for top normal ESR for men is age divided by two. For women, the top normal ESR is age + 10 divided by 2. C-reactive protein level may also be measured. Finally, a temporal artery biopsy should be performed if giant cell arteritis is suspected from the symptoms, signs, or ESR. Incidentally, the ESR may not necessarily be increased in all cases. Histopathological tissue changes in giant cell arteritis include the occluded lumen and multiple giant cells. Prompt recognition and initiation of steroid therapy may prevent loss of vision; if ischemia is complete, treatment may prevent loss of vision in the opposite eye. The patient should be warned that treatment is not invariably effective. The management of this disease is best undertaken as a joint effort between ophthalmologist and internist.

Cranial arteritis should be distinguished from ischemic and hypertensive optic neuropathy. In classic ischemic neuropathy, no treatment is effective. In hypertensive neuropathy, reduction of blood pressure is indicated. Neither condition shows an elevated ESR, and both tend to occur in a somewhat younger age group (late middle life). Low-tension glaucoma and shock optic neuropathy must also be kept in mind.

**Transient Ischemic Attacks**

Transient ischemic attacks are fleeting episodes of focal neurological deficits lasting minutes to hours. An attack that lasts longer than 24 hours is treated as a completed stroke. Recognition of transient ischemic attacks is important in the prevention of stroke.

The pathogenesis of ischemic attacks is complex and varied. Causes might include stenosis of the carotid and vertebrobasilar systems, embolism (atheromatous, platelet, or myxomatous), decreased cardiac output (from failure, arrhythmias, dehydration, anemia, or overcontrol of hypertension), compression of vessels in the neck, hypoglycemia, hypercoagulation states, cranial arteritis, migraine, and reverse flow in cerebral vessels (e.g., steal syndromes).

Clinical features depend on whether the carotid (anterior) or vertebrobasilar (posterior) distribution is involved. The importance of this differentiation is that carotid disease is potentially subject to surgical treatment, whereas the posterior distribution is usually not.

Signs and symptoms of carotid system disease include monoparesis, hemiparesis, hemiparesthesias, and contralateral visual loss. Vertebrobasilar diseases produce brainstem symptoms, including monoparesis, alternate-side paresis, facial numbness on one side and motor loss on the other, diplopia, dysarthria, vertigo, drop attacks, and dysphagia. Loss of consciousness, confusion, amnesia, and tonic-clonic activity are not usually caused by transient ischemic attacks, and the practitioner should suspect mass lesions.

Examination might include testing the blood pressure in each arm, auscultating carotids, determining the pulse rate, palpating temporal arteries, taking the temperature of limbs, and looking for signs of congestive heart failure. Compression of neck vessels is never performed as a provocative test. The laboratory workup may include a complete blood count (CBC), carotid Doppler examination, electrocardiogram, echocardiogram, lipid profile, glucose tolerance, chest x-ray for cardiac configuration, and computed tomographic (CT) scan of the brain if the patient's condition permits.

Ophthalmic manifestations occur in 40% of patients with carotid disease and are the result of transient hypoxia of the retina rather than of the higher visual pathway. Monocular visual loss is therefore more common than transient episodes of hemianopia. Amaurosis fugax may be described by the patient as blur-outs, gray-outs, visual field contractions, a curtain or window shade phenomenon, or a cloud or mist in the field of vision. If the clinician has a chance to observe the patient during the attack, he or she may observe nonreactive pupils, narrowed retinal arteries, perhaps an embolus at the bifurcation of an artery and, occasionally, Horner's syndrome. Cotton wool spots and hemorrhages are features of retinal ischemia. Two types of emboli are commonly seen: orange, scintillating cholesterol flakes (Hollenhorst's plaques) and dull white platelet emboli.

Ophthalmic signs of vertebrobasilar insufficiency may include transient visual loss, but it tends to be mild and is often unreported. Oculomotor palsies, including nystagmus, are important eye symptoms. Attacks may be precipitated by turning the head to one side or using one arm. Diplopia is uncommon with carotid insufficiency.

Ophthalmodynamometry is a noninvasive, but not completely innocuous, procedure. If performed incorrectly, it may result in severe ischemia or even central retinal artery occlusion. Several techniques are available: compression, suction, oculoplethysmography, Doppler flow sonography studies, and oculocerebrovasculometry. The principle involves elevation of intraocular pressure with a tension-recording instrument while observing the pulsation of the central retinal artery ophthalmoscopically. Carotid stenosis must exceed 50% to become hemodynamically significant. Observation of diastolic pressure is safer than increasing tension to the point of total collapse of the artery. Diagnosis is based on noting a pressure difference of the two sides.

The significance of emboli in producing transient episodes of visual loss is apparently related to fragmentation and dissolution of plugs on the one hand and passage to smaller vessel branches on the other. Another mechanism appears to be a transient circulatory arrest within the eye followed by reactive vasodilation. In some cases no emboli are found, and the mechanism may be transient optic nerve ischemia.

The time sequence has some diagnostic value. Vascular ischemic attacks last 5 to 15 minutes and are unilateral. Attacks lasting seconds, occurring in both eyes, and repeated many times during the day may be attributable to chronic papilledema. Migraine attacks may be accompanied by photopsias and headache and can last up to 30 minutes. Short episodes that alternate from one eye to the other may be hysterical. In auscultating the carotid system, a pediatric bell endpiece should be placed over the angle of the jaw, the middle of the neck, and the heart. The absence of a bruit can mean normal flow, less than 50% stenosis, or total stenosis.

**Thyroid Ophthalmopathy**

Thyroid ophthalmopathy can be discussed equally well under neuro-ophthalmic disorders because eye manifestations are often independent of the endocrine course, motility disorders are a common presenting symptom, and the chief visual risk of the disease is compression of the optic nerve.

Graves' disease may occur at any age but is most common in the fourth decade. It has a greater prevalence in women and in those with other autoimmune disorders. The disease results from thyroid-stimulating hormone receptor antibodies causing an increase in thyroid hormone production. Clinical manifestations of hyperthyroidism include goiter, weight loss, fine tremor, nervousness, excessive sweating and heat intolerance, palpitations, arrhythmias, tachycardia, and cardiac failure.

Ophthalmic features include a characteristic frightened appearance caused by proptosis and lid retraction, lid lag on downgaze, infrequent blinking, convergence insufficiency, and restriction of ocular movements (exophthalmic ophthalmoplegia). In rapidly progressive exophthalmos, there is chemosis, conjunctival injection, corneal exposure with ulceration, and optic nerve compression leading to atrophy. The proptosis is usually bilateral, but it may be unilateral. The differential diagnosis includes orbital masses, hemorrhage, vascular malfunctions, inflammation, uremia, and Cushing's syndrome. The disease is characterized by an inflammatory infiltrate of orbital contents with water, connective tissue, lymphocytes, plasma cells, and mast cells. Infiltration of extraocular muscles may simulate tumors on computerized tomography and is responsible for the ophthalmoplegia. Neural and myopathic ophthalmoplegias may be confused with this. Lid retraction and lid lag are important signs and are attributed to excessive innervation of Müller's muscle. If the levator muscle is infiltrated, exposure keratopathy is possible. Bell's phenomenon should be checked. Other causes of lid retraction are uncommon (aberrant third nerve regeneration, pineal tumors, myotonic dystrophy, and ptosis on the opposite side).

The most common motility disorder is a double-elevator palsy (an old orbital floor fracture should be considered). Forced ductions may help identify mechanical restrictions. The most serious complication is optic nerve compression. Danger signals are a central scotoma, color defects, afferent pupil sign, and disc edema. Such findings require emergency decompression of the orbit to save vision.

The course of the disease is unpredictable; ophthalmopathy may progress despite resolution of hyperthyroidism, and radioiodine therapy may aggravate it. After reaching a plateau, the eye findings may subside spontaneously, with variable recovery.

### Neuro-ophthalmic Disorders

Neurological diagnosis is unique in three ways; it logically follows anatomy, requires minimal equipment, and demands the most systematized reasoning. A practical plan of examination consists of an appropriate history, a specific workup, and pertinent laboratory tests. If a diagnosis is still needed, either nature cures the patient or autopsy reveals the exact disorder.

The history is fundamental because many neurological symptoms have no physical manifestations (e.g., headache, pain, photopsias, parethesias, or obscurations). Patients must convey what they see or feel—or, indeed, whether they can see at all. Moreover, the history is a therapeutic as well as diagnostic tool.

Diminished smell, hearing, and sight contribute to sensory deprivation in older adults. Hearing loss (presbycusis) increases with age and is usually sensorineural. Speech sounds become distorted and unintelligible, although patients know when they are being spoken to. People with hearing loss naturally must rely more on visual cues; hence concurrent visual impairmant greatly compounds the sense of isolation.

Dizziness is a common complaint of older patients. True vertigo is characterized by a sensation of motion or rotation, either of self or the environment. It is often accompanied by nausea and blurred vision, hearing loss, tinnitus, and nystagmus, perhaps aggravated by head turning and upright posture. True vertigo should be differentiated from lightheadedness, faintness, nervousness, or spatial disorientation precipitated by new glasses. Labyrinth disease is the most common cause of vertigo. Menière's disease, on the other hand, is an endolymphatic hydrops characterized by vertigo, unilateral fluctuating sensorineural deafness, and tinnitus. Toxic labyrinthitis may follow the use of drugs (streptomycin, sedatives, phenytoin, or diuretics), heavy metals, or alcohol. Common motion sickness may be precipitated by sudden movements of the head in older adults. Lesions of the vestibular nuclei cause severe vertigo and may result from demyelinating disease, vascular insufficiency, tumors, and edema. Central vertigo is usually associated with headaches, diplopia, vomiting, and elevated intracranial pressure. Vertigo may be a prodrome of migraine, epilepsy, or transient ischemic attacks. Vertigo associated with facial, trigeminal, and auditory signs may be caused by acoustic neuromas.

Trigeminal nerve disease can be caused by aneurysm; mass lesions; or inflammation of the orbital apex, the superior orbital fissure, the cavernous sinus, or the gasserian ganglion outside or within the brainstem. The chief ocular symptom is corneal anesthesia. Local corneal anesthesia also occurs with herpes simplex infection and after a variety of intraocular surgical procedures. The combination of facial nerve palsy, insufficient tear production, and corneal anesthesia is part of the cerebellopontile angle tumor syndrome.

Trigeminal neuralgia is a disease of older people characterized by attacks of intense pain in the distribution of any of the three branches of the ganglion; its cause is unknown. Surgical relief may be complicated by corneal anesthesia. Neuroparalytic keratitis may result in perforation in a matter of days unless the cornea is properly protected.

Headaches are probably universal, but the patient who presents with headache as the chief complaint deserves special attention. Because physical signs are usually absent, a meticulous history is essential. The key question is, "In what way are these headaches different from those you usually experience?" Any headache of sudden onset, incapacitating severity, or increasing frequency or duration that is not relieved by previously successful therapy or that is accompanied by focal neurological signs or mood changes should have an ophthalmic workup, including pupil evaluation, intraocular tension, funduscopy, visual field, blood pressure, carotid auscultation, temporal artery palpation, and whatever laboratory tests are indicated by the examination. As a checklist, headaches may be conveniently classified as vascular (including migraine), muscle contraction, traction, inflammatory, and psychogenic (especially in depression).

Approximately 60% of patients with brain tumors report headaches. The pain may be dull, intermittent, and interrupt sleep. Pain often worsens by factors that increase intracranial pressure (coughing, stooping, or straining). Mass lesions in older adults may include abscess, aneurysm, and tumor. The tumors are frequently metastatic and may be symptomatic before the primary lesion. The diagnosis of mass lesions depends on correlating signs and symptoms with neuroradiological findings. The most common symptoms are headache, seizures, personality changes, and motor and speech disturbances. Diagnosis has been markedly facilitated by computerized tomography (greater than 90% detection by this method). Angiography is indicated in planning surgery.

The chief ophthalmoscopic sign of increased intracranial pressure is papilledema. Its features include the loss of a previously noted venous pulse, hyperemia, blurring of the disc margin, venous congestion, peripapillary edema with concentric traction lines, and hemorrhages. Filling in of the physiological cup is not a reliable sign, and an enlargement of the blind spot is of no help except in following the course of the disease. In contrast to optic neuritis, the vision is generally good, Marcus Gunn pupil is not present, no inflammatory cells are in the vitreous, and no pain results from eye movement. Color vision is not affected. Patients with increased intracranial pressure are often ill, with nausea, vomiting, headaches, and even fluctuating levels of consciousness. Chronic papilledema may cause transient obscurations of vision. When conduction in the nerve is compromised, the signs and symptoms of neuritis appear. Odd-looking discs may be confused with papilledema. These include congenital anomalies, staphylomas, hyperopia, and optic nerve drusen. Drusen are often familial, are rare in black individuals, and have an incidence of almost 0.5%. Disc margins may be blurred with a scalloped contour. Drusen tend toward a yellow translucent color and may be elevated several diopters. Buried drusen are invisible but become more superficial with age. Occasionally they erode peripapillary capillaries (causing hemorrhages) or compress optic nerve fibers (causing atrophy). Optic nerve drusen can be associated with any ocular disease, including papilledema.

Perimetry plays a major role in neuro-ophthalmic diagnosis because of the long course of visual sensory fibers from one end of the skull to the other. The concept of the field as an island of vision in a sea of blindness is useful in understanding that the field can be approached from the side (kinetic perimetry) and from above (static perimetry). The use of targets of different sizes (or differing luminances and colors) is called quantitative perimetry. Although it takes time, the temptation to omit or postpone the test must be resisted. Regarding automated instruments, Traquair's admonition that visual fields are tested by the perimetrist, not the perimeter, should be kept in mind. At least two isopters are always plotted to confirm validity and reliability. In many disorders field defects are the only clue to the presence of disease. Unilateral field abnormalities suggest a careful search for defects in the "normal" eye because bilaterality is not always symmetrical. A bilateral anomaly usually places the problem in the chiasma or beyond. Recall that lesions of the optic tract and anterior radiation tend to be incongruous, whereas posterior lesions are congruous; this rule is of no value once the hemianopia is complete.

Acquired diplopia is a serious, potentially life-threatening condition in older adults. The causes may be traumatic, infectious, vascular, metabolic, or neoplastic. In a certain proportion of cases no cause can be discovered. True diplopia can be distinguished from monocular diplopia by asking the patient to close one eye. Neural disorders can be differentiated from mechanical restrictions by forced duction tests; from myopathies by lack of innervational pattern; and from strabismus by history, old photographs, and presence of amblyopia. Diagnosis is based on accompanying features so that the disease can generally be traced to the orbit, the orbital apex, the cranial cavity, or the brainstem. For example, a painful sixth nerve palsy associated with a hearing loss on the same side may suggest Gradenigo's syndrome or an angle tumor. Bilateral sixth nerve palsies with papilledema suggest intracranial pathology. Isolated fourth nerve palsies are often traumatic. Third nerve palsies may result from aneurysm, diabetes, migraine, and tumors. Aberrant regeneration is found after aneurysm and trauma, rarely with tumors, and never with infarcts or diabetes. Multinerve involvement is often neoplastic. Lesions of the base of the brain may show visual field defects or other signs of vascular insufficiency. Supranuclear palsies are characterized by disturbances of saccadic, pursuit, vergence, or vestibular eye movement systems; diplopia is rare. Brainstem lesions often involve adjacent nerves (facial, auditory, vestibular, or trigeminal), the pupils, and the medial longitudinal fasciculus. Unlike strabismus in the young, diagnosis is simplified by the absence of suppression, anomalous correspondence, and eccentric fixation. The workup should include specification of the timing, direction, and magnitude of the deviation in different cardinal positions. Note head tilt, ptosis, proptosis, pupil involvement, visual field defects, lid retraction, papilledema, orbital and carotid bruits, tenderness of temporal arteries, facial and auditory nerve function, corneal sensation, mechanical restriction, periorbital anesthesia, nystagmus, blood pressure, and evidence of aberrant regeneration. Pertinent laboratory tests, in addition to radiological investigations, may include blood sugar level, sedimentation rate, serology, and hematocrit. When indicated, the Tensilon test, angiography, lumbar puncture, biopsy, and neurosurgical consultation are helpful.

Transient diplopia occurs in multiple sclerosis, vertebrobasilar insufficiency, epilepsy, myasthenia, parkinsonism, minor strokes, phoria decompensation, and intermittent squint. The presence of a head tilt means fusion is present in some directions of gaze. Mechanical mechanisms of diplopia have no neural pattern. Peripheral neuropathies may involve any nerve branch.

Involvement of the extrapyramidal system is common in the aged, evident as rigidity, hypokinesia, flexed posture, and tremor. The tremor exists at rest, is coarse, and is aggravated by voluntary movements and stress. In contrast, the tremor of parkinsonism exists at rest but subsides on willed movements. In its fully developed form, the clinical picture of paralysis agitans is highly characteristic: stooped posture, stiffness, slow movements, fixed facial expression, festinating gait, and no sensory changes. Postencephalitic parkinsonism may be indistinguishable from the primary disease. Drug-induced parkinsonism should be ruled out. Disturbances of vertical gaze and lid movement, oculogyric crises, and blepharospasm are the usual ophthalmic findings.

Myasthenia gravis is a muscular disease that can occur at any age and in both sexes. In men the peak incidence is in the sixth and seventh decades. The mechanism appears to be an increase in circulating antibodies to acetylcholine receptors on an autoimmune basis. Pathologically, muscles are infiltrated with small, round cells. Ophthalmic findings occur early because of the high nerve/muscle ratio of extraocular muscles. Clinically, the onset is chronic and often insidious. Bilateral ptosis or other extraocular muscle weakness occurs in 90% of cases. Weakness progresses with exercise or during the day. Pupils are never affected. Choking and food aspiration may be caused by weakness of palatal muscles, and the voice may have a nasal quality. Infections, large meals, and alcohol aggravate the symptoms. The incidence of thyroid disease, arthritis, and cancer is higher in these patients. Diagnosis is based on the history and the improvement of muscle function with the Tensilon (edrophonium chloride) test.

Joint and muscular disease in older adults is frequently treated with corticosteroids. Steroid-induced glaucoma and cataracts therefore deserve special mention. Tonometry reveals a rise in pressure, and funduscopy may show disc changes. The crystalline lens often exhibits posterior capsular opacities, and the patient may report glare, halos, and monocular diplopia. A disproportionate loss of reading vision compared with distance vision can be misinterpreted as progressive presbyopia. Finally, the presenting symptom may be a red eye caused by bacterial, fungal, or herpetic infection exacerbated by steroids.

The clinical syndrome of dementia is characterized by deficits of memory, judgment, language, and other cognitive functions as well as changes in personality and behavior. The causes are varied; some are treatable, such as drug reactions, metabolic dysfunctions, infections, trauma, nutritional deficiencies, or benign neoplasms. Unfortunately the most frequent causes of dementia are progressive despite symptomatic treatment. These include Alzheimer's disease and multiinfarct dementia. Alzheimer's disease is a senile dementia of unknown etiology; its diagnosis is based largely on exclusion. Current research focuses on correcting possible neurotransmitter imbalances and preserving the function of surviving neurons. Treatment is symptomatic. Multiinfarct dementia may occur after repeated cerebrovascular accidents, and the diagnosis is based on a history of recurrent strokes. Dementia must be differentiated from functional and emotional disturbances. Apathetic patients may fail to respond to questions regarding orientation in time, place, and events. Loss of remote memory carries a more grave prognosis than loss of recent memory. All organic brain syndromes have a functional overlay because patients react emotionally when aware of intellectual deterioration.

## SUGGESTED READINGS

### General Texts

Allingham RR, Damji KF, Freedman S, et al: *Shields' textbook of glaucoma*, Philadelphia, 2005, Lippincott.

Duane T: *Clinical ophthalmology*, Philadelphia, 2002, Lippincott.

Duke-Elder S: *System of ophthalmology*, 15 vols, St. Louis, 1956-1976, C.V. Mosby.

Kasper DL, Braunwald E, Fauci AS, et al, editors: *Harrison's principles of internal medicine*, New York, 2005, McGraw-Hill.

Kline L, Bajandas F: *Neuro-ophthalmology review manual*, Thorofare, NJ, 2000, Slack.

### Special Texts

Blodi FC, Allen L, Frazier O: *Stereoscopic manual of the ocular fundus in local and systemic disease*, St. Louis, 1970, C.V. Mosby.

Cogan DG: *Ophthalmic manifestations of systemic vascular disease*, Philadelphia, 1974, W.B. Saunders.

Gass JDM: *Stereoscopic atlas of macular diseases*, St. Louis, 1997, C.V. Mosby.

Harrington DO: *The visual fields*, St. Louis, 1976, C.V. Mosby.

Reichel W, editor: *Clinical aspects of aging*, Baltimore, 1978, Williams & Wilkins.

Sekuler R, Kline D, Dismukes K, editors: *Aging and human visual function*, New York, 1982, Liss.

Yanoff M, Fine BS: *Ocular pathology*, St. Louis, 2002, Mosby.

# CHAPTER 7

# The Optometric Examination of the Older Adult

**IAN L. BAILEY**

Older adults are a special group within optometry's patient population. Many of their visual characteristics and their varied needs make them different from the younger segments of the clinical population. This chapter focuses on the special considerations commonly required in the provision of vision care for the older patient. Inevitably, a chapter such as this is laden with generalizations because it emphasizes features that may be relatively common in older adults even though they are by no means universal within, or unique to, this group.

Visual needs are often changed by retirement or by changes in lifestyle imposed by physical or sensory limitations acquired through aging. Aging brings inevitable changes to the visual system, such as loss of accommodation, reduced transmittance of ocular media, and pupillary miosis. The visual system is also affected by age-related ocular pathological conditions, the most notable of which are maculopathy, cataracts, glaucoma, and retinopathy. Changes in the visual needs and normal and pathological changes in the visual system create a wide diversity of special clinical problems. The eye care practitioner becomes obliged to apply special emphasis and techniques, and special optical treatment or other rehabilitative attention often is essential.

The diversity of vision needs and characteristics distinguishes older adults from the rest of the patient population. Therefore, when dealing with older patients, practitioners must use more imagination and flexibility in structuring the examination and treatment to suit these diverse individual needs.

## CASE HISTORY

The goal of all case history taking is to obtain an understanding of the patient's problems and needs. The case history shapes the sequence and emphasis of examination and assessment procedures, the design of treatment programs, and the presentation of recommendations and advice. The rapport developed in the case history interview can be a crucial factor in determining the success of any treatment. The optometrist must develop and display a genuine strong concern for the patient's needs that are motivating the investigative procedures and treatment considerations.

The patient's demands should be given some overt attention, but the optometrist should remain conscious of the possibility of an unspoken hidden agenda that might be harbored by either the patient or the eye care practitioner. The practitioner should mentally take stock and ask three questions: (1) What does this patient want? (2) What, in my opinion, does this patient need? (3) What is the real reason for the patient's being here today? These three questions will sometimes give rise to the same answer; in older adults especially, however, any differences in these answers can be important in making and presenting decisions and recommendations.

The case history should begin with the patient being asked to identify the main visual problem or problems. The optometrist should encourage a full elaboration of the presenting complaint by asking questions motivated by a genuine curiosity and a desire to understand fully the patient's problem. After the major presenting complaint has been adequately explored, the patient should be asked if other problems are present, and each of these should be pursued in turn. Some older patients, especially those who are lonely or have some doubts about their self-worth, may relish being the focus of attention, and the interview might become quite diverted. The clinician should be sensitive and tolerant toward such digressions.

When the patient exhausts the self-generated list of problems, some important topics should be raised if they have not been covered already. These areas can be divided into the following four categories:

1. *Distance vision.* Patients should be asked about the adequacy of their distance vision for particular tasks, among which are recognizing faces, watching television or movies, and reading signs. Mobility tasks such as driving, using public transportation, and walking in familiar and unfamiliar environments can be important. Reactions to different illumination conditions may be included here.

2. *Near vision.* Reading is typically identified as the most important near vision task. The optometrist should establish whether the patient can satisfactorily read books and magazines, private and business correspondence, and labels and price tags. Patients should be asked about the use of computers and any optical or electronic magnifiers or special lighting conditions that are important to reading tasks. Other near vision tasks such as handicrafts, maintenance chores, self-grooming tasks, and food preparation also warrant attention.

3. *Ocular and general health history.* Current and previous ocular health and general health conditions or treatment should be investigated. The practitioner should determine whether the patient is currently taking any medications and, if so, consider any possible side effects. The patient's experience with glasses or other optical aids should be investigated, and any problems or shortcomings of previous optical treatment should be identified. When some loss of vision has occurred, the pattern of development of the loss should be established. The practitioner should ask patients about their perception of the cause, prognosis of the ocular condition, and the treatment that has been given.

4. *Lifestyle.* Some major changes in the activities of daily life occur with aging. Some changes will be forced by age-related changes in health and deficits in motor, sensory, or cognitive functions. The living environment may change; interests, aspirations, and habits may be altered; the capacity of independent travel and independent home management may be curtailed; and dependence on relatives, friends, or rehabilitation personnel may develop. The practitioner should be alert to such changes because they can significantly influence the needs of the patient.

Aging patients often have special fears and prejudices that require consideration. Most people have some fear of vision loss occurring in their advancing years. This fear becomes heightened when peers experience vision loss or begin to require attention or treatment for cataracts, maculopathy, or glaucoma. Older patients commonly and strongly fear impending blindness or serious vision loss, but they rarely admit this fear. The practitioner should therefore be careful to read between the lines during the history and identify such fears. In recent years the public's awareness of health care issues has rapidly increased. The practitioner should stay abreast of the latest developments in current and emerging treatments, including nutritional supplements, particularly as they relate to disorders affecting vision. Through the Internet, patients and their families now have easy access to medical information and opinions, and consequently clinicians now have to be prepared to answer more sophisticated questions.

A partial or total vision loss is inevitably an emotionally traumatic experience for the individual concerned. After the initial shock, a sequence of emotional reactions can involve depression, anxiety, disbelief, grief, denial, and anger. In time, however, the individual's emotional state stabilizes. Practitioners dealing with patients who have a recently acquired loss of vision should be aware of the probability of changing emotional attitudes. Sometimes delaying the finalization of prescription decisions until the patient comes to reasonable terms with having visual limitations is warranted.

Patients who already have some loss of vision commonly fear that total blindness or substantially worse vision is inevitable. Patients should be encouraged to discuss these fears. Often associated with the fear of blindness is a concern that some past abuse of the eyes is the cause of their vision loss and will soon produce dreaded injurious consequences. Excessive reading, excessive fine work, poor illumination, wearing glasses, failure to wear glasses, wearing the wrong glasses, sitting too close to the television, using fluorescent lamps, or watching color television are all believed to ruin vision, and such mistaken beliefs are more prevalent in older adults. Patients with these concerns should be given appropriate advice and reassurance. Patients who have already suffered some vision loss are particularly likely to be influenced by erroneous but commonly held beliefs that may lead them to expect a dismal visual future. Furthermore, low vision patients may sometimes proudly claim great virtue and restraint because they do not sit too close to the television, do not read any more than is essential, and do not use strong light, when, in fact, the avoided behaviors pose no threat to remaining vision and could provide the means for a broader and more enjoyable range of activities. Thus practitioners should take special care to counsel their older patients about their future eye care needs and the prognosis for changes in their vision and ensure that the patients really understand the status of their own vision.

When an individual retires, interests and priorities often change. Especially if some age-related disability has occurred, older people often curtail their social, vocational, and recreational activities. Withdrawal from social and other pleasurable activities can be passive and unconscious. The eye care professional should understand the patient's range of current daily visual activities. When some vision loss has occurred, the extent to which the vision loss is restricting activities or aspirations should be determined. A useful approach is to ask patients to describe their typical daily activities. Ask what they do from the time they get out of bed in the morning until they go to bed at night. Such questioning often reveals the range of visual demands and, when restricted vision is present, often indicates the extent to which people are modifying their lives because of vision difficulties. The frustration and regret associated with a vision loss is often revealed by the question, "What things could you do when you had good vision that you cannot do now?"

In bringing the introductory interview to a close, the careful optometrist will summarize the priorities for the examination process that is to follow: "So, if I understand things correctly, the most important thing for us to concentrate on is your reading, especially for bank statements. And we should thoroughly check the health of your eyes. Is this right?"

Reminding the patient that mutually agreed upon goals have been established and that these goals motivate all the examination procedures can be reassuring. Advising the patient of the purpose of various tests and relating them to the patient's symptoms emphasizes the clinician's concern and develops a stronger spirit of participation in the patient.

## OCULAR HEALTH EXAMINATION

A thorough inspection of the external and internal aspects of the eyes with appropriate instrumentation is especially important in older patients. Statistically they are much more likely to have significant ocular and general health diseases and disorders.

The inspection of the interior of the eye can be more difficult than in younger patients because of small pupils and lack of media clarity. Unless contraindicated, the pupils should be dilated to enable the examination. However, postponing the instillation of the mydriatic and the full ocular inspection until after the visual abilities have been tested is beneficial. When ophthalmoscopy remains difficult, easier observation is possible by using small-diameter ophthalmoscope systems and perhaps reducing the illumination level. Slit lamp examination of the eyelids, conjunctiva, cornea, anterior chamber, iris, and lens requires more attention in older patients because of the relatively high prevalence of aging changes affecting these tissues.

Tonometry should be performed routinely on older patients because of the higher incidence of raised intraocular pressure and glaucoma.

During the examination of the eyes, the practitioner should explain what is being done. Older patients are almost invariably aware of cataract, glaucoma, and macular degeneration, and they should be reminded that these and other ocular diseases are being given close attention. They should be fully and clearly advised of the state of their own ocular health. This is part of the clinician's basic responsibility and also reinforces the message that regular eye examinations are important to older individuals. The details of discussion about ocular disease will vary according to the patient, the examiner, and their previous interactions. Even though the examiner can grow tired of giving essentially the same routine explanations to patient after patient, this responsibility should not be neglected or conveniently curtailed.

## REFRACTION

The older population experiences significant changes in refractive error.[17] Commonly a shift toward more against-the-rule astigmatism occurs, and the spherical component of refraction shifts in the direct of hyperopia. The prevalence of oblique astigmatism and anisometropia increases. Cataractous changes in the lens may precipitate rapid changes in refraction. Often an individual's refractive status is changed substantially as a result of cataract surgery.

### Objective Refraction

Retinoscopy can be more difficult in older patients because of small pupils and media irregularities and opacities. However, it remains an important technique and the examiner should make every effort to obtain a retinoscopic estimate of refractive error. When retinoscopy becomes unusually difficult, however, the clinician should be prepared to vary techniques. Moving to closer than usual observation distances or moving off axis may provide an "easier" retinoscopic reflex; Mehr and Freid[25] described this as radical retinoscopy. If a useful retinoscopic reflection cannot be obtained with the standard procedures, the clinician should

first move closer and thus reduce the working distance, perhaps to as close as 5 cm in search of a satisfactory reflex. This technique is useful with unsuspected high myopia. If moving closer still provides no useful retinoscopic reflection, high hyperopia could be responsible. Placing a high positively powered lens (e.g., +14.00 D) at the patient's eye, beginning with a standard working distance and gradually reducing the distance, might enable the clinician to find a difficult retinal reflection in patients with high hyperopia. Of course, when the retinoscopic working distance is changed, an appropriate allowance must be made in estimating the power of the refractive correction. Furthermore, moving off axis may produce some inaccuracy in both the spherical and astigmatic components; thus this procedure is used only when axial viewing does not provide an adequate reflex.

When substantial lenticular irregularities are present because of cortical or posterior subcapsular cataract, obtaining consistent or accurate results may be impossible because the apparent movement of the reflected light seems to be fragmented (moving in different directions or at different speeds). In these circumstances, a spot retinoscope is sometimes more useful than a streak retinoscope.

Objective optometers or automated refractors depend on light being reflected from the retina. Again, the small pupils and media opacities commonly found in older patients often lead to less-reliable results. Sometimes no result at all can be obtained.

Keratometry or keratography to estimate total astigmatism becomes more important when retinoscopy or objective optometer measurement fails. A record of corneal curvature can be useful in quantifying any future changes.

Patients with low vision are often unable to make accurate judgments in subjective refraction procedures. Thus more than usual reliance on objective refraction results may be necessary.

### Subjective Refraction

Subjective refraction often requires more time with older patients. Their sensitivity to blur may be reduced because of small pupils or because of media or retinal changes that affect visual discrimination. Judging changes of image clarity in response to small refractive changes becomes difficult. Slower presentation of alternatives and sometimes repeated presentations can become necessary. However, older patients, lacking accommodation, do have a stable refractive state, which can improve the reliability of refractive error measurement.

When visual acuity is expected to be normal or near normal, a phoropter and the usual range of refractive techniques may be used. The biochrome (or duochrome) test, which is sometimes unreliable in younger patients, can be a more reliable test in older individuals. Again, small pupils may make discriminating the relative clarity of the red and green targets more difficult. The yellowing of the crystalline lens with age may cause the brightness of the green background to be reduced more than the red. Importantly, clarity of the letters rather than the brightness of the red or green background is the criterion.

When the observation distance is 4 m or closer, an appropriate dioptric allowance (obtained by changing the refraction result by 0.25 D for a 4-m distance) should be made if clearest distance vision is being sought. With older patients, the binocular balancing of the spherical refraction becomes easier because of the stability of the accommodative state. Standard binocular balancing techniques may be used.

Astigmatism may be determined by using crossed-cylinder techniques; the clock dial or related techniques also may be used. In the presence of media irregularities, however, the crossed-cylinder method is preferred. Clock dial, sunburst, paraboline, and similar techniques involving judgment of the relative clarity of lines in particular orientations all can produce anomalous results when refractive irregularities in the media are present. Similarly, the stenopeic slit method for determining astigmatism may be less appropriate for patients with significant lens or corneal irregularities.

### Refraction of Patients with Low Vision

Patients with low vision often require different refraction techniques. The phoropter should not be used. Patients should be free to move the head and eyes to any preferred positions; they should not be artificially shielded from the ambient illumination; their eye movements and eye position should be observable by the clinician; and they should be aware that improvements achieved are attributable to simple lenses rather than the "magic box" that the phoropter might represent.

Trial lenses supported in trial frames, or in lens clips attached to the patient's current glasses, should be used. However, trial frames tend to be clumsy and often require repeated readjustment and repositioning. Furthermore, the vertex distance they provide is often larger than the eventual spectacle-lens vertex distance. These factors all become more bothersome when the refractive error is large. In general, therefore, trial lens clips (Halberg, Bernell, Jannelli, or other clips) that attach to existing glasses are easier to use. With trial lens clips used over the patient's current glasses, the frame usually sits securely and the lenses have a more appropriate vertex distance and pantoscopic tilt. These together enable a more accurate determination of the required refractive correction.

Working over the current glasses, the practitioner typically has to use only relatively low-powered lenses. This is useful because low-powered lenses are easier to insert and remove from trial lens mountings and are usually available in finer steps of power.

Astigmatism can usually be measured more accurately when trial lens clips are used. For either retinoscopic or subjective determination of astigmatism, the practitioner should first completely ignore an astigmatic correction that may be in the old glasses. The astigmatic component of the overrefraction is determined as though it were completely independent. The axis and power of the overcorrecting cylinder does not have to bear any relation to the cylinder present in the glasses over which the refraction is being performed.

When the overrefraction has been completed, the glasses—with lens clips and trial lenses still attached—are taken to a lensometer, and the back vertex power of the combination is measured. This gives the total power required to optimally correct the refractive error. For example, a patient may be wearing a correction of 0.00 DS −4.50 DC × 35, and the overrefraction in the trial lens clips may be +0.75 DS −1.25 DC × 160. The examiner could do laborious calculations to determine the resultant power, but measuring the back vertex power of the combination with a lensometer is easier. The resultant power will be found to be 0.00 DS −4.25 DC × 27. Note that the axis of the overrefraction cylinder (160 degrees) is different from the axis of the original (35 degrees) or the final (27 degrees) cylinder and that a moderate over-refraction cylinder power (1.25) gives rise to a very small 0.25 change in the final astigmatic correction. This method becomes particularly valuable when the lens powers are high.

In any new glasses the pantoscopic tilt of the lenses and the vertical positioning of the optical centers will probably be similar to those in the previous glasses. Any power errors that may have resulted from the aberrational effects created by tilt and position of the lens will be compensated for by the overrefraction, and a more appropriate refractive correction determination will be obtained.

Patients with low vision are often less sensitive to refractive changes. In general, the poorer the acuity, the poorer the sensitivity to change. However, this is far from being a universal rule. Sometimes patients with visual acuities of 20/500 will be able to respond reliably to 0.50 D of change, and some patients with 20/60 acuity may not be able to respond to 1.50 or 2.00 D of change. The clinician should not have a fixed expectation of the patient's sensitivity to refractive changes based of the visual acuity. Beginning the refraction with an open mind and waiting for the patient's responses to reveal the individual sensitivity to blur is best.

### Refraction Procedures

Subjective refraction with a low vision patient begins with directing the patient's attention to visual acuity chart letters at, or close to, the patient's limit of resolution. The best estimate of refractive error should already be in place; this might be the retinoscopic finding or the patient's previous correction. Initially the steps of dioptric power should be large enough to be certain that recognizing changes in clarity will be easy for the patient.

Begin with a strong plus lens in one hand and a minus lens of equal power in the other (e.g., +6.00 D and −6.00 D). Once the patient can make confident responses to dioptric changes, the size of the changes should be systematically reduced in the process of pursuing the refractive error. When using handheld lenses, fabri-

cating the plano presentation is often advisable by holding lenses of equal and opposite power together rather than using no lens at all. Some patients have already decided whether they want a change of correction, and this can influence their responses to "with" to "without" comparisons.

When large steps of dioptric power are being used, the clinician can be guided by the strength of the patient's response. This may be revealed by the patient's choice of words, tone of voice, or quickness of response. Encouraging patients to describe what they see is better than simply indicating whether they prefer the "first" or "second" view. For example, upon the introduction of a +6.00 D lens, the patient is asked, "What happens with this lens? Does it make it worse, better, or no difference?" The patient might respond, "That's blurry." Upon switching to the −6.00 D lens, the patient says firmly, "That's much worse." To a plano presentation (+6.00 D combined with −6.00 D) the same patient responds, "Ah! That's better." From this sequence, the examiner has learned that plus is preferred to minus and the patient has a solid preference for 0.00 D over +6.00 D. The refractive error appears to be positive: closer to 0.00 D than +6.00 D, but it is not very close to 0.00 D because of the strong difference between +6.00 D and −6.00 D. At this stage a reasonable guess at the spherical refraction error would be in the range of +1.25 D to +2.25 D. This process is called "bracketing," which means obtaining "rejections" from both an excess of plus and an excess of minus.

At this stage the patient's spherical refractive error is contained within a ±6.00 D bracket, and it appears to be on the hyperopic side of plano. Next, a reasonable estimate of the spherical refraction (e.g., +2.00 D) is added to the trial frame and a new pair of handheld bracketing lenses are used. A +1.50 D and a −1.50 D might be chosen. The clinician should expect the patient to "reject" both limits of the new bracketing range (+0.50 D and +3.50 D) and indicate a preference for the central region of this range. With the +1.50 D over the +2.00 D, the patient might say "That makes it blurred." Switching the +1.50 D to the −1.50 D the patient may say, "That's a bit better," and when the +1.50 D and −1.50 D are combined, the patient may say, "That's better still." This sequence of responses first indicates that the refractive error is closer to +0.50 D than to +3.50 D, which means it is less than +2.00 D. Second, it is closer to +2.00 D than +0.50 D, which means it is more than +1.25 D. If the responses have been reliable, the only logical possibilities remaining are that the refractive error is +1.50 D or +1.75 D. Changing the lens power in the trial frame to one of these two alternatives, and using a +0.75 D and −0.75 D, for example, to create a tighter bracket might lead to a final decision. If the +1.50 D lens is in the trial frame and the +0.75 D handheld lens is preferred to the −0.75 D, then the answer is +1.75 D. The answer is +1.50 D if no preference between the ±0.75 D is stated. The spherical refraction is finalized when changing from plus to minus in the finest discriminable step elicits a response indicating that both presentations appear slightly, but equally, blurred.

On completing the initial spherical power determination, the optometrist can begin the astigmatic determination with some knowledge of the patient's responsiveness to refractive blur. This knowledge can guide the practitioner in choosing the power of the Jackson cross cylinder to be used. In a general optometric office, ±0.25 D and a ±0.75 D handheld cross cylinder should be available. The lower power cross cylinder is useful for normally sighted patients, and the ±0.75 D cross cylinder will be strong enough for most low vision patients with poorer discrimination. The test target observed during the Jackson cross-cylinder refraction is usually a selected letter or letters on the Snellen chart at, or close to, the limit of the patient's acuity. Remember that the flip cross-cylinder test works best when the spherical equivalent of the test lens combination is kept constant. Again, bracketing approaches are recommended. Begin using large steps of power to obtain strong rejections of powers that are too strong and too weak. When determining axis, elicit strong rejections by presenting alternative axis orientations that are substantially to one side or the other of the predicted true axis of astigmatism.

After the astigmatism has been measured, recheck the spherical component. If any significant spherical change is necessary, the power of the cylindrical correction should be rechecked.

## VISUAL ACUITY MEASUREMENT

Visual acuity measurement requires a little more care in older patients than in younger ones. Older patients are more affected by the luminance of the test chart and the distribution of light within the luminous environment. Thus more care than usual should be taken to ensure that the chart illumination is at a standard level (80 to 320 cd/m$^2$) and that potentially troublesome glare sources are eliminated from the field of view.[12] Illumination conditions may need to be changed while visual acuity is being measured. Because older patients are more likely to have ocular changes that affect their vision, for reference purposes the best practical measure of visual acuity should be made and the viewing conditions kept the same.

When visual acuity is reduced, nonstandard techniques become necessary. Projector charts, which are suitable for the measurement of normal or near-normal visual acuity, should not be used for low vision patients. Most projectors do not provide the high contrast or the simple and broad range of luminance adjustability that is available with printed panel or transilluminated charts. Also, projector charts lack flexibility to extend the range to larger angular sizes to measure poorer acuities. With printed panel charts, altering the observation distance over a wide range is easy.

For all visual acuity measurement, recording acuity by giving partial credit for rows that were only partially read correctly (20/20 −2, or 20/25 +1, etc.) is important. Practitioners who do not always use the same chart should always make note of the chart that was used.

### Visual Acuity Measurement in Low Vision Patients

Chart design can influence the visual acuity score, which can become most important when macular function is disturbed. The number of letters per row and the relative spacing between letters and between rows can cause substantial variations in visual acuity scores. Many low vision patients require a reduced observation distance, and the practitioner should be aware that, with some charts, changing observation distances can influence the acuity scores obtained.

First, scaling may change. Many charts have a size sequence of 200, 100, 80, 60, 50, 40, 30, 25,

20, and 15. At 20 feet, an acuity of 20/200 might be recorded, indicating that the patient read the 200-foot symbols but failed to read the 100-foot symbols. On changing to a 10-foot observation distance, the practitioner might first anticipate that the acuity score will be 10/100 because that is consistent with the 20/200 result. Consistency with the 20-foot measurement only requires that the acuity be at least 10/100, but not as good as 10/50. Thus the acuity score could be measured as 10/100, 10/80, or 10/60 and still be fully consistent with the 20/200 finding. Only when the chart follows a logarithmic (or constant proportion) size progression can this scaling problem be avoided.

Second, changing to a closer observation distance often alters the nature of the task at threshold. The number of letters per row may increase, and the relative spacing between optotypes may change. With macular dysfunction, contour interaction and crowding become much more important than usual, and increasing the number of letters per row or reducing spacing can significantly reduce the acuity score that can be obtained.[14] A patient who reads a single 20/200 letter with ease might not be able to read any of three closely spaced letters on a 100-foot row when the viewing distance has been changed to 10 feet.

Visual acuity scores will be more valid and more impervious to change with changing observation distance if the task is made essentially the same at each size level. This requires that almost equally legible symbols be used, that the same number of symbols be in each row, that the spacing between symbols and between rows be proportional to symbol size, and that size follow a geometric (or logarithmic or common multiplier) progression. Bailey-Lovie logMAR charts and their derivatives follow these principles.[6,13,32]

The Bailey-Lovie design principles were developed to avoid problems often encountered in low vision work. Their original size range extended from 200- to 10-foot letters (60 m to 3 m). With the chart as close as two feet, acuities of 2/200 (equivalent to 20/2000) can be measured. The Feinbloom visual acuity chart is a popular chart designed for low vision work. The size progression is irregular, and wide variation exists in spacing and the number and legibility of symbols at the different size levels.

These features together reduce the reliability of visual acuity measurement and the consistency of scores when viewing distance or magnification is changed. Nevertheless, the Feinbloom chart does have attractive features: the size range extends to a 700-foot symbol, and the symbol size sequence progresses in relatively small but irregular steps. The page-turning mode of presentation can be psychologically encouraging to patients who have become accustomed to reading few letters correctly when tested on more common charts. The Feinbloom chart also uses numbers rather than letters. Numbers can be useful optotypes for patients who are not familiar or facile with the English alphabet. Landolt rings and the tumbling E are alternative optotypes that do not require any level of literacy from the patient.

Low vision patients may have their visual acuity significantly altered by relatively minor changes in illumination. Thus the recommended procedure is to make the first measurement of acuity at the standard or customary illumination level. Then, referring the patient to the smallest letters that can be read, ask if any change is perceived when illumination is increased or decreased. When externally illuminated panel charts are being used, the illumination may be controlled by increasing or decreasing the room light, moving a light closer to or further from the chart, or using masks to shield the chart from light.

When central or paracentral scotomas are present, the manner in which the patient reads the chart may be informative. Many patients perform much better when reading letters at the start or the end of rows and perform poorly when attempting to read more central letters. At other times a pronounced hesitancy and difficulty reading the letters in sequence are present. These behaviors usually indicate problems from central scotomas and may lead the clinician to expect some limitation of the patient's potential to read efficiently.[11] When evidence or suspicion of macular disturbance is present, encouraging eccentric viewing is useful by directing the patient to fixate above, below, to the right of, or to the left of a row of letters that has been found to be difficult. Any reported changes in visibility can indicate whether eccentric viewing strategies may facilitate reading the chart. For some patients the scotoma size and its effect on the ability to read the chart will vary substantially with relatively modest changes in chart luminance.

## ASSESSMENT OF NEAR VISION

Some aspects of the near vision assessment become much easier with older patients. Because older patients lack accommodation, their working distance becomes highly predictable from the power of the addition being used. The range of clear near vision depends on pupil diameter and the size of the test target detail. If the target is newsprint, or something of similar legibility, the range of clear vision is commonly measured to be approximately 1.00 D in older patients. Using charts with print sizes that go smaller than the patient's resolution limit, and providing that the patient always looks at the smallest print that can just be read, the range of clearest vision is often found to be reduced to approximately 0.25 D in patients with good visual acuity.

For patients with normal distance visual acuity, an equivalent near-vision letter chart visual acuity usually will be achieved. Occasionally, near visual acuity may be significantly worse if central lenticular opacities are present that have a more harmful effect on vision when the pupil constricts in response to viewing near objects. More rarely, acuity can improve at near distances because peripheral lens opacities are rendered less important by pupillary constriction.

The quantity and quality of illumination should be optimized, and older patients generally should be given advice on how to arrange their lighting for prolonged near visual tasks. An adjustable lamp with a compact lamp or bulb (60 or 100 W) provides an almost universally useful means of controlling the task illumination. The illumination on the task can be increased by moving the lamp closer to the page. The lamp or bright spots from the reflector of the lamp should not be directly visible to the patient.

The most appropriate near-vision addition can be determined in various ways, but the desired viewing distance dominates the decision for the typical older patient. A variety of methods can be used to determine the power of the addition; the range of clear vision, biochrome, or cross cylinder at near techniques

all can work satisfactorily on older patients. After the clinician has determined the power of the required addition while using test charts at the desired working distance, performance should be tested by using magazines, newspapers, bank statements, or whatever represents the patient's most common or most important near vision tasks.

If a change in the power of the addition is to be considered, the clinician should be conscious of the magnitude of resolution improvement that can be expected. Almost all distance visual acuity charts use a size progression ratio of approximately 5:4 in the region of 20/20 (50, 40, 30, 25, 20, and 15). Changing viewing distance by a 5:4 ratio (50 cm to 40 cm, 40 cm to 32 cm, etc.) should proportionally increase resolution capacity equivalent to one line of improvement on the test chart. Because dioptric power is inversely proportional to viewing distance, the addition must be increased by a ratio of 5:4 to achieve improvements that may be thought of as one line of acuity. Thus 1.50, 2.00, 2.50, 3.25, 4.00, and 5.00 D is a series of lens powers in which each step represents approximately one line of acuity improvement. Note the close similarity between the numbers in this sequence and the size progression in the 20/20 region of the distance visual acuity chart. With this sequence as a reference, the clinician can deduce that if an addition is increased from +2.50 D to +2.75 D, only a marginal improvement will occur (one third of a line). A +3.25 D addition would be required to provide a resolution improvement that could be described as "one full line."

Optometrists usually measure and record the near visual acuity. Near visual acuity may be measured with a letter chart, similar to the kind used for distance visual acuity, or a reading chart that uses typeset print. The near visual acuity record should specify both the observation distance and the size of the smallest print that may be read. Specifying print size in M units or points is preferable. M units express the distance in meters at which the height of the lowercase letters subtends 5 minutes of arc. Points indicate print size according to the units used by printers and typesetters. Charts from the United Kingdom usually specify print size with the letter N followed by a number (e.g., N.8). The N indicates the font is Times New

Roman, and the number indicates the size of the print in points. Expressing print size as a reduced Snellen equivalent, a fraction that expresses the equivalent distance visual acuity required to read that particular print when it is viewed from 40 cm, is common but not appropriate. This method is clearly inappropriate when the viewing distance is other than 40 cm. Recording 20/20 at 30 cm is confusing and inaccurate because this expression, as it is most commonly used, is intended to indicate that the visual acuity is in fact less than or equivalent to 20/20.

Print that is truly equivalent to 20/20 at 40 cm can be said to be 0.40 M units in size. By using the M unit notation, near visual acuity can be expressed as a true Snellen fraction. Print that is 0.40 M (20/20 at 40 cm) viewed at 40 cm would demand an acuity of 0.40/0.40 M; if the same print were just legible at 30 cm, the acuity would be 0.30/0.40 M. The M unit system is far more appropriate and more consistent with the methods traditionally used to measure distance visual acuity. Another alternative system for indicating print size is the Jaeger notation, which is favored by many ophthalmologists. Print sizes are labeled with a letter J followed by a number, with smaller numbers associated with smaller print sizes. The Jaeger system is not standardized and, between different charts, substantial differences in the size of print that have the same J label can occur—J.3 print on one chart may be as much as twice the size of J.3 on another. Fortunately, the Jaeger system is becoming less commonly used, and its lack of standardization is becoming well known.

In patients with normal or near-normal vision, close concordance between the near and distance visual acuities usually exists. The visual task for the near visual acuity measurement usually involves reading typeset print, which is more complex than reading the fairly widely spaced letters found on the distance visual acuity charts. Such differences in complexity do not have much influence on acuity scores in the normally sighted eye. In patients with disturbed macular function, however, task complexity can cause major inconsistencies in acuity scores. Patients with macular degeneration commonly have a near or reading acuity score that is twofold worse than the distance letter chart acuity.

Near visual acuity measurements with reading charts often serve as a basis for determining the magnification that a low vision patient might require to perform a complex task at near satisfactorily. Distance visual acuity measurements taken with letter charts are much less reliable for this purpose.

Reading efficiency or speed is often assessed, usually qualitatively during the assessment of near vision needs. Clinicians should be aware that, even when the patient has good visual acuity, reading speed is likely to be reduced in older patients because of contrast, motor, and attention deficits.[24]

Many satisfactory reading charts are available for testing normally sighted patients. Reading charts with larger size ranges and more systematic design features have been designed by Keeler,[21] Sloan,[30] Bailey and Lovie,[7] and Legge et al.[22]

## ASSESSMENT OF BINOCULAR VISION

As patients grow older, they are more likely to have some ocular motor difficulties because of changes affecting the neuromuscular mechanisms and the structural tissues around the eyes. In examining binocular coordination, care should be taken to observe the version movements of the eyes as they move in the six cardinal eye movement directions (right, left, up and right, down and right, up and left, and down and left). A relative lagging of on eye indicates an oculomotor dysfunction that warrants a more detailed evaluation of the noncomitancy.

The cover test should be carefully and routinely performed at distance and near for older patients. Older patients lack accommodation and have no stimulus to accommodative convergence; thus they show more exophoria at near. Vertical deviations are also more common in older adults. Phorias or tropias should be measured at both distance and near by using loose prisms. When large near exophoria is found, the strength of the fusional vergence mechanism can be judged by the facility and speed with which the patient makes vergence eye movements to obtain fusion when a base-out prism (e.g., 10 prism diopters) is introduced before on eye. Poor fusional responses tend to indicate a need to consider prescribing prisms.

Although measuring the near phoria with the test target close to eye level is common practice, having the target lower so that downgaze is required is more appropriate. This is more representative of the habitual reading eye posture, particularly if the patient holds or touches the near fixation target.

A variety of subjective tests are available for measuring heterophoria in younger patients, and these often provide different measures of the heterophoria. However, more consistency is found in older patients because of the absence of accommodation, so the choice of method for measuring heterophoria becomes less important.

When a heterophoria is potentially significant, the practitioner must decide if a prism is to be prescribed and, if so, how much. Many reasonable approaches to these decisions are available (see Chapter 13). Fixation disparity, rules involving fusional reserves, and rules based on phoria magnitude can all be useful in indicating how much prism should be prescribed. Checking the advantage obtained from the prism can be prudent by introducing the prism of the indicated power and orientation and asking the patient to report on the clarity or comfort of vision while observing fine print. The prism is then removed and reintroduced after a pause, but with the base direction changed 180 degrees. If a patient with exophoria does not prefer base-in to base-out prisms, judged by changes in clarity or by relative difficulty in adapting to the change, the decision to prescribe prisms should be carefully reconsidered. With vertical prism, the prism power magnitudes are usually smaller, and making this kind of change may be more convenient by keeping the prism in the same orientation but transferring it to the other eye, changing from 2 BUR to 2 BUL, and so forth.

Anisometropia creates special problems, especially relating to vertical phorias. Younger patients with anisometropia can use a forward or backward head tilt to achieve viewing through the optical centers of the lenses, which avoids differential prismatic effects. Older patients wearing bifocals must move their eyes in downgaze to view through the bifocal segment when they read. When patients are already wearing a bifocal correction for anisometropia, decision making is easier. Unless refractive error has substantially changed, the patient's need for vertical prismatic correction can be tested at distance and at near with methods, such as those previously described, using the patient's old glasses. Many patients with anisometropia may exhibit significant vertical heterophoria at near, but they do not have symptoms or show a strong preference for having a correcting prism in place. Each case should be considered individually. When the anisometropia is newly acquired, perhaps because of a myopic shift in one eye, symptoms and adaptation difficulties are more likely. Some practitioners prefer to prescribe some overall vertical prism to minimize such vertical phoria problems at near. Others choose to prescribe bifocals with no special prism compensation, but they may warn the patient of possible symptoms and adaptation difficulties; this strategy avoids prescribing a special prism until the patient fails to adapt.

The remedies for the bifocal problems in anisometropia are to use slab-off or other prism-controlled bifocals, executive bifocals where no prism is present at the dividing line, Franklin split-lens bifocals, or asymmetrical bifocal segments (e.g., a round segment in one eye and flat top in the other) or to revert to separate distance and reading glasses. Fresnel press-on prisms can be cut so they are confined to the bifocal segment region. Although they are not often used as a permanent solution, they can be useful in investigating the potential value of a prismatic correction in the bifocal segments.

Several tests can determine whether a patient truly does have binocular vision in a particular situation. Good stereoacuity, the ability to see both monocular targets on a fixation disparity test, and fusion with the Worth four-dot test are useful standard criteria. The simple bar-reading test is sometimes overlooked; holding a pen midway between the eyes and the page of print should not obscure any point if simultaneous binocular vision is present.

## VISUAL FIELD MEASUREMENT

Visual field losses are more common in older patients. Field defects may come from glaucoma, chorioretinal disease, optic atrophy, and visual pathway disorders. Also, visual sensitivity is reduced with age and, for a given visual stimulus strength, the measured visual field becomes reduced in size for older patients.[8,31]

When measuring visual fields, the clinician should be conscious of the purpose of conducting the test (Box 7-1).

The stimulus parameters and testing strategies will vary accordingly. Today most visual field testing is done with automated perimetry instruments that present lights at various luminosities at selected locations in the visual field following computer controlled sequences. The presence of risk factors and symptoms associated with glaucoma and other neurological and retinal diseases guides the clinician's choice of which field tests and what testing strategies should be used. The Humphrey Visual Field Analyzer (Carl Zeiss Meditec AG, Jena, Germany) and the Octopus (Bio-Rad, Cambridge, Mass.) are the two most widely used automated perimeter instruments. They both offer a wide range of options for selecting different sets of stimulus locations by using different strategies for determining thresholds in given locations. They can also check the consistency of the patient's responses and their maintenance of fixation. The visual field testing programs for screening are of relatively short duration (often 2 or 3 minutes), with fewer points tested and fewer presentations at each location, whereas more extensive and longer routines ranging from 7 to 20 minutes per eye may be used for monitoring and for more thorough diagnostic purposes. The results for a given eye can be analyzed in different ways. Summary statistics, such as the mean deviation, provide an index of the average reduction in visual sensitivity compared with value to normal visual field for the age-matched population. Graphic display printouts typically show the regional variations in visual sensitivity with gray scales to indicate the severity of reductions in visual sensitivity. Such plots may show absolute threshold values, reductions relative to the thresholds for an age-matched normal population (commonly called "total deviation"), and regional reductions relative to the individual's overall sensitivity level ("pattern deviation"). Most of the automated perimetry devices concentrate on testing the central 25 to 30 degrees of the visual field. The characteristics of field loss in glaucoma have influenced many of the testing and analysis strategies. The glaucoma hemi-field test analyses threshold data and compares the relative sensitivity of selected regions in the superior and inferior visual fields, looking for patterns characteristic of glaucomatous field loss.

Display technology and advances in visual science have lead to the development of new visual field tests that specify properties of visual processing of information originating in different regions of the visual field. They attempt to identify deficits in specific neural processing mechanism that may be especially vulnerable to certain diseases. Again, the central visual fields receive the most attention. The frequency-doubling perimetry test is a central visual field test in which a large area (5 degrees square) of flickering grating is presented in one of 17 different locations. The grating has a spatial frequency of less than 1 cycle per degree, and when presented in rapid counterphase flicker (more than 15 Hz), there is an illusion that twice as many stripes are in the target pattern.[20] This frequency-doubling illusion depends on the sparse large-diameter magnocellular nerve fibers, which are believed to be especially vulnerable to damage from glaucoma. The visual system is more sensitive to contrast at the higher spatial frequency. The test measures contrast thresholds for detecting the grating in each of the selected locations. This test is reported to be sensitive for the early detection of glaucoma. The visibility of the stimulus is relatively unaffected by optical defocus, ambient illumination, pupil diameter, or media clarity. Another test that shows good sensitivity to early losses in glaucoma is the short wavelength automated perimetry (SWAP), in which the a large blue target is presented on a bright yellow background.[19] Some automated perimetry procedures use temporal variations and involve detection of flickering stimuli or detection of motion or displacements. High-pass resolution perimetry is performed on a display screen, and the patient's task is to see rings that have a light central region with a dark region on either side. The average luminance of the dark and light regions is equal to the luminance of the background. The diameter of the rings and the widths of the dark and light components are gradually increased until the ring can be seen in different regions of the visual field.

Automated perimeters do include some programs that present stimuli beyond the central 30 degrees, typically testing out to 60 degrees. Testing in these more peripheral regions is obviously important in some diseases (e.g., retinitis pigmentosa, retinal detachment, visual pathway disorders).

The automated visual field testing procedures have special advantages that come mainly from consistent control of the test stimuli, the test procedures, and the computerized analysis of the results. They are not as useful for mapping out the detailed shape of scotomas or for testing the more peripheral parts of the visual field. Detailed information about the shape and location of scotomas across the entire visual field can be very important for predicting functional abilities.

The classic perimetric techniques of tangent screen and bowl perimeter examination for fields are less commonly used today, but they remain the best methods for determining the shape and location of scotomas. The targets may be spots of various sizes or lights of various luminosity and sizes at the end on a handheld wand, or they may be projected spots of light, usually with variable luminance and size. Illumination conditions such as luminance of the illuminated perimeter bowl, or the ambient illumination on the tangent screen, need to be controlled and a record should be kept of the test conditions. Usually most of such testing is done with kinetic perimetry, in which the clinician moves the chosen target across the visual field. Sometimes static perimetry techniques are used; a target location is chosen and the clinician turns the target on and off while the patient reports when the target is seen.

The test parameters (target size and luminance as well as background luminance) and strategies for presentation will vary according to the purpose for conducting the test.

For screening, test spots should be just comfortably detectable, and a systematic broad search should be made of the whole visual field. For confirming tentative diagnoses, the test targets should be just detectable—and only just detectable in the region where the field defect is most likely to occur. The test target presentation should be confined largely to this region of the visual field, and the motion of dynamic targets should be such that the direction is approximately at right angles to the probable border of the scotoma. Results are more reliable and the scotoma shape becomes better defined if the direction of motion goes from nonseeing to seeing.

To monitor the progression of visual field defects with tangent screen or bowl perimetry techniques, the stimulus conditions should be identical (or as similar as possible) to those previously used. Again, any target motion should be orthogonal to the known border of the scotoma.

For functional evaluation of the visual fields, binocular observation may be more relevant then the monocular fields.[23] Relatively easy to see targets (large or bright) should be used.

Special problems may be associated with visual field measurement in low vision patients. If a central scotoma is present, two alternative strategies may be used. One is to have the patent look at the fixation spot by eccentric viewing. Patients with central scotomas often develop a preferred retinal locus (PRL) that they use for giving direct visual attention to an object. This may be many degrees away from where the anatomical fovea was located. Allowance for this displacement must be made when interpreting the visual field results. The central scotoma region will be located to one side of the fixation point. The second alternative is to use a fixation cross centered on the fixation point. Elastic cord, masking tape, or chalk may be used on the tangent screen to provide a cross through the central point. The patient is instructed to look toward the center of the cross, even though he or she may not see the actual intersection. Flashing the target can make it easier for the patient to maintain central fixation because patients are less tempted to move their eyes to check on the presence of the target when it is flashing.

Functional visual field testing is important in low vision patients. Whenever frank scotomas are found on the tangent screen or bowl perimeter, a much coarser test of functional detection ability should be made by using larger and more visible targets. A hand or piece of paper may be used as a target against a black screen to establish whether the scotoma is truly absolute.

Coarse screening for peripheral field loss may be performed by using confrontation or similar techniques.[10] With confrontation testing, the patient's visual field is compared to that of the clinician. The clinician closes one eye, the patient closes the opposite eye, and they each look toward the open eye of the other. In a vertical plane midway between their eyes, the clinician introduces the test stimulus, which may be a handheld target or the clinician's fingers. It is though the clinician and the patient are looking at clear glass screen from opposite sides, and the anatomical limitations of the peripheral fields from the brow, nose, and cheek should project to similar locations for the patient and the examiner. If no substantial peripheral field deficits are present, the point of appearance and disappearance of the test target should be at approximately the same location for both clinician and patient. An alternative technique is to move the target along an arc beginning from behind the patient and simulating a sweep across a bowl perimeter. This pseudoperimeter technique enables better testing of the more peripheral regions of the field, especially on the temporal side.

The Amsler grid can be a useful test of central visual function, characterizing disturbances of central vision.[29] Patients may report absences, fading, or distortion in parts of grid pattern while they maintain fixation on its center. When patients report observable changes, the practitioner may gain insights into the nature of the visual disturbance and perhaps may be better able to predict or understand the patients' functional difficulties. However, a patient often will not recognize scotomas because "filling in" seems to occur. Indeed, the normal physiological blind spot usually cannot be observed on the Amsler grid pattern. Useful information is obtained about the patient's vision function when visual disturbances are reported on the Amsler grid test. When no visual disturbance is observed by the patient, however, no definite conclusion should be made about the presence or absence of scotomas.

## COLOR VISION TESTING

The purpose of testing color vision is twofold. First, the identification of color vision anomalies can assist in the diagnosis or detection of pathological changes in the visual system. Second, altered color vision can cause some difficulties with color discrimination tasks, and the possibility of such functional difficulties should be discussed with the patient.

Color discrimination usually changes slightly as the patient ages because of yellowing of the crystalline lens and physiological and pathological changes in the macular region. Such acquired defects tend to be tritanopic, the most obvious manifestations being a reduction of color discrimination ability for the blue and blue-green regions of the spectrum. The congenital color defects found in approximately 8% of the male population (0.5% in women) are almost always of the deuteranopic or protanopic types, and the main color discrimination difficulties are in the "tomato" region of the spectrum (green, yellow, orange, red). The congenital color vision defects do not cause new functional problems in older patients.

The test of choice for the routine assessment of color vision in older patients is the Farnsworth Panel D-15 test, in which 15 colored chips are arranged so that they appear to be in order according their chromatic similarity. Patients with normal aging changes affecting color vision typically make only a few small-magnitude errors of the tritanopic type. When retinal disease is present, however, the number and magnitude of errors in arranging the D-15 targets are greater. In cases of substantial retinal pathology, the magnitude of errors in arranging the D-15 test targets is large, and the pattern of the errors is more random (see Chapter 2 for further discussion of age-related vision changes).

## OTHER TESTS OF OCULAR OR VISUAL FUNCTION

A variety of clinical tests of visual functions can be useful in identifying the presence of ocular pathological changes, for making diagnostic distinctions, or for explaining functional difficulties resulting from the disease. Contrast sensitivity losses of small magnitude are common in older adults, and more severe losses of contrast sensitivity accompany many of the ocular and visual pathway disorders associated with aging. No close relationship between visual acuity and contrast sensitivity exists; sometimes one function may be significantly reduced while the other may be scarcely affected. Mobility and driving performance and many other tasks of daily living are more affected by impaired contrast sensitivity than by impaired visual acuity.

Contrast sensitivity measurements are mainly useful for predicting functional abilities, but they can also have value in making diagnostic decisions and in understanding the nature of a person's vision loss. Three basic approaches for measuring contrast sensitivity are taken. The traditional method is to present sinusoidal grating targets at selected spatial frequencies. Then contrast is varied to determine the minimal contrast required for detection of the striped grating pattern for each of the selected spatial frequencies. The contrast sensitivity function is a graph showing how contrast sensitivity varies with spatial frequency (see Chapter 2). The grating displays may be presented on oscilloscope or video screens or on printed chart displays.[16] The second method is to measure visual acuity with low-contrast letter charts that effectively determine the spatial frequency limit for resolution at selected contrast levels.[27] The third method is to present a sequence of large targets, such as large letters or edge targets, in which a progression of reducing contrast is shown, and the lowest contrast at which the target can be recognized is the measure of contrast sensitivity.[4,26,34] The most widely used contrast sensitivity test is the Pelli-Robson chart, which has a series of large letters (49-mm high) with a progressive reduction in contrast in which each successive set of three letters becomes lower in contrast by 0.15 log units (70%). Patients read as far as possible down the chart until reaching their threshold contrast.

Disability glare is more of a problem in older patients because all develop increased intraocular light scatter as a result if inevitable aging changes in the lens of the eye. Light scatter becomes more pronounced with the development of cataract or with disorders affecting the cornea or the vitreous. Tests of disability glare can be useful for monitoring the development of cataract or other medical opacities or for the

prediction of functional difficulties that may be experienced under glare conditions. The common feature is that all glare tests measure a visual function, visual acuity or contrast sensitivity, tested with and without the presence of a glare source. The Brightness Acuity Tester is a device that has a 6-cm diameter hemispherical bowl of controlled luminance held over the eye.[18] The patient observes a visual acuity or contrast sensitivity chart through an aperture in the center of the bowl. A more analytical assessment of light scatter and glare can be made by a method introduced by Van den Berg[33] in which scattered light from a flashing bright annulus of light can induce a flickering appearance in a steady, central, spot target. Introducing counterphase flicker of variable intensity into the central spot provides a means of nulling the flickering appearance induced by the light scattered from the annulus. This effectively quantifies the scattered light. Low-contrast letter charts with a surrounding field of glare have been shown to be sensitive measures of disability glare.[5,28] Most clinicians do not have glare tests at hand, and a less-controlled assessment of disability glare can be made by shining a penlight at the patient's eye as a visual acuity chart is being read.

Retinal adaptational mechanisms may be impaired by some age-related eye diseases, and dark adaptation and glare recovery tests may identify such losses. Sophisticated instrumentation is available for testing dark adaptation and glare recovery, but some relative or functional assessments may be made by testing the patient's ability to see objects in very dim light or by measuring the time taken for maximal visual acuity to return after exposure to a strong light such as from a penlight held close to the eye. Differential diagnosis of pathological conditions may be facilitated by the use of electroretinograms, electro-oculograms, fluorescein angiography, measurement of responses to flicker, special tests of color vision function, and visually evoked cortical potentials.

## PRESCRIBING SPECTACLES FOR THE NORMALLY SIGHTED

Most older patients require optical corrections for both distance and near vision tasks. Driving, watching television and movies, watching public events, and referring to distant informational signs cause good distance vision to be important for most individuals. At near, tasks ranging from writing and reading personal and business correspondence; reading labels on foods and medicines; reading price tags; reading directories; and recreational or educational reading of books, newspapers, and magazines are all commonly encountered as part of regular daily life for most people. Obviously most people want easy access to clear distance and near vision.

Progressive addition lenses, bifocals, or trifocals are worn by older patients. Small in number are the emmetropes who do not need distance glasses, myopes who never need near vision glasses, and people who choose to use only single-vision glasses and switch spectacles when they change from distance to near viewing.

Progressive addition lenses have two benefits. One is that they are preferred by people who do not like the appearance of, or are distracted by, the sharp dividing line of standard bifocal or trifocal segments. Progressive addition lenses also provide a channel of progressively increasing power between the distance viewing point and the near viewing point. In effect, this provides a continuous sequence of focus for all possible intermediate distances. Objects at intermediate distances will be seen in good focus when the head and eyes are positioned so that the most appropriate portion of the lens is being used. The patient can experience some diminished clarity and some spatial distortion when viewing through the areas in the lower half of the lens that are outside the channel of progressive power change. Many patients are not bothered by this. Others find it annoying and distracting, but most adapt in a few days or weeks.

In optical corrections for presbyopia, the practitioner's starting point is usually a consideration of the dioptric range of clear vision. What is the near point of the patient's range of clear vision with the best "distance" correction? What will be the far and near limits of the range of clear vision through the best "near" portion of the lens? What working distances are most important for the patient? What is the closest working distance required for the patient?

Whether that presbyopic correction is to be in the form of a progressive addition or a bifocal or trifocal lens, a fundamental decision must be made about the power of the addition. This, combined with the depth of focus and any remaining accommodation, determines the closer viewing distances at which best visual acuity may be obtained. The "distance" portion of the spectacles may be designed for a distance that is significantly closer than optical infinity, especially for glasses to be used in office environments.

Providing good vision within the intermediate space between the clear vision ranges for the "distance" and" near" portions of the lens can be most easily handled by choosing progressive addition lenses. For patients with no accommodation, bifocal lenses might leave a relatively deep range of intermediate distances over which vision will be blurred. Trifocals typically have an intermediate segment that is half the power of the stronger reading segment, and best (or close to best) visual acuity will usually be obtainable at all intermediate distances.

For progressive addition lenses, the intermediate portion of the lens is necessarily a relatively narrow channel; thus the lateral extent of the field of good vision will be somewhat limited, and more exacting head movements may be required for many tasks. Trifocals and bifocals provide wider fields of clear near vision than do progressive additions.

The size and position of bifocal or trifocal segments should be chosen to suit the patient's functional needs and particular wishes. The width of the field of clear near vision, prismatic jump, and chromatic effects can influence the recommendations made (see Chapter 11 for a further discussion of vision corrections for the older adult).

Monovision solutions for enabling good vision for both distance and near tasks have become more common in recent years. Cataract surgery, contact lens corrections, and sometimes refractive surgery deliberately correct one eye for distance vision and the other for near.

Older patients are more likely to have ametropia of high magnitude. In progressive myopia, the magnitude of refractive error can continue to increase throughout life. Also, fairly large myopic shifts can occur from changes in the crystalline lens. At the other end of spectrum, some older patients become highly hyperopic in cases where intraocular lens implants are not used after cataract extraction.

Correction of high refractive errors requires special consideration. When performing the refraction, care should be taken to ensure that the vertex distance and pantoscopic angle of the lenses being worn are similar to those expected to be present in any new glasses that might be worn in the future.

The position of the optical centers relative to the patient's pupil can become much more significant when lens powers exceed approximately 8.00 D. A basic principle guiding lens positioning is that the optic axis of the lens should point toward the center of rotation of the eye. Lens designers assume this when lens design parameters are chosen to avoid unwanted aberrational effects. The center of rotation is typically approximately 27 mm behind the spectacle plane. Pantoscopic tilt of the spectacle plane is a relevant factor in determining the vertical placement of the optical centers. The greater the pantoscopic angle, the lower the centers should be. A simple method for measuring pantoscopic tilt is to take a protractor with a plumb line (or a straightened paper clip) attached to its center. The base of this protractor can be held so that it is against or parallel to the spectacle place. With the patient's head in its natural or habitual posture, the plumb line will indicate the most usual pantoscopic tilt. To compensate for the effects of pantoscopic tilt, the optical centers should be made lower than the center of the pupils by 1 mm for each 2 degrees of pantoscopic tilt. Ten degrees of pantoscopic tilt is common, and for this the height of the optical centers should be 5 mm below the pupil center. This will be about level with the corneal limbus. The correctness of the optical alignment can be verified by having the patient tilt his or her head back while fixating a bright light at an appropriate distance. The optometrist, with the eye close to the light, should observe the reflex from the cornea being in line with those from the lens surfaces.

Aphakic spectacle corrections, though currently uncommon, require special lens design considerations. Bifocals, and rarely trifocals, become virtually essential. The prescribing practitioner is obliged to consider a number of lens design options. For example, should the lens material be plastic to minimize weight? Glass because of its scratch resistance? Or high-index material to minimize thickness? Aspheric lens surfaces are likely to be used, and the purpose may be to enhance appearance by reducing thickness and sagittal depth or provide imagery of better quality when the patient views through more peripheral regions of the lens. Some aspheric lenses available today have been primarily designed to achieve a better cosmetic appearance. Others are designed to minimize aberrational effects. In general, this kind is a little less effective in minimizing thickness. The responsible optometrist stays abreast of developments in lens designs and is prepared to consider the weight, appearance, durability, and aberrations of the lenses. Of course, many of the problems associated with spectacle lenses of higher power can be avoided or minimized by the use of contact lenses.

## PRESCRIBING FOR PATIENTS WITH LOW VISION

Most older patients with low vision can benefit from optical aids to enhance their visual performance. The low-vision aids for individual patients depend on the range and relative importance of the visual tasks they want to perform, their vision characteristics, and their psychological attitudes toward their disability and the use of optical aids. Patients who need low vision aids usually need more than one special optical aid. In prescribing optical aids, the magnification effect is usually the first optical parameter considered. The field of view, distribution of image quality, image brightness, adjustability of focus, appearance, portability, convenience, cost, working distance, and maintenance requirements are other factors that enter the decision-making process.

Optical low vision aids can be placed in three categories: (1) magnifiers for distance vision (telescopes), (2) magnifiers for near vision, and (3) nonmagnifying aids to vision (see Chapter 14 for a discussion of vision care of the older adult who is visually impaired).

### Magnification for Distance Vision: Telescopes

Telescopes are commonly used by low vision patients to enhance the resolution of detail in signs, distant faces, television, movies, or other visual displays and scenery. Many older patients with low vision need to travel independently; if their vision is not adequate for driving, however, they may have to rely on public transportation. Dependence on public transportation, in turn, necessitates reading bus numbers, street signs, and traffic signals.

Prescribing a telescope (or telescopes) for a low vision patient involves first determining the required magnification and then selecting an appropriate telescope.

### Achieving the Required Acuity

The practitioner first determines visual acuity with best spectacle correction and estimates the resolution performance required to meet the patient's specific needs. Most commonly, an acuity performance of 20/30 to 20/40 is set as a practical and useful goal for visual acuity with the telescope, but higher resolution is some-times sought. When acuity is poor, the goal may be reduced to approximately 20/60. If accept-able telescopes do not improve visual acuity to 20/80 or better, the value of a telescope pre-scription becomes questionable.

Calculating the required magnification is simple; it is a matter of ratios. For example, a patient with a visual acuity of 20/200 who wishes to read bus numbers might require a 6× magnification to reach an approximate 20/32 level of performance.

Most low vision patients do obtain the expected improvement in resolution. Exceptions may occur when using acuity charts that make the task more difficult (more letters, closer spacing, or both for the smaller letters). In these cases the improvement may be less than simple theory predicts. The optometrist should verify that the patient does, in fact, obtain the expected visual acuity with the magnification originally predicted. Occasionally some modi-fication of the magnification value will be necessary.

Certain techniques are important when testing patient performance with telescopes, especially with older patients. For best vision, the telescope must be focused properly. The greater the magnification, the more critical this becomes. If the patient has only a small refrac-tive error, the clinician may focus the telescope for his or her own eye, observing the chart from the correct viewing distance. Then only small-focus adjustments should be required of the patient. When patients have higher refractive error and remove their spectacles to use the telescope, then the clinician may use a trial lens to simulate the patient's refractive error and

again adjust the telescope. Thus, for a 6.00 D myope, the clinician should look through a telescope while holding a +6.00 D lens between the telescope eyepiece and his or her own eye (or glasses, if worn) and, being careful to be at the correct observation distance, focus to obtain clearest vision. The telescope should then be close to correct adjustment for the patient. Remember that increasing the telescope length adds plus power to either correct hyperopic refractive errors or to focus for closer viewing distances. Shortening the telescope length adds minus power.

Some telescopes of 6× or greater magnifica-tion do not provide enough focusing range to enable a focus for the commonly used 20- or 10-foot distances. This is especially true for binocular telescope systems. If the range of focus on the chart is insufficient, the clinician can effectively simulate optical infinity by moving the chart to 4 m (12.5 ft) and then hold a +0.25 D trial lens against the objective of the telescope. A chart observation distance of 2 m with +0.50 D lens in front of the telescope achieves the same effect.

Ensuring in-focus vision is necessary when determining whether the patient will achieve the resolution goal sought. The clinician should always verify that the prescribed telescope does indeed focus at the distance required. The patient's actual working distance should be established and simulated in the office or local environment. The patient's required observa-tion distance may be 30 ft (e.g., a lecture theater) or 8 ft (an overhead menu at a fast-food restau-rant); whatever this observation distance is, however, it should be simulated, and the clini-cian should be sure that the telescope's focusing range is adequate.

When more than one viewing distance is required, prescribing a removable lens cap of appropriate power may be necessary to achieve the shift in focus. Today, most series of monoc-ular telescopes that have been designed for low vision patients provide wide focusing ranges extending from infinity to distances well within arm's length.

Another important optical parameter is the exit pupil of the telescope, which defines the size of the beam of rays that can emerge from the telescope. The exit pupil can be calculated by dividing the diameter of the objective lens by the magnification of the telescope. Thus an $8 \times 20$ telescope has an $8\times$ magnification and a 20-mm objective lens diameter; the exit pupil size is $20 \div 8 = 2.5$ mm. An $8 \times 40$ telescope has a 40-mm objective, and thus has a 5-mm exit pupil. Telescopes of $4 \times 20$, $6 \times 30$, $8 \times 40$, and $10 \times 50$ all have 5-mm exit pupils.

The exit pupil can determine image brightness. If the exit beam is smaller than the eye pupil diameter, the image brightness is reduced as though the eye pupil had constricted to become the same size as the exit pupil of the telescope. An $8 \times 20$ telescope with a 2.5-mm exit pupil used by an eye with a 5-mm pupil will cause a fourfold decrease in retinal image illumination. In this example, the effective diameter of the pupil is reduced by a factor of 2, so the effective area is reduced by a factor of 4. If the exit beam of the telescope is larger in diameter than the eye pupil, the image brightness should not be reduced except for the small loss by reflectance and absorption. Lens coatings can reduce this kind of light loss.

The discussion of image brightness and telescopes applies to the observation of most objects. Different arguments and conclusions apply to the observation of stars, because for point sources the size of the retinal images is not affected by the magnification of the telescope, but image brightness is.

Telescopes with smaller exit beams are generally more difficult to use, especially if the patient is inexperienced or has unsteady hands. Maintaining a small exit beam in alignment with the eye pupil can be difficult.

Older patients who have difficulty using telescopes to view the visual acuity chart are helped if the magnification is lower, the exit pupil is larger, or the field of view is larger. Sometimes developing the patient's skills gradually by starting with telescopes of lower magnification is necessary. Patients with alignment difficulties can be assisted by reducing the room lighting and increasing the illumination on the chart. If the telescope is not aligned properly, the exit beam will be visible to the clinician as it illuminates the iris, sclera, or eyelids. The patient can be guided so that the exit beam enters his or her pupil. Even when the telescope is aligned, it may be necessary for the clinician to continue to help maintain alignment and assist with the focus adjustment. In general, older patients need significantly more training and guidance to become proficient at using telescopes.

### Selecting a Telescope

Once it has been verified that a patient can achieve the desired visual acuity with the use of a telescope of a particular magnification, the clinician must select the type of telescope that produces the required magnification and most conveniently satisfies the patient's needs. The prescribed telescope may be monocular or binocular. Binocular telescopes may be preferred when the visual acuity is similar for the two eyes. Some patients find binocular telescopes easier to hold because the two eyecups can touch the eyebrows and provide some support or tactile feedback to help the patient maintain proper alignment. However, binocular telescopes are bulky and heavy, which detracts from their portability and comfort, and their focusing range can be limited.

Patients who use telescopes to assist in their independent travel abilities typically prefer monocular telescopes that are lightweight, concealable, easily carried in a pocket or purse, and easy to use. Wrist straps, neck cords, or small finger-ring mountings may help keep the telescope easily accessible for use as needed. Difficulties in holding a higher powered telescope with adequate steadiness can sometimes by reduced or eliminated by the use of a tripod, monopod, or other supporting structure.

Telescopes mounted in a spectacle frame or similar mounting have their advantages. They can prove most useful when observation with the telescope is used for protracted periods (for example, when watching sporting events, stage presentations, or movies). Ready-made sports glasses, which are a pair of adjustable telescopes mounted in a spectacle-style frame, can be relatively inexpensive. Hook-on monocular telescopes can be attached to existing distance spectacles, thereby simultaneously correcting the refractive error and providing magnification.

Patients often request a head-mounted telescope system for viewing television. In general, the patient is better off moving closer to the television. Because telescopes restrict the field of view, in many television-viewing situations telescopes will not allow the patient to see the whole screen at one time. Keplerian telescopes provide wider fields of view, with the field widths usually being about equal to the equivalent viewing distance (EVD). For telescopes, the EVD is equal to the viewing distance divided by the magnification. For example, a 4× Keplerian telescope and a viewing distance of 2 m will create an EVD of 50 cm; the expected field of view will be approximately 50 cm. The field of view for Galilean telescopes is typically substantially smaller than the EVD. Many older patients resist sitting close to the television because they believe it is harmful to the eyes. Such misconceptions should be corrected.

Bioptic telescopes are spectacle-mounted telescope systems that are arranged to enable a quick transition from viewing through the telescope portion to viewing through the lens in which the telescope is mounted. These systems are more commonly prescribed for younger adults, but some older patients benefit from them. Bioptic telescopes can be used in driving, permitting the wearer quick access to telescope viewing for short-term observation of signs and traffic signals. Many states permit driving with bioptic telescopes provided that the usual visual acuity standard is met when the wearer views through the telescope. Some states have requirements regarding the visual acuity through the nontelescope portion of the bioptic telescope system. Drivers wearing bioptic telescopes may have some general or individual restrictions on their driver's licenses. Older patients who use a bioptic telescope system for driving might want a bifocal addition for viewing the speedometer and other gauges and displays. Some telescopes have auto-focus that quickly adjusts the focus when the telescope is pointed toward objects at different distances.

Spectacle-mounted bioptic telescope systems are available in magnifications up to 8×, but 3× and 4× seem to be most useful. For high-magnification bioptic telescopes, the small field and difficulties with steadiness and aiming the telescope make the system harder to use.

Older patients, who are often self-conscious about their visual handicap, may be reluctant to even consider the use of any kind of telescope. Most patients with a visual acuity of 20/60 or poorer should be given information about telescopes so they can understand their potential advantages. Encouraging patients to borrow a telescope for use at home for a week or so can produce some appreciation of the benefits and may change attitudes about telescopes.

**Magnification for Near Vision**

Magnification devices to provide low vision patients with assistance for near vision tasks can be grouped into six categories: (1) high-addition reading glasses, (2) handheld magnifying glasses, (3) stand magnifiers, (4) head-mounted loupes, (5) near-vision telescopes, and (6) video magnifiers.

Three basic steps are involved in prescribing a magnifier to provide a level of resolution that will meet the patient's visual needs:

1. Determining the magnification or the EVD required
2. Deciding what kind of magnifier (e.g., handheld, stand) would be most appropriate
3. Given the required EVD and the kind of magnifier, determining which of the available models has the best combination of features to satisfy the patient's requirements

*Determining Magnification Requirements*

Magnification for near vision can be a difficult topic to discuss many conflicting definitions of magnification are used. To illustrate the difficulty, a 5.00 D lens held at a full arm's length might produce an apparent magnification of 5×, and the resolution could be 2× better than that obtained with a previous 2.50 D addition that gave clear vision at 40 cm. However, the manufacturer likely has this magnifier labeled 2.25×; in addition, the clinician may recall a simple formula ($M = F/4$) that suggests the magnification should be 1.25×. The word magnification implies a comparison and demands the question, magnified compared with what? Because this question has several alternative answers, several alternative definitions of magnification are used, and which definition is most appropriate is not always clear. The example above shows four magnification values arising from four different definitions.

Much of the potential confusion surrounding the use of the term magnification can be avoided by using the concept of EVD to quantify the magnifying effect that optical systems provide. The EVD is the distance at which the object would subtend the same angle as that being subtended by the image seen with the magnifying device. For example, a 4× photographic enlargement of a sample of print that is viewed from a distance of 40 cm presents the observer with an image whose angular size is equivalent to that obtained if the original print sample was viewed from a distance of 10 cm; that is, the EVD is 10 cm. Similarly, a video magnifier giving an image that is 50 cm from the eye and enlarged 10 times provides an EVD of 5 cm.

Many optical magnifiers can be used to create an image at optical infinity, in which case the EVD is equal to the equivalent focal length of the magnifier. Thus a +20 D lens being used to give an image at infinity will provide an EVD of 5 cm.

Frequently optical magnifiers create an enlarged image that is located not at infinity, but at a finite distance. The EVD is then the eye-to-image distance divided by the enlargement ratio (or transverse magnification). For example, consider a fixed-focus stand magnifier that gives an image that is enlarged by a factor of 3 and is located 20 cm behind the lens of the magnifier. If the patient uses this magnifier so the separation between the eye and magnifier is 10 cm, this will achieve an EVD of (10 + 20)/3 = 30/3 = 10 cm. For a given patient, systems that provide the same EVD will enable the same visual resolution if, of course, the image is in satisfactory focus.

A patient with presbyopia would be expected to obtain the same resolution with each of the optical systems listed in Box 7-2.

---

**BOX 7-2**

### Providing an EVD of 8 cm by Several Different Means

A +12.5 D spectacle addition; print at 8 cm.

A +12.5 D handheld magnifier regardless of how far it is held from the eye while the patient uses distance vision glasses (the lens-page separation will be 8 cm).

A 2.5× telescope with a +5 D cap to provide a 20-cm working distance.

A stand magnifier with a +20 D lens whose image is 20 cm (5 D) below the lens with the patient using a +2.50 D addition. The separation between the object and the magnifier must be 4 cm (25 D), and the enlargement ratio will be 5×. If the eye-lens separation is 20 cm, the eye-to-image distance is 40 cm.

A video magnifier giving an enlargement of 10× when the viewing distance is 80 cm (+1.25 D addition).

---

All five systems provide an EVD of 8 cm (or equivalent viewing power of +12.5 D). All afford a resolution equal to that expected if the patient were to hold the object of interest 8 cm from the eye while maintaining a clear image by accommodation or using an addition. In any evaluation of near-vision performance, the patient should wear an appropriate addition and hold the test material so that it is in good focus.

### Determining the Equivalent Viewing Distance Required

Although using distance visual acuity to estimate how much dioptric power is required to enable a patient to read print of a certain size is possible, this is not the surest approach. Letter charts used for distance vision and reading cards used for near vision present tasks of different complexity; no strong concordance exists between letter chart acuity and reading chart acuity, especially when macular disturbances are present. Patients with presbyopia almost invariably have a reading correction, and the most convenient and appropriate way to begin the power determination is to measure the patient's reading acuity while he or she uses an existing reading correction. For example, a patient might have eyeglasses that incorporate a +3.00 D addition. Holding the test card at 33 cm, this patient may be able to read 2.5 M print (which could, on some charts, be labeled 20 points or 20/125).

The EVD required to reach a resolution goal then can be determined by simple ratios or proportions. For example, the clinician might decide that the resolution goal should have the patient able to read text of newsprint size (1 M, 8 points, or 20/50 in size) with the same level of confidence or difficulty exhibited when the patient read the 2.5 M print at 33 cm. Whatever units are used, a 2.5× improvement in resolution is required. The required improvement in resolution can be achieved by changing the viewing distance from 33 cm by a factor of 2.5×, so that an EVD of 13 cm is indicated. For this presbyopic patient, the power of the addition needs to be increased from 3.00 D to 7.50 D. The clinician should then verify that the patient does, in fact, achieve satisfactory reading of the 1 M print (8 points or 20/50) that had been set as the goal. This testing is usually done with spectacle lenses in a trial frame or trial lens clip.

When working over existing bifocals, the lens clip might not allow full access to the bifocal portion of the lens. In such a case, the lens clip can be raised so that only the distance portion of the lens is being used, and the full required addition can be introduced into the lens clip. Special care must be taken to ensure that an appropriate working distance is being used because some older patients strongly resist working at close distances.

### Selecting the Magnifying Aid

Once the EVD needed to provide the desired reading resolution performance has been determined, the optometrist must decide which of the various aids should be used to provide the required EVD.

Spectacle lens corrections afford the widest fields of view, leave both hands free to support or manipulate task materials, are convenient to carry, and are relatively inconspicuous. Their disadvantage is the close working distance they may impose. If a spectacle prescription is to be issued, the lens form must be considered. Will it be single-vision lenses, bifocals in a standard configuration, bifocals with high placement of the segments, special series lenses, or aspheric lenses? Binocularity issues should be addressed. If binocular vision is to be achieved (it is usually achievable if addition powers are +8.00 D or less), the prism or decentration must be considered. Fonda[15] recommends as a rule of thumb that, relative to the distance prism, 2 mm of total decentration be given for each diopter of addition power. Thus 8 mm of total decentration should be present for a 4.00 D addition, 16 mm for an 8.00 D addition, and so on. This method provides a small net amount of base-in prism.

Many patients with low vision must perform near-vision tasks monocularly, either because there is substantial inequality between the two eyes or because the required lens powers are too high. Even though the other eye might not be used during the main reading tasks, some attention should be given to the lens that will be worn in front of the second eye. A simple balance lens may be indicated. Often monovision possibilities should be considered. Having a single-vision lens before the poorer eye to give in-focus distance vision or provide clearest focus for intermediate or near vision may be useful. A bifocal or trifocal lens before the poorer eye might best satisfy the patient's overall visual needs and convenience.

Handheld magnifiers have as their main advantage the adjustability of working distance. In one extreme, the patient can hold the magnifying glass in the spectacle plane, in which case the reading material will need to be in the appropriate focal plane, usually relatively close to the lens. At the other end of the scale, the magnifier may be held at a full arm's length; again, the object of regard will need to be in the proper focal plane. The further the lens is held from the eye, the smaller is the field of view. The field of view is equal to the EVD multiplied by the ratio of the lens diameter to its distance from the eye. For example, a +12.5 D lens held 8 cm from the page and 50 cm from the eye will give an EVD of 8.0 cm. If, in this example, the lens diameter is 5 cm, the diameter-to-distance aspect ratio is 5/50 cm, then the field of view—8.0(5/50)—is 0.8 cm. Provided patients are using their distance glasses, the resolution expected from a handheld magnifier can be determined directly from the equivalent power of the lens. The EVD will simply be the focal length of the magnifier. Bifocal wearers should not view through their bifocal segments unless the magnifier is being held close (i.e., closer than one of its focal lengths) to the spectacle lens. Holding the magnifier against the reading addition in spectacles effectively provides the sum of the two powers. The combination then will act as a strong spectacle lens.

Handheld magnifiers provide portability and flexibility. They are ideally suited for looking at price tags, reading maps, and checking labels on containers in a store.

Stand magnifiers are most commonly used for short-term reading tasks. They can be particularly helpful to older patients because steady hands are not necessarily needed. If strong dioptric powers are required, and even if no hand steadiness problems are present, stand magnifiers provide a level of easy and reliable control not attainable with spectacles or handheld magnifiers. For reading tasks of limited duration (e.g., reading telephone books and television schedules, checking bills, and reading greeting cards), stand magnifiers can be of value. Most incorporate a light to illuminate the task. Stand magnifiers may be somewhat bulky and therefore less convenient to carry, and the working situation becomes much more rigidly defined.

The practitioner must understand a few basic optical principles to prescribe stand magnifiers intelligently. First, fixed-focus stand magnifiers produce images that are relatively close to the lens of the magnifier. Rarely is the image farther than 50 cm behind the magnifying lens, and most image locations are in the range of 3 cm to 40 cm behind the lens surface. Consequently, patients with presbyopia must wear a reading correction to obtain a clear view of the image. The image location and the power of the spectacle addition determine the separation required between the magnifier and the spectacles. If the image of the magnifier is 10 cm below its surface, and the patient is focused for 40 cm because of a +2.50 D reading addition, then the required separation between the eye and the magnifier is 30 cm. Had the spectacle addition been 5.00 D, the required eye-to-image distance is 20 cm so the required eye-to-magnifier distance becomes 10 cm for a stand magnifier. The practitioner needs to know the image location for the stand magnifier being used.

The second basic optical principle to be understood is that the image produced by the stand magnifier is larger than the original object by a fixed ratio. The net effect of the magnifier is to produce an image that is both larger and more remote than the original object. The power of the magnifier lens and the object-lens separation determine the size of the image. The enlargement ratio (which may also be called transverse magnification) is constant for a given magnifier, and the enlargement ratio should be known to the clinician because it influences the final resolution.

Third, when the patient views the enlarged image formed by the magnifier, the resulting EVD can be determined by dividing the eye-to-image distance by the enlargement ratio. Some clinicians prefer to consider the EVD in dioptric units; then the equivalent viewing power may be determined by multiplying the accommodation demand by the enlargement ratio. If a stand magnifier forms an image that is 20 cm below the lens and the enlargement ratio is 3×, then a patient whose eye is 10 cm above the lens will have eye-to-image distance of 30 cm, so the EVD is 10 cm. The accommodation demand is 3.33 D, so that the equivalent viewing power

**TABLE 7-1**

**Comparison of Two Stand Magnifiers**

| Magnifier | COIL 5289 | Lighthouse PowerMag 9528 |
|---|---|---|
| Labeled power/ magnification | +28.00 D/8.0X | +28.00 D/8X |
| Equivalent power | +23.40 D | +27.40 D |
| Image position | 25 cm | 53 cm |
| Enlargement ratio | 6.9X | 14.6X |

is 10 D. The EVD can be used in predicting the resolution that the patient will be able to achieve with the system.

The following demonstrates some of the important considerations that should be made when using stand magnifiers. Two widely used stand magnifiers, one from COIL (Slough, England) and one from the Lighthouse PowerMag series (Optelec, New York, NY), have the same magnification ratings assigned by the manufacturers. However, comparison of their optical properties shows how they have different optical effects (Table 7-1).

If the patient's eye were 15 cm from the lens, then the eye-to-image distances would be 40 cm and 68 cm for these two magnifiers, and the ideal additions would be +2.50 D and +1.50 D, respectively. The EVDs that would be achieved would be 40/6.9 = 5.8 cm and 68/14.6 = 4.7 cm. The visual acuity difference would be equal to one row on the chart. If, however, the eye were placed 5 cm from the lens, the eye-to-image distances would be reduced by 10 cm and the EVDs would become 4.3 cm and 4.0 cm, respectively.

Unfortunately most, but not all, manufacturers do not specify image location or the enlargement ratio; even their nominal lens powers or magnification ratings are often inappropriate or wrong. However, simple in-office methods are available for measuring these key optical parameters.[1-3,9]

Head-mounted loupes are positive-powered lenses mounted so they sit in front of the spectacle plane. They are mainly used for viewing manipulative tasks. A variety of such devices are available. Some are single lenses that attach to the spectacle frame or spectacle lens, and the lens generally is mounted on a pivoting bracket that allows it to be conveniently removed from or inserted into the line of vision. These can provide monocular viewing, and lens powers usually range from 10.00 D to approximately 30.00 D. Binocular loupes, which are available in powers up to approximately 10.00 D or 12.00 D, usually incorporate some prism or decentration to reduce the convergence demand. Some binocular loupe systems attach to spectacles, but most are mounted on a headband that positions the lens bracket 2 cm or so in front of the spectacle place. Many can be flipped up and down as needed. Another potential advantage of head-mounted loupes is that mounting the lenses a few centimeters away from the spectacle means the object of regard may be moved a few centimeters further from the face. For some manipulative tasks, this modest change in viewing distance is useful.

Near-vision telescopes (sometimes called telemicroscopes) are commonly prescribed for older patients, but they have distinct advantages that sometimes make them essential. Near-vision telescopes are called for when a certain level of dioptric power is necessary to provide the EVD required to achieve a given resolution goal, but the patient is compelled to have a long working distance and unrestricted or bimanual access to the task. Performing surgery and viewing computer terminals are two examples of tasks for which near-vision telescopes might be considered. The advantage of near-vision telescopes is the increased working distance, but this must be balanced against the principal disadvantage: the reduced field of view. The depth of field is also quite small, so the working distance must be accurately maintained. The small fields of view almost invariably make near-vision telescopes unsuitable for use at computer screens.

Near-vision telescopes can be created most simply by adding a lens cap to the objective lens of a distance telescope. The EVD achieved by the system can be computed easily; it is simply the focal length of the lens cap divided by the telescope magnification. For example, a system made from placing a 4.00 D lens cap on the front of a 2.5× telescope creates a focus for 25 cm. The EVD = 25/2.5 = 10 cm (equivalent viewing power = 4.00 × 2.5). This will provide the same resolution as any other system that achieves an EVD of 10 cm. In this example, the working distance is 25 cm because it is set by the focal lens of the lens cap. Other near-vision telescope systems to achieve an EVD of 10 cm could be created by combining a 2.00 D lens cap and a 5× telescope (working distance, 50 cm), a 3.00 D cap and a 3.3× telescope (working distance, 33 cm), a 5.00-D cap and a 2.0× telescope (working distance, 20 cm), or many other combinations. Many near-vision telescope systems are created by taking a distance-vision telescope and increasing its optical path length to achieve a near-vision focus. The EVD can be determined from the formula EVD = $u/M - f_{oc}$, where u is the telescope-to-object distance, M is the magnification of the telescope, and $f_{oc}$ is the focal length of the ocular. For most Keplerian telescopes the value of $f_{oc}$ is approximately 1 cm. The critical optical parameters for prescribing near-vision telescopes are the working distance and the EVD that the system provides.

### Electronic Display Systems

Computer displays and video magnifiers are becoming more widely used by older people to compensate for visual impairments. The use of electronic systems will continue to increase rapidly as information technology becomes more user friendly and as technophobia becomes less prevalent.

### Video Magnifiers

In video magnifier systems (often called CCTVs), the image from a video camera is imaged on a cathode-ray tube or flat-panel display screen. The size and other characteristics of the image can be manipulated by adjusting the optical or electronic components of the system. Most commonly the camera is in a stand pointing down toward an x-y table on which printed material is placed. The table surface may be easily moved left and right and back and forth to position the required area of the reading material under the camera. The height of the image of the print on the screen depends on the size of the screen and the characteristics and state of adjustment of the camera system. Almost all systems use color cameras, and easy controls enable the image to be changed to high-contrast black-on-white or reversed-contrast with white-on-black. Typically a variety of combinations of background and foreground colors are available. The range of magnification changes by a factor of approximately 10 or 12 times in most cases. For most stand-mounted cameras, at minimal magnification the field of view has a width of 10 to 15 cm. At maximal magnification, the displayed print becomes so large that only a few letters are seen across the width of the screen. The enlargement ratio is equal to the screen width divided by the field of view. The equivalent viewing distance is equal to the eye-to-screen distance divided by the enlargement ratio. That is, EVD = d/(W/FoV), where d is viewing distance, W is screen width, and FoV is field of view. Patients typically sit closer when the screen is smaller. The patient typically adopts a viewing distance that is approximately equal to the width of the display screen. If the viewing distance is equal to the screen width, then the EVD becomes equal to the width field of view. When the viewing distance is equal to half the screen width, the EVD will be half of the field of view. Given that the magnification levels are easily adjustable with a knob or a lever, and some scope can change viewing distance, patients can easily balance enlargement ratios, fields of view, and EVDs according to the size of the print they are reading. The special advantage that video magnifiers have over optical magnifiers is that they can give a larger field of view when strong magnification is required. The field of view of optical magnifiers is usually equal to or less than the EVD, but for a video magnifier giving same EVD, the field of view may exceed the EVD, provided the viewing distance is less than the screen width.

The most widely used video magnifiers have a camera with an easily adjustable zoom lens mounted above a moveable x-y table; the display screen sits above the camera stand. Other camera systems are available. Handheld cameras, some as small as a computer mouse, can be moved over the page. Some cameras mounted on stands or movable carriages allow the axis of the camera to be rotated and redirected from pointing down at the tabletop to distant objects or displays. The output of some of the small handheld camera systems can be fed into a standard television or computer display. Some specialized systems have the camera head mounted so that hat shifts in the point of regard are achieved by moving the head.

Display screens have traditionally been cathode-ray tube video monitors separated from the tabletop by the camera system, a work space, and the x-y table. Such models are relatively heavy and bulky, and they require a dedicated workstation. Flat-panel displays have enabled more portability and more flexible screen placement. A few systems have used head-mounted displays that have a small digital display screen and a high-powered viewing lens mounted within a goggle or visor device. A recent addition to the armamentarium of electronic magnifiers are small units that have a 10- to 15-cm wide display screen and a camera system built into a small, thin box that rests on the page. Such systems currently have limited adjustability of magnification, but this will change and they are likely to become a popular replacement for optical hand and stand magnifiers (see Chapter 15 for further discussion of video magnifiers).

### Computers

Computer display systems create their displays by taking stored digital information that can be manipulated to provide outputs with the possibility of a diverse range of characteristics. The display outputs can use senses other than vision. Auditory and tactile displays are readily available in the form of synthesized speech and Braille outputs. With the visual displays, the size and appearance of printed material can easily be selected to suit the patient's needs. Some modifications can be made to enhance the accessibility of information from graphic or pictorial displays. The input of the information into the computer may come from the keyboard and mouse; from scanning hard copy documents; or to the computer already in digital form accessible over the Internet by e-mail, web browsers, or a variety of modes of storage media ranging from floppy disks to compact disks. Voice-recognition software convert's a user's speech to digital text documents that can be stored or displayed as needed.

With electronic visual displays the size, font, style, spacing, and foreground and background colors can all be manipulated by the user to optimize the appearance of displayed text. When the print needs to be large, the amount of information than can be displayed on the screen is reduced. For a patient with low vision, some of the simplest ways of enhancing the visibility of the screen displays may come from choosing to use a large screen or from using standard control panel options to reduce the number of pixels displayed on the screen. Modern computer operating systems offer ways of easily changing the visibility of the cursor and making simple adjustments to the size and color and contrast features of the screen images. Speech output options are also available. Most current word processing or spreadsheet programs have options for making the printed material within the document smaller or larger by a ratio that the user may select.

For some patients, more sophisticated enhancements of displayed material are needed, and special software may be required. Dedicated programs to enhance access to computer information may facilitate quick changes in magnification or other visual display characteristics over the whole screen or parts of the screen. Speech or other nonvisual outputs may be readily engaged or disengaged. The display layout characteristics may be changed to a horizontal streaming mode, by which the text is presented in a single row that moves from right to left across the screen; a vertical streaming mode, in which the column width is made equal to the screen width at all print sizes; or the "rapid serial visual presentation" mode, in which the words appear one at a time in one location on the screen. For each of these presentation modes, the user controls the speed of presentation, and a facility exists for switching back to the original display layout to ascertain place or shift to a new region of the document.

Display technology will continue to develop rapidly, and the older population, especially those with visual impairment, are sure to benefit from enhanced and simplified access to information technology, from more flexible flat-panel and head mounted visual displays, and from nonvisual input and output systems mediated through touch and sound.

### Nonmagnifying Aids to Vision

For all near-vision magnification systems, care should be taken to adjust the illumination to suit the patients' needs. Most older, low vision patients require more illumination than usual, but they are more susceptible to problems with glare. Consequently, more than the usual attention should be paid to positioning the light and

the task material so that potentially troublesome glare is avoided.

A device that has long been useful for glare control is the typoscope, or reading mask. This is a black card with a rectangular aperture that is usually made large enough to accommodate three lines of one-column-width print. The typoscope can enhance reading acuity and comfort by reducing glare from white paper close to the immediate fixation point. This device also serves as a line guide and helps patients with field defects maintain their place when reading.

Yellow filters also are beneficial to some patients, who report that they make vision clearer and more comfortable. Illumination control by varying the quantity and quality of the task and ambient lighting should be routinely included in the assessment of the patient's near-vision magnification needs.

Filters also can be beneficial to many older patients. For reasons that are not fully understood, many patients with retinal disorders and some with cataracts report seeing better when yellow filters or some other "minus blue" filter is worn (see Chapter 2). Older patients, especially those with visual disorders, tend to be more sensitive to bright light; thus sunglass filters (sometimes very dense ones) are often required. The approach to prescribing tints is largely empirical. Decisions are based on reported symptoms and the patient's perception of the effect of the filters.

Contact lenses can offer special advantages to some low vision patients. They can substantially reduce the effect of corneal irregularities caused by corneal or anterior eye scarring or dystrophies. When the corneal distortion is more pronounced, soft contact lenses are not as effective because some of the corneal distortion may be translated to the front surface of the lens. Rigid lenses can be more effective in nullifying the optical effect of distortion, but they are more likely to cause potentially troublesome pressure spots on the distorted cornea. The other major optical benefit of contact lenses is that they substantially reduce aberration and prismatic effects that can produce vision difficulties with the use of stronger spectacle lenses. Because the contact lenses move with the eye, the visual axis of the eye is always close to the optic axis of the correcting lens; this means that peripheral aberration problems are eliminated or at least greatly reduced. Differential prismatic effects that occur with spectacle corrections for anisometropia are much better controlled with contact lenses. Patients with aphakia often have perceptual and depth judgment difficulties when they are introduced to spectacle corrections, and they may be bothered by the field restriction and the "jack-in-the-box" effect created by the high plus spectacle lens. These effects are avoided or minimized by using contact lenses. Many older patients have impaired manual dexterity or reduced vision that may create difficulties for handling and caring for contact lens, thus making them contraindicated (see Chapter 12 for further discussion of contact lenses and the older adult).

Visual field defects accompanying pathological changes can produce functional difficulties for patients, especially in mobility tasks. Three kinds of optical devices can help patients with particular kinds of visual field defects: reversed telescopes, hemianopic mirrors, and partial prisms.

Reversed telescopes can be useful for some patients who have a concentric loss of visual field such as what occurs in advanced retinitis pigmentosa or glaucoma. Reversed telescopes minify and obviously reduce visual acuity, but they can provide an enlarged visual field. Most patients who use reversed telescopes only do so for navigational purposes, and then only when the local environment contains repetitive or potentially confusing details. An example of such a situation is an intersection at which many roads or paths meet. Most reversed telescopes are handheld and are of a moderate range of magnification (2× to 6×). A handheld minus lens positioned 30 to 50 cm from the eye can achieve a similar minification, field-expanding effect.

Partial prisms are prisms that cover only part of the spectacle lens area and can be prescribed to help patients with field problems. Their main use is in hemianopsias, but they are sometimes used for a concentric loss of visual field. Partial prisms are usually in the form of Fresnel membrane prisms of high deviation (15 to 40 prism diopters) that are most commonly placed on the lens so that they are totally within the blind field when the patient looks straight ahead. The base direction of the prism is always away from the primary line of sight. When the patient makes an eye movement toward a blind part of

the field, the prism will be encountered after a certain degree of eye rotation. The prism optically shifts things in from the periphery. This means that smaller eye movements will be required to view more peripheral objects on the blind side. Stated another way, an eye movement of a given magnitude allows the patient to see further to the periphery when viewing through the prism. The prism, however, creates a blind spot, and the patient may be distracted by the apparent jumping or disappearance of objects when eye movements traverse the edge of the prism. The prisms are placed so they will remain unnoticed within the patient's blind field most of the time when relatively normal, small-magnitude lateral eye movements are being made. When the patient wants to inspect more peripheral regions briefly, larger eye movements are called for and are supplemented by the effect of the prism.

A fairly typical configuration of the partial prisms for a patient with right hemianopsia would be a 30 prism diopter base-out prism mounted on the right lens so that it covers the full vertical height of the lens beginning at a point approximately 6 mm to the right of the primary viewing point. Partial prisms are sometimes used for both eyes; for the case presented here, the left lens would have 30 prism diopter base-in, and it would be smaller in area. Again, the vertical edge of the prism would be approximately 6 mm from the primary viewing point. Because Fresnel membrane prisms can be removed and replaced easily, experimenting with this kind of correction is not difficult or expensive. An alternative arrangement of partial prisms is to have a horizontal strip of prism across the width of the lens above or below (or even both) the primary line of sight.

Vision through these strong prisms is necessarily degraded by chromatic aberration and other contrast reductions. The purpose of these various partial prism systems is to make the patient more aware of objects of potential interest that are off to the blind side. Once located, the patient makes appropriate head and eye movements to look at the object of interest directly so he or she is not looking at it through the prism.

Hemianopic mirrors can occasionally help patients with homonymous hemianopia. A mirror is mounted on the nasal eyewire of the spectacles in front of the eye that is on the same side as the field loss. The mirror is angled so that it is approximately 5 or 10 degrees with respect to the primary line of sight and approximately 20 mm to 40 mm in width. For a patient with a right homonymous hemianopia, the mirror would therefore be mounted on the nasal portion of the right eyewire and angled slightly toward the right eye. By reflection, this mirror will present part of the right-hand field of view to the right eye. This segment from the blind field seen through the mirror will seen by the right eye to be reversed and unstable, and it will be projected so that it seems to be superimposed on the left-hand field. The purpose of the mirror is to provide some awareness of events and hazards on the blind side. The patient must learn not to give close attention to detail seen in the mirror. When the patient becomes aware of an object or event deserving attention, the head should be turned so that the full inspection and any decision making can be made with benefit of direct vision. Few patients with hemianopia actually have mirrors prescribed, but optometrists nevertheless should be aware of them as a possibility.

Some have advocated prisms for patients with central scotomas to "relocate" the image that would normally fall on the fovea and position that image on a more central or paracentral region of the retina. Such relocation is logically impossible with simple prisms. However, these prism systems may have some advantage through encouraging changes in habitual head and eye postures that might somehow facilitate eccentric viewing.

### Training in the Use of Optical Aids

Adaptation, practice, and training are often necessary if patients are to receive maximal benefit from their low vision aids. Many aids demand that new skills be learned. Older patients are generally less able to adapt, and they require more training. For example, structured, guided practice in techniques for sighting and focusing with telescopes can be vital to success. Furthermore, initial training with telescopes that have lower magnification and larger exit pupils is beneficial because they are easier to use.

A variety of skills may need to be developed for reading, including positioning the head, the eyes, the aid, and the material to achieve clear focus and then making the required relative movements to enable the most fluent reading. Sometimes only brief instruction is needed, whereas other situations may require extensive training and supervision.

Many low vision patients have central scotomas, and their visual performance and efficiency may improve if they can learn eccentric viewing strategies. Similarly, many patients may need training to develop more efficient scanning and search techniques.

Ensuring that a patient has reasonable proficiency with any optical aid before it is issued is a good policy. Training the patient to be efficient in the use of an aid or the eyes can be the key to success.

### ADVICE AND RECOMMENDATIONS

When all the clinical data have been collected, the practitioner should pause and take stock. Has all the relevant information been uncovered? Again, the following questions should be asked: "What does the patient really want?" "What do I want the patient to have?" "Really, why did the patient come to see me?"

The clinician should decide on the treatment options and then consciously consider the strategy for presenting recommendations and advice. For example, should others be present when the advice is given, and to what extent should they be involved? What issues need to be given strongest emphasis, and what should be sidestepped or downplayed? How strongly should the various treatment recommendations be advocated? What does the patient really need to know? What will the patient like to hear, and what will not be accepted easily?

The advice and recommendations the optometrist submits to older patients need not be confined to optical, visual, and ocular health matters. As a health care practitioner, the optometrist has a responsibility to the patient's general health, and any need for rehabilitative attention that may contribute to the patient's overall well-being should be discussed. The optometrist can be a critical link in the health care chain by taking the initiative in directing patients toward appropriate and broadly based care for their health and well-being.

Eye care professionals need to stay abreast of new developments in the treatment and understanding of eye disease. New scientific advances in treatment of eye disease often get considerable publicity, but the reports in the media are commonly exaggerated or wrong. The public access to technical and medical information through the Internet adds to health care practitioners' responsibility to stay well informed so that they can offer appropriate advice and opinion to their well-informed, as well as misinformed, patients. Optometrists should remain well informed about health care and other supporting services available in the local community. In particular, the practitioner should maintain contacts with the medical community and rehabilitation counselors or social workers as well as be familiar with the activities and services of organizations serving persons who are visually impaired.

## REFERENCES

1. Bailey IL: Locating the image in stand magnifiers, *Optometric Monthly* 71:22-4, 1981a.
2. Bailey IL: The use of fixed-focus stand magnifiers, *Optometric Monthly* 71:37-9, 1981b.
3. Bailey IL: Verifying near vision magnifiers, *Optometric Monthly* 72:34-8, 1981c.
4. Bailey IL: Mobility and visual performance under dim illumination. In *Night vision: current research and future directions,* Washington, DC, 1987, National Academy Press, pp. 220-30.
5. Bailey IL, Bullimore MA: A new test of disability glare, *Optom Vis Sci* 68:911-7, 1991.
6. Bailey IL, Lovie JE: New design principles for visual acuity letter charts, *Am J Optom Physiol Opt* 53:740-5, 1976.
7. Bailey IL, Lovie JE: The design and use of a new near-vision chart, *Am J Optom Physiol Opt* 57:378-87, 1980.
8. Bedwell CH: *Visual fields,* London, 1982, Butterworth.
9. Dickinson C: *Low vision: principles and practice,* Oxford, 1998, Butterworth-Heinemann.
10. Elliott DB, North I, Flanagan J: Confrontation visual field tests, *Ophthalmol Physiol Optics* 17(suppl 2):S17-24, 1997.
11. Elliott DB, Patel B, Whitaker D: Development of a reading speed test for potential-vision measurements, *Invest Ophthalmol Vis Sci* 42:1945-9, 2001.
12. Ferris FL, Bailey IL: Standardizing the measurement of visual acuity for clinical research studies, *Ophthalmology* 103:181-2, 995-6, 1996.
13. Ferris LA, Kassoff A, Bresnick GH, et al: New visual acuity charts for research purposes, *Am J Ophthalmol* 94:91-6, 1982.
14. Flom MC, Weymouth FW, Kahneman K: Visual resolution and contour interaction, *J Opt Soc Am* 53:1026-32, 1963.
15. Fonda GE: *Management of low vision,* New York, 1981, Thieme-Stratton.
16. Ginsburg AP: A new contrast sensitivity vision test chart, *Am J Optom Physiol Opt* 6:403-7, 1984.
17. Haegerstrom-Portnoy G, Schneck ME , Brabyn JA, et al: Development of refractive errors into old age, *Opt Vis Sci* 79:643-9, 2002.
18. Holladay JT, Prager TC, Truillo TC, et al: Brightness acuity tester and outdoor visual acuity in cataract patients, *J Cataract Refract Surg* 13:67-9, 1987.
19. Johnson CA, Adams AJ, Casson EJ: Blue-on-yellow perimetry: a five-year overview. In Mills RP, editor: *Perimetry update,* Amsterdam, 1993, Kugler & Ghedini, pp 459-67.
20. Johnson CA, Samuels SJ: Screening for glaucomatous visual field loss with frequency-doubling perimetry, *Invest Ophthamol Vis Sci* 38:413-28, 1997.
21. Keeler CH: On visual aids for the partially sighted, *Trans Ophthalmol Soc UK* 76:605-14, 1956.
22. Legge GE, Ross JA, Luebker A: Psychophysics of reading. VIII. The Minnesota low-vision reading test, *Optom Vis Sci* 66:843-53, 1989.
23. Lennie P, Van Hemel SB, editors: *Visual impairments: determining eligibility for Social Security benefits,* Washington, DC, 2002, National Academies Press.
24. Lott LA, Schneck ME, Haegerstrom-Portnoy G, et al: Reading performance in older adults with good acuity, *Opt Vis Sci* 78:316-24, 2001.
25. Mehr EB, Freid AN: *Low vision care,* Chicago, 1975, Professional Press.
26. Pelli DG, Robson, JG, Wilkins AJ: The design of a new letter chart for measuring contrast sensitivity, *Clin Vis Sci* 2:187-99, 1988.
27. Regan D: Low-contrast charts and sine wave grating tests in ophthalmological and neurological disorders, *Clin Vis Sci* 2:235-50, 1988.
28. Regan D: Specific tests, specific blindnesses: keys, locks and parallel processing. The 1990 Prentice Award lecture, *Optom Vis Sci* 68:489-512, 1991.
29. Schuchard RA: Validity and interpretation of Amsler grid reports, *Arch Ophthalmol* 111:776-80, 1993.
30. Sloan LL: New test charts for the measurement of visual acuity at far and near distances, *Am J Ophthalmol* 48:807-13, 1959.
31. Spry PGD, Johnson CA: Senescent changes of the normal visual field: an age old problem, *Optom Vis Sci* 78:436-41, 2001.

32. Strong G, Woo GC: A distance visual acuity chart incorporating some new design principles, *Arch Ophthalmol* 103:44-6, 1985.

33. Van den Berg TJTP: Importance of intra-ocular light scatter for visual disability, *Doc Ophthalmologica* 61:327-33, 1986.

34. Verbaken J, Johnston AW: Population norms for edge contrast sensitivity, *Am J Optom Physiol Opt* 63:724-32, 1986.

# CHAPTER 8

# *Factors That Complicate Eye Examination in the Older Adult*

**LYMAN C. NORDEN**

Aging adults undergo and adjust to many physical and emotional changes. Although many of these changes may be unrelated to their eyes or vision, they can make an eye examination more difficult and more time-consuming than is customary for younger patients. The widely varying reasons for this are broadly classified in Box 8-1.

Knowing how to recognize and overcome these problems can make the examination both more effective and more efficient. This chapter describes eye examination techniques adapted specifically to older patients.

## HEARING IMPAIRMENT

Hearing impairment is a common problem associated with aging. It is more prevalent among older patients than is visual impairment, and it can greatly impede the clinical assessment of vision.[16] Depending on the population being served, 25% or more of those 65 years or older and 50% or more of those older than 80 years are hearing impaired.

Hearing impairment associated with aging usually manifests as difficulty with higher pitched sounds that is made worse by background noise. Simply speaking louder does not always work with hearing-impaired older adults, especially if a louder voice results in a higher pitch. It also means that assistive listening devices may not work as well as expected by not adequately screening out background noise or helping isolate desired frequencies. These may be among the reasons why older adults who have hearing aids sometimes choose not to wear them.

Whether or not the patient is wearing a hearing aid, communication can always be improved by reducing background noise, facing the patient, and speaking with deliberate clarity. Close the door and eliminate as much ambient noise as possible. Leave the room lights on so the patient can see the examiner's face and lips. Use as few words as possible, with as few syllables as possible. Add slight emphasis to word sounds that are easy to hear and slight pauses to separate word sounds that are hard to hear. Sounds associated with the letters *h*, *t*, and *d* are relatively easy to emphasize with a little extra push from the diaphragm. Softer sounds associated with the letters *z*, *sh*, *r*, *m*, and *n* are hard to emphasize but become easier to hear when followed by a slight pause. A good example of this is heard in the way a sergeant calls a room full of soldiers to attention. He does not shout, "Room, attention." He shouts, "Hroomm… ahTenn… Hutt." Of course this extreme is not necessary with patients, but clinicians can speak purposefully from the diaphragm, adding emphasis to hard sounds

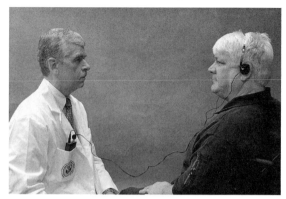

**Fig. 8-1** Pocketalker used to amplify examiner's voice for hearing-impaired patient.

possible to the mouth to selectively amplify the voice. Lightweight headset earphones are available for added convenience and for use over a patient's existing hearing aids if necessary (see Chapter 9 for further discussion of auditory impairments in the older adult).

## COGNITIVE IMPAIRMENT

The prevalence of cognitive impairment among older patients is not as easily determined as is hearing impairment. Depending on methods and criteria used, reports range that from 1% of persons aged 60 years and younger have a cognitive impairment to 33% of persons older than 60 years have a cognitive impairment.[5,9,22] One study of community-dwelling older adults found that 3% to 11% have dementia.[4] Unlike the hearing impaired, the cognitively impaired do not self-report their condition and usually respond to questions as though they both hear and understand—but they may not respond reliably.

Neuropsychologists are able to detect and categorize cognitive impairment with a highly specialized battery of tests, such as the Wechsler Adult Intelligence Scale. Less specialized but highly popular is the Mini-Mental Status Exam, with test items such as "Spell *world* backwards." More basic are three simple questions testing orientation to person, place, and time: (1) "What is your name?" (2) "Where are we now?" or "What is this place called?" and (3) "What day is this?" Questions such as these, however, seem out of place in an eye examination. They are time-consuming, and some patients would understandably be offended at their implication. The practical solution to this problem is to incorporate elements that require

and pauses to soft sounds. A clinical example of this technique is "Hwhitch is PbeTTer… Hwon… or Two (Box 8-2)?"

If despite these measures a hearing problem persists, a readily available assistive listening device known as the Pocketalker can be kept in the examination room for use as needed. The Pocketalker (Williams Sound Co., Eden Prairie, Minn.) is a small, single-unit amplifier and microphone that fits in the pocket and assists hearing in noisy backgrounds. It amplifies the higher frequencies and picks up sound closer to its source, providing a better speech-to-background-noise ratio. As Figure 8-1 shows, the user places it in a breast pocket as close as orientation to person, place, and time into questions that also supply useful ocular information.

The first question or request of the patient could be, "Tell me your full name." Although this is actually a command, presenting it more as a question—raising the voice slightly on the last word—sounds better and is easier for the hearing impaired to hear. This answers the "orientation to person" question and serves to verify that the right patient data are destined for the right patient's chart. Mistaken patient identity is a potential problem in busy clinics and institutional settings.

If the patient is seriously cognitively impaired, he may be accompanied by a family member or significant other who preempts the patient with correct answers. As a practical matter, and as a matter of courtesy, never begin the interview by addressing that person instead of the patient. Rather, ask the patient, "Who is this with you today?" If the patient answers, you gain whatever information comes with the answer, and you avoid offending anyone. If, however, the other person provides an answer such as, "I'm his daughter and I'm here with him because he has Alzheimer's," the patient's cognitive status is quickly determined.

If serious cognitive impairment is not clearly established by the first question, continue with the following questions. Look directly at the patient and ask, "How long has it been since your last eye examination?" This calls for a calculation that represents a fairly high level of mental ability. Despite their ability, however, many patients will reply by naming a year or a month and year, which, if correct, indicate orientation to time. The immediate follow-up question of "Where was that [eye examination] done?" indicates orientation to place.

This brief line of questioning provides useful information on both cognitive status and ocular history. The next question to ask is, "Did the doctor say whether you have any eye disease?" Most older adults remember terms such as "cataract" or "glaucoma," and this question leads into the medical/ocular history phase of the interview.

## DEPRESSION

Another potential barrier to communication with older patients is depression. Depression can easily be mistaken for subcortical dementia or simply normal aging because all three have similar neurobehavioral manifestations.[3] Approximately 2% to 14% of community-dwelling older adults have depression.[2] Symptoms of depression include anxiousness, agitation, irritability, sadness, and loss of interest. When some of the problems common to older patients are considered, such as loss of a spouse or close friends, chronic pain and illness, decreased mobility, frustration with normal memory loss, and need to adapt to changing living circumstances, the difficulty in making distinctions between normal sadness and clinical depression can be perceived. In either case, some difficulty communicating with, and subjectively examining, some older adults will occur (Boxes 8-3 and 8-4).

Understanding the impact and the signs of both dementia and depression is the first step toward making the eye examination as effective and efficient as possible. Recommended examination techniques for working around these problems are essentially the same as for normal older adults. Ask brief, directed questions and offer clear, discrete choices.

---

**BOX 8-3**

### Symptoms of Depression in Older Adults

- Persistent, vague, or unexplained somatic complaints
- Memory complaints or problems
- Difficulty with concentration
- Confusion, delusions, or hallucinations
- Social withdrawal
- Loss of interest in normally pleasurable activities
- Persistent sadness, hopelessness
- Decreased appetite
- Sleep disturbances
- Irritability or demanding behavior
- Lack of attention to personal care

---

**BOX 8-4**

### Signs of Dementia

- Changes in memory, personality, and behavior
- Asking the same questions repeatedly
- Getting lost in familiar places
- Inability to follow directions
- Disorientation to time, people, and places
- Neglecting personal safety, hygiene, and nutrition

## COMPLEX MEDICAL/OCULAR HISTORY

Older patients have had many years to compile a lengthy medical/ocular history and often are willing to relate every detail that any clinician wants to hear. In some cases the information being offered is unrelated or too outdated to help determine the patient's current needs. For these reasons, using brief and structured interview questions is recommended so that judgment is required of the patient. The three medical/ocular history questions presented earlier are designed to do that specifically, and the next question does the same. Ask, "What bothers you most about your eyes [today]?" If the patient responds with multiple problems, ask, "Which one would you like to have me to start with?" Listen for all problems but try to narrow them down to one at a time.

Once the patient has focused on a single problem, ask, "When did that problem start?" Then ask, "Is it worse now than when it started?" If the patient says "yes," ask if it is worse now than it was half the reported time interval ago (e.g., 6 months ago for a problem that started 1 year ago). If the patient says "yes," ask, "Is it worse now than it was 1 month ago?" If "yes," ask, "… 1 week ago?" Finally, ask: "Is there anything that makes it better? …worse?" If clinician and patient are unable to narrow a chief complaint in this way, the subjective examination and resulting treatment will probably be equally unsuccessful.

## LIMITED MOBILITY/EXAMINATION ENVIRONMENT

Mobility of older patients can greatly influence the course of an eye examination, as can a limiting examination environment (e.g., nursing home). Patients may generally be classified as ambulatory, wheelchair, or bedridden. Most of these examination techniques can be useful for all three, although some described below as screening procedures may apply to patients restricted to wheelchairs, gurneys, or otherwise limiting environments.

### Ambulatory Patients

Most older patients are able to move about on their own, although some require a cane or walker. The fact that they move more slowly than younger adults, however, can influence the course of their eye examination. It may be impractical to move patients from pretest station to examination chair to waiting area (for pupil dilation) and back to the chair for examination completion, as is often done with more mobile, younger patients. For this reason, leaving the patient in the examination chair the entire time and starting pupil dilation as early as possible may be preferable. Whether pupil dilation adversely affects the subjective refraction of patients with absolute presbyopia is a debatable question, but no published data are available to provide the answer and many eye care providers have found it acceptable. Early pupil dilation is discussed later.

### Wheelchair Patients

Not all wheelchair patients are wheelchair bound. Many can transfer to the examination chair with minimal assistance. This can be facilitated by parking the wheelchair as close to a right angle as possible at the front of the examination chair. Once in position, lock the wheels and raise the footrests on both the wheelchair and the examination chair to provide a clear path for the patient.

If the patient cannot easily transfer to the examination chair, he or she can be examined while seated in the wheelchair. Specially designed examination chair glides or wheelchair-accessible stand-and-chair sets are available for such applications. If the examination chair cannot be moved back to allow wheelchair access to the stand-mounted phoropter and slit lamp, the examination can still be conducted with handheld instruments and trial frame. Techniques for this are described below.

### Bedridden Patients

Bedridden patients can be examined only with handheld instruments, and the following techniques described as screening procedures can be applied to bedside examination as needed (see Chapter 18 for a more complete discussion of the delivery of vision care in nontraditional settings).

## DIMINISHED QUALITY OF VISION

Diminished quality of vision can result from a variety of age-related conditions ranging from media opacity to reduced contrast sensitivity. Because these conditions are not resolved by optical correction, the eye examination process may be more difficult than usual. The following examination procedures are designed to help overcome these difficulties and make the examination both more effective and more efficient.

## EXAMINATION PROCEDURES

Patient flow is often less smooth and efficient with older patients. Therefore examination techniques that move instruments and test procedures to the patient instead of moving the patient to them are generally preferable. For the same reason initiating pupil dilation earlier in the examination sequence than is customary with younger patients is helpful. This discussion of examination procedures therefore begins with early pupil dilation and emphasizes procedures that can facilitate early pupil dilation. After those topics (beginning with confrontation fields) the emphasis shifts to examination techniques that simplify the patient's task and improve subjective reliability.

### Early Pupil Dilation

Early pupil dilation means instillation of mydriatic eye drops as early in the examination process as possible before subjective refraction. Safe, early pupil dilation calls for three preliminary steps: (1) assess entering visual acuity, (2) rule out preexisting angle closure, and (3) rule out pupil abnormality. The acuity screening method described later can be completed far more quickly than formal acuity measurement and can actually make its later measurement more efficient. Ruling out preexisting angle closure is more applicable and reliable than predicting its occurrence, as is generally attempted in a slit lamp examination. Assessing pupils is often more difficult in older patients because of small pupil size and minimal reactivity. The anterior segment screening method described later is useful for those circumstances in which a slit lamp examination is not possible.

### Visual Acuity Screening

The two objectives of this method of screening visual acuity are (1) to determine how well the patient is able to function visually in the average room environment, regardless of whether one or both eyes are used in producing that vision; and (2) to determine how well each eye functions on its own, as an indicator of possible ocular disease. Efficiently accomplishing these two objectives calls for a special adaptation of

the popular Rosenbaum visual acuity screener and a +2.50 DS, alternate occluding flipper, as further described below. Acuity screening thresholds are 20/50 and 20/25 at both distance and near. Distance acuity testing is actually performed at 10 feet instead of 20 for two reasons: (1) most rooms are less than 20 feet long and (2) communication with older patients is more effective at 10 feet than at 20 feet (Boxes 8-5 and 8-6).

As previously stated, the objective in this type of acuity screening is to estimate quickly the level of useful vision in each eye before instilling mydriatic eye drops. More precise measurement of acuity occurs during subjective refraction.

---

**BOX 8-5**

### Making the Visual Acuity Screener

1. Order a Rosenbaum Pocket Vision Screener and a +2.50 DS alternate occluding flipper (Fig. 8-2) from a preferred equipment supplier.
2. Spray paint a standard tongue depressor flat black.
3. Cut out the Rosenbaum 20/400 "7" and "4," leaving as much white margin around each as possible. This character size of 10.5 mm is equivalent to 20/50 at a 9.5-foot test distance.
4. Cut out the 20/200 "8" and "3," again leaving ample white margins. This character size of 5.25 mm is equivalent to 20/25 at a 9.5-foot test distance.
5. Cut out the 20/40 "4 2 8" and "3 6 5" number sets. This character size of 1.5 mm is equivalent to 20/50, or 1 M, at 16 inches. (Disregard the printed statement on the card about using a 14-inch test distance.)
6. Cut out the 20/20 "4 2 8" and "7 3 9" number sets. This character size of 0.75 mm is equivalent to 20/25, or 0.5 M, at 16 inches.
7. On one side of the tongue depressor, and at opposite ends, glue the larger number sets: the "7" and "4 2 8" and the "4" and "3 6 5" as shown in Figure 8-3. (Fingernail polish works well for this.)
8. On the other side of the tongue depressor, glue the smaller number sets as shown in Figure 8-3.

---

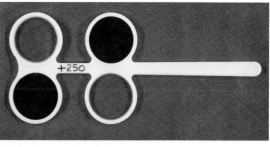

**Fig. 8-2** +2.50/occluder flipper bar for efficient monocular acuity screening at near.

**BOX 8-6**

## Using the Visual Acuity Screener

1. Start with the eyeglasses the patient is already wearing (Fig. 8-4). Do not ask the patient to look for or put on eyeglasses he or she might be carrying. This usually takes more time than it is worth.
   a. If the patient relies on eyeglasses for distance vision, he or she will most likely be wearing them.
   b. If the patient has eyeglasses and is not wearing them, they can be retrieved and neutralized later while waiting for the pupils to dilate.
2. Hold the acuity screener up approximately 10 feet from the patient, with the larger numbers facing the patient, and ask the patient to read the number at the top ("7" or "4").
   a. If the patient reads it, turn the side with the smaller numbers toward the patient and ask the patient to read the number at the top ("8" or "3").
      i. Record the acuity accordingly as either "OU 20/50" or "OU 20/25."
      ii. Technically, the acuity is "10/25" or "10/12.5," but recording its 20-foot equivalent simplifies data recording and later analysis.
   b. If the patient is unable to read the larger number at 10 feet, gradually move closer until the patient is able to and record it as "(test distance)/25 = 20/(25 × 20/test distance)." For example, if the large number had to be moved in to 5 feet for recognition, the acuity would be recorded as "OU 5/25 = 20/100." Again, recording the 20-foot equivalent simplifies more formal acuity measurement later.
3. Use the +2.50/occluder flipper to assess near acuity for each eye.
   a. If the patient is wearing bifocals, trifocals, or progressives, have the patient look only through the distance portion with the +2.50 flipper lens held in front. Regardless of the type of spectacle worn by the patient, save time by having the patient use only the area slightly above the vertical midpoint of the lens.
   b. If the patient is able to read the smaller number set with the right eye, record it as "OD 0.5 M." If the patient is unable to read the larger number set with the left eye, for example, record it as "OS worse than 1 M."

### Anterior Segment Screening

Screening the anterior segment involves using the binocular indirect ophthalmoscope and 20 D lens as an illuminated loupe (Fig. 8-5). This is accomplished by positioning both the condensing lens and examiner closer to the patient than the usual working distance for indirect ophthalmoscopy. The resulting magnification

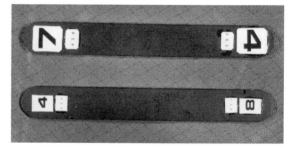

**Fig. 8-3** Visual acuity screener. 20/50 numbers are on one side and 20/25 on the other.

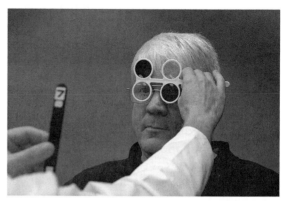

**Fig. 8-4** Use of the +2.50/occluder flipper over a patient's existing eyeglasses. Always direct the patient's gaze through upper half of the spectacle lens in case he or she is wearing multifocals.

of anterior structures is similar to that produced by the slit lamp at low power. The only thing not produced is a parallelepiped/optic section coming from a focused light source. This rules out the van Herrick angle assessment technique but still leaves the shadow test using a separate, handheld light source at the temporal canthus.

Predicting that an angle will close with pupil dilation is difficult at best, with or without a slit lamp. More important in anterior segment assessment is ruling out an already established, asymptomatic angle closure. Discovering a closed angle later in the examination raises the troubling question of whether the examiner closed the angle when he or she dilated the pupils. If the clinician can confidently say no signs of angle closure were present before dilation, the diagnosis and need for treatment will be clear. If, on the other hand, a closed angle is discovered before dilation, the diagnosis will

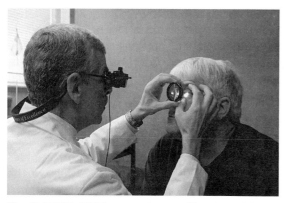

**Fig. 8-5** BIO-20D lens used as an illuminated loupe by shortening the distance between both the examiner and lens and the patient and lens.

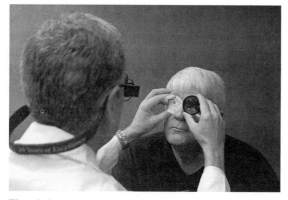

**Fig. 8-6** Swinging flashlight test with condensing lens positioned to observe the left pupil as the BIO-20D loupe light is swung from right eye to left eye.

not be acute-angle closure and the treatment may not have to be emergent. Signs of angle closure that can easily be seen with the BIO-20D loupe include venous congestion; steamy cornea; and fixed, distorted, mid-dilated pupil.

The next most important part of the anterior segment assessment is pupillary reactions, especially if reduced acuity of one eye is present, because this calls for a careful swinging flashlight test (Fig. 8-6). This, too, is easily done with the BIO-20D loupe by holding the lens in place before the suspect eye and swinging the BIO light from eye to eye. Then repeat, holding the lens before the opposite eye. The magnification produced by the condensing lens and the bright illumination provided by the light beam make even small pupil movements more visible.

## Slit Lamp Examination

If the examination environment permits more comprehensive assessment, a portable slit lamp is highly recommended. The focused slit beam enables better assessment of corneal integrity, anterior chamber features, and clarity of the media (e.g., cataracts). Current examples of readily available portable slit lamps include Zeiss HSO-10 (Carl Zeiss Meditec AG, Jena, Germany), Kowa SL-14/15 (Kowa Optimed, Inc., Torrance, Calif.), Clement Clarke 904 (Clement Clarke International, Harlow, England), Heine HSL 150 (Heine Optotechnik, Herrsching, Germany), and Scan-Optics SO-850 (Scan-Optics, Manchester, Conn.). The Zeiss, Kowa, and Clement Clarke instruments offer similar features, including rechargeable batteries for added portability; nevertheless, they will occupy considerable space in a trunk used to transport portable eye care instruments. The Heine and Scan-Optics instruments are smaller but offer fewer options for control of the slit beam.

## Tonometry

Tonometry before pupil dilation is highly recommended to avoid the problem of later discovering an elevated intraocular pressure with a normal-appearing anterior chamber. A portable tonometer is suitable for this, and an added benefit is that the use of an anesthetic at this point usually enhances the effect of mydriatic eye drops. Current examples of readily available portable or handheld tonometers include Perkins (Clement Clarke International Ltd, Harlow, United Kingdom), Kowa HA-2 (Kowa Optimal Inc., Torrance, Calif.), Tono-Pen (Reichert Ophthalmic Instruments, Depew, NY), Keeler Pulsair (Keeler, Windsor, England), Reichert PT100 (Reichert Ophthalmic Instruments, Depew, NY), and Schiotz (Sklar Instruments, West Chester, Pa.). Each has its unique advantages and disadvantages. The Perkins requires subdued room lighting and proximity, sometimes awkward, to the patient. The Pulsair and PT100 are electronic, noncontact instruments that are heavier and less portable than the others. The Schiotz is the least expensive and most portable but requires the patient to be reclined, is hard to sterilize, and measures by indentation rather than applanation. A clinical study comparing all but the

PT100 to standard slit lamp Goldmann tonometry showed acceptable reliability for all instruments.[21]

## Combining Mydriatic Eyedrops

Instilling eyedrops in an older adult's eyes can be a remarkably time-consuming process. The older adult has considerable difficulty in tilting the head back, and the cul-de-sac is usually able to hold only a small amount of instilled fluid. This means that using both tropicamide and phenylephrine hydrochloride (Neo-Synephrine) would normally call for at least two instillations per eye, requiring a longer than usual waiting time between instillations. This problem can be overcome by pre-mixing the tropicamide and phenylephrine hydrochloride in a single, appropriately marked bottle. This can be done by a compounding pharmacist. A less expensive option is to use the hydroxyamphetamine-tropicamide combination, Paremyd (*www.akorn.com*).

## After Mydriatic Instillation

Once the mydriatic eye drops have been instilled, attention can shift to completing the rest of the examination. At this point, the following test items have already been completed and may be recorded: (1) preliminary history (as with any patient, the history continues throughout the examination), (2) preliminary acuities, (3) external examination to include lids, lashes, conjunctiva, cornea, and anterior chamber, and (4) pupils. The examination can now proceed with visual field screening.

## Confrontation Fields

When field screening methods for the older adult are decided, the significant patient health risks and the potential yield from testing should be considered. Disorders that may manifest only as visual field defects and otherwise be hidden to physical examination are hemispheric cerebrovascular disease (stroke) and chiasmal disease (pituitary or compressive vascular disease). Stroke damage manifests as homonymous hemianopsia, which can reliably be detected with confrontation fields.[13] Chiasmal disease usually manifests as either bitemporal or junctional pattern field defects, both more apparent superiorly than inferiorly.[11,19]

Disorders that may not be easily detectable by physical examination (i.e., ophthalmoscopy) but may manifest as a confrontation field defect include chronic glaucoma, anterior ischemic optic neuropathy, and branch retinal artery occlusion. These disorders manifest as differential visual field sensitivity across the horizontal midline, either as an altitudinal hemianopsia or a wide nasal step defect.

Efficient screening for these types of visual field defects calls for a confrontation technique in which the examiner, not the patient, occludes the eye not being tested (Fig. 8-7). One of the examiner's hands provides the occlusion while the other provides the traditional finger counting stimulus. Time is saved by first testing the patient's right visual field of each eye (the right eye's temporal field followed by the left eye's nasal field) and then the left visual field of each eye (the left eye's temporal field followed by the right eye's nasal field). Save more time by first turning the patient's head toward the right before testing the right field, and then toward the left before testing the left field. This will keep the patient's nose from obstructing the inferior nasal field. When turning the patient's head, hold it gently with both hands until the patient properly resumes fixation on the examiner's nose. If an apparent depression is found in either eye's temporal field, check for differential sensitivity across the vertical midline. If an apparent depression is found in either eye's nasal field, check for differential sensitivity across the horizontal midline. Some patients have great difficulty understanding questions about differential sensitivity. Try asking the patient, "Is my hand *easier* to see here, or here?" (quickly moving the hand from one quadrant to the other). Then say, "Tell me *when* it becomes easier to see" (while moving the hand across the midline in question).

Confirming and classifying an apparent visual field depression can often be problematic. The examiner's hand may be less visible to the patient in one area because of poorer contrast against a nonuniform background. Moving the hand from one area to another and asking the patient to compare what was seen often raises the question of subjective reliability. These problems can be minimized by using a pair of 20/200 tumbling E's for simultaneous presentation (Fig. 8-8). The stark black-and-white contrast of the E is not affected by a nonuniform background behind the card, and having the

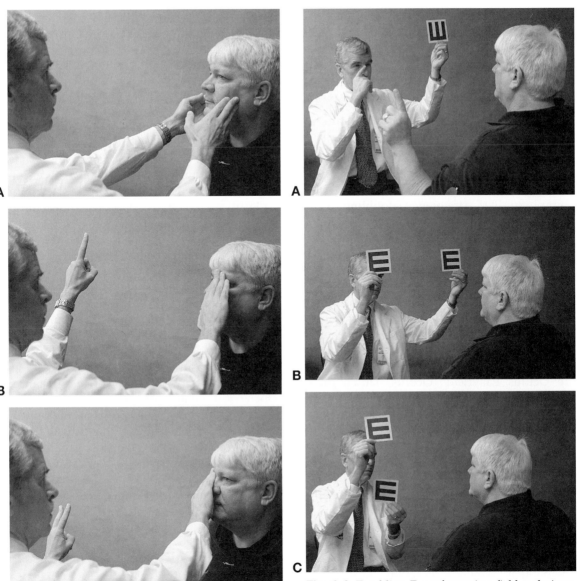

**Fig. 8-7** Finger count confrontation field technique. **A,** The patient's head is turned slightly to the right so his nose will not obstruct the right hemifield of the left eye. The right and left hemifields of both eyes are quickly screened with this technique. **B,** Testing of the right eye's superotemporal field. **C,** Testing of the left eye's inferonasal field. Turn the patient's head slightly to the left to screen each eye's left hemifield.

**Fig. 8-8** Tumbling E confrontation field technique. Subjective reliability is improved by having the patient indicate the direction of the letter's legs (**A**). Simultaneous presentation of two high-contrast targets provides more reliable comparisons across *vertical* (**B**) *and horizontal* (**C**) midlines.

patient state the direction of the E provides a better indication of subjective reliability. Each quadrant can be tested with a single E, and paired quadrants can be compared with simultaneous presentation of two Es. Change on crossing either a vertical or horizontal midline

is also easier for a patient to see when a large, tumbling E is used. The examiner will need both hands free so that if the patient is unable to occlude his or her own eye reliably, a tie-on eye patch can be applied.

Unfortunately, some patients cannot understand the simple instruction, "Look at my nose and tell me which way the E [off to the side] is pointing." If the patient erroneously but accurately looks *at* the E in each quadrant, his or her fields are probably full to confrontation. If the patient seems to ignore movement of the E in one quadrant but responds as soon as it is moved into another quadrant, the first quadrant is typically depressed.

### Specialized Field Screening Instrumentation

Visual field screening instruments may be useful in the examination of older patients if mobility and cognition are not a problem. One widely used field screening instrument, the Humphrey FDT (frequency doubling technology) (Carl Zeiss Meditec AG, Jena, Germany), is table mounted and must either be moved to the patient or the patient moved to it. The FDT perimeter is specifically designed to detect glaucomatous field defects and has been shown to miss neurological defects such as hemianopsia and quadranopsia.[8,20] Consequently, it may be a useful adjunct to confrontation field screening but should not be relied on to replace it.

A similarly portable visual field instrument, the Oculus Easyfield (Oculus, Dutenhofen, Germany), uses a more conventional, Goldmann III stimulus that should be more likely to detect neurological disorders than the FDT, but no reliability studies have been published to confirm this. Unlike the FDT, the Easyfield requires an auxiliary lens to neutralize refractive error, and the eyepiece design requires accurate and steady positioning of the patient—often a problem with older patients.

### Visual Acuity Measurement

The popular method of presenting a full acuity chart and asking, "What is the smallest line you can read?" does not work well with many older adults. Often, the older adult will simply start at the top and attempt to read every letter in turn, presumably expecting the examiner to decide which is the smallest line that can be read. The patient may in fact be seeing none of the letters clearly enough to say which can be correctly identified. To save time, isolate a vertical line of letters arrayed with the top letter being the size the patient was able to read in the preliminary acuity screening. Then isolate a horizontal line of letters of the size the patient was just able to read in the vertical array. Consider this the threshold line for refinement by subjective refraction.

Standard Snellen acuity charts have a few practical limitations that may influence examination of older patients. The progression of letter size is not uniform, and unequal numbers of letters are used on each line. Also, the recording system does not accurately account for a patient's ability to read most but not all of the letters on one line, some of the letters on the next line, and sometimes one or two letters on a third line. These factors combine to cause some inconsistency in measuring change in vision over time. The logMAR (log of the minimum angle of resolution) chart design helps minimize these errors by maintaining consistency in visual demands from one line to the next. Clinical considerations in adopting a logMAR chart system include the need to learn a new recording system and a slight increase in test time.[15] Regardless of which acuity system is preferred, an important feature for examination of older patients is the ease with which letters can be isolated.

Precise measurement of threshold acuity at near requires careful control of test distance, which is difficult with older patients. More important, however, than precisely measuring near acuity is determining the patient's preferred working distance. Let the patient hold the near point card and ask what working distance he or she prefers. Make note of the patient's preferred working distance so that, assuming no visual impairment, an add power corresponding to that distance can be later prescribed.

### Contrast Sensitivity

Standard visual acuity measurement can give a misleading impression of the older patient's visual status. The patient may be able to read 20/20 size letters in the clinic but still report worsening vision in everyday life. Much of this may be attributed to contrast sensitivity, which is known to decline with advancing age.[17,18] Contrast sensitivity can be measured in the clinic with specially designed charts such as the Vistech Vision Contrast Test System (Vistech Consultants, Dayton, Ohio), the Pelli-Robson test, or the Bailey-Lovie chart. Measuring low-contrast acuity in the clinic offers some reassurance to the patient that his or her visual symptoms are understood, and research suggests that impaired low-contrast acuity is predictive of impaired standard acuity in later years, but an optical prescription is still best determined by using standard, high-contrast acuity charts.[10] Most important, 20/20 visual acuity does not always mean "normal" vision for the older patient, and new eyeglasses that improve Snellen acuity may not improve the patient's overall quality of vision as hoped.

### Subjective Refraction

Emphasis on threshold acuity is important in subjective refraction of the older adult. Many older adults have difficulty saying whether progressive lens changes actually make vision progressively better, as occurs with standard refraction technique. A classic example of this is seen in refraction of the patient with a nuclear sclerosis cataract. The patient reports gradually worsening blur and with current spectacles sees 20/30. Subjectively the patient accepts incremental steps of −0.25 sphere totaling a diopter or more of additional minus over the habitual prescription, but he still sees only 20/30. Then when asked to compare the new refraction to his habitual prescription, he says it looks approximately the same. As Figure 8-9 shows, this method of subjective refraction accomplished little more than moving a succession of similar-appearing blur circles across the fovea. The effect on refraction is similar in other cases of blurred retinal imagery from age-related causes ranging from hazy media to macular degeneration. The way to overcome its adverse effect on subjective refraction is to make lens changes in steps consistent with the patient's threshold level of acuity.

For a younger adult starting with a threshold acuity of 20/30 because of myopia, a −0.25 D lens change would be expected to improve vision slightly and with another −0.25 D to

improve it a little more—the expected end point being 20/20 or better with no further improvement on further lens changes. For an older adult with a threshold acuity of 20/30 not due to refractive error, a progression of 0.25 D lens changes produces incremental changes in focus too small to appreciate in subjective refraction. For a threshold acuity of 20/30 (regardless of its cause), lens changes in 0.50 D steps are more likely to produce a useful subjective response. If the 20/30 acuity is caused by myopia, −0.50 DS will likely correct it to 20/20 and +0.50 DS will likely degrade it to approximately 20/50.[6,7] If the 20/30 acuity is caused by something other than refractive error, neither lens is likely to improve vision. Similarly, for a 20/50 threshold acuity, either +1.00 DS or −1.00 DS should quickly isolate refractive error from whatever else may be limiting vision.

This method of subjective refraction is similar to the Humphriss immediate contrast technique of presenting lens choices on opposite sides of the presumed refractive end point.[12] In this adaptation, the technique is referred to as "bracketing" instead of "immediate contrast" and the principle is applied to both cylinder power and axis as well as to sphere. If at least some of the subjective blur is attributable to refractive error, some subjective improvement should occur with either one or the other opposing lens options. Also, if one lens change produces a subjective improvement, its opposite should produce a subjective decline. This is a good way to verify subjective responses when patient misunderstanding, disinterest, or cognitive impairment may be present.

Integral to the Humphriss technique is the immediacy between opposing lens presentations. This is not possible with a phoropter

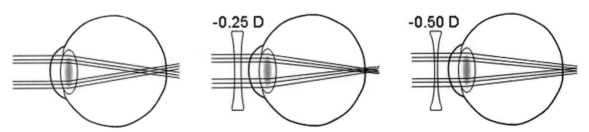

**Fig. 8-9** Effect of nuclear sclerosis cataract on subjective refraction. Small, incremental spectacle lens changes serve only to move similar-appearing blur circles across the fovea, making refractive end points hard to establish.

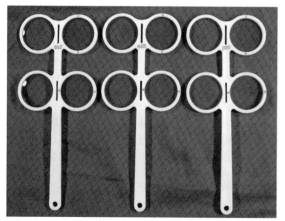

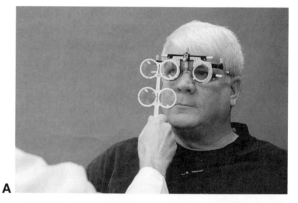

A

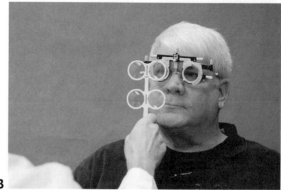

B

**Fig. 8-10** ±, Sphere/cylinder flippers used for bracketing refraction. Cylinders are mounted at right angles to one another. The 0.25 D flipper should be used for 20/20 to 20/25 threshold acuity, the 0.50 D for 20/30 to 20/40 threshold acuity, and 1.00 D for 20/50 or worse.

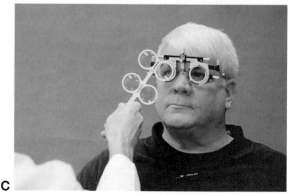

C

because of intervening lenses between the two intended choices. Three lenses are between the ±0.50 choices and seven lenses are between ±1.00. Just as with the well known Jcc test, the ± bracketing technique works best when the interval between presentations seems, to the patient, almost immediate. This requires the use of handheld lenses in front of either the phoropter or the trail frame. The ±0.50 Jcc and ±0.25, 0.50, and 1.00 sphere/cylinder lens flippers (Fig. 8-10) can easily be obtained from an ophthalmic equipment supplier.

Because the introduction of an additional test lens sometimes degrades vision from that produced by the base lens correction already in the phoropter or trial frame, giving the patient three choices is sometimes helpful ("Which is better, one, two, or three?"), with one of the choices being without the additional test lens device (Fig. 8-11).

The bracketing refraction method enables two useful verification steps: (1) if one test lens improves vision, its opposite should degrade it, and (2) if a given test lens choice leads to a change in the base lens, a new threshold acuity line should accompany that change. Isolating that new line then facilitates the next ± bracketing choice.

Cylinder power and axis are refined with the Jackson Cross Cylinder when flipper bar refrac-

**Fig. 8-11** Bracketing refraction method using ± lens flipper and trial frame. Flipper lens strength is chosen to correspond with the patient's threshold acuity. First check the sphere (**A**), then the cylinder in the four major meridians (**B** and **C**).

tion produces no further improvements in threshold acuity. With the Jackson Cross Cylinder, it may be necessary to select a new, slightly bigger threshold line and isolate the roundest letter on that line. The objective is to encourage a response of "better or worse" rather than an attempt to read all the letters. Some acuity charts, such as the Marco CP 670

(Marco, Jacksonville, Fla.), offer a pattern of round dots for this purpose.

Although the emphasis in this section is on reliability and efficiency in reaching a subjective refraction end point, a brief discussion on establishing a starting point is in order. The initial base lens selection can be derived from any, or a combination, of the following: current prescription, retinoscopy, or autorefraction. The current prescription is often the most reliable place to start, assuming the patient is not borrowing someone else's eyeglasses. Spectacles can easily be neutralized outside the normal office setting with a portable lensometer. Portable lensometers are lightweight, battery powered, and easily obtained through Internet sources, if not available from current ophthalmic suppliers (Fig. 8-12).

Retinoscopy is traditionally the preferred method for establishing a starting point for subjective refraction and is understandably more difficult with handheld lenses than with a phoropter. Several types of handheld retinoscopy lens bars are available for nonphoropter applications, but they have some important limitations. The larger ones consist of multiple pieces that must be individually manipulated. The smaller ones consist of fewer pieces, but the small lenses are hard to keep in proper alignment with the patient's pupil. Both large and small retinoscopy bars require mental transposition of an optical cross into a spherocylinder equivalent for the trial frame. For some this can be difficult if only done infrequently. If so, using the trial frame and individual lenses (first

sphere, then cylinder) directly from the trial case may be easier. When the retinoscopy end point is reached, remove the working lens power (1.50 D if using the standard 67-cm retinoscopy distance) from the base sphere and start the subjective refraction. If retinoscopy is made difficult by small pupils, media opacities, eye movements, and so forth, its accuracy will improve with pupil dilation.

Autorefraction is an increasingly popular method for establishing a starting point for subjective refraction. Although validation studies have shown autorefraction outcomes to be comparable to both retinoscopy and subjective refraction, for young adults no known comparisons have been made with older subjects.[1,14] Factors common in older patients that appear to diminish accuracy in autorefraction include small pupils, media opacities, and unsteady fixation. Reliance on autorefraction in such cases can be improved by immediately following the initial test with a retest. Paired readings that match are more likely to provide a reliable starting point for subjective refraction. Table-mounted autorefractors in an office setting with efficient wheelchair access and sufficient ancillary staffing can be useful in the examination of older patients. Portable autorefractors are also available for use in other settings where inherent limitations of the examination environment must be weighed against accuracy in refraction.

**Trial Frame Verification/Demonstration**

When the distance refraction is completed, the patient can best understand its effect by seeing it in a trial frame. The patient can easily compare it to his or her current eyeglasses and more easily understand cases in which a new prescription does not provide the level of vision expected. The patient can actually see firsthand when lens changes in either direction fail to improve vision. Unfortunately, such demonstrations are sometimes necessary when the patient presents with the expectation that a simple visit to the optometrist will result in restoration of good vision—as may have been the case for many years before.

With the distance correction in a trial frame, arriving at a suitable near point addition by using another set of specially designed lens flippers is a useful clinical method (Figs. 8-13 and 8-14).

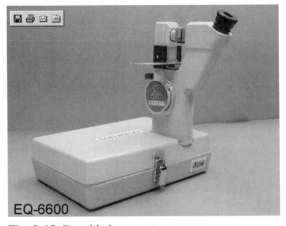

EQ-6600

**Fig. 8-12** Portable lensometer.

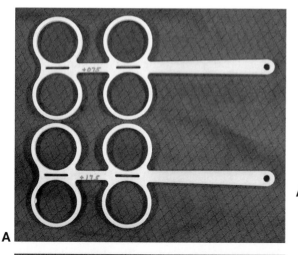

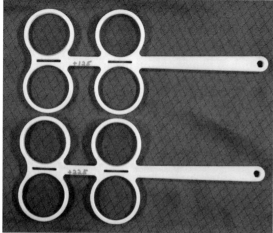

**Fig. 8-13** Bifocal add flippers for use with trial frame. **A** and **B,** Opposite sides with the label indicating the lens strength below. Higher adds, up to +3.50, can be obtained by overlapping the two flippers.

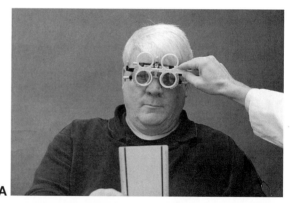

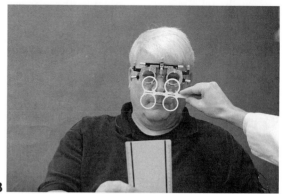

**Fig. 8-14** Bifocal add flippers used with trial frame to determine the best prescription for the patient's customary working distance (**A**). The flipper can also be used to show first-time bifocal wearers how to use them (**B**).

## Trial Frame Refraction

In some cases, trial frame is the only possible means of refraction; in others it may be preferable to phoropter refraction. Box 8-7 lists several reasons why it may be preferable. Box 8-8 lists several recommendations for making trial frame refraction more efficient.

If the patient's vision is impaired, requiring a higher add and closer working distance, some additional time will probably need to be set aside for patient education and possible low vision rehabilitation.

These examination techniques are designed to help the patient understand and make his or her own choices from the available treatment options. They can be used for patients of all ages but are particularly helpful for older patients with multiple age-related health problems.

## REFERENCES

1. Allen PM, Rodhakrishnan H, O'Leary DJ: Repeatability and validity of the PowerRefractor and the Nidek AR600-A in an adult population with healthy eyes, *Optom Vis Sci* 80:245-51, 2003.
2. Beekman AT, Copeland JR, Prince MJ: Review of community prevalence of depression in later life, *Br J Psychiatry* 174:307-11, 1999.
3. Blackmun S: Is it depression or is it dementia? *Psychiatric Times* 15:2, 1998.
4. Bristani M, Peterson B, Hanson L, et al: Screening for dementia in primary care: a summary of the evidence for the U.S. Preventive Services Task Force, *Ann Intern Med* 138:927-37, 2003.
5. Busse A, Bischkopf J, Riedel-Heller SG, et al: Mild cognitive impairment: prevalence and incidence according to different diagnostic criteria. Results of the Leipzig Longitudinal Study of the Aged (LEILA75+), *Br J Psychiatry* 182:449-54, 2003.
6. Crawford JS, Shagass C, Pashby TJ: Relationship between visual acuity and refractive error in myopia, *Am J Ophthalmol* 28:1220-5, 1945.
7. Eggers H: Estimation of uncorrected visual acuity in malingerers, *Arch Ophthalmol* 33:23-7, 1945.
8. Fong KC, Byles DB, Constable PH: Does frequency doubling technology perimetry reliably detect neurological visual field defects? *Eye* 17:330-3, 2003.
9. Grigsby J, Kaye K, Shetterly SM, et al: Prevalence of disorders of executive cognitive functioning among the elderly: findings from the San Luis Valley Health and Aging Study, *Neuroepidemiology* 21:213-20, 2002.
10. Haegerstrom-Portnoy G: Vision in elders—summary of findings of the SKI study, *Optom Vis Sci* 82:87-93, 2005.
11. Halle AA, Drewry RD, Robertson JT: Ocular manifestations of pituitary adenomas *South Med J* 76:732-5, 1983.
12. Humphriss D, Woodruff EW: Refraction by immediate contrast, *Br J Physiol Opt* 19:15-20, 1962.
13. Johnson LN, Baloh FG: The accuracy of confrontation visual field test in comparison with automated perimetry, *J Natl Med Assoc* 83:895-8, 1991.
14. Jorge J, Queiros A, Almeida J, ET AL: Retinoscopy/autorefraction, which is the best starting point for a noncycloplegic refraction, *Optom Vis Sci* 82:64-8, 2005.
15. Laidlaw DAH, Abbott A, Rosser DA: Development of a clinically feasible logMAR alternative to the Snellen chart: performance of the "compact reduced logMAR" visual acuity chart in amblyopic children, *Br J Ophthalmol* 87:1232-4, 2003.
16. Lichtenstein MJ: Hearing and visual impairment, *Clin Geriatr Med* 8:173-82, 1992.
17. Owsley C, Sekuler R, Siemsen D: Contrast sensitivity throughout adulthood, *Vision Res* 23:689-99, 1983.
18. Owsley C, Sloan ME: Contrast sensitivity, acuity, and perception of "real world" targets, *Br J Ophthalmol* 71:791-6, 1987.
19. Trobe JD, Tao AH, Schuster JJ: Perichiasmal tumors: diagnostic and prognostic features, *Neurosurgery* 15:391-9, 1984.
20. Wall M, Neahring RK, Woodward KR: Sensitivity and specificity of frequency doubling perimetry in neuro-ophthalmic disorders: a comparison with conventional automated perimetry, *Invest Ophthalmol Vis Sci* 43:1277-83, 2002.
21. Wingert TA, Bassi CJ, McAlister WH, et al: Clinical evaluation of five portable tonometers, *J Am Optom Assoc* 66:670-4, 1995.
22. Yesavage JA, O'Hara R, Kraemer H, et al: Modeling the prevalence and incidence of Alzheimer's disease and mild cognitive impairment, *J Psychiatr Res* 36:281-6, 2002.

# CHAPTER 9

# Auditory Impairment in the Older Adult

PAIGE BERRY, JOHN MASCIA, and BERNARD A. STEINMAN

Referring to the effects of combined vision and hearing loss, Helen Sloss Luey said, "Hearing loss interferes with understanding people's words, getting clues from tone of voice, and quick recognition of who is speaking. Vision loss makes it difficult to know who is present, who is talking, and what feelings might be attached to words."[17] On the basis of her extensive work with individuals with dual sensory loss, Luey coined the term "double trouble" to describe the impact that combined loss of vision and hearing may have on an individual's socialization, communication, and ability to live independently.

Among older adults, the risks associated with dual sensory loss are prominent concerns because of the increased likelihood of experiencing hearing and vision difficulties among this population. As individuals age, vision and hearing declines can stem from normal age-related changes and pathological conditions that attack the sensory organs. In addition, vision and hearing losses are often associated with other chronic health problems such as diabetes, hypertension, and cardiovascular conditions, which further increase the risks shared by older adults.

This chapter addresses the issues faced by older individuals who are hard of hearing or deafened in old age. Common causes and implications of hearing loss are discussed, as well as what can be done to ameliorate the negative impact of sensory loss on socialization, communication, and independent living among older people. By illuminating these issues for professionals and concerned others, this chapter may reduce the "double trouble" that those facing dual sensory impairment late in life may otherwise face.

## OVERVIEW OF PREVALENCE DATA

Reduction in sensory function increases sharply with age. Across an array of studies, age has been implicated as a major predictor of declines to both visual[12,24,26] and auditory[4,7,10] sensory function. As the large number of baby-boomers begins to reach age 55 years and older, and demographic trends shift toward a population that is older and living longer, the incidence of primary sensory impairment in the United States is projected to increase at an unprecedented rate. In congruence with this rising incidence of sensory impairment among the population in general will come an increased concern for the communication and socialization needs of those it affects, particularly the needs of older Americans who have begun to experience hearing and vision losses.

Prevalence estimates are not simple to make. Researchers who are concerned about the functional abilities of older people may rely on definitions that emphasize self-reports or proxy reports that state a person's ability to hear or see clearly.[15,20,25] Individuals are categorized into groups based on a subjective sense of their own aural or visual perception. This type of measure is useful for assessing issues related to communication and socialization because it reflects the individual's awareness and willingness to recognize and address the impairment. In contrast, researchers who are interested in acquiring an objective measure of sensory impairment often use clinical methods of assessment. Clinical tests for aural functioning are used to categorize individuals along a spectrum ranging from normal hearing through mild, moderate, severe, or profound hearing impairment.[8] Visual measures are used to distribute individuals along a spectrum of objectively defined degrees of impairment (e.g., low vision, legal blindness, totally blind). These types of measures are useful in conjunction with subjective measures because they allow the professional to assess the accuracy of the individual's self-awareness and report.

In general, prevalence figures do support the claim that sensory loss is disproportionately experienced by persons in the latter quarter of their lives. According to Raina,[23] among persons with disabilities older adults are more likely than younger adults to experience a sensory disability because they are at greater risk for the diseases that cause them (e.g., cataracts or macular degeneration). Furthermore, factors inherent in the aging process itself may foster the development of sensory disabilities in older people. For example, Raina cites decreased spectral and temporal resolution as a major age-related cause of hearing impairment. Similarly, natural, age-related changes in the malleability of the eye's lens increase the difficulty of focusing on objects. Whatever the causes, older persons experience the lion's share of the disabilities that affect their ability to function comfortably and normally in everyday settings.

Currently national census data estimate that nearly 8 million working and retirement-age Americans report difficulty or an inability to hear; more than 7.7 million are disabled because of their vision difficulties or the inability to see.[27] Of those with impaired hearing, more than half (4.3 million) are aged 65 years or older; older visually impaired persons make up 3.9 million of all reported cases. Lighthouse International[16] used data from the Longitudinal Study of Aging to arrive at prevalence figures for persons aged 70 years and older who have both impairments concurrently. Dual sensory impairment was found to affect one in five persons older than 70 years (21%) in the United States.

Taken together, these figures are astounding considering that just 12% of the population is aged 65 years or older.[1] Nevertheless, although these figures serve well to accentuate the extent to which age is related to the decline of sensory functions, they do not directly spell out the social and personal implications to which many older Americans choose, simply, to become accustomed. Fortunately, alternatives to living quietly with sensory impairments are available. Training in the use of techniques and technology can reduce the negative effects of hearing loss, which otherwise would have a profound and detrimental affect on the individual's ability to interact with the world. Family members and professionals who serve older individuals must be aware of the behavioral signs of hearing loss, what functional ramifications may occur because of sensory loss, what can be done to facilitate interactions with older impaired individuals, and where rehabilitation and independent living services can be obtained.

## HEARING LOSS AND THE OLDER ADULT

Hearing loss that occurs because of aging is called presbycusis. Current theories about why presbycusis occurs with such frequency are represented by both environmental and genetic points of view. Environmental theorists suggest that the auditory system simply breaks down over time due to wear and tear. As in any mechanical system, environmental factors and events such as exposure to loud noise, infections, toxins, and trauma over time begin to take their toll on the effectiveness of the auditory system to respond to the environment. Genetic theorists, on the other hand, believe that hearing loss from aging can be primarily attributed to hereditary processes. Gradual retrogressive changes in cell function, cell structure, and the number of total cells may occur because of natural genetic factors in each individual.[11]

Age-related physical changes in the auditory system may occur throughout the system.[13] In the outer ear, hearing loss may occur because of compounded earwax or growths within the ear canal that block incoming sound waves; the ear

**TABLE 9-1**

**Causes of Hearing Loss**

| Outer ear | Middle ear | Inner ear |
|---|---|---|
| Wax | Infection | Head trauma |
| Growths | Head trauma | Drugs (e.g., aspirin, furosemide) |
| Decreased elasticity | Growths on the ossicles | Heart disease |
| | Damage to the eardrum | Diabetes |
| | | High blood pressure |
| | | Noise trauma |
| | | Tumors |
| | | Kidney failure |
| | | Chemical toxins |

canal may also narrow because of the reduced elasticity of the skin (Table 9-1). Losses that begin in the middle ear can occur when age-related changes to the ossicles (small bones in the middle ear) reduce their ability to relay vibratory data to the inner ear or because of the reduced flexibility of the tympanic membrane, which communicates information, in the form of vibrations, from the outer ear.[11] Changes to the outer and middle ear are typically not serious and may frequently be ameliorated by using amplification devices. Although hearing aids are widely prescribed by audiologists for hearing losses associated with outer and middle ear problems, medical and surgical options are usually initially pursued.

Age-related changes to the structure of the inner ear are more serious. The atrophy of receptors on the basal end of the cochlea may make processing high-frequency sound waves difficult, especially among older men.[28] Language decrements may vary according to the specific area of damage within the cochlea. Because impairments in the inner ear involve a complex system of electrochemical conversion and transmission of sound waves to the brain, they are much more difficult to treat. In healthy systems, hair cells within the cochlea convert vibrations into signals that pass along the auditory nerve, through substructures of the brainstem and thalamus, before being processed by higher structures in the cortex. When any of these complex structures is absent or damaged, hearing loss may occur. Audiologists are particularly sensitive to these differences between individuals when prescribing hearing aids. Microscopic digital technology, embedded in modern hearing aids, allows the hearing specialist to adjust the device specifically for the individual. Analog hearing aids function primarily to amplify sounds; modern digital hearing aids can provide better sound quality, greater flexibility and, although imperfect, can improve performance in "noisy" listening environments.

## ANATOMY OF THE EAR: A PRIMER

Researchers and workers in the field of deafness and the hard of hearing typically discuss age-related losses in relation to their areas of origin. For example, conductive hearing loss occurs when barriers such as earwax or growths block the flow of sound waves in the outer or middle ear.[18] In general, these types of hearing losses are the least serious, and hearing aids can often be prescribed to increase amplification when conductive losses occur. Sensorineural hearing losses, caused by damaged cells in the cochlea and the auditory nerve, are more serious. Cell damage may occur from the aging process itself or from other factors, including genetic syndromes such as Usher's syndrome or Alström syndrome; diseases such as maternal rubella or mumps; tumors[6]; or by certain drugs such as aspirin, cisplatin, streptomycin, kanamycin, or tobramycin. Central hearing losses are caused by damage to areas in the brain where auditory stimuli are processed. A person may have "normal hearing" sensitivity but still be hearing impaired, nevertheless, because of central processing disorders.

Figure 9-1 shows the three sections of the ear: the outer and middle ear sections, which funnel and transmit vibratory sound waves to the inner ear, where they are changed into neural-electrical messages that are sent to the brain for processing.

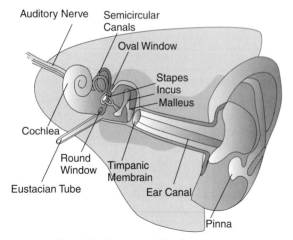

**Fig. 9-1** Diagram of the human ear.

## Outer Ear

The outer ear is composed of two parts: the pinna and the ear canal. The pinna is the fleshy part of the ear that makes up the lobe. Although unnecessary for hearing, the pinna serves an important function in gathering sound. As sound waves make their way through the environment, the pinna helps locate the source of a sound. The ear canal, which is divided into two sections, is less than an inch long. The first half of the canal is made of cartilage that is lined with wax (cerumen)-producing cells. The second half of the canal is carved out of bone and terminates at the tympanic membrane, or the eardrum, marking the beginning of the middle ear.

## Middle Ear

The middle ear is composed of the tympanic membrane, the ossicles, the outer membrane of the oval window, and the Eustachian tube. The eardrum is an elastic membrane that receives vibratory sound waves, like the head of a drum, from the outer ear. Sound vibrates the eardrum at varying frequencies, setting the three ossicles, individually called the malleus (hammer), the incus (anvil), and the stapes (stirrup), into motion. The ossicles transfer sound mechanically from the environment to the inner ear by vibrating against a membrane on the cochlea called the oval window. The middle ear is particularly prone to changes in pressure, to which the eardrum is highly sensitive.[21] The Eustachian tube keeps pressure stabilized by

functioning as a pressure-release valve to the middle ear.

## Inner Ear

The inner ear is made up mostly by a pea-sized, snail-shaped organ called the cochlea, which is encased in bone deep within the skull. For its small size, the complexity of the cochlea, and its importance for the transduction of vibratory sound waves into electrochemical messages that can be processed by the brain, is impressive. As the stapes from the middle ear moves against the outer membrane of the oval window, vibratory waves from the outer environment are transferred to fluid contained within the cochlea. The fluid shifts along the basilar membrane, activating the auditory nerve by causing chemical reactions to occur between hair cells on the basilar membrane and the auditory nerve fibers. Hair cells are arranged along the basilar membrane in order of the sound frequencies that they process.[22] If, for example, the cochlea were unrolled, hair cells nearest the base end of the cochlea would process high-pitched sounds, whereas cilia nearest the unfurled tip would process low-frequency sound waves.

Also encased in the inner ear are the semicircular canals—organs that are important to the vestibular system. Their purpose is to provide proprioceptive information about the individual's movement in space and changes in balance and posture. Thus systems within the inner ear contribute to orientation and motor coordination as well as hearing processes.[13]

## DEGREES OF HEARING LOSS

Along with classification by location or type, hearing loss may also be classified by degree. Degree of hearing loss is determined by tests that quantify the level of loudness (decibel) at which an individual begins to hear a specific pitch (frequency). The degree of hearing loss is usually classified by the thresholds recorded in the speech range (500 Hz to 4000 Hz). For instance, an individual may have a mild loss in the very low frequencies (250 Hz), a moderate loss in the speech range, and a severe loss in the high frequencies (8000 Hz). Table 9-2 shows range of loss (in decibels) at each classification and the effects of various degrees of hearing loss.

**TABLE 9-2**

### Degrees of Hearing Loss

| Level of Loss | Description | Effect | Hearing Aid Need |
|---|---|---|---|
| 25 to 40 dB | Mild | Difficulty understanding normal speech | In specific situations |
| 41 to 55 dB | Moderate | Difficulty understanding loud speech | Frequently |
| 56 to 80 dB | Severe | Can understand amplified speech only | In all communication |
| ≥81 dB | Profound | Difficulty understanding amplified speech | Possible supplemental speech reading, aural rehabilitation, or sign language |

**BOX 9-1**

### Behavioral Signs of Hearing Loss

- Changes in the volume of the television, or radio, especially an increase in volume and sitting closer than usual
- Leaning closer to the speaker during conversations or cupping the hand over the outer ear
- Difficulty understanding speech on the telephone
- Difficulty understanding conversations in noisy environments, such as a restaurant
- Inappropriate responses to questions or comments unrelated to the general discussion
- Repeated requests to speak louder
- Difficulty in the ability to hear high-pitched sounds such as door bells, a ringing telephone, or a smoke detector, or the inability to locate the source of a sound
- Decrease in sociability or friendliness
- Increase in time spent alone, (isolation and inactivity)
- Uncharacteristic outbursts due to frustration (person experiences more and more difficultly doing familiar tasks that have been taken for granted)
- Any dramatic change in behavior or subtle change in long-standing habits should be investigated.

## BEHAVIORAL SIGNS OF HEARING LOSS

Behavioral responses to a hearing loss are likely to vary between individuals; however, the behavioral changes in Box 9-1 may indicate that an older person is having difficulty hearing.

## FUNCTIONAL IMPLICATIONS OF A HEARING LOSS

Age-related changes to hearing are likely to be as heterogeneous or unique as the individuals who experience them. Hearing losses occur on a wide spectrum. The extent of these changes depends on factors such as heredity, illness,

accidents, and exposure to environmental noise. Because of damage to hair cells in the cochlea, older people may lose their ability to hear certain pitches. In most cases, high-pitched sounds are lost first. A common characteristic of age-related hearing loss is the inability to hear high-frequency sounds (particularly *th* and *f*), resulting in reduced speech discrimination or recognition.

Presbycusis may cause speech to sound distorted, particularly in noisy or acoustically poor environments. Indeed, the most difficult problem facing older adults with age-related hearing loss is their reduced ability to discriminate speech. Such difficulties understanding speech often lead to the common complaint, "I can hear you but I can't understand you."[19] Speech may not sound clear and may be difficult to understand. For example, similar sounding words may be confused, like "pat" and "bat" or "dinner" and "thinner." Speaking loudly or increasing the volume on a television may not help make speech easier to understand. In fact, increased volume may cause greater distortion to the sound.

Many older adults may also experience tinnitus concomitant with hearing loss. Tinnitus is characterized as a ringing, buzzing, swishing, or clicking sound even when no sound exists in the environment. Possible causes of tinnitus range widely in their severity and include damage to the inner ear, earwax, or high (or low) blood pressure. Tinnitus is difficult to treat and may be hard to diagnose, especially in individuals with developmental disabilities who may have difficulty verbally expressing themselves. Research regarding treatments that offer hope to patients who can be taught to better cope with tinnitus is ongoing.

## DUAL SENSORY LOSS AND INDEPENDENCE

The acquisition of both hearing and vision loss at any age does not preclude the ability to live independently or guarantee a reduced quality of life. It likely does mean, however, change and challenges for individuals who experience them. Loss of vision and hearing can tax an individual's ability to cope with day-to-day tasks that are normally taken for granted. Because of the varying nature of individuals, these imminent challenges will be met head on by some and with reluctance by others.[3]

Nevertheless, independence is closely tied to the individual's ability to make information-based choices. Without information to provide an understanding of alternatives, choices are limited and thus independence may be in jeopardy. When the two major avenues for acquiring information (i.e., vision and hearing) are drastically reduced, family members may view the resulting difficulty in communication as an inability to function predictably and rationally. Older people may become anxious about their family's beliefs that they have lost the ability to function independently and handle their own affairs. Other feedback and reactions may cause older adults to begin to doubt their own abilities and may elicit concern that certain responsibilities will be taken away from them.[9]

Confusion, inappropriate responses to questions, and apparent disorientation may all result from age-related hearing and vision losses. Because sensory declines often develop slowly, a problem may not be recognized until a great deal of hearing or vision is lost. The gradual development of sensory losses may contribute to the family's misunderstanding and result in inappropriate assumptions about the individual's behavioral changes. Sensitivity to behavioral change and patience to rule out sensory problems before assuming a "mental" problem will prevent needless loss of functioning and decreased quality of life.[2]

Family, friends, caregivers, service providers, and medical specialists must be careful not to take the right of choice from older adults with sensory decline. By encouraging participation in rehabilitation and independent living programs and fostering the use of adaptive techniques, aids, and devices, many older adults may be able to maintain full or partial independence. Although an age-related hearing loss cannot be slowed, maintaining good general health, avoiding external factors that will adversely affect hearing, and using hearing aids and assistive listening devices will aid in maintaining the remaining hearing for as long as possible.

Undoubtedly many sensory-impaired individuals could benefit from vision and hearing rehabilitation services that would enable them to maximize their potential and remain functionally independent and active members of their communities. The benefits of services to blind or visually impaired older adults that include instruction in orientation and mobility, activities of daily living, and preparation for reintegration into the workforce or the community have been shown by evaluations of current programs funded under Title VII, Chapter 2 of the Rehabilitation Act of 1973, as amended.[5] A listing of state vocational rehabilitation agencies serving older individuals who are blind or visually impaired can be found on the Website maintained by the Rehabilitation Research and Training Center on Blindness and Low Vision at Mississippi State University (*www.hknc.org/images/FieldServicesOlderBlindProgs.htm*). Although no equivalent federal program designed specifically for hearing-impaired older adults exists, general independent living programs offer training aimed at minimizing or eliminating the barriers that hearing impairments may foster.[28] Other services and information for older people with vision and hearing loss are available through the Older Adults Program at the Helen Keller National Center for Deaf-Blind Youths and Adults (*www.hknc.org*).

## ACCOMMODATING FOR COMBINED HEARING AND VISION LOSS

Clinicians who suspect that a patient has an undiagnosed hearing loss should recommend that the patient have his or her hearing tested by a certified audiologist. Once hearing and vision losses are identified, adaptations and accommodations can be made to make communication and visual tasks easier. A variety of devices and adaptive techniques are available. Included among these devices are hearing aids or assistive listening devices to help better discriminate sounds and speech; amplified door-bells; amplified voice and telephone ringers; vibro-tactile alerting devices for the door, telephone, smoke alarm, and other sound sources; and large print or Braille telecommunication devices. Magnifiers or other low vision devices are used to assist visually impaired individuals in reading print. Distance devices such as telescopes may be useful for viewing television, reading street signs, and spotting objects at greater distances. Tactile markers for appliances, clothing, and cooking utensils can ease the difficulty of household tasks. Environmental adaptations such as color contrast and lighting may improve safety conditions around the home.

## OPTIMIZING COMMUNICATIONS AND INDEPENDENCE THROUGH TECHNOLOGY

Assistive technology available for persons with vision and hearing loss generally fall into two categories. Low vision aids, including prescriptive magnification aids for both near and/or distant vision, may enhance visual functioning by enabling the individual to read mail, watch television or read captions on the television, identify objects, or perform other visual tasks. Recommendations for low vision aids are discussed in Chapters 14 and 15.

To enhance aural functioning, a person may benefit from hearing aids or assistive listening devices, including telephone amplification, personal communication devices, and room amplification systems with individual receivers. Technologically advanced hearing aids dispensed with the appropriate counseling can be effective tools for many people who have communication difficulties as result of hearing loss. Unfortunately, most hearing aids work well only in quiet environments, whereas most social situations involve background noise. Communication, even with a hearing aid, can be a frustrating experience. For instance, a hearing-impaired person dining at a restaurant may pick up unwanted noise and conversations from nearby tables because of the microphone in the hearing aid. Some of these problems can be reduced with more advanced hearing aid technology (i.e., directed microphone), but more so with the use of assisted listening devices (ALDs). An ALD can be used with or without hearing aids and functions by pro-

viding the individual with direct access to pickup from a microphone placed near the source of the desired sound. ALDs work in one-to-one conversations or in small or large groups. In the home ALDs can be directly connected to the television, radio, or a voice output of a computer. Audiologists can be helpful in determining which ALDs are appropriate for helping an individual function more efficiently in noisy environments.

Loss of central vision can make receptive communication difficult for deaf and hard of hearing individuals who rely on lip reading. Additional technology, such as the Communication Access Realtime Translation (CART) system and TypeWell Educational Transcription System (CodeWell LLC, Arlington, Mass.), can provide a computerized real-time, large-print display of speech communication. For the deaf individual who uses manual communication or American Sign Language, an interpreter who is skilled in tactile sign language may be needed to enhance communications. The deaf individual with restricted visual fields, or tunnel vision, may need the interpreter to sign in a small space or to sit at a distance for signs to be perceived. At social gatherings or during personal tasks, a support service provider can work one on one with the impaired person to make sure that he or she is able to communicate effectively, travel safely, and be aware of environmental concerns.

## INTERACTING WITH AN INDIVIDUAL WITH HEARING LOSS

Socialization of older sensory-impaired adults can be maximized by creating the best possible environment and by adjusting communication style to fit the needs of the individual. Communication can also be enhanced by considering the dynamic cognitive status of the older adult.[14] For example, optimized communication will occur when the individual is most alert and by keeping meetings brief when attention is low. Other tips for communicating effectively with dual sensory-impaired older adults are provided in Box 9-2.

Given the growing demographic of older individuals, issues related to the visual and auditory functioning of this group will soon be at center stage, if they are not already. Gerontologists, advocates, and other professionals who work with aged individuals need

**BOX 9-2**

## Tips for Effective Communication

- Before speaking, get the listener's attention.
- Introduce yourself. Not everyone recognizes voices.
- Pick a well-lit, quiet place to communicate. Avoid noisy areas.
- When in doubt, ask the person what to do to improve communication.
- Use facial expressions.
- Face the patient with no obstructions.
- Speak more slowly and with a lower pitched voice.
- *Do not* shout. Shouting can distort the voice and facial expressions.
- Remove objects from the mouth.
- Speak clearly and at a moderate rate of speed. Take slightly longer pauses between phrases and sentences.
- Rephrase if the message is misunderstood.
- Reconfirm important points.
- Stay in the same room with the listener.
- Be patient and positive. Allow the person to do tasks at his or her own pace.

to face issues related to communication, functional capacity, and rehabilitative options as these issues relate to sensory-impaired older adults. Given their wide prevalence among this age group, sensory impairments will one day affect the lives of most people, either directly or in the role of caregiver for someone who is experiencing a sensory loss. Sensory impairment and its ramifications must be understood by professionals who have the ability to affect the quality of life and well-being of older individuals with whom they work. With appropriate knowledge about issues related to sensory impairments, clinicians help ensure that older adults do not find themselves in the state of "double trouble."

## REFERENCES

1. Administration on Aging: *A profile of older Americans,* accessed July 29, 2002, from http://www.aoa.gov/prof/statistics/profile/2002/profiles2002asp.
2. Bagley M: *Vision and hearing losses among older adults: strategies and resources,* Sands Point, NY, 1989, Helen Keller National Center.
3. Bagley M: *Helen Keller National Center Confident Living Program Manual,* Sands Point, NY, 1994, Helen Keller National Center.
4. Blanchfield BB, Feldman JJ, Dunbar JL, et al: The severely to profoundly hearing impaired population in the United States: prevalence estimates and demographics, *J Am Acad Audiol* 12:183-9, 2001.
5. Cavenaugh BS, Steinman B, Butler S: *LIFE: living independence for elders, state of Arkansas title VII, chapter 2 evaluation report 2001,* Starkville, MS, 2002, Mississippi State University.
6. Everson JM: *Supporting youths with deaf-blindness in their communities: a guide for service providers, families and friends,* Baltimore, 1995, Paul H. Brooks.
7. Gates GA, Cooper JC, Kannel WB, et al: Hearing in the elderly: the Framingham cohort, 1983-1985, *Ear Hearing* 11:247-56, 1990.
8. Heller KW: Etiologies and characteristics of deaf-blindness. In *Teaching research assistance to children experiencing sensory impairments,* Monmouth, OR, 1994, Western Oregon State College.
9. Hull R: Hearing evaluation of the elderly. In Katz J, editor: *Handbook of clinical audiology,* ed 2, Baltimore, 1978, Williams & Williams.
10. Ives DG, Gonino P, Traven ND, et al: Characteristics and comorbidities of rural older adults with hearing impairments, *J Am Geriatr Soc* 43:803-6, 1995.
11. Jerger S, Jerger J: *Auditory disorders: a manual for clinical evaluation,* Boston, 1988, Little, Brown.
12. Kahn HA, Leibowitz HM, Gangley JP, et al: The Framingham eye study: outline and major prevalence findings, *Am J Epidemiol* 106:17-32, 1977.
13. Katz J: *Handbook of clinical audiology,* ed 3, Baltimore, 1985, Williams and Wilkins.
14. LeJeune BJ, Steinman B, Mascia J: Enhancing socialization of older people experiencing loss of both vision and hearing, *Generations* 27:95-7, 2003.
15. Lighthouse International: *Prevalence of vision impairment,* accessed March 10, 2006, from http://www.visonconnection.org/content/research/epidemiologyandstatistics/default.htm.
16. Lighthouse International: *Dual sensory impairment among the elderly,* accessed November 18, 2003, from http://www.visionconnection.org/content/forprofessionals/patientmanagement/dualsensoryloss/default.htm.
17. Luey HS: Understanding age-related hearing loss among older adults. In Watson D, Boone S, Bagley M, editors: *The challenge to independence: vision and hearing loss among older adults,* Little Rock, AR, 1994, University of Arkansas.
18. Martin FN: *Introduction to audiology,* ed 4, Englewood Cliffs, CA, 1991, Prentice Hall.
19. Mascia J: Understanding age-related hearing loss among older adults. In Watson D, Boone S, Bagley M, editors: *The challenge to independence:*

*vision and hearing loss among older adults,* Little Rock, AR, 1994, University of Arkansas.

20. Mor V, Wilcox V, Rakowski W, et al: Functional transitions among the elderly: patterns, predictors, and related hospital use, *Am J Public Health* 84:1274-80, 1994.

21. Northern JL: *Hearing disorders,* ed 2, Boston, 1984, Little, Brown.

22. Northern JL, Downs MP: *Hearing in children,* ed 4, Baltimore, 1991, Williams and Wilkins.

23. Raina P: Prevalence, risk factors and self-reported medical causes of seeing and hearing related disabilities among older adults, *Can J Aging* 19:260-78, 2000.

24. Rudberg MA, Furner SE, Dunn JE, et al: The relationship of visual and hearing impairments to disability: an analysis using the longitudinal study of aging, *J Gerontol* 48:M261-5, 1993.

25. Slawinski EB, Hartel DM, Kline DW: Self-reported hearing problems in daily life throughout adulthood, *Psych Aging* 8:552-61, 1993.

26. Tielsch JM, Sommer A, Witt K, et al: Blindness and visual impairment in an American urban population, *Arch Ophthalmol* 108:286-9, 1990.

27. U.S. Census Bureau: *Americans with disabilities: current population reports,* accessed November 11, 2003, from http://www.census.gov/hhes/www/disability/disability.html.

28. Weinstein BE: A primer on hearing loss in the elderly, *Generations* 27:15-9, 2003.

# CHAPTER 10

# Pharmacological Aspects of Aging

**SIRET D. JAANUS**

Patients aged 65 years and older are estimated to represent approximately 13% of the population and take approximately 30% of all prescription medications in the United States.[1] Approximately 60% of older adults take at least one prescription drug a day, but most take an average of three to five medications.[2,12] Older adults are prescribed more medications than other age groups, are the major consumers of nonprescription (over-the-counter, or OTC) drugs, and many (approximately 40%) also use some form of dietary supplement.[11]

Numerous factors influence the efficacy and safety of drug therapy in older adults, including the physiological effects of aging and pathological conditions. Multiple illnesses can result in visits to several health care professionals.[15] Noncompliance with prescribed drug therapy in older patients has been estimated to range from 21% to 55%.[9] Multiple medication use, complicated dosage regimens, improper adjustment of dosages, and increased sensitivity to drugs leading to adverse reactions are among the reasons for noncompliance.[5,14]

Adverse drug events are a common cause of iatrogenic illness in older adults. One study revealed that adverse effects are the cause of hospitalization in 25% of patients aged 80 years and older.[15] Among the drug classes most frequently implicated are the nonsteroidal antiinflammatories (NSAIDs) and cardiovascular and psychotropic agents (Table 10-1).

Prevention of drug reactions requires understanding of both the physiological changes that take place in the aging patient and the pharmacological characteristics and disposition of drugs that tend to cause reactions (Table 10-2). An awareness of pharmacological principles as they related to geriatric drug effects is important to the vision care provider to help prevent and minimize age-related adverse drug effects.

## PHARMACOKINETIC AND PHARMACODYNAMIC FACTORS

### Absorption

Clinical studies generally have failed to demonstrate significant age-related effects on drug absorption from the gastrointestinal tract (see Table 10-2). Gastric acid secretion may decrease by as much as 40% in older adults, and gastric pH is elevated. However, the onset of action of certain drugs may be slowed. The lack of effect of age on drug absorption may be related to the fact that most drug absorption is passive and dependent on drug concentration gradients. However, studies do suggest that agents absorbed by active transport mechanisms, such as calcium, organic iron, and certain vitamins, are absorbed to a lesser extent in older adults.[20] Disease conditions, the presence or absence of food in the stomach, and concurrent use of drugs are more likely important factors in drug absorption than is age.[32]

**TABLE 10-1**

## Most Frequently Prescribed Medications for Older Adults

| Drug | Indication | Adverse Effects | Key Drug Interactions |
|---|---|---|---|
| **Diuretics** | | | |
| Furosemide<br>Hydrochlorothiazide<br>Triamterene | Hypertension, edema in<br>CHF, hepatic and renal<br>disease, diuresis | Dry mouth<br>Increased thirst<br>Metabolic disturbances<br>(hypokalemia, hyponatremia,<br>hypomagnesemia), orthostatic<br>hypotension, nausea,<br>dizziness, photosensitivity,<br>hyperglycemia, dehydration<br>Confusion, nervousness,<br>numbness in hands and<br>feet (triamterene) | Corticosteroids: ↑<br>electrolyte imbalance<br>NSAIDs: ↓ antihypertensive<br>effect |
| **ACE Inhibitors** | | | |
| Enalapril, lisinopril | Hypertension, CHF,<br>diabetic nephropathy,<br>idiopathic edema | Orthostatic hypotension, fatigue,<br>dizziness, headache, insomnia,<br>dry hacking cough, skin rashes<br>Neutropenia, agranulocytosis<br>Taste changes, oral ulceration,<br>dry mouth, angioedema | Alcohol, phenothiazines: ↑<br>hypotensive effect<br>NSAIDS: ↓ hypotensive<br>effect<br>Antacids: ↓ ACE absorption<br>Digoxin: ↑ serum digoxin<br>levels<br>Tetracycline: ↓ tetracycline<br>absorption |
| **Calcium Channel Blockers** | | | |
| Nifedipine | Vasospastic, chronic<br>stable angina;<br>hypertension;<br>hypertrophic<br>cardiomyopathy | Dysrhythmia, edema, CHF,<br>nausea, polyuria, giddiness,<br>headache, fatigue, drowsiness,<br>slurred speech, constipation,<br>gastroesophageal reflux, flushing | May ↑ phenytoin and<br>digoxin serum<br>concentrations<br>Cimetidine: may ↑<br>nifedipine (serum) |
| **Antianginals** | | | |
| Nitroglycerin | Acute/chronic stable<br>angina pectoris,<br>CHF, prophylaxis of<br>angina pain | Orthostatic hypotension,<br>bradycardia, headache, flushing,<br>dizziness, nausea, vomiting,<br>restlessness, tachycardia | Benzodiazepines,<br>phenothiazines, calcium<br>channel blockers: ↑<br>hypotensive effect |
| **Beta-blockers** | | | |
| Propranolol,<br>metoprolol | Hypertension, chronic<br>stable angina,<br>dysrhythmias, migraines | Orthostatic hypotension,<br>bradycardia, bronchospasm,<br>depression, fatigue, lethargy,<br>dizziness, nausea, dry mouth | Sympathomimetics:<br>hypertension,<br>bradycardia |
| **Cardiac Glycosides** | | | |
| Digoxin | CHF, atrial dysrhythmias,<br>atrial fibrillation | Headache, confusion,<br>disorientation, fatigue,<br>depression, nausea, anorexia,<br>blurred vision, muscular<br>weakness, dry mouth | Antacids: ↓ digoxin<br>absorption<br>Erythromycin: ↑ digoxin<br>levels |
| **Anticoagulants** | | | |
| Warfarin | Peripheral thrombus,<br>pulmonary embolism,<br>myocardial infarction,<br>dysrhythmia, CHF,<br>thromboembolitic<br>disorders, atrial<br>fibrillation with embolism | Rash, fever, anorexia, hematuria,<br>hemorrhage, gingival bleeding | NSAIDs, cimetidine,<br>ketoconazole,<br>corticosteroids,<br>erythromycin: ↑ effects<br>of warfarin |

**TABLE 10-1—cont'd**

## Most Frequently Prescribed Medications for Older Adults

| Drug | Indication | Adverse Effects | Key Drug Interactions |
|------|-----------|-----------------|----------------------|
| Dipyridamole | Prevention of transient ischemic attacks, inhibition of platelet aggregation to prevent myocardial reinfarction, long-term management of angina | Hypotension, headache, dizziness, weakness, syncope, rash, gingival bleeding | Aspirin and other NSAIDs: increased anticoagulant effect |
| **NSAIDs**<br>Ibuprofen | Inflammatory diseases and rheumatoid disorders, mild to moderate pain, fever, gout, osteoarthritis | Fluid retention, arrhythmias, drowsiness, vertigo, dizziness, fatigue, hyperglycemia, hypoglycemia, dyspepsia, heartburn, constipation, tinnitus | Probenecid: ↑ NSAIDs (serum)<br>Digoxin, methotrexate, lithium: may ↑ (serum) |
| **Gastrointestinals**<br>$H_2$-blockers:<br>Ranitidine, cimetidine | Duodenal ulcers, gastroesophageal reflux, hypersecretion | Bradycardia or tachycardia, edema, headache, dizziness, agitation, confusion, anxiety, depression, insomnia, diarrhea | ↓ Absorption of ketoconazole and diazepam<br>May ↑ warfarin clearance, ↑ anticoagulant effect<br>Antacids: ↓ absorption<br>Aspirin, NSAIDs: gastrointestinal ulceration, bleeding<br>May ↑ blood levels of benzodiazepines, alcohol, lidocaine |
| **CNS agents**<br>Antianxiety agents<br>Diazepam | Anxiety, skeletal muscle spasm, adjunct in seizure disorders (long-acting)<br>Anxiety, panic disorders, anxiety with depression | Dizziness, drowsiness, Hypotension, blurred vision, dry mouth, ulcerations | All CNS depressants, alcohol: ↑ effects of diazepam |
| Alprazolam | Anxiety, panic disorders, anxiety with depression | Dizziness, drowsiness, hypotension, blurred vision, dry mouth | Alcohol, CNS depressants: ↑ CNS depression<br>Erythromycin: ↑ CNS effects |
| *Sedative/Hypnotics*<br>Triazolam | Insomnia | Headache, lethargy, drowsiness, daytime sedation, dry mouth | Erythromycin: ↑ CNS effects<br>Alcohol, CNS depressants, opioid, analgesics or anesthetics: ↑ sedation<br>Avoid use with ketoconazole |
| *Antidepressants*<br>Fluoxetine | Major depression | Headache, nervousness, insomnia, fatigue, sedation, poor concentration, agitation, anorexia, nasal congestion, hot flashes, palpitations, dry mouth | Alcohol, all CNS depressants: ↑ CNS depression<br>Highly protein bound drugs (e.g., aspirin): ↑ side effects, ↑ half-life of diazepam |
| Sertraline | Major depression, antiobsessional effects | Insomnia, headache, dizziness, nausea, dyspepsia, dry mouth | |

*Continued*

**TABLE 10-1—cont'd**

## Most Frequently Prescribed Medications for Older Adults

| Drug | Indication | Adverse Effects | Key Drug Interactions |
|------|-----------|-----------------|----------------------|
| **Endocrine Agents** | | | |
| Glyburide | Stable adult-onset diabetes mellitus | Hypoglycemia, headache, weakness, anxiety, confusion, drowsiness, nervousness, leukopenia/ thrombocytopenia | NSAIDs, salicylates, ketoconazole: ↑ hypoglycemic effects<br>Corticosteroids and thiazides: ↓ action of glyburide |
| Estrogen, conjugated | Estrogen replacement | Hypotension, dizziness, migraine, depression, nausea, rash, folic acid deficiency | Oral anticoagulants: ↓ effect<br>Glipizide: glucose tolerance changes<br>Vitamin C may ↑ effects (serum) of estrogen<br>Increases action of corticosteroids |

*CHF,* Congestive heart failure; *ACE,* angiotensin converting enzyme; *CNS,* central nervous system; ↑ = increase; ↓ = decrease
Adapted from Diamond JP: Systemic adverse effects of topical ophthalmic agents, *Drugs Aging* 11:352-60, 1997.

**TABLE 10-2**

## Physiological Factors and Pathological Conditions Affecting Drug Action in Older Adults

| Physiological Change | Possible Influence on Drug Effect |
|----------------------|-----------------------------------|
| **Absorption** | |
| Increased gastric pH | Increased absorption of drugs inactivated by stomach acid |
| Reduced GI blood flow | Minor effect |
| Reduced absorptive surface | Minor effect |
| Reduced GI motility | Minor effect |
| **Distribution** | |
| Decreased cardiac output | Impaired delivery of drugs to organs of elimination |
| Decreased total body water | Increased concentration and effect of drugs distributed in body water |
| Reduced lean body mass | Increased concentration and effect of drugs distributed in lean body mass |
| Reduced serum albumin | Increased effect of, and interaction between, drugs extensively bound to albumin |
| Increase alpha-1 acid glycoprotein | Minor effect |
| Increased body fat | Increased sequestration of lipophilic drugs in fat |
| **Metabolism** | |
| Reduced mass and enzyme activity | Decrease phase 1 metabolism of some drugs |
| Reduced hepatic blood flow | Decreased metabolism of drugs normally rapidly cleared by the liver |
| **Excretion** | |
| Reduced renal blood flow | Decreased renal elimination of water-soluble drugs and metabolites |
| Reduced glomerular filtration rate | Decreased renal excretion of water-soluble drugs and metabolites |
| Reduced tubular secretion | Decreased renal elimination of drugs and metabolites actively secreted into urine |

*GI,* Gastrointestinal.
Adapted from Heft MW, Mariotti AJ: Geriatric pharmacology, *Dent Clin N Am* 46:869-85, 2002.

## Distribution

After absorption, the distribution of drugs in the body depends on body composition, plasma protein binding, and blood flow to the organs.[14] Body weight generally decreases and body composition, particularly adipose and muscle tissue mass, changes with age (see Table 10-2). The percent of body weight contributed by fat increases from 18% to 36% in men and 33% to 45% in women. Lead body mass decreases by 20%. Total body water also decreases with age between the ages of 30 and 80 years by 10% to 15%. These factors can alter the volume of drug distribution in older adults. Fat-soluble drugs, such as the barbiturates (e.g., phenobarbital), benzodiazepines (e.g., diazepam), and anesthetics, may be stored in fatty tissue to a greater extent in older adults, who may exhibit undesirable effects at the usually prescribed dosages because of longer half-lives of drug elimination. Because water-soluble drugs are primarily distributed in lean body tissue, the volume of drug distribution of hydrophilic drugs such as ethanol, digoxin, and cimetidine is smaller, but initial plasma concentrations can be high, leading to unexpected adverse effects.[20,22]

## Protein Binding

Effects of certain drugs on target organs may be altered if changes occur in protein binding (see Table 10-2). After drug administration, a certain percentage is bound to serum proteins, primarily albumin. The bound drug is in equilibrium with the unbound drug. Only the free drug is pharmacologically active. While bound, drug molecules cannot cross the blood-brain barrier, and metabolism and elimination of the drug cannot take place at the usual rates. Because of decreased hepatic production, serum plasma proteins, including albumin, have shown a decrease of up to 25% in older adults. Reduced protein binding of drugs can lead to a more intense clinical effect and greater risk of adverse effects, as is the case with the highly protein-bound anticoagulant drug warfarin and the anticonvulsant phenytoin. Conversely, in the presence of inflammation, an acute phase reactant alpha-1 glycoprotein maybe released that can increase the protein binding of certain drugs.[14]

Although the exact relation between the free drug level and the clinical effect of most drugs is not well established, the data do imply that alteration in drug dosage or measurement of plasma free drug concentration during long-term drug therapy may be beneficial in older patients.[8,20]

## Metabolism

The liver is the major site for biotransformation of drugs. The metabolism of drugs by the liver depends on the activity of microsomal enzyme mixed-function oxidase system, which includes cytochrome P-459 (phase I) and conjugation of drug molecules with glucuronide or other moiety (phase II) and also on the hepatic blood flow. Hepatic blood flow has been estimated to decrease by 40% from age 25 to 65 years. In the case of drugs with rapid rates of metabolism, the rate-limiting step appears to be blood flow, and certain drugs with high hepatic extraction ratios show decreased clearance in older adults. In the case of drugs metabolized by the hepatic enzyme systems, several enzymatic reactions of the cytochrome P-450 system are slowed significantly with age (see Table 10-2). Biological variations among subjects as well as other factors such as smoking, for example, may also be factors in drug metabolism.[8,14,20,22]

## Drug Elimination

The kidneys eliminate drugs from the body in the polar, water-soluble form. Age-related changes in renal function include decreases in renal blood flow and glomerular filtration rate (see Table 10-2). The rate of clearance of creatinine is an indication of the rate of renal drug elimination. Although individual variations exist, creatinine clearance can decrease by approximately 35% between the ages of 20 and 90 years in patients without evidence of renal disease.[8] Plasma levels of drugs with predominant renal elimination should be monitored, particularly with long-term therapy in older adults. Such drugs include digoxin, chlorpropamide, cimetidine, and lithium.[31] For establishing dosage schedules, pharmacokinetic principles, particularly renal and hepatic factors, should be combined with clinical response of the patient to the established drug regimens, particularly for those agents in which age-related changes in their clinical actions have been observed.[19] Box 10-1 lists some drugs that have been associated with age-related changes in pharmacokinetic parameters.

### Environmental Factors

Dietary intake can be an important factor in drug metabolism. Protein and certain micronutritional deficiencies, such as lack of vitamin C, can impair the metabolism of drugs. Cigarette smoking induces hepatic microsomal enzyme activity but the effect on drug metabolism is variable.[18]

### Drug-Receptor Interactions

The mechanisms involved in age-related changes in drug responses are not well understood. In addition to altered pharmacokinetics, changes in receptor density or affinity and altered biochemical responses have been suggested. The effect of drugs on target sites has been studied less extensively than the pharmacokinetic parameters. Both heightened and reduced drug effects, which have not been related to altered pharmacokinetic variables, have been suggested to be caused by changes in tissue sensitivity, altered homeostasis, or complications associated with chronic disease states in older adults, such as altered vascular tone.[14] Enhanced clinical responses at drug levels below the therapeutic range have been observed with analgesics, psychoactive agents, and anticoagulants. In contrast, beta-adrenergic blocking agents and the calcium channel blockers show decreased receptor sensitivities.[31] Some guidelines for drug use are presented in Box 10-2.

## SPECIFIC DRUG GROUPS AND AGE-RELATED RISKS

A number of drugs are more frequently used in the geriatric population (see Table 10-1). To prevent adverse reactions associated with polypharmacy or improper use of medications, patient education, close monitoring of drug use, and dosage reduction when necessary are part of the guidelines for safe and effective drug utilization in older adults (see Box 10-2).[21,32]

### Cardiovascular Drugs

Cardiovascular disease accounts for the majority of hospital admissions in older adults, and hypertension, especially systolic pressure, increases after age 50 years.

#### Diuretics

Diuretics are commonly used in older adults to treat hypertension above the age-corrected norm and congestive heart failure. Although the basic principles of therapy are not different, cautions resulting from altered pharmacokinetics and possible drug sensitivity do apply in older adults. Thiazide diuretics often show a decreased natriuretic effect, particularly in patients with renal impairment when creatinine clearance drops below 20 mL/min.[8] Potential for volume depletion may lead to decreased cardiac output and electrolyte imbalance. Risk of hypokalemia is greater, which may increase the potential for digoxin toxicity. Use of any diuretic in an older patient should be monitored closely, particularly if the patient is on multiple drug therapy.[3,7] Visual effects can include a sudden onset of myopia or changes in refraction.[4]

### Cardiac Glycosides

Preparations of digitalis have been used for more than 100 years for the management of congestive heart failure and atrial arrhythmias. Dosage levels between therapeutic and toxic effects are narrow, and the half-life of elimination of digoxin is increased by approximately 40% in older adults.[24] Several classes of drugs can affect digoxin serum levels when taken concurrently. Diuretics and certain calcium channel blocking agents, such as verapamil, have been observed to enhance the effects of digoxin.

Close monitoring is essential to avoid potential side effects, which can include gastrointestinal, cardiac, neurological, and visual disturbances. Nausea, anorexia, fatigue, depression, and confusion can be early signs of toxicity. The vision care practitioner should pay particular attention to possible visual effects, especially alterations in color vision.[4,15]

### Beta-Adrenergic Blocking Agents

Beta-adrenergic blocking agents are widely used in cardiovascular disease. Studies have shown that older adults exhibit a decreased clinical response to beta-blocking agents such as propranolol and timolol.[30] The decreased responsiveness of this class of drugs in the older adult population is presumed to be the result of their reduced interaction with cell receptors. Side effects are also higher. Depression is more common in older adults, as are confusion and falls.[15]

### Calcium Channel Blocking Agents and Angiotensin Converting Enzyme Inhibitors

Calcium channel blockers are being used with increasing frequency to treat angina, supraventricular tachyarrhythmia, and hypertension. Geriatric patients with hypertension appear to respond well to these agents. Dosage and frequency of administration should be monitored carefully in patients with renal or hepatic insufficiency. Dosage reduction based on renal function has been suggested with the angiotensin converting enzyme inhibitors because acute renal failure, hypotension, and hyperkalemia have been associated with their use.[6]

### Nonsteroidal Antiinflammatory Drugs

Approximately half of the population older than 65 years is estimated to have symptomatic arthritis.[7] NSAIDs are frequently prescribed and are also self-administered for pain and various rheumatic problems. Aspirin, ibuprofen, naproxen, and ketoprofen are available OTC. Aspirin, although an effective analgesic and antiinflammatory agent, can cause serious gastrointestinal irritation and bleeding and may be of limited usefulness as an antiinflammatory agent for long-term use. NSAIDs exert their pharmacological effects by interference with prostaglandin synthesis. Although prostaglandins appear to play a major role in the inflammatory response, they also play a vital role in the protective mechanism of the gastric mucosa and the autoregulation of renal blood flow. A significant incidence of gastrointestinal disease and renal impairment has been observed in older patients when therapeutic dosages of NSAIDs are used.[22,26]

Acetaminophen can be an effective alternative if the patient has no history of hepatic dysfunction or alcohol abuse. The nonacetylated salicylates, which do not affect renal blood flow, or an NSAID such as sulindac, which is inactivated by the kidney, may be used in patients at risk.[26]

In general, use of NSAIDs in older adults should be monitored carefully for dosage and possible adverse effects, particularly in patients with chronic disease and those taking multiple medications.[17] The dose of NSAID has been recommended to be reduced initially and increased slowly to the desired clinical effect.

Misoprostol, an analog of the E series prostaglandins with antiulcer properties, has been found useful in patients at risk for gastrointestinal complications.[13]

## Central Nervous System Agents

Use of agents for psychological disorders produces an enhanced effect in older adults.[29] The half-lives of the barbiturates and benzodiazepines increase with age, particularly during the decade from 60 to 70 years. Benzodiazepines, with relatively shorter half-lives, such as alprazolam, lorazepam, and temazepam, should be used because an increase in falls has been associated with benzodiazepines whose half-lives are prolonged with aging. Daytime drowsiness and ataxia are indications of excessive benzodiazepine dosage.[7,23,29]

The antipsychotic agents have been used extensively in older adults, particularly in those who demonstrate agitated and disruptive behavior. However, full control of the patient's behavior is not always possible, and dosage should not be increased because side effects become prominent. Before prescribing these agents, practitioners should ascertain that the patient's condition is not already the result of drugs being administered for other disease entities. The incidence of extrapyramidal effects, particularly akathisia, should not be mistaken as insufficient drug administration.[7] Haloperidol can be effective in the treatment of symptoms associated with agitation, combativeness, and paranoia, but serious adverse effects, particularly extrapyramidal symptoms, are common.[29]

Depression is often misdiagnosed and untreated in older adults. The symptoms associated with psychiatric depression, such as apathy and social withdrawal, may be mistaken as senile dementia.[29] Again, before beginning therapy with an antidepressant drug, the possible effects of other medications that the patient may be taking must be considered. When an antidepressant drug is chosen its sedative, anticholinergic, and cardiac side effects must be considered. According to these criteria, desipramine and trazodone are often the drugs chosen for geriatric depression.[7,27]

## H$_1$-Blocking Agents

The classic H$_1$ antihistamines, such as diphenhydramine and chlorpheniramine, are available OTC. They are distributed to all tissues and are highly lipophilic, so they also cross the blood-brain barrier. The central nervous system effects of these drugs can manifest as stimulation or depression, with depression more common in adults, particularly older adults. Sedation is generally the most common side effect. Older adults are also more sensitive to the cognitive effects of these agents, and care must be taken in their use to minimize the anticholinergic effects. When used in older adults the dosage should generally be lowered and the drug administered at bedtime if possible.

The second generation of H$_1$ receptor antagonists such as fexofenadine, loratidine, and cetirizine do not penetrate the blood-brain barrier, and central nervous system depression is not a prominent side effect. The second-generation antihistamines are also available in combination with the sympathomimetic pseudoephedrine, an antihistamine-decongestant. Caution is advised because sympathomimetics are more likely to induce adverse reactions such as palpitations, headache, and insomnia in older adults.[22]

## H$_2$-Blocking Agents

Available OTC, the H$_2$ blockers have been useful in controlling various peptic and duodenal disorders. Their use is generally safe, but headaches and mental confusion can occur. Drug interactions with these agents are of concern, particularly with cimetidine, a potent inhibitor of cytochrome P-450.[28,29] Drugs metabolized by the oxidative cytochrome P-450 system, such as certain benzodiazepines, phenytoin, theophylline, and warfarin, may have their serum levels altered to potential toxic levels when administered with an H$_2$ blocking agent.

## Anticholinergic Drugs

Anticholinergic drug toxicity is of concern, particularly in older adults because they appear more susceptible to impaired autonomic effects on organ systems such as the bowels, bladder, and central nervous system. Older adults may be especially sensitive to the cognitive effects caused by anticholinergic drugs or drugs in general that have atropinelike effects. Loss of memory and delirium are common features of anticholinergic toxicity in older adults. Use of scopolamine transdermal preparation has been associated with sudden loss of memory and delirium.[25] Box 10-3 lists drugs with anticholinergic properties.

## Antimicrobial Drugs

Mortality rates from infection are generally higher in older patients because of various factors, including reduced host-defense mechanisms and reactions to antimicrobials.[33] Broad-spectrum antibiotics generally are preferred in older adults, and the basic principles of therapy are the same as for younger patients. The age-dependent factor that must be considered is possible decrease in renal function. This is an important consideration with the use of anti-infective agents such as fluoroquinolones and amantadine. Tetracyclines, with the exception of doxycycline and minocycline, are excreted by glomerular filtration and tend to accumulate in the presence of renal failure.[19] In most older patients with normal renal function, antiinfectives such as the penicillins, cephalosporins,

and trimethoprim-sulfamethoxazole combination may be prescribed in standard doses.

## Nonprescription Drugs

Approximately $12 billion is spent annually in the United States on OTC drugs. The geriatric population is believed to be a major consumer of OTC drugs, and most of this use is without prior consultation with a health care provider.[29,32] Because nonprescription drugs such as analgesics, antacids, cough and cold remedies, laxatives, and vitamins can contribute to adverse drug reactions and drug interactions, all health care practitioners should monitor patients for OTC drug use. Table 10-3 lists some possible clinical effects with concomitant prescription and OTC drug use.

Antacids are frequently used for symptomatic relief of upset stomach, heartburn, and peptic ulcers. The sodium content of these products varies and should be considered in patients with congestive heart failure and decreased renal function. Antacids can affect the absorption and elimination of drugs taken concurrently. By altering intestinal pH, absorption of acidic drugs can be increased and those of basic drugs decreased. By delaying gastric emptying, drug absorption from the intestine also may be altered. The use of these products should be ascertained and their use monitored as closely as possible.[16]

Cough and cold preparations offer relief from symptoms associated with accumulation

---

**BOX 10-3**

### Drugs with Anticholinergic Properties

Antipsychotics
Antidepressants
Antiepileptics
Antispasmodics
Antihistamines
Hypnotics

---

**TABLE 10-3**

## OTC Drug Interactions

| OTC Drug | Prescription Drug | Possible Clinical Effect |
|---|---|---|
| Alcohol | CNS depressants | Enhanced depression |
| | Aspirin | Gastrointestinal bleeding |
| Antacids | Phenothiazines | Inhibition of phenothiazine absorption |
| | Tetracycline | Divalent cations (e.g., calcium present in formulations impairs absorption of tetracycline) |
| Aspirin | Methotrexate | Enhanced clinical effects of methotrexate |
| | Anticoagulants | Enhanced anticoagulant effects |
| | Probenecid | Reduced uricosuric effect |
| Agents with anticholinergic effects (e.g., antihistamines, cold and cough preparations) | CNS depressants, anticholinergics | Enhanced anticholinergic effects |
| Phenylephrine Pseudoephedrine | Monoamine oxidase inhibitors | Enhanced effects of these and other adrenergic agonists (e.g., possible hypertensive crisis) |

*CNS,* Central nervous system.
Adapted from Lamy PP: *Prescribing for the elderly,* Littleton, MA, 1980, PSG Publishing Co.

of secretions in the bronchial passages. These preparations may also contain alcohol, antihistamines, bronchodilators, and decongestants. Alcohol can potentiate the central nervous system effects of antipsychotics, sedatives, and $H_1$ antihistamines. Older patients with asthma, glaucoma, and urinary tract problems generally are advised against the use of products containing antihistamines or anticholinergic agents.

Laxative use is more common among older adults. Disease, poor nutrition, diminished physical activity, and emotional factors can be possible causes of constipation. Long-term use of laxatives should be evaluated because it can lead to adverse effects such as disturbances in electrolyte and water balance.[16] Bulk formers and stool softeners have been recommended as the safest laxatives for chronic constipation.

Vitamin supplementation appears to be common in older adults. Although evidence for large-scale vitamin deficiencies is lacking, excessive intake appears common. Megadose intake of certain vitamins has been associated with renal and central nervous system effects.

Niacin can alter liver function and raise blood levels of uric acid and glucose. Vitamins A and D can interfere with some laboratory tests.[16] Vitamin supplementation may be necessary in older patients with long-term drug use, certain disease states, and excessive stress.

## Topical Ophthalmic Agents

Topical ophthalmic drug-induced systemic side effects are most likely to occur with long-term therapy. Older patients undergoing long-term ophthalmic drug therapy, such as for glaucoma, are also more likely to have other medical conditions.[10] Cardiac and respiratory conditions may be induced or exacerbated by topical ophthalmic agents, and polypharmacy, more common in older adults, increases the risk of drug interactions. Because patients may not associate systemic symptoms with ophthalmic medications, the eye care provider needs to question the patient directly.[4,10]

The most frequently reported systemic effects of ocular drugs are listed in Table 10-4. Among the adrenergic agonists, topical use of

**TABLE 10-4**

## Systemic Effects of Ocular Drugs

| Ocular Drug | Example | Systemic Side Effect |
|---|---|---|
| Adrenergic agonist | Apraclonidine | Dryness of upper respiratory passages |
| | Epinephrine | Headache, anxiety, tachycardia, hypertensive crisis |
| | Dipivefrin | |
| | Phenylephrine | Hypertension, reflex bradycardia, tachycardia, subarachnoid hemorrhage, occipital headache |
| Adrenergic-blocking agents | Timolol | Bradycardia, conduction arrhythmias, hypotension, bronchospasm, asthma, depression, confusion, impotence, diarrhea, nausea |
| | Levobunolol | |
| | Betaxolol | |
| | Carteolol | |
| Cholinergic agonist | Pilocarpine | Headache, bradycardia, hypotension, bronchospasm, gastrointestinal disturbances, marked salivation, profuse perspiration |
| | Echothiophate | |
| Cholinergic antagonist | Atropine | Allergic dermatitis, thirst, fever, somnolence, urinary retention, tachycardia, excitement, hallucinations, convulsions |
| | Cyclopentolate | Drowsiness, ataxia, disorientation, incoherent speech, restlessness, visual hallucinations |
| Local anesthetics | Proparacaine | Allergic dermatitis, nervousness, tachycardia, hypertension, hypotension, tremors, respiratory depression, convulsions |
| | Benoxinate | |
| | Tetracaine | |
| | Cocaine | |
| Antiinfective agents | Chloramphenicol | Aplastic anemia |
| | Neomycin | Contact dermatitis |
| | Sulfonamides | Contact dermatitis, photosensitization, erythema multiforme, exfoliate dermatitis |

phenylephrine for mydriasis has been associated with cardiac and central nervous system effects. The incidence of adverse effects with the cholinergic agonist used for mydriasis and uveitis is generally dosage dependent and least likely occur with tropicamide. However, idiosyncratic dosage-independent reactions have been reported.[10]

Use the alpha-2 adrenergic agonists apraclonidine and brimonidine for control of intraocular pressure may induce oral dryness, fatigue, and ocular allergic reactions. Systemic adverse effects with the use of topical nonselective adrenergic-blocking agents such as timolol may range from relatively common bronchial effects to cardiovascular and central nervous system effects, including fatigue, depression, and confusion. Prostaglandin receptor agonists appear to be generally well tolerated in older patients with controlled bronchial or cardiovascular disease.

## REFERENCES

1. AARP Administration on Aging: *A profile of older Americans 1999*, Washington, DC, 1999, AARP.
2. ASHP Research Report: *American Society of Health System Pharmacists. Snapshot of medication use in the U.S.*, Washington, DC, 2000, ASHP.
3. Baldwin T, Vacek J: Use of cardiovascular drugs in the elderly, *Postgrad Med* 85:319-30, 1989.
4. Bartlett JD, Jaanus SD: Ocular effects of systemic drugs. In Bartlett JD, Jaanus SD, editors: *Clinical ocular pharmacology*, Boston, 2001, Butterworth, pp 309-48.
5. Beyth RJ, Shorr RI: Epidemiology of adverse drug reactions in the elderly by drug class, *Drugs Aging* 14:231-3, 1999.
6. Brawn LA, Castleden CM: Adverse drug reactions: an overview of special considerations in management of the elderly patient, *Drug Safety* 5:421-8, 1999.
7. Buechler JR, Malloy D: Drug therapy in the elderly, *Postgrad Med* 85:87-99, 1989.
8. Chutka DS, Evans JM, Fleming KD, et al: Drug prescribing for elderly patients, *Mayo Clin Proc* 70:685-93, 1995.
9. Coons SJ, Sheahan SL, Martin SS, et al: Predictors of medication noncompliance in a sample of older adults, *Clin Ther* 16:110-7, 1994.
10. Diamond JP: Systemic adverse effects of topical ophthalmic agents, *Drugs Aging* 11:352-60, 1997.
11. Fugh-Berman A: Herb-drug interactions, *Lancet* 355:134-38, 2000.
12. Giron MS, Wang MS, Bersten C, et al: The appropriateness of drug use in an older nondemented and demented population, *J Am Geriatric Soc* 49:277-83, 2001.
13. Graham DY: Prevention of gastroduodenal injury induced by chronic nonsteroidal, antiinflammatory drug therapy, *Gastroenterology* 675-81, 1989.
14. Heft MW, Mariotti AJ: Geriatric pharmacology, *Dent Clin N Am* 46:869-85, 2002.
15. Kane RL, Ouslander JG, Abrass I: Drug therapy. In Kane RL, Ouslander JG, Abrass I, editors: *Essentials of clinical geriatrics*, ed 4, New York, 1999, McGraw-Hill, pp 379-411.
16. Lamy PP: *Prescribing for the elderly*, Boston, MA, 1980, Littleton PSG.
17. Lamy P: Renal effect of non-steroidal antiinflammatory drugs: heightened risk in the elderly? *J Am Geriat Soc* 34:361-7, 1986.
18. Luisi AF, Owens NJ, Hume AL: Drugs and the elderly. In Gallo JJ, Reichel W, editors: *Reichel's care of the elderly: clinical aspects of aging*, ed 5, Philadelphia, 1999, Williams & Wilkins, pp 59-87.
19. Mallet L: Age-related changes in renal function and clinical implication for drug therapy, *J Geriat Drug Ther* 5:6-29, 1991.
20. Montamat SC, Cusack BJ, Vested RE: Management of drug therapy in the elderly, *N Engl J Med* 321:303-9,1989.
21. Montamat SC, Cusack B: Overcoming problems with polypharmacy and drug misuse in the elderly, *Clin Geriatr Med* 8:143-58, 1992.
22. Paunovich ED, Sadowsky JM, Carter P: The most frequently prescribed medications in the elderly and their impact on dental treatment, *Dent Clin N Am* 41:699-726, 1997.
23. Ray WA, Griffin MR, Downey W: Benzodiazepines of long and short elimination half-life and the risk of hip fracture, *JAMA* 262:3303-7, 1989.
24. Reuning RH, Geraets R: Digoxin. In Evans WE, Schentag SS, Creasey H, et al, editors: *Applied pharmacokinetics: principles of therapeutic drug monitoring*, ed 2, Spokane, WA, 1986, Applied Therapeutics, pp 570-623.
25. Rozzini R, Inzoli M, Trabucchi M, et al: Delirium from transdermal scopolamine in elderly women, *JAMA* 260:478-82, 1988.
26. Sack KE: Update on NSAIDs in elderly, *Geriatrics* 44:71-90, 1989.
27. Salzman C: Geriatric psychopharmacology, *Ann Rev Med* 36:217-35, 1985.
28. Sawyer D, Conner CS, Scalley R, et al: Cimetidine: adverse reactions and acute toxicity, *Am Hosp Pharm* 38:188-97, 1981.
29. Steiner JF: Pharmacotherapy problems in the elderly, *J Am Pharm Assoc* 36:431-67, 1996.

30. Vestal RE, Cusack BJ: Pharmacology and aging. In Schneider EL, Rose WW, editors: *Handbook of the biology of aging,* New York, 1990, Academic Press, pp 349-83.

31. Vestal RE, Dawson GW: Pharmacology and aging. In Finch CE, Schneider EL, editors: *Handbook of the biology of aging,* ed 2, New York, 1985, Van Nostrand Reinhold, pp 744-89.

32. Williams CM: Using medications appropriately in older adults, *Am Fam Physician* 66:1917-24, 2002.

33. Yoshikawa TT: Antimicrobial therapy for the elderly, *J Am Geriatr Soc* 38:1353-72, 1990.

# CHAPTER 11

# Vision Corrections for the Older Adult

**ROBERT J. LEE and ROD TAHRAN**

According to AARP some 18 million older adults (defined as people older than 55 years) are currently in the workforce. A recent AARP survey suggests that number will continue to grow.[6] Currently 63.2 million older adults live in the United States, which represents 29% of the entire population.[4] What are some of the visual challenges and opportunities eye care practitioners can expect when prescribing spectacles for this patient population? How can their visual well-being be better served?

## LIFESTYLE CHANGES

Millions of older, active Americans are trying new careers, launching new businesses, volunteering, and returning to school.[6] For eye care practitioners to prescribe effectively and learn more about their diverse visual needs, a lifestyle questionnaire may be useful. The lifestyle questionnaire should ask about each of these activities along with details about sports and hobbies. An ideal questionnaire has patients check off activities they regularly participate in and rank the importance of these activities from "important" to "very important." Vision enhancement recommendations based on activities most important to the patient should be well received (Fig. 11-1). An area on the questionnaire that asks about the likes and dislikes of the patient's present eyewear can also provide valuable information to discuss features and benefits of lens materials, design, and treatments. Secondary

questions should be asked about working distance, field of view, and visual acuity requirements based on each task and an explanation of unfamiliar occupations or hobbies.

## SPECTACLE PRESCRIPTION CHANGES

Because of normal age-related changes to the ocular media, crystalline lens, and retina, changes in the spectacle lens power are often necessary for older patients. An increase in distance minus power caused by media changes such as cataracts or systemic changes from diabetes can be unnerving to the patient, especially if the prescription change is greater than 1.00 D. Patient education and trial framing of the new prescription are beneficial to aid in adaptation and visual comfort. Patients with unstable blood glucose levels require a referral as well as patient education on expected spectacle lens changes until their glucose levels are stabilized. An increase in plus add power is especially difficult because near and intermediate working distances will both be reduced. The shortened working distances will also necessitate more positive fusional convergence by the patient. This demand is compounded by the higher add power, which results in a more exophoric posture at near. Symptomatic patients may be made more comfortable by the decentration of the multifocal segment inward to create a base in prism effect at near. The segment width should be increased to compensate for the decentration effect. Consider a flat top 35 or 45 segment,

## PATIENT LIFESTYLE QUESTIONNAIRE

*This questionnaire has been developed to assist us in prescribing and recommending the best eyewear suited for your work and recreational needs. Please check the sections that apply to you and the way you use your eyes.*

Patient Name: _____ Date _____

1.  What do you like the **MOST** about your present eyewear?
    _____

2.  What do you like the **LEAST** about your present eyewear?
    _____

3.  Do you currently have more than one pair of glasses?    ☐ Yes   ☐ No

4.  If yes, is your second pair for a special application such as *(check appropriate one)*:
    ☐ Occupational eye protection      ☐ Home or leisure eye protection
    ☐ Sunwear      ☐ Computer      ☐ Other: _____

5.  Explain any special visual needs or requirements you have (such as magnifiers, scuba lenses, welders mask): _____
    _____

6.  Check any activities below in which you are involved and their importance to you:

| Activity | Importance of activity to you | |
|---|---|---|
| ☐ Computers | ☐ Somewhat Important | ☐ Very Important |
| ☐ Typewriters, Calculators, etc. | ☐ Somewhat Important | ☐ Very Important |
| ☐ Musical Instrument _____ | ☐ Somewhat Important | ☐ Very Important |

☐ Sports *(circle ones that apply)*:

Baseball, Biking, Boating, Fishing, Football, Golf, Hiking, Horses, Motorcycling, Racquetball, Running, Skin Diving, Snow/Water Skiing, Soccer

☐ Hobbies *(please list)*: _____

☐ I am involved in work or leisure activities where impact resistant lenses would help protect my eyes:

Explain: _____

**Fig. 11-1** Sample lifestyle questionnaire. (Courtesy Southern California College of Optometry Eye Care Center.)

noting that the segment "ledge" will be more apparent as the width of the segment increases.

## LENS MATERIALS

A thinner, lighter lens with good optical performance is a goal of lens designers, eye care professionals, and patients. Are both comfort and good vision possible with today's lens materials? Polycarbonate has gained a U.S. market share of greater than 25% because of a relatively high index of refraction (n = 1.586), low specific gravity (1.20 g/cm³), and superior impact resistance compared with CR-39 resin (n = 1.498) specific gravity (1.32 g/cm³).[3] Polycarbonate also offers good value to the patient with its inherent scratch-resistant coating and ultraviolet (UV) blocking properties (blocks 97% of UV radiation up to 400 nm). Lenses can be surfaced to 1.0 mm center or edge thickness, which reduces edge thickness and weight. Because of an Abbe value of 30, color fringes caused by lateral chromatic aberration can sometimes be seen by patients, especially when viewing off the lens optical center. Although chromatic aberration can be expected and is a factor with all high-index materials, it can be distracting for the patient. A reduction in contrast and peripheral acuity is a function of the prismatic effect and the nu value of the lens material.[18] To minimize these unwanted effects, polycarbonate should be limited to corrections less than 4 D.

A lens material called Trivex (Younger Optics, Torrance, Calif.) is a viable alternative to polycarbonate. Marketed under the Trilogy name, it combines the best attributes of thermoplastics (polycarbonate) and thermosets (CR-39). The Abbe value is similar to CR-39 with a specific gravity less than polycarbonate. Trivex is a mid-index lens (n = 1.53) and has a specific gravity of 1.11 g/cm³. Its Abbe value of 43 to 46 (depending on the manufacturer) rivals CR-39's Abbe of 30. Trivex can also be surfaced down to 1.0-mm center or edge thickness for dress lenses. These lenses are especially suited for rimless and three-piece applications because of reduced distortion and stress at the drill holes (Table 11-1).

## LENS DESIGNS

The maturing patient with presbyopia typically already has a habitual vision correction. This correction may take the form of store-bought reading glasses, lined multifocals, or progressive addition lenses.[2] These patients are experienced spectacle wearers and may have minimal or no complaints with their habitual multifocal lens design. How does the practitioner decide what lens design is most appropriate for the patient? Should the patient be kept in the same style lens as before? Certainly a well-adapted bifocal wearer may subjectively be free of visual complaints. As previously mentioned, a lifestyle questionnaire and additional questions may uncover visual needs that the patient never considered. Consider the vision requirements of diverse hobbies and interests such as a home workshop, piloting a plane, playing billiards, surfing the Internet, painting at an easel, and playing the piano. They all have something in common: the need for clear, comfortable, intermediate vision. Although reduced amplitudes of accommodation as presbyopia increases are inevitable, the loss of intermediate vision ranges can be maintained by prescribing trifocals or progressive addition lenses (PALs).

Restrictions with vertical and lateral head or eye movements may limit the patient's ability to use a trifocal or PAL effectively, especially for extended periods of reading. The trifocal design lowers the near segment in the lens because of the position of the intermediate segment. The progressive lens wearer may also be affected because the full add power is also lower in the

**TABLE 11-1**

### Comparison of Lens Materials

|  | n | Abbe | Specific Gravity (g/cm3) | Edge Thickness* |
|---|---|---|---|---|
| CR-39 | 1.498 | 58 | 1.32 | 4.50 mm |
| Polycarbonate | 1.586 | 30 | 1.20 | 3.13 mm |
| Trivex | 1.530 | 45 | 1.11 | 3.36 mm |

*-4.00 D sphere prescription, 50 mm round lens. CR-39: 2.0 mm center thickness. Polycarbonate and Trivex: 1.0 mm center thickness.

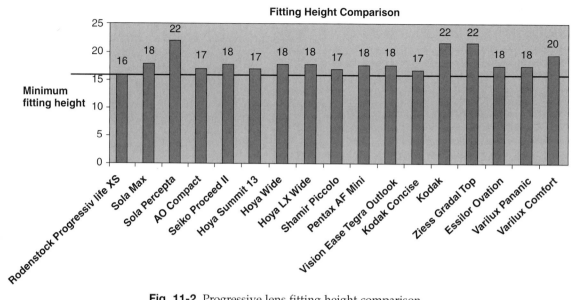

**Fig. 11-2** Progressive lens fitting height comparison.

lens. A vertical head movement is necessary to access the near reading zone of the PAL. Consider a short-corridor progressive addition lens for these patients. The progression of plus power for near is reached faster because the corridor length is shorter. By reaching the full add power sooner, vertical excursions of the head and eyes are reduced (Fig. 11-2).

Trifocal wearers may be satisfied with their current lens style: three defined areas of stable, clear vision. The intermediate power of a trifocal is typically 50% of the add power. Trifocals are also offered with intermediate powers of 40% and 70% of the add power. For those patients desiring a larger vertical field of view through their intermediate segments, consider the 14 × 35 trifocal. Also consider an occupational trifocal; the vertical height of the intermediate segment is 14 mm—twice the height of a conventional trifocal (Fig. 11-3).

Progressive addition lenses (PALs) have come a long way since the Varilux 1 was introduced in 1959 and should be considered for all mature patients. Progressive lenses are especially appropriate for add powers greater than +1.75 D because these patients benefit from the intermediate working distance afforded by a PAL. Patients who have tried the older generation progressives did not have the benefit of today's advanced technology. Past strategies suggested fitting an established multifocal

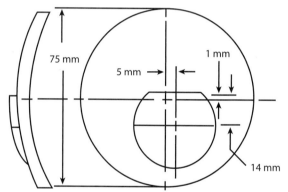

**Fig. 11-3** 4 × 35 trifocal. The vertical intermediate height is twice the height of traditional flat top trifocals. (Courtesy Vision Ease, Ramsey, Minn.)

wearer with a "hard" design PAL. Hard designs have their unwanted peripheral astigmatism in concentrated areas below the 180 line of the lens, mainly on either side of the progressive corridor. Patients accustomed to viewing through a lined segment were thought to adapt to the hard design's defined corridor and near zone.

For older patients desiring to wear PALs, today's "soft" designs have their advantages. Unwanted astigmatism is spread over larger areas of the lens, including above the 180 line of the lens. This results in a smoother transition from distance to near, making adaptation easier. Studies have shown that more than 90% of lined multifocal wearers successfully adapt to PALs [1,14]

## VARIABLE FOCUS LENS

Patients who are effectively emmetropic at distance may only wear single-vision reading glasses. The practitioner often has to address the complaint of "blurry vision when I look up with my readers." Another scenario is the lined multifocal wearer who reports blurred vision and neck and shoulder discomfort after surfing the Internet for several hours. Yet another scenario is the PAL wearer who works on the computer and desires a wider intermediate field of view. Could the lens design be contributing to these patients' complaints?

Variable focus lenses are an all-purpose lens for vision tasks in the near to intermediate range. Because of its design, the lens has unwanted astigmatism like a progressive. However, because the lens has only intermediate and near power, the unwanted astigmatism can be moved farther out in the lens periphery, away from the patient's field of view. This results in wider intermediate and near zones compared with a traditional progressive lens (Fig. 11-4). Although these lenses are not designed for driving, the reduction in plus power from the bottom of the lens toward the top allows acceptable distance vision up to 6 to 10 feet. This lens design can address the complaint of blur through single-vision lenses when looking up from reading.

According to Liz Kelleher, content development manager for AARP Services, Nielsen/NetRatings found that in 2002 the fastest growing population for broadband Internet access in the United States was composed of 55- to 64-year-olds, which surged 78% to approximately 2.9 million.[9] Computer use has obviously become commonplace in the lives of many older adults. However, the visual demands of using a computer are different from the demands of reading printed text (Box 11-1).

Variable focus lenses position the lens power at the correct height and distance for a computer monitor. These lenses virtually eliminate the awkward head posture required of traditional bifocal wearers. Because the lens provides only near and intermediate vision, the unwanted astigmatism can be distributed to a more peripheral part of the lens, thereby increasing the field of view.

Variable focus lenses should not be restricted to only computer use and reading. They are a viable option for eye care practitioners as well. Entrance tests are easier to observe with variable focus lenses, including the cover test, motility, and external adnexa. The phoropter is in clear focus along with the patient's chart (Table 11-2).

---

**BOX 11-1**

### Issues Causing Vision Problems for Computer Users

The monitor is higher and farther away compared with printed text.

The monitor is self-illuminated.

The text viewed on the monitor has poor contrast compared with printed text.

Traditional bifocals do not provide clear vision unless the user leans forward and elevates the chin to view through the bifocal segment.

Traditional trifocals and progressive lenses intermediate viewing zones are narrow, necessitating lateral head movement.

---

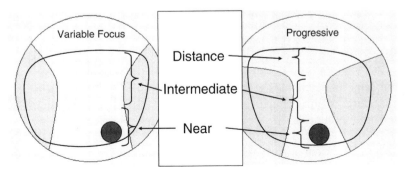

**Fig. 11-4** Variable focus versus progressive lens viewing zones.

**TABLE 11-2**

### Examples of Variable Focus Lenses

| Brand Name | Description |
| --- | --- |
| AO TruVision Technica | CR-39, small distance window above the fitting cross |
| Sola Access | CR-39 and polycarbonate, power shifts of 0.75 D and 1.25 D |
| Sola Continuum | Spectralite and polycarbonate, power shift of 1.00 D |
| Essilor Interview | CR-39, power shift of 0.80 D |
| Prio's Prio | CR-39, with four power shifts: 0.75 D, 1.25 D, 1.75 D, and 2.25 D |
| Prio Browser | CR-39, with two power shifts: 1.00 D and 1.50 D |
| Rodenstock Cosmolit Office | CR-39, power shifts of 1.00 D and 1.75 D |
| Zeiss Gradal RD | CR-39, lab increases distance power by 0.50 D and reduces add power by 0.50 D |

## LENS APPEARANCE, PERFORMANCE, AND WEIGHT

Patient adaptation and comfort may further be hindered by the physical appearance and weight of a new prescription. Weight is perhaps the biggest consideration in choosing frame and lens materials for the older patient. When lens weight is a factor, both Trivex and polycarbonate are available in aspheric designs in flat top and progressives. These lenses can be surfaced to 1.0 mm thickness, further reducing weight.

The older patient has the same concerns of lens appearance relating to their eyewear as any patient would. The three tips listed in Box 11-2 can be given to patients when selecting frames.

To minimize the temporal and nasal thickness of the finished lens, select a frame in which the frame PD (box system "A" measurement added to the distance between lenses) equals the patient's pupillary distance. This will reduce the need for decentration of the optical centers of the lenses, reducing weight and lens edge thickness.

If the correction exceeds 4.00 D, recommend a higher index aspheric lens to reduce the lens center or edge thickness. The cosmetic improvement is especially apparent with hyperopic corrections. The surface curves of aspheric lenses flatten toward the periphery of the lens. This flattening reduces the sagittal depth of the lens, allowing the lens to be fit closer to the eye. Reducing this vertex distance reduces the magnified image of the hyperopic eye. Because of the geometry of the lens, decentering the optical center to induce prism is not recommended. Prescribed prism, however, can still be ground.

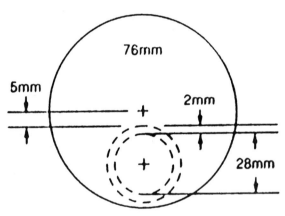

**Fig. 11-5** Blended 28-mm bifocal. Note the 2-mm blended annular ring. (Courtesy Sola International, San Diego, Calif.)

Complaints of flat top segments being too visible can be helped by prescribing round, blended, or curved top bifocal designs. A slight hint of tint in a skin-enhancing color such as pink or beige renders the segment almost invisible. Be aware that the blended segment has an annular ring of blur of 2 mm surrounding the segment (Fig. 11-5). This blur area may be disconcerting to some patients.

Field of view through the segment can be expanded by increasing the segment width, decreasing the vertex distance, and increasing pantoscopic tilt. A dedicated pair of glasses available for any prolonged task in which sharp vision and a larger field of view are required may be beneficial to the patient. Suggest single-vision reading or variable focus lenses for traditional progressive lens wearers who enjoy reading in bed or a recliner.

The well-adapted multifocal wearer will not typically have complaints adapting to their lined multifocal lens design. Potential adaptation problems may occur, however, when attempting to increase field of view or cosmesis by changing segment styles. Image jump is the prismatic effect produced when the wearer is not viewing through the optical center of the segment. The jump is most bothersome at the top of the segment where the distance from the segment optical center is greatest. Patients often perceive image jump as a shift or altered position of the image as their line of site passes from the distance portion of the lens to the reading segment, or vice versa. The amount of image jump is independent of the distance prescription. This prism effect is calculated by Prentice's

rule, which is equal to the add power (F) multiplied by the distance (in centimeters) the segment optical center is from the segment top. Executive bifocals in which the segment optical center is located on the segment line have zero image jump. Round and Ultex segments[6a] with lower optical center locations have the greatest amount of image jump. As shown in Figure 11-6, this is a base-down prismatic effect, resulting in a scotoma as the eye traverses the segment top.

## TINTS AND COATINGS

As the eye ages the amount of useful light reaching the retina may be attenuated by fluorescence and increased scatter. Morgan[10] reported that light levels reaching the retina of a healthy 60-year-old are approximately one third of the light reaching the retina of a 20-year-old. Thus older patients require more light to achieve the retinal illumination of younger patients. Kelleher[9] also found that visual performance in the home is significantly worse compared with the clinical setting because of insufficient lighting. Light transmission is reduced to 92.06% viewing through clear CR-39 resin, 91.4% through clear crown glass, and 89.4% through clear polycarbonate. This reduction in light transmission is caused by inherent surface reflections found in all lens materials. As the index of refraction increases, so does the surface reflection. Prescribing an antireflective coating (ARC) can increase light transmission up to 99% by reducing these spectacle lens surface reflections (Table 11-3). Other strategies to reduce reflections are changing the pantoscopic tilt or face form of the spectacles. Often this adjustment moves the reflection to a peripheral lens area away from the visual axis. Patients with myopia sometimes are bothered by the presence of myopic rings—multiple reflections within the lens of the roughened, semiopaque

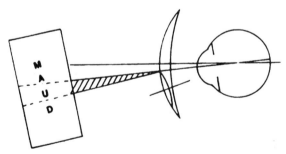

**Fig. 11-6** Image jump. The base-down prism effect causes a scotoma. The letter U is in the scotoma, resulting in the word "MAD" being read. (Reprinted from Fannin TE, Grosvenor T: *Clinical optics*, ed 2, Newton, MA, 1996, Butterworth-Heinemann.)

**TABLE 11-3**

### Light Transmission

| Lens Material | Index of Refraction | Without ARC (%) | Including Multilayer ARC (%) |
|---|---|---|---|
| CR-39 | 1.50 | 92.06 | 99.1 |
| Glass | 1.52 | 91.4 | 99.2 |
| Polycarbonate | 1.59 | 89.4 | 99.0 |
| High-index plastic | 1.60 | 89.4 | 99 |
| Super-high-index plastic | 1.67 | 87.8 | 98.2 |

lens bevel (Fig. 11-7). A light tint may also provide a solution to multiple reflection complaints. Pink tints have traditionally been used to reduce the glare from fluorescent lights. The pink tint serves to reduce some of the blue light emitted from the fluorescent lights. This decreases brightness and fluorescence within the eye.

## ANTIREFLECTIVE COATINGS

The use of ARCs can reduce glare from an oncoming car's headlights, thereby improving night vision (Fig. 11-8). The glare from car headlights behind the driver can also be reduced with ARCs. Swanson[16] reported that disability glare during driving at night can be so burdensome that many older drivers voluntarily stop driving during evening hours. ARCs can also reduce annoying surface reflection from surrounding objects reflecting on the spectacle

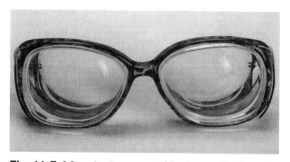

**Fig. 11-7** Myopic rings caused by internal reflection.

lenses. This improves comfort and reduces fatigue while viewing a computer monitor.

Avoid prescribing a single-layer ARC because it is optimal for only one particular wavelength, and resulting reflections will be strongly colored. Modern ARCs are multilayer coatings reflecting little, if any, light at any wavelength. A secondary benefit of ARCs is enhanced cosmetic appearance of the eyes. ARCs minimize lens reflections that hide the eyes, in turn making eye contact easier to establish when communicating with other people. The ocular surface of a sunglass lens may act as a mirror, often resulting in patients complaining that they see a reflection of their own eyes. Sunglass lenses should have a backside ARC to reduce these annoying reflections.

## GLARE

Two types of glare exist: discomfort glare and disabling, or veiling, glare. Discomfort glare has been reported to typically start at approximately 3000 lumens (Table 11-4).[17] The response of the unprotected eye to low levels of glare is a squint. This glare can occur in any weather, including overcast days. Glare from higher luminance sources causes pupil constriction, eye closure, and head turnaway from the offending source.

Disabling glare occurs at 10,000 lumens and causes lower contrast. An example of direct disabling glare is looking toward a sunset or automobile headlights at night. Reflective disabling

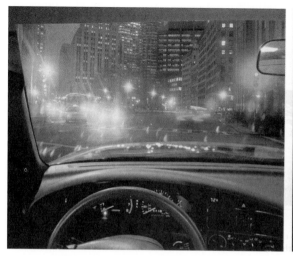
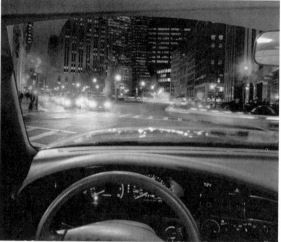

**Fig. 11-8** Glare reduction while driving at night with antireflective coatings. (Reprinted from Giammanco F: Vision care product news, *Essilor Product News* 2002.)

TABLE 11-4

## Illumination of Typical Environments

| Environment | Illumination (lumens) |
|---|---|
| Indoor, with artificial light | 400 |
| Sunny day, in the shade | 1000-14,000 (optimal lighting) |
| Sunny day, on the grass | 3500 (comfort limit) |
| Concrete highway | 6000-8000 |
| Beach or ski slopes | 10,000-12,000 |
| High-altitude snowfield | >12,000 |

glare occurs when light is reflected off an object (e.g., a windshield) on a sunny day. The glare is intense enough to overwhelm the eye with light, masking what is behind the glare. It can have a drastic effect on vision and create dangerous situations when driving. Two or more glare sources in the field of vision have also been shown to be additive.[17] Increased light scatter within the lens is largely responsible for the clinical complaint of glare experienced by the older driver.

## PHOTOCHROMIC LENSES

The first commercially available ophthalmic photochromic lenses appeared in the late 1960s. The best-known photochromic glass products were Photogray Extra, Photobrown Extra, and Photosun developed by Corning Glass Works. With the introduction, proliferation, and acceptance of plastic lenses, market share of glass lenses has declined to 5%. Plastic photochromic lenses were introduced in the early 1990s. Early plastic photochromic lenses were not recommended for older adults because the lenses never became clear. A slight reduction of light transmission occurred when worn indoors and at night. This presented a potential problem for older eyes after dark. With new photochromic technology, modern plastic photochromics are virtually clear indoors and at night. These lenses are indicated for nearly all older patients because of their ability to adjust to varying light levels. Photochromic lenses block up to 100% of UVA and UVB.

There are two methods of incorporating photochromic technology in the lens material. The earlier "in-mass" method mixed photochromic compounds into the lens monomer. The limitations of this technique led to "bull's-eye" or "raccoon" effects for high plus or high minus lenses, respectively, because of the thickest part of the lens having the most photochromic compounds present. In-mass technology also had the limitation of lenses not being truly clear indoors because of excessive photochromic dye. Transitions Optical developed and commercially introduced Imbibition or Trans-Bonding photochromic technology. With Imbibition, photochromic compounds are driven into the lens surface. The compounds become permanently imbedded to a depth of 150 to 200 microns. The photochromic compounds cannot be scratched or peeled off and do not exhibit the bull's-eye or raccoon effect. The Trans-Bonding process makes it possible to offer photochromic technology in desirable lightweight, impact resistant, and durable materials such as polycarbonate and Trivex.

Plastic photochromic lenses, such as Transitions, automatically darken and lighten in response to varying degrees of UV exposure. Visual comfort and function are maintained, ranging from virtually clear indoors, to semi-dark under cloudly or overcast conditions, to sunglass dark under direct high illumination.

Night vision has been shown to be affected by an individual's previous exposure to sunlight during the day.[17] Visual acuity, contrast, and overall sensitivity can be reduced up to 50% from the sun's sustained bleaching of the retinal photochemical rhodopsin. A 2- or 3-hour exposure to sunlight delays the initial phase of dark adaptation as much as 10 minutes. After 10 daily exposures, visual acuity and contrast discrimination show a 50% elevated threshold. To maintain night vision, contrast discrimination, and visual acuity, lenses with 20% transmission or less should be worn when participating in activities of 2 hours or longer in bright sunlight. These can be fixed-tint or photochromic lenses.

## POLARIZED LENSES

Fixed-tint and photochromic lenses attenuate glare, but polarized lenses eliminate glare from reflected surfaces. Delamination issues in the past have been addressed by suspending the polarizing film within the lens mold. The film then becomes an integral part of the finished lens. Polarized lenses should be prescribed for any patient who spends time out of doors and desires visual comfort and clarity. They are available in virtually any lens material and multifocal lens design. A more compelling

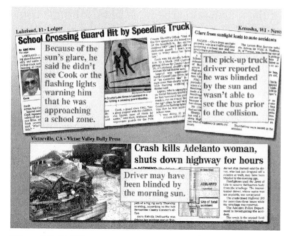

**Fig. 11-9** Glare as a causative factor in automobile accidents. (Courtesy Younger Optics, *www.youngeroptics.com/news/mur3.html*.)

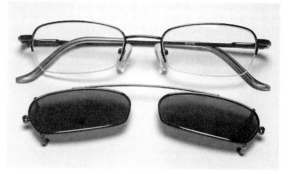

**Fig. 11-10** Clip-on sun lens.

reason to prescribe polarized lenses to the older patient is driving safety. In 1999 a 100-car pile-up on Highway 10 near San Bernardino, Calif., was attributed to drivers who simply could not see ahead of them because of intense sun glare (Fig. 11-9).[12] Morgan,[10] among others, reported that older adults are more sensitive to glare than are younger patients. This is indicated by an increase in reaction and redetection time in the presence of a glare source. Karr[8] reported that although they are involved in fewer accidents than younger people because they drive less often, individuals older than 65 years are the most likely to die in car accidents according to the National Highway Traffic Safety Administration.

## PROTECTING THE EYE FROM GLARE AND ULTRAVIOLET RADIATION

Ocular changes from aging and various pathological conditions can make the eyes hypersensitive to what normal eyes see as moderate glare. This glare is often disabling glare, generally within the eye because of blue light scatter. Patients may report hazy vision and loss of contrast. Prolonged adaptation time and photophobia often occur. Glare and loss of contrast may arise from developing cataracts, aphakia or pseudophakia, diabetic retinopathy, albinism, retinitis pigmentosa, and aniridia. Patients should visually test the lenses to ensure they can distinguish traffic color signals before driving.[5]

The mechanism of damage from UV radiation (UVR) is photochemical and thermal. The photochemical mechanism is primarily in the UVC and UVB wavelengths. As UVA is approached, the thermal mechanism is involved. Pitts[11] reported that UVR risk factors include aphakia, pseudophakia, cataracts, photosensitizing drug use, and sun exposure more than 8 hours daily as well as vocations or avocations rich in UVR such as arc welding, electronic chip assembly, snow skiing, or mountain climbing. The phakic retina is more sensitive to UVR at 325 nm by a factor of 2.5. Strategies to control UVR exposure include wearing ophthalmic lenses with UVA- and UVB-blocking properties such as polycarbonate and Trivex. For maximal protection these lenses should be larger and worn close to the eyes. Although UV-absorbing soft and gas-permeable contact lenses and intraocular lenses protect the cornea, lens, and retina against UVR, UV-blocking ophthalmic spectacle lenses are necessary to protect the eyelids and surrounding skin. Rosenthal et al[13] found that wearing a hat with a 4-inch brim in sunlight reduced ocular exposure to UVR by approximately 50%.

For the patients who would rather not have a dedicated pair of sunglasses, alternatives do exist. Clip-on sunglasses are popular because of the convenience of not having to carry two pairs of glasses. They are most beneficial when polarized lenses are dispensed. Clip-on sunglasses are attached to the frame with traditional clips or sturdy magnets. The magnets provide a strong point of attachment but do add minimal additional weight to the clip (Fig. 11-10). An additional option is a pair of over-the-counter sunglasses. Up to 52% of people with corrected

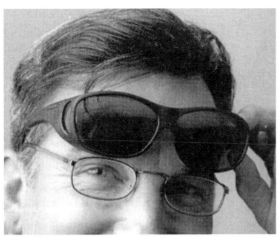

**Fig. 11-11** Plano sunglasses that fit over prescription spectacles. (Courtesy of Live Eyewear, San Luis Obispo, Calif.)

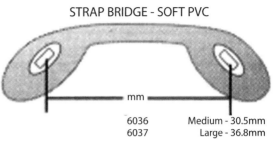

**Fig. 11-12** One-piece strap bridge. (Courtesy of Sadler Optical Tools and Findings, South Attleboro, Mass.)

vision are reported as not electing to purchase prescription sunglasses, photochromic lenses, clips, or plano sunglasses. Polarized sunglasses that quickly slip over prescription eyewear are an extremely popular option for prescription eyeglass wearers (Fig. 11-11).

## FRAME CONSIDERATIONS FOR OLDER ADULTS

As people age, the fatty tissue between the nose and the nose pads thins, resulting in less cushioning for glasses. This can result in pressure sores on the bridge of the nose. A temporary solution is to remove the glasses to relieve the pressure. This may be a poor solution for patients who depend on glasses. Larger nose pads may be helpful because the larger surface of the pads distributes the weight over a larger surface area. Silicone pads can also be used to minimize frame slippage. Nylon suspension or drill mount frames offer minimal weight while almost disappearing on the face, especially with the addition of an antireflective coating. Nickel is a common material used as the base material for metal frames. Patients who are bothered by allergies and cannot wear costume jewelry or need to use hypoallergenic makeup may also be sensitive to nickel. This sensitivity can be seen by examining the inside of the frame's temple. A patient's skin oils or perspiration may corrode the electroplating, exposing the underlying nickel. Look for roughened, dry, irritated areas where the temples make contact with the

skin. Consider titanium and titanium alloy frames that offer corrosion resistance as well as high tensile strength, durability, and light weight. Plastic frames that offer light weight include polyamide and copolyamide materials. These are a blend of nylons with reduced weight and flexibility. Optyl is another good choice because of its light weight (30% lighter than zylonite) and hypoallergenic properties.

A round eyewire is the ideal frame shape to minimize weight. When minimal weight is desired, frame shapes that depart from a round or oval increase the weight of the lens. Steer patients away from goggle shapes, which add unwanted lens mass at the frame's inferior nasal corner. A strap bridge is a one-piece nose pad that acts like a saddle bridge of a zylonite frame. These can often be retrofitted to a metal frame, increasing the weight-bearing area of the frame and minimizing pressure points (Fig. 11-12).

## PRESCRIBING STRATEGIES FOR PATIENTS WITH ANISOMETROPIA

Anisometropia has been defined as "a condition of unequal refractive state for the two eyes, one eye requiring a different lens correction than the other."[7] These patients can present with anisometropia as a consequence of unilateral intraocular lens or refractive surgery procedures, asymmetrical refractive error shifts from cataract progression, or blood glucose shifts in unstable diabetic patients. They may be symptomatic because of vertical prism being induced when they view below the distance optical centers of their glasses. This typically occurs when the patient reads through multifocal segments. Often a Fresnel prism is of diagnostic value to determine the subjective amount of vertical prism to alleviate symptoms. These "press-on" plastic membranes are applied to the ocular side of the bifocal segment (Fig. 11-13). The top of the prism should coincide with the segment top. Patients should be made aware that the Fresnel prism will reduce acuity by approximately one line and can be cosmetically dis-

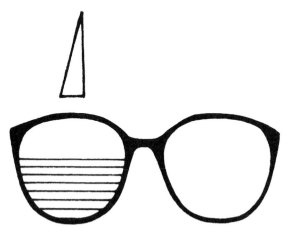

**Fig. 11-13** Diagnostic Fresnel prism. The prism should be placed with a base-down prism orientation on the lens, with the most plus or least minus vertical power. (Courtesy 3M Health Care, St. Paul, Minn.)

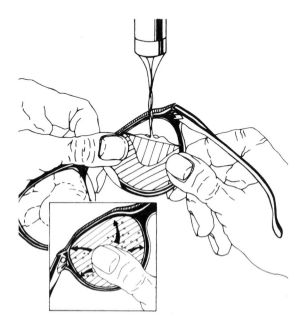

**Fig. 11-14** Fresnel prism application. (Courtesy 3M Health Care, St. Paul, Minn.)

tracting because of its striated appearance. They should also be instructed how to apply the prism if they are inadvertently removed during routine cleaning of the lenses (Fig. 11-14).

Optometrists have several prescribing options to address the vertical prism imbalance: (1) separate pairs of glasses for distance and reading, (2) prescribe dissimilar bifocal segments to neutralize the vertical prism induced by the distance correction, or (3) prescribe slab-off or reverse slab-off lenses. The advantage of prescribing distance and near glasses is that the optometrist can control the vertical optical center height of both pairs of lenses. As long as the patient views through the optical centers, no prism effect is induced. As a rule the optical centers of the reading glasses should be lowered 5 to 10 mm compared with the distance optical centers. The disadvantage, however, is the inconvenience of juggling two pairs of glasses.

## PRESCRIBING DISSIMILAR BIFOCAL SEGMENTS

A vertical difference in location of the segment optical centers exists between dissimilar bifocal segments. This difference in vertical location induces a prism effect equal in power but opposite in base direction compared with the prism induced by the distance correction (Fig. 11-15). The segment that has its optical center farthest from the segment top induces base-up prism because of the segment. The base-up prism neutralizes the base-down prism caused by the distance correction. For example, consider a prescription of OD –5.00 DS and OS –2.00 DS. If the patient reads 10 mm below the distance

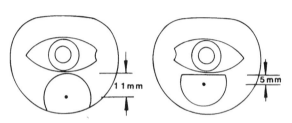

**Fig. 11-15** Dissimilar bifocal segments. The segment with its optical center farthest from the segment top is prescribed for the most minus lens. (Reprinted from Fannin TE, Grosvenor T: *Clinical optics,* ed 2, Newton, MA, 1996, Butterworth-Heinemann.)

optical centers the vertical prism effect OD is 5 prism diopters base down. The OS prism effect is 2 prism diopters base down. Prescribe the flat top bifocal for the lower minus left eye and the round 22 bifocal for the more minus right eye. In theory this works very well optically. Patient education is crucial because cosmesis will be an obvious concern.

## SLAB-OFF

Slab-off lenses are indicated when the vertical prism imbalance is 1.5 prism diopters or greater. A slab-off lens is made by bicentric grinding. This procedure results in the removal of base-down prism in the lower portion of the lens. Note this prism removal does not change the refractive power of the lens below the slab-off line. Because slab-off removes base-down prism, it should be prescribed for the lens that induces the most base-down prism from viewing below the distance optical center. Thus it should be placed on the lens having the least plus or most minus power in the vertical meridian. Bicentric grinding results in a horizontal line across the entire width of the lens. The line is best concealed when the line coincides with the segment top of a straight top bifocal (Fig. 11-16).

A high degree of skill is necessary to grind plastic slab-off lenses. Precast or molded, semi-finished reverse slab-off lenses are now available. These lenses have base-down prism in the segment rather than removing base down prism by bicentric grinding. This lens is placed on the lens that induces the least base-down prism or the most plus or least minus power in the vertical meridian. Reverse slab-off lenses can be inventoried by the laboratory as semi-finished lenses. The optometrist can realize both reduced cost and faster delivery times compared with individually produced slab-off lenses.

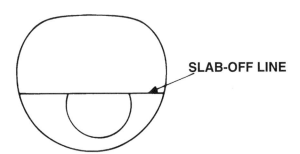

**Fig. 11-16** Reverse slab-off lens. Prescribe reverse slab-off for the lens with the least minus vertical lens power. (Reprinted from Fannin TE, Grosvenor T: *Clinical optics,* ed 2, Newton, MA, 1996, Butterworth-Heinemann.)

## REFERENCES

1.  Borish IM, Hitzeman SA, Brookman KE: Double masked study of progressive addition lenses, *J Am Optom Assoc* 51:933-43, 1980.
2.  Boroyan HJ, Cho MH, Fuller BC, et al: Lined multifocal wearers prefer progressive addition lenses, *J Am Optom Assoc* 66:296-300, 1995.
3.  Bruneni JL: Poly goes global, *Eyecare Business* April 2001: 64-7.
4.  Bruneni JL: Going grey, *Eyecare Business* December 2002:32-7.
5.  Defranco LM: Spectacle lens options for light-sensitive patients, *Refractive Eyecare for Ophthalmologists* November/December 1998, 2:22-6.
6.  Duka W, Nicholson T: Retirees rocking old roles, *AARP Bulletin* December 2002, pp. 1-2.
6a. Fannin TE, Grosvenor T: *Clinical optics,* Boston, 1996, Butterworth-Heinemann, pp. 229-30.
7.  Hofstetter HW, Griffin JR, Berman MS, et al: *Dictionary of visual science and related clinical terms,* Boston, 2000, Butterworth-Heinemann, pp 26-7.
8.  Karr A: *States find ways to aid older drivers,* AARP Bulletin, *www.aarp.org/bulletin/yourlife/Articles/a2001-06-26,* accessed October 2003.
9.  Kelleher L: *Breaking the stereotype of older adults online,* AARP, *www.aarp.org/olderwiserwired/Articles/a2003-02-20,* accessed October 2003.
10. Morgan MW: Normal age-related vision changes. In Rosenbloom A, Morgan M, editors: *Vision and aging,* Boston, 1993, Butterworth-Heinemann, pp 184, 189.
11. Pitts DG: Ocular effects of radiant energy. In Pitts DG, Kleinstein RN, editors: *Environmental vision: interactions of the eye, vision and the environment,* Stoneham, MA, 1993, Butterworth-Heinemann, p 161.
12. Rips JD: Driving and sun glare—a lethal combination, *LensTalk* April 2000.
13. Rosenthal FS, Phoon C, Bakalian AE, et al: The ocular dose of ultraviolet radiation to outdoor workers, *Invest Ophthalmol Vis Sci* 29:649, 1988.
14. Spaulding DH: Patient preference for a progressive addition multifocal lens (Varilux2) vs. a standard multifocal lens design (ST-25), *J Am Optom Assoc* 52:789-94, 1981.

15. Swanson MW: The elderly. In Benjamin W, editor: *Borish's clinical refraction,* Philadelphia, 1998, W.B. Saunders, p 1200.

16. Transitions optical monograph: light, sight, and photochromics, Pinellas Park, FL, 2002, Transitions Optical, Inc., pp 42-3.

17. Tunnicliffe AH: Dispensing single vision lenses: part one—minus lenses, *Br J Optom Dispens* 5:104-14, 1997.

# CHAPTER 12

# Contact Lenses and the Older Adult

## EDWARD S. BENNETT, BARRY A. WEISSMAN, and MELVIN J. REMBA

Contact lenses have assumed an important, if not vital, role in the visual treatment of patients of all ages because they address a wide variety of ocular conditions. Contact lens practitioners traditionally focus primarily on fitting and management of healthy, young patients with myopia and hyperopia. These individuals are typically easier to manage, with stable tear films and uncomplicated refractions. They are dexterous in handling lenses and possess good motivation for lens wear. However, ruling out any patient because of age is both unfair and unwise. The visual benefits of cosmetic contact lens wear lead to enhancement of the quality of life and subsequent patient satisfaction at almost any age. Many clinicians see a current trend in prescribing and fitting both younger and older patients with contact lenses. Reasons for expansion in the older adult population are listed in Box 12-1.[5,74]

This chapter discusses ocular conditions common to the older patient population and the role of contact lenses in correction of these conditions. Patient selection, lens design alternatives, fitting considerations, problem-solving, and psychological aspects of contact lens use by older adults are discussed. Conventional contact lenses are not within the scope of this chapter, although many older patients use such lenses well. Instead, those specific areas in contact lens practice that pertain particularly to more senior patients are emphasized: presbyopia and therapeutic applications.

## PATIENT SELECTION

Patient selection is always an important component of eventual success in contact lenses; this is especially true with older patients. Before fitting the practitioner must perform the necessary subjective and objective procedures to assess the patient's suitability and potential for successful contact lens wear and consider any contraindications. If these prefitting procedures are not performed or are performed inadequately, contact lens–induced complications and patient dissatisfaction with lens wear can result. Box 12-2 provides a checklist for the initial selection of the older patient.[63]

Obviously, some of these factors pertain more to individuals wearing cosmetic lenses (i.e., daily wear and presbyopic lenses), whereas others pertain more to the extended wear/bandage/therapeutic contact lens wearer.

Patient motivation is an extremely important factor for success because perseverance is an essential part of both physical and visual adaptation necessary with any contact lenses, especially presbyopic correction. Not only must first-time wearers be patient during the 2- to 4-week adaptation process, something with which they have not been concerned for their previous 50, 60, or more years of life experience, but they also have to learn how to handle and care for the lenses and, in some cases, they have to adapt to multiple imagery that is inherent in most bifocal lens designs. The younger patient is usually motivated solely by cosmetic factors, but the older patient may have additional motivating factors, including visual and medical considerations. A patient with monocular aphakia with good phakic vision in the opposite eye, for example, is likely to be highly motivated to wear a lens successfully to gain binocularity. Even more common now, a patient with modest myopia with evolving cataracts may be able to achieve vision with contact lenses

good enough to delay the need for surgery for several months to years.

Many older patients express anxiety about possible inability to care for the lenses; therefore encouragement and reinforcement by the practitioner and staff members are vital. The practitioner often may balance the patient's visual or medical requirements with his or her motivation, temperament, physical disabilities (if any), degree of activity, and ability to handle difficulties. In particular, patients already wearing contact lenses usually make the transition to a presbyopic contact lens correction much easier than do first-time presbyopic candidates.

The importance of comprehensive patient education cannot be underestimated. Many older patients have little idea of what a contact lens is and what options are available to them. The practitioner must take great care in explaining to the patient exactly what is involved in lens care, including handling, cost, and follow-up office visits. If the patient is quite old a spouse, child, or other family member present both at the initial discussion and, at minimum, the first few visits may be beneficial to ensure that advice and instruction are understood completely and later reinforced. In addition, older or infirm patients may benefit from assistance from family members for insertion, removal, and disinfection of contact lenses. A person who lives alone or is in any form of care facility may therefore not be a good candidate for contact lens wear, especially if manual dexterity is poor.

## ANATOMICAL AND PHYSIOLOGICAL CHANGES

General anatomical and physiological changes in the older eye are discussed in Chapter 2. Several important changes should be considered in this discussion because they specifically pertain to the prospective contact lens–wearing older patient.[5,74]

### Eyelids

With age a reduction occurs in muscle tone, amount of orbital fat, and elasticity of the eyelids. The lower lids of older individuals may not retain sufficient elastic memory to resume their customary place against the surface of the globe. This can be particularly disadvantageous in the case of alternating bifocal contact lenses, in which it is important that the prism ballasted and truncated inferior edge of the lens rest against the lower lid margin and not sag into the lower fornix. The upper eyelid also loses elasticity as a patient ages. Blepharochalasis is often present, and tonic retraction of the upper lid by Müller's muscle is diminished so that ptosis is likely. Because the superior eyelid has an important role in contact lens centration and movement, especially with rigid lenses, evaluation of lid tension before fitting is important. If rigid (non–prism ballasted) lenses are indicated, the use of both a lenticular construction with rounded edges and optimal peripheral thickness profile are important to facilitate removal. Loss of lid elasticity, common with many older patients, often requires alternative methods of lens insertion and removal (discussed later).

It is important to rule out appositional abnormalities a priori that would interfere with lens wear—such as ectropion, entropion, and lagophthalmos— although the latter two conditions are occasionally treated with bandage soft lenses that blanket the cornea to protect it from eyelash-induced foreign body irritation.[62] Trichiasis should be ruled out, or, if present, addressed with epilation before fitting.

Evidence of chronic blepharitis (e.g., irregular lid margins, seborrheic discharge, collarettes, ulcerations, or chalazia) may discourage (but not contraindicate) contact lens wear. Treatment of lid disease and subsequent tear abnormalities is usually a long-term part of contact lens care of most older patients.

### Tear Film

Tear flow is known to gradually reduce with age. Aging tends to decrease both the number and function of secretory cells responsible for lubricating the corneal surface. Goblet cells of the conjunctiva and the mass of the lacrimal glands decrease with age, resulting in a progressive reduction of tear production.[91] This decrease may be as much as a factor of four, resulting in one form of dry eye. Reduced tear flow can also result as a complication of autoimmune disease (such as rheumatoid arthritis) in the form of Sjögren's syndrome. In addition, overnight ocular exposure resulting from incomplete lid closure also compromises the lacrimal lubrication system by evaporation effects.[5] Therefore these

patients, especially if an extended-wear schedule is prescribed, should be advised to not sleep under a ceiling fan and avoid any forms of air drafts during the day, which typically act to evaporate tear fluid.

Careful evaluation of the tear film quality and quantity is essential and aids in selecting the best lens type. Because reduced tear flow results in an increase in the amount of lens surface deposition, leading to blurred vision, discomfort, and possible papillary hypertrophy, the selection of a wettable lens material and a wearing schedule compatible with tear-film function are important. Frequent use of ocular lubricants is often necessary. If a soft lens is selected, a planned replacement or disposable lens program is indicated. Unless absolutely necessary, extended wear is particularly contraindicated in cases of dry eye or lacrimal dysfunction.

Treatments beyond just palliative artificial tears and lid hygiene include both punctal occlusion and immune-modulating topical agents (e.g., steroids, cyclosporin A).

### Conjunctiva

Slit-lamp examination of the conjunctiva will determine whether it is thickened and insensitive. The presence of pingueculae and other elevations of the conjunctiva can physically lift the lids away from complete contact with the cornea, creating "lid gap." This accelerates corneal desiccation in the case of rigid lens wear (potentially inducing dellen), and pingueculae may be irritated further by soft lens wear. Therefore the bulbar conjunctiva and peripheral cornea need to be monitored in these patients. In addition, as a result of the reduction in elasticity of the conjunctival tissue, "conjunctival drag" is more apparent, making assessment of soft lens movement with the blink misleading if not carefully evaluated (i.e., the lens appears to be moving more than it actually is).

### Cornea

With aging, the cornea itself also undergoes changes that can affect contact lens wear. Corneal desiccation, manifested by a localized superficial punctate keratitis, often inferiorally, may occur as a secondary effect of reduced tear layers. Drying of the soft lens surface promotes mucoprotein and lipid lens deposition and contamination, and a tertiary diffuse epithelial staining is possible from the trapped debris. A fluorescein evaluation of the cornea under filtered (cobalt blue) slit-lamp magnification is vital before and during the fitting process with all contact lens–wearing patients, especially older adults.

A second corneal change with age is a progressive decrease in corneal sensitivity; this process is accelerated after cataract surgery and penetrating keratoplasty. Reduced corneal sensitivity can be beneficial in some cases; for example, a nervous, older, first-time wearer may discover that rigid contact lenses are not as "painful" as feared. Conversely, reduced corneal sensitivity may be detrimental in not alerting the patient early in the event of an ocular complication that should prompt medical treatment. Superior lid ptosis can decrease oxygen supply to the superior cornea.[5,6] This can become a clinically significant problem because most bifocal designs and all aphakic lenses are much thicker than conventional, or nonaphakic, lenses, further depressing oxygen supply to the cornea. Finally, degeneration of subepithelial tissues, including Bowman's membrane, and their replacement by other connective-like tissue, can result in pterygia.

The aforementioned corneal changes make selecting an oxygen-transmissible contact lens and maintaining sufficient lens lag/movement imperative to maximize tear interchange and flushing. Although high oxygen transmissibility can now be achieved with either rigid or soft materials, the "metabolic pumping" action of gas-permeable lenses may be especially advantageous. If the patient can handle the lenses and is motivated to do so, a daily wear schedule should be recommended rather than overnight wear, except for special therapeutic indications (discussed later).

## Visual Function

Older patients have to adjust to retinal luminance and contrast sensitivity decline over time as well as the loss of accommodative amplitude. Contrast needs to be increased by approximately 3× in 70% of the 60-year-old population to restore visual performance to that found in 20-year-olds.[15] Therefore, with additional reduced pupil size and opacification of the ocular media with age, older patients require

more illumination to perform near visual tasks. Target illumination may need to be doubled every 13 years over the age of 20 years to achieve equivalent dark-adapted vision.[40] This effect is compromised even further by any uncorrected errors of refraction. For mesopic vision, 1.00 D out of focus may require two to three times the amount of light, whereas a 2.00 D uncorrected error may necessitate five to six times the light.[5] Precise optical correction therefore becomes most important in the older patient to minimize the effect of reduced visual functions.

For these reasons, first performing an accurate refraction is even more important in older contact lens candidates than in younger individuals, as is performing a careful overrefraction to be incorporated in the proposed contact lens upon diagnostic fitting. In addition, contact lens wearers with presbyopia should be advised to increase the normal level of background illumination used in near tasks, especially if simultaneous vision bifocals (discussed later) have been fitted.

## Patients with Presbyopia

Any eye care professional can attest that by far the most prevalent condition generating patient concern and complaints in the middle to older age group is the loss of visual function from presbyopia. These patients also represent the largest growing segment of the population in the United States as the so-called post-WWII baby-boomers age. With approximately 78 million baby-boomers (i.e., individuals born in the United States between 1946 and 1964), a large group of potential bifocal contact lens wearers exist.[84] Of these individuals, only approximately 3% wear some form of presbyopic contact lens correction.[82,99] This age group represents the largest untapped segment of the contact lens market. Despite changes in tear volume that can result in greater symptoms of dryness with contact lens wear, patients with presbyopia remain quite viable candidates for contact lens wear.[29]

Manufacturers are attempting to meet this anticipated demand by introducing several new gas-permeable (GP) and soft bifocal designs, with others being patented and under clinical investigation. As a result of such factors as cost, perceived design and fitting complexity, limited success, and the wealth of spectacle lens advertising, the numbers of bifocal or multi-focal contact lenses fitted have traditionally been low. However, this is beginning to change as new and better designs replace older ones, manufacturing technology improves, and consumer confidence in the improved lenses and fitting skills of practitioners is established.

Several contact lens options are available for the patient with presbyopia, including single-vision contact lens wear and overreading glasses, monovision, and bifocal contact lenses. Many bifocal philosophies and designs exist, both in GP and hydrogel materials.

## SINGLE-VISION CONTACT LENS WEAR AND READING GLASSES

The use of single-vision lenses (hydrogel or GP) in combination with reading glasses affords the benefits of simplicity of fit, optimal and binocular vision at both distance and near, and limited expense. Overspectacles are usually single-vision plus add lenses but may be progressive addition, especially to assist with intermediate correction. In some cases minimal add powers are used to enhance the reading ability of patients with emerging presbyopia. However, patients with varied near and distance tasks will complain of the inconvenience of frequently putting on and removing supplemental spectacles. In addition, many patients choose contact lenses with the intent or wish of cosmetically eliminating the need for spectacles. Nevertheless, the single-vision/overspectacles option should be presented to all potential presbyopic contact lens wearers. Some patients prefer to begin with this most basic option; however, at a later date, they may change to one of the other presbyopic contact lens systems mentioned to them at the original fitting and consultation visit.

## MONOVISION

Monovision is defined as contact lens correction of one eye for distance vision and the other eye for near vision. Monovision represents the most commonly used method of presbyopic contact lens correction and is used in approximately 70% of all presbyopic fittings.[49] This form of correction has many advantages when compared with bifocal contact lenses, including (1) the use of conventional lenses because special lens designs are rarely necessary; (2) decreased professional time; (3) less expense for the patient;

(4) thinner lenses, which are more physiologically acceptable to the cornea; (5) the requirement that only one contact lens be changed for continuing distance vision lens wearers; and (6) avoidance of many of the patient symptoms/compromises present with bifocal contact lenses, including ghost images, reduced illumination, reduced contrast sensitivity, and fluctuating vision related to pupil size.

Several possible problems, however, are observed and reported from this mode of presbyopic contact lens correction, including reduced stereopsis, spatial disorientation, decreased contrast sensitivity, difficulty in resolving critical distance vision tasks, and possible liability considerations.[50] Glare and haloes contributed to decreased satisfaction with monovision under mesopic and scotopic conditions.[31] Although reduced measurable stereopsis has been found to be present as a result of monocular blur, whether this effect is often transferred into subjective problems with depth perception is arguable.[65] Therefore any reduced stereopsis compromising contact lens performance would be contraindicated if stereoacuity is occupationally important.[50] Some monocular suppression of blur occurs in monovision, which is desired; however, the blurred eye will still contribute to binocular summation.[94] The degree of suppression usually increases as the add increases.[23] Residual astigmatism has also been observed to cause a significantly greater reduction of binocular visual acuity in the monovision condition than in normal binocular conditions. This effect appears to be related to a process of meridional interocular suppression.[23] Development of anisometropia occurred significantly more often among monovision wearers than in spectacle- or contact lens–wearing control subjects. Changes in anisometropia greater than or equal to 0.50 D, with amounts up to 1.25 D, occurred in 29% of monovision wearers.[95] Contrast sensitivity function is reduced in monovision and, in high adds, binocular summation is difficult to achieve.[21,60,78] Although visual performance of patients with monovision is comparable to that of patients with non–absolute presbyopia with balanced binocular corrections, in photopic conditions blurring one eye for distance, especially in advanced presbyopia, can result in significant compromise in critical distance vision–related tasks, including night driving

---

**BOX 12-3**

## Monovision Fitting and Prescribing Considerations

- Fit patients who do not require long periods of critical distance vision.
- Perform binocular function testing to determine the effect of monovision on stereopsis.
- Demonstrate the add power effect to the patient; the patient could wear a trial frame to simulate this effect on vision. Subjective reaction to adding a plus factor to one eye can help determine the preferred distance-corrected eye.
- Select the proper eye for near; because distance vision should be less impaired, the near eye typically represents the nondominant eye or the eye in which vision is reduced relative to the other. Often, but not always, this is the left eye. This may be reversed if the patient's job involves prolonged close work or if a subjective preference is indicated during the diagnostic visit. If the patient is anisometropic, the higher myopic eye should be considered for near, with all other factors being equal.
- Prescribe the full amount of correction; it is tempting to undercorrect the near eye and overcorrect the distance eye to lessen the anisometropia. However, for optimal near and distance vision, prescribing the full add amount is preferable.
- Strongly encourage (if not require) patients with monovision to purchase either a pair of driving spectacles (i.e., minus power over near eye) or a second distance contact lens for use while driving. The patient should also be encouraged to first be a passenger in the car to experience the monovision effect before driving.[10,98]
- An informed consent that discusses the benefits and limitations of monovision as well as alternative forms of presbyopic correction (contact lens and spectacles) should be reviewed and signed by the patient.
- A handling tint in the contact lenses also is recommended to aid lens location and application.
- Although most patients adapt to monovision within 2 weeks, they nevertheless should be told 4 to 6 weeks may be required for complete adaptation. If they have difficulty in adapting, consider changing lenses (e.g., distance lens on previous near eye, and vice versa). If problems persist, refit the patient into one of the other available methods (bifocal contact lenses, single-vision contact lenses, or reading glasses).

---

and some occupations.[47,78] Finally a practitioner could possibly be held liable for any injury for which a monovision prescription could be a contributing factor.[43] The report of an aviation accident with a pilot wearing a monovision correction—which is prohibited by the Federal Aviation Administration—heightened consumer awareness of possible compromise with this form of correction.[70]

The philosophy of monovision must first be discussed with the patient. Some patients require assurance that no damage to their sight will occur. The likelihood of the need for supplementary spectacles also should be emphasized to prevent later misunderstandings. The best monovision patients have been found to be those who are driven to do their best and are conscientious, determined, cooperative, and realistic.[28]

Box 12-3 includes some fitting and prescribing considerations for monovision.[10,11]

## BIFOCAL CONTACT LENS DESIGNS

### Use

Of the 1 million presbyopic patients wearing a presbyopic contact lens correction, only 30% wear bifocal contact lenses; the other 70% wear monovision lenses.[82,99] Several reasons exist for why this figure is so low. First, a certain level of practitioner apprehension exists about the complexity and expense of the designs and potential length of time for the fitting, refitting, and adaptation. Two of the most frequently stated consumer concerns posted at a popular contact lens website (*www.contactlenses.org*) are the inability to find a practitioner to fit these lenses and reports that patients are informed that bifocal contact lenses either do not work or are not very successful.[9] Bifocal contact lens fitters can certainly argue that the visual performance of these designs, in addition to the visual freedom enjoyed by lens wearers, is a powerful benefit if the patient is aware of this option and the practitioner is willing to provide it.

### Definitions

Bifocal contact lenses are typically defined as lenses that provide two corrections: distance and near. Multifocal lenses provide a correction for more than two distances, often in a progressive manner. These designs use either the simultaneous vision or alternating vision technique and are available in soft and GP lens materials.

#### Simultaneous Vision

Simultaneous vision (also termed bivision or selective image) pertains to the vision achieved

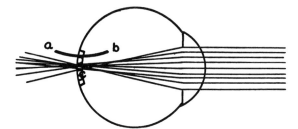

**Fig. 12-1** Ray tracing diagram showing the optical caustic formed on the retina by central and paraxial rays passing through an aspheric contact lens on the cornea.

# Concentric Bifocals

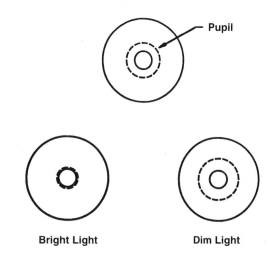

**Fig. 12-2** Relation of the pupil, in bright and dim illumination, to the fixed distance segment zone of a concentric bifocal, making this bifocal pupil dependent.

when the distance and near-power elements are positioned within the pupillary opening at the same time; light rays from both distance and near targets are therefore imaged on the retina. The patient will selectively suppress the most blurred images that are not desired for a given visual task. This concept functions on the basis of blur interpretation and blur tolerance of superimposed multiple images on the retina, which are formed by the various powers of the lens (Fig. 12-1).[5] For true simultaneous vision, the two primary segments must remain within the pupillary boundary in all positions of gaze and, to give equally bright images, the distance and near areas of the lens should cover nearly equal areas of the pupil. Three designs using the simultaneous vision concept are aspheric, concentric/annular (or target), and diffractive. Aspheric lens designs have a gradual change of curvature along one of their surfaces based on the geometry of conic sections. This rate of flattening (or eccentricity) is much greater than with aspheric single-vision lenses and creates a plus add power effect. In some aspheric multi-focals, eccentricity is located on the posterior surface and increases in plus power from the center to the periphery. Conversely, center-near aspheric lenses have their maximal plus power at the center, which then gradually decreases away from the geometrical center. Concentric or annular lens designs are structured with a small (typically two thirds to three fourths the size of the pupil in normal room illumination) annular central zone that, in most designs, provides the distance vision correction; the near correction is ground on the annulus that surrounds the distance zone (Fig 12-2). Reverse centrad concentric bifocals are constructed so that the near add

occupies the central 2- to 3-mm segment portion of the lens. Diffractive lenses function through a central diffractive zone plate that focuses images at distance by refraction of light and near through diffraction principles created by the zone eschelettes. This design is pupil independent because equal amounts of light pass through both the distance and near-power elements of the lens for all normal pupil opening diameters. All three of these simultaneous vision lens designs must center.

### Alternating Vision

Alternating vision pertains to lens designs and function in which vertical movement or translation results in only one power zone to position in front of the pupil (or visual axis) at any one time (i.e., ideally the distance zone is in front of the pupil when viewing at a distance and the near zone when viewing is at near). Essentially an intentional shifting of lens position occurs in which separate, discrete images formed by the two power segments in the lens focus on the retina with a change of gaze from distance (up) to near (down) or vice versa. Typically these designs are nonrotating by prism ballast construction, sometimes in combination with inferior truncation, which stabilizes the lens and allows a smooth translation from the superior distance zone to the inferior near zone when lowering the gaze to read. Several types of GP prism ballast lenses have been developed through the years, including decentered concentric, one-piece segmented, and fused crescent and segmented. These nonrotating segmented designs are similar to spectacle bifocals: executive and flat-top segments. They are most commonly used with rigid lens materials, although several attempts have been made to create translating ballasted hydrogel bifocals with very limited success. Alternating bifocal lenses must translate sufficiently when the patient shifts gaze from one distance to another, and this translation is attained much more easily with rigid lenses than with hydrogels. For these reasons, simultaneous image designs have been more successful when incorporated in soft lenses; translating designs are rarely used today and are not discussed in this chapter.

## GAS-PERMEABLE BIFOCAL DESIGNS

As a result of advancements in manufacturing technology, a number of new and improved lens designs have been introduced in recent years. These have included higher add aspheric multifocal designs, monocentric optics alternating designs, and alternating designs with an intermediate aspheric correction. As a result, a trend toward GP multifocal and bifocal lens fitting and away from monovision was demonstrated in the results of a recent survey of Diplomates in the Cornea and Contact Lens Section of the American Academy of Optometry.[14]

### Simultaneous Vision

Although a few GP concentric designs are still available, the most common form of simultaneous vision correction is aspheric multifocals. These designs are not strictly "simultaneous" vision. Aspheric multifocal lens designs must exhibit some upward shift or translation on downward gaze to be successful. Good candidates include any of the anatomical characteristics listed in Box 12-4.

Numerous presbyopic designs have an entirely (not peripheral only) aspheric back surface geometry. The peripheral flattening of the back surface provides a continuously variable near addition. To provide the maximal near addition, a high degree of peripheral curvature

flattening or asphericity must be used. This departure from spherical shape is known as eccentricity, or e factor. These lenses are commonly fit approximately 1.00 to 1.50 D steeper than flat corneal curvature (or K). As a result of the aspheric geometry and rate of flattening, however, an alignment or slight central clearance fluorescein pattern will be present (Fig. 12-3). High eccentricity lens designs also fit approximately 2.5 D to 3.00 D steeper than K. The best candidates for these lenses are individuals who are not good candidates for translating design bifocals. With aspheric GP lenses, generating the necessary add power within the pupillary zone is difficult without inducing disturbing aberration effects on distance vision; therefore early or emerging presbyopic patients are the best candidates. Several lens designs now incorporate higher add powers, often by a modification of the front surface resulting in increased plus power and a smaller effective distance optical zone. Achieving greater than a +1.75 D to +2.00 D effective add power is still difficult. Other candidates include any of the anatomical characteristics listed in Box 12-4.

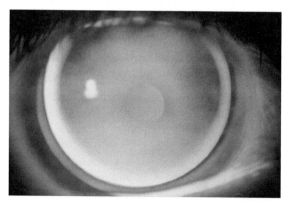

**Fig. 12-3** An optimum fitting aspheric GP multifocal.

**BOX 12-4**

### Good Aspheric GP Candidates

- Small-to-average pupil size; a larger than normal pupil size is a contraindication because of the aberrations induced, particularly at night.
- Lower lid margin well above or below limbus.
- Steep corneal curvatures.
- Loose lids that will not support prism ballast lenses.

The benefits of aspheric designs include the absence of prism and truncation in their construction. Therefore the thickness profile is similar or better than conventional single-vision lenses, which makes them a good option for the single-vision GP lens wearer who has become presbyopic. Likewise, because these lenses, if fit properly, exhibit little movement, the presbyopic athlete can benefit from them. Good intermediate vision is often obtainable because of the progressive add feature, which benefits the computer user. This design is not recommended for patients who have very critical distance vision demands, a large pupil size, or are not motivated for a GP lens design.

When fitting these lenses, a well-centered fitting relationship with minimal movement with the blink is desired. With the ease of fitting these lenses, an empirical method has been recommended.[1] This has the benefit of allowing the new multifocal wearer to experience the potential visual benefits immediately, which in turn may lessen the perception of initial awareness. The use of a topical anesthetic at the initial application will also be beneficial in enhancing the initial experience.[12] The use of either loose trial lenses or ±0.25/0.50 D flip lenses is preferred to a phoropter for overrefracting. Likewise, it is important to have the patient walk around the office and perform common tasks (e.g., look at a magazine, computer, off at a distance) to determine the initial level of satisfaction and perhaps what improvements may be necessary.

Excessive decentration or excessive movement will result in variable and generally unsatisfactory vision at all distances. When this occurs, steepening the base curve by, at minimum, 0.50 D may solve the problem. Increasing the overall diameter may likewise be beneficial. Another problem pertains to the patient with presbyopia who requires a higher effective add power than the lens is able to provide. Many designs now provide multiple add powers. For example, a popular design is the Essentials Multifocal (Blanchard Laboratories, Manchester, NH), which has Series I (low add), Series II (medium add), and Series III (high add) lens designs. Conforma Laboratories (Hampton Roads, Va.) manufactures a popular high-eccentricity design (VFL 3), which is also available in the model SuperAdd. Nevertheless, particularly for

---

**BOX 12-5**

**Modified Bifocal Candidates**

- Slightly overcorrect one eye for optimal near vision while only slightly compromising distance vision.
- Use a lower add bifocal on one eye (e.g., Series II) and a higher add on the other eye (e.g., Series III). Low plus power reading spectacles for occasional use (e.g., small print, low illumination).

---

advanced presbyopic individuals and those exhibiting a smaller than average pupil size, achieving a sufficient effective add for near work is often difficult. Therefore a modified bifocal approach is recommended. This could include any one of the approaches listed in Box 12-5.

### Alternating Vision

Two types of alternation (translating) bifocal GP designs are available. These are more commonly used than the simultaneous type bifocals. These include concentric and segmented lens designs.

#### Annular/Concentric

The front or back surface concentric designs are also know as target bifocals. These designs typically have a 3- to 5-mm central distance zone that is decentered to the superior part of the lens, and prism and truncation are present to prevent lens rotation and facilitate translation when shifting gaze. For example, a common design incorporates 1 to 1.5 prism diopters with a small amount of truncation. The distance zone is decentered 1 to 2 mm superiorly.

When the patient shifts gaze inferiorly to read, the near zone of the lens should translate into the proper position in front of the pupil as the lens is held by the lower lid margin, and the eye rotates downward. Thus the term "alternating vision" is used. This is the mechanism by which all translating lenses function.

Good candidates for this design, as well as for all other prism ballast segmented bifocals, include patients with a lower lid margin tangent to, or slightly above, the limbus; an 8.5-mm or larger vertical fissure size; normal (not loose) lid tension; and myopic/low hyperopic refractive powers. The benefits of these lenses include the ability to achieve precise correction and good vision at distance and near unaccompanied by secondary images, assuming proper

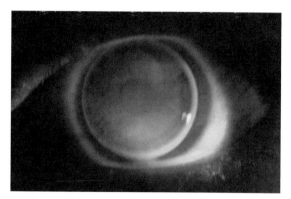

**Fig. 12-4** The Mandell Seamless Bifocal.

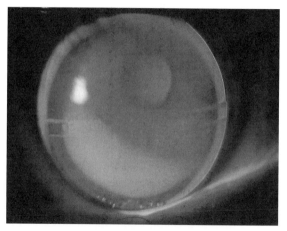

**Fig. 12-5** Tangent Streak trifocal design.

fit, minimal lens rotation, and consistent translation. In addition, any amount of presbyopic adds can be successfully corrected. The disadvantages may include the increased center thickness required with a prism ballast, although the translating concentrics are the thinnest of the prism ballast bifocals. With annular segments, specification of a distance zone large enough to minimize distance flare is important. Finally, image jump, due to prismatic effects resulting from the bicentric construction of these lenses, can result in patient problems during gaze shift with concentric, translating bifocals. Some representative fitting problems and methods of managing them are listed below. These are applicable to all types of prism ballast, including segment type bifocal GP lenses.

These lenses are often fitted slightly flatter than K because heavy GP lenses tend to decenter inferiorly when a flat base curve is selected, a desirable characteristic with a translating lens design because the inferior edge should position adjacent or very close to the lower lid. A new concentric annular design, the Mandell Seamless Bifocal (Con-Cise, San Leandro, Calif.), provides an aspheric transition zone between the distance and near annular zones. It is a front surface concentric design with central distance zone diameters ranging from 3.0 to 3.8 mm and an average overall diameter of 9.8 mm (Fig. 12-4).[24,42,61,85]

### Segmented

Although more complex in design, perhaps the most successful bifocal contact lenses from a visual standpoint are the GP segmented translating designs. These lenses have had a long history of development and refinement during the "polymethylmethacrylate years," 1960 to 1980. Segmented one-piece GP bifocals are now available with monocentric optics. Monocentric means that the optical centers of the lens power zones are coincident and image jump when viewing from one section of the lens to another is eliminated. This benefit was, at one time, limited to fused bifocal designs. However, because of the difficulty in fusing the softer GP lens materials, the near and distance optical centers were manufactured to be coincident at a tangent at the segment line—as a result of the pioneering work of George Tsuetaki of Fused Kontacts. Thus the introduction of the Tangent Streak (Firestone Optics, Kansas City, Kan.) lens in the 1980s repopularized segmented translating bifocals. The Tangent Streak, like all prism ballasted designs, is typically provided in a high oxygen permeability material to provide sufficient oxygen transmission. A full range of powers and geometries is also available because the lenses are custom designed by the clinician. It is heavily prism ballasted (1.75 to 4.00 prism diopters available) and truncated. The segment shape is similar to an "executive" bifocal; the seg can be ordered at any height, and a trifocal version of this lens is also available (Fig. 12-5).

The following diagnostic lens specifications are recommended (20 lenses) by the manufacturer:

| | |
|---|---|
| Base curve radius (BCR): | 41.00 D to 45.50 D |
| Seg height: | 4.2 mm |
| Optical power: | ±2.00 D |
| Add: | +2.00 D |
| Overall diameter (OAD) | 9.4/9.0 mm |

Some of the same fitting principles (e.g., anesthetic use [for a new wearer], loose trial lenses, or flipper bars) used with aspheric patients also apply to the patient requiring an alternating design. However, these lenses, like all alternating designs, are fit slightly flatter than K. The lens rests on the lower lid during distance gaze and the seg line should be positioned at or slightly below the lower pupil margin (Fig. 12-6). The lens must decenter (translate) 2 mm or more on downward gaze to obtain near point add. The position typically varies between 1.75 and 3.00 prism diopters and increases with increases in minus power and increased add power.

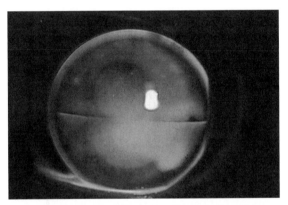

**Fig. 12-6** An optimally fitting Tangent Streak lens.

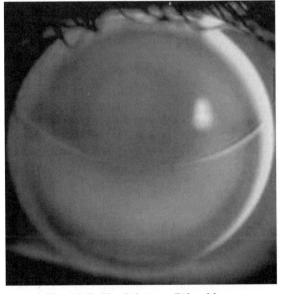

**Fig. 12-7** The Solutions Bifocal lens.

The lens should ride with its lower edge supported by the lower lid margin. With the patient fixating straight ahead, the lens is usually picked up 1 to 2 mm on the blink and then quickly drops back to the lower position. This phenomenon of prism ballasted lens movement is termed lens "lift and recovery."

Several popular segmented lens designs are available, including Metro-Seg (Metro Optics, Austin, Tex.), Solitaire II (Tru-Form Optics, Dallas, Tex.), and Solutions (X-Cel, Atlanta, Ga.). The latter design is a representative example of current efforts to make these designs easy to fit. It is a crescent design that is fit similarly to the Tangent Streak in terms of base curve radius and seg position (Fig. 12-7). However, it is available in only three prism amounts (low, medium, and high) and five seg heights. The standard design is not truncated and the diagnostic set has medium prism, an intermediate seg height, a 9.6-mm overall diameter, and similar distance and near powers as the Tangent Streak diagnostic set.

Good candidates for this design are similar to other translating bifocals and are listed in Box 12-6.

Patients with high hyperopia may have more difficulty because of the increased thickness of the prism ballasted plus lenses. Individuals with loose lids may not be able to maintain proper alignment of the thicker inferior edge on the lower lid margin with downward gaze. The advantages of this design are the same as for the translating concentric designs; however, the segmented designs have the advantages of having a larger distance zone and the absence of image jump. The disadvantages primarily pertain to the thickness inherent in their construction and the importance of achieving

---

**BOX 12-6**

**Candidates for Segmented Bifocal GP Lenses**

- Early and advanced presbyopia
- Lower lid above, tangent to, or no more than 0.5 mm below the limbus
- Myopia and low hyperopic powers
- Normal to large palpebral fissure sizes
- Normal to tight lid tension

## Potential Problems with Segmented GP Lens Designs

- Insufficient or lack of translation. This may be resolved by increasing the amount of edge clearance to allow the lens edge to exhibit more contact with the lower lid. This can be accomplished by selecting a flatter base curve lens or, alternatively, flattening the peripheral curve radius. If this change is not beneficial and the lens is still not translating, it is most likely the result of a flaccid lower lid, which becomes more problematic with age.
- Excessive rotation with the blink. This is often the result of a base curve radius that is too steep. Flattening the base curve radius by 0.50 D will often allow the lens to fall quicker to the lower lid and not be prone to the rotational effects of the upper lid.
- The lens exhibits excessive movement with the blink. If the lens is picked up too superiorly with the blink, increasing the prism should result in less upward displacement.

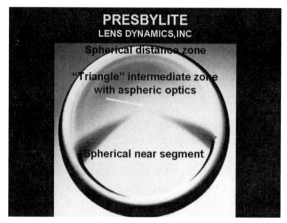

**Fig. 12-8** The Presbylite segmented multifocal lens design.

translation with downward gaze. Potential problems are listed in Box 12-7.[8]

Another problem with segmented translating designs is the absence of an intermediate correction for the patient with advanced presbyopia. A few of the segmented bifocal lens designs are also available in a trifocal (Tangent Streak Trifocal from Firestone Optics and both Llevations and Solitaire I from Tru-Form Optics). Several recently introduced lens designs have also eliminated this problem. The Presbylite lens (Lens Dynamics, Golden, Colo.) is a nontruncated lens design with 1.5 $^\Delta$. This lens design incorporates a spherical distance zone, spherical near zone, and a unique triangle-shaped aspheric intermediate zone (Fig. 12-8).[24] The Solitaire II (Tru-Form Optics) is a nontruncated executive design that incorporates a small aspheric zone on the front of the lens between the near and distance zones for intermediate vision. The X-Cel ESSential-Solution segmented aspheric multifocal is the result of a combined effort of two of the leading GP bifocal manufacturers (X-Cel and Blanchard).[71] The posterior geometry of this design generates approximately 1.00 D of add power. The front surface is similar to the X-Cel Solutions Bifocal with a crescent-shaped segment configuration.

Translating GP lenses yield the highest success rate of any contact lens bifocals available today, but their fitting requires precise measurement of anterior eye anatomy, familiarity with the translating concept, use of a reliable diagnostic lens, and a willingness to consult with the experts at the fabricating laboratory. Many resources are available (e.g., clinical management guide, laminated pocket card, fitting and problem-solving videotape and C/D-ROM) as well as a listing of all of the Contact Lens Manufacturer's Association member laboratories and the bifocal and multifocal lens designs they manufacture available from the GP Lens Institute (*www.gpli.info*).

## SOFT BIFOCAL/MULTIFOCAL DESIGNS

Soft bifocal and multifocal lens designs have certain limitations compared with their GP counterparts. The quality of vision is somewhat compromised as a result of both the water content and the specific multifocal design. In fact, the term "20/Happy" has been ascribed to these lenses because their best corrected vision may be reduced compared with their best spectacle corrected acuity, but the patient is satisfied. Some individuals with presbyopia are so motivated not to wear spectacles that they are satisfied with a multiple-line Snellen acuity reduction; however, this becomes an ethical issue for the practitioner. Likewise, the inability of these designs to translate negates an important benefit for optimizing near vision with GP designs. However, numerous improvements in both lens design and replacement have resulted in greater use and success with soft lenses than in the past. Perhaps the most important change has been the availability of these designs in frequent replacement and disposable modalities. As tear volume decreases with age, the impact of deposits should be minimized, both on ocular health and quality of vision. In addition, although these designs use the simultaneous vision principle, the ability to vary the design between eyes to optimize vision at various distances is present. This is important because of the large number of single-vision soft lens wearers who would prefer to continue soft lens wear as they become more presbyopic.

Good candidates for soft bifocal lenses include the current single-vision soft lens wearer who has become presbyopic, dissatisfied monovision wearers, those with low (or no) refractive astigmatism, and individuals who do not have a critical distance vision demand.

Several lens designs are currently available. The easiest method of differentiating commonly used soft bifocal and multifocal designs is by whether the design is center distance or center near.

### Center-Distance Design

Center-distance lens designs can be either aspheric or concentric, although most are concentric in design. Common designs in this category include the Acuvue Bifocal (Vistakon, Jacksonville, Fla.), Frequency 55 Multifocal (CooperVision, Fairport, NY), and UltraVue (Acuity One, Scottsdale, Ariz.).

A popular center-distance concentric design is the Acuvue Bifocal. In lieu of a more conventional two-zone design, this lens is multizone with five alternating distance and near zones (Fig. 12-9).[13,36] The multizone design enhances distance and near power coverage of the pupil as it dilates or constricts with contact lens movement. It is available in 0.25 D increments from +4.00 D to -6.00 D with +1.00 D to +2.50 D adds in 0.50 D increments. The lenses are replaced every 2 weeks.

The benefits to this lens design, as with other frequent replacement lenses, includes the ability to fit directly from inventory and to allow the

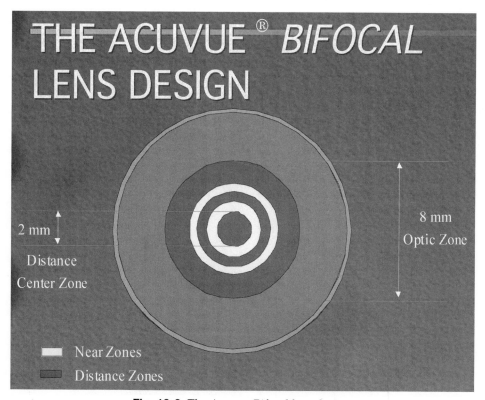

**Fig. 12-9** The Acuvue Bifocal lens design.

patient to try the lenses for a designated period (often 1 week). The lens can be fine tuned at that time if a change is indicated. According to Rigel,[81] 51% will be successful with the full binocular approach. A total of 32% were successful with a modified bifocal approach (adding plus power to the distance prescription of the nondominant eye to enhance near vision). A total of 17% were fitted with the enhanced monovision approach (fitting the nondominant eye with a single-vision lens for near and

reducing the add power of the Acuvue Bifocal in the dominant eye). Lee[54] recommends the guidelines listed in Box 12-8 for problem solving reduced vision with the Acuvue Bifocal. Importantly, 75% of successfully fitted patients have a distance prescription within ±0.25 D of the best corrected sphere.[59]

The Frequency 55 Multifocal is derived from the UltraVue lens design from Acuity One. This design combines multifocal optics with monovision. A center distance lens, which transitions through an aspheric intermediate to an outer near zone, is placed on the dominant eye. A center near lens, which transitions through an aspheric intermediate to a spherical peripheral distance zone, is placed on the nondominant eye (Fig. 12-10).[46,76,90] Binocular summation is expected, providing acceptable vision at all distances under binocular conditions. The central zone sizes are different between the distance lens (2.3 mm) and near lens (1.7 mm) to emphasize the visual performance at the emphasized vision demand zone. As with the Acuvue Bifocal, it is available in one overall diameter and base curve. It is available in +1.50 D, +2.00 D, and +2.50 D Adds and is recommended to be replaced monthly. In a multicenter study, on average patients had 0.12 D greater Add with the Frequency 55 Multifocal nondominant lens compared with their vision with spectacles in the same eye.[46] The patient should be advised about possible shadowing and ghost images,

---

**BOX 12-8**

### Acuvue Bifocal Problem-Solving

■ Distance single-vision Acuvue on dominant eye and Acuvue Bifocal on nondominant eye for patients with critical distance vision demands

■ Acuvue Bifocal on the dominant eye and Acuvue single-vision lens in dominant eye for patients with extremely fine near work

■ Both eyes wearing Acuvue Bifocals with less add on the dominant eye to provide greater intermediate correction if needed

■ Fit Acuvue Bifocals on both eyes but increase the distance plus power on the nondominant eye (modified monovision) to increase the effective add

■ Use a single Acuvue Bifocal contact lens on the dominant eye of patients with low myopia or on the nondominant eye of those with low hyperopia.

(Adapted from Lee WC: Factors for fitting success, *Contact Lens Spectrum* 14:7a, 1999.)

---

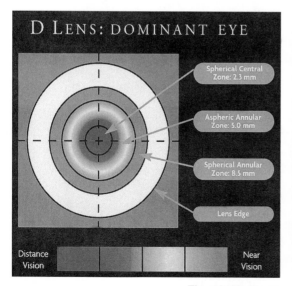
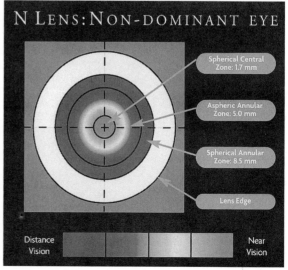

**Fig. 12-10** The Frequency 55 Multifocal.

which may be adaptational, and to return in 4 to 7 days.[90] Changes in lens design can be expected with 20% to 40% of the patients at the first follow-up visit.

The UltraVue lens design is similar to the Frequency 55 lens. The Ultravue P lens (add in the periphery) is designed for the dominant eye and has a spherical central zone for distance vision.[16] The central zone is surrounded by an aspheric, annular zone that creates a gradual refractive shift toward plus power and offers intermediate and near visual function. The UltraVue C lens (add in the center) is designed with a spherical central near vision zone surrounded by an aspheric, annular zone that creates a gradual refractive shift toward minus power and offers intermediate and distance visual function. The goal is to achieve 20/20 distance vision and 20/40 near vision from the UltraVue P lens and vice versa from the UltraVue C lens.

### Center-Near Design

Several aspheric or progressive near-center lens designs are available. An example of this design is the Focus Progressive (Ciba Vision, Duluth, Ga.). This is a center-near aspheric lens design with a 2-week to 1-month replacement schedule (Fig. 12-11).[13,85] It is approved for up to six nights of extended wear and has two base curve radii. The add is reported to be a nominal add that could provide up to 3.00 D, although patients with advanced presbyopia do not often need to add +0.50 to 0.75 D over the nondominant eye.[77] In a comparison study, the Focus

Progressive resulted in significantly better distance vision and was rated higher in comfort and handling by patients when comparing its performance to the Acuvue Bifocal.[32] These results were not consistent, however, with a recent study by Guillon et al.[39] Ciba Vision recently unveiled Focus Dailies Progressive, which is available in one base curve and discarded daily.

### Diffractive Bifocals

The only diffractive bifocal lens design available today is the Echelon (Ocular Sciences, Concord, Calif.). This design uses a diffraction zone plate to separate light rays equally to both the distance and near focal images. The distance power is refracted, and the near power is achieved by the diffractive principles. The major advantage of this design is pupil size independence. The near diffractive power is achieved through the circular annular grooves (echelettes) on the back surface of the lens and the refractive index of the tear layer that pools behind the grooves. The radii and spacing of the annular grooves determine the add power of the lens. This posterior diffractive zone is approximately 4.00 to 4.5 mm in diameter, located at the center of the line, and the entire lens contains the distance power. The central zone plate can easily be observed against the dark background of the pupil with biomicroscopy. When fitting this lens, the use of trial lenses to assess fit, centration, and power determination by overrefraction is essential (Fig. 12-12).[89] If only slight decentration is present, the patient can still achieve success with the Echelon lens; however, more add power may be required in this case. In addition as, at

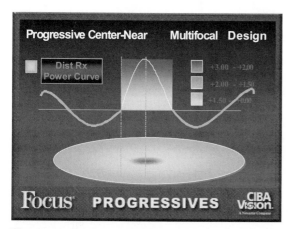

**Fig. 12-11** The Focus Progressive multifocal design. (Courtesy Ciba Vision, Duluth, Ga.)

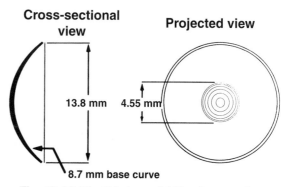

**Fig. 12-12** The Echelon soft bifocal contact lens.

minimum, half of the illumination is lost to higher orders of diffraction, the illumination should be high when the patient is performing near tasks. However, whereas the Echelon and other simultaneous vision soft bifocal/multifocal lenses compromise distance binocular contrast sensitivity, two experimental diffractive/refractive soft multifocal lens designs from Austria were recently found to result in no compromise in this function.[87]

A limitation to the aforementioned lens designs is the correction of astigmatism. Several lens designs are available, although they are custom and not available in planned replacement or disposable forms. The Horizon 55 BiCon Toric (Westcon Contact Lens, Grand Junction, Colo.) is a concentric center-near lens that can correct as much as 5.00 D of astigmatism and +3.00 D of add.[13,42] The UCL Multifocal Toric (United Contact Lens, Everett, Wash.) has an aspheric back surface that results in a center-distance design. The Essential Soft Toric Multifocal (Blanchard Laboratories) has a front aspheric, center-near design with posterior astigmatic correction and anterior double slab-off for stability. The UltraVue 2000 Multifocal Progressive Toric (Opti-Centre Laboratories, Sherbrooke, Quebec, Canada) is available with a center-distance design and a center-near design for the dominant and nondominant eyes with up to +3.50 D add power.

## LENS SELECTION

### Success Rates

The low lens cost, ease of fitting, and relatively high success rates (often 70% to 90%) achieved with monovision have made it a popular technique for presbyopic contact lens correction among practitioners.[22,50,92] A comparable, if not higher, success rate (75% to 86%) appears to be present with GP multifocal and bifocal lens designs.[18,52,57,80,97] Most traditional soft bifocal studies resulted in only a 40% to 50% success rate.[27,30,41,44] However, with the introduction of innovative new designs and frequent replacement modalities, this success rate is currently higher.[73] Nevertheless, the need to screen patients and use an adequate and reliable diagnostic set of the desired bifocal lens design is imperative.

Comparison studies have shown, however, that when given a choice bifocal contact lenses are often preferred to monovision and exhibit improved objective performance. Kirschen et al[53] found that Acuvue Bifocal lenses provided a lower interocular difference in visual acuity than monovision, which resulted in improved stereoacuity and a lower prevalence of suppression at distance and near. Johnson et al[48] fit subjects with GP monovision for 6 weeks followed by 6 weeks of the Boston Multivision GP aspheric design (or vice versa). At the conclusion of the study 75% of the subjects preferred the multifocal design. Therefore, if given the choice, patients will likely prefer a multifocal/bifocal lens design. Experts in the field are recommending that bifocal contact lenses be positioned ahead of monovision when presenting presbyopic contact lens options to interested patients.[4,14]

Rajagopalan[79] assessed the contrast sensitivity function of subjects wearing GP multifocals, soft bifocals, and GP monovision lenses. The results showed that GP multifocal lens wearers exhibited the highest contrast sensitivity function at all spatial frequencies. Soft bifocal wearers exhibited a significantly lower contrast sensitivity function: however, their performance was significantly improved compared with monovision. Several recent studies have found subjective preference to be similar between soft bifocals and monovision, with the latter requiring fewer lenses to achieve an optimal fit.[33,38]

Extended wear is not recommended for older patients, particularly because complication rates for all extended wear soft lenses is approximately four to six times that of daily wear.[75]

### Factors Important to Patient Success

A summary of important factors in the fitting of contact lens multifocal and bifocal designs is shown in Box 12-9. The most important considerations are the visual demands and expectations of the patient.[19] The first lens of choice for those individuals who lower their gaze to perform their work is a translating GP segment design. Patients who need intermediate or near vision while viewing in the primary position of gaze would benefit from a simultaneous bifocal such as an aspheric, or annular, design. Aspheric GP multifocals or soft lens designs, often used in some form of modified bifocal technique, are

**BOX 12-9**

## Bifocal/Multifocal Contact Lens Fitting Guidelines

- Be sure to indicate to the patient the differences between the selected contact lens bifocal and spectacles. Some vision compromise may exist, and a few lenses may be required to achieve the best fit and quality of vision.
- When possible, provide lenses in their prescription so they can comment on perceived strengths and weaknesses. Likewise, have the patient walk around the office and determine if any commonly performed task is being significantly compromised by the lenses.
- Use trial lenses or flip lenses as opposed to a phoropter to overrefract.
- Determine what the patient's primary visual goals are and attempt to meet them; although not typically necessary, the patient should be told that spectacles may be necessary for occasional tasks. The goal is to meet, at minimum, 80% of visual needs and goals.
- Emphasize the bifocal option compared with the other contact lens options.
- Allow sufficient time (15-20 minutes) for the lenses to settle before assessing the lens-to-cornea fitting relation.
- Be willing to try different types (GP and soft) to achieve success.
- Do not hesitate to prescribe unequal Adds.
- Check vision binocularly to simulate a real-world environment.

popular for most patients who do not have a critical distance vision demand and perform tasks (e.g., computer use) that require intermediate correction. The anatomical considerations, such as pupil size and lower lid position, are critical when fitting a GP lens design. Simulating the patients' working environment during the screening visit is preferable when determining the type and powers of a presbyopic contact lens correction with the aid of trial lenses. At minimum, one translating GP trial set, one aspheric GP trial set, and two or three different soft simultaneous design trial sets or inventories should be sufficient for good patient screening and success assessment. Ordering lenses on a warranty basis is preferable initially; once experience has been gained with a particular GP bifocal lens, the additional fee for a warranty may not be necessary. For the many patients who are beginning presbyopia and are long-term, successful single-vision con-

tact lens wearers, staying with the same lens material, GP or soft, is best when refitting with a multifocal lens.

What about the role of monovision? Certainly the controversy continues regarding how monovision should be positioned in the practice, whether as a first or last choice. Although monovision is a viable option, unless definite contraindications are found, assessing patient response to a bifocal diagnostic lens fitting before choosing monovision empirically as the first presbyopic contact lens option is preferable.

## PATIENT EDUCATION AND LENS CARE

Patients with presbyopia, especially new contact lens wearers, need to be thoroughly educated about proper lens care and handling. Contact lens wear can be intimidating for the patient who has never worn contact lenses and who also may have been exposed to negative experiences or complications from friends and relatives. In addition, these individuals need to be monitored closely because of possible complications that may arise from the physiological changes of the aging eye and to reinforce compliance with lens care procedures.

### Care and Handling

The keys for successful handling of contact lenses by the patient with presbyopia are patience and reassurance. These older individuals, especially the novice wearer, will be apprehensive and lack confidence. No matter how frustrated the individual performing the instruction may feel, that emotion must not be conveyed to the patient. The instructions must be provided slowly and on a one-to-one basis. The patient should never have the perception that the optometrist has lost confidence in his or her ability to handle the lenses properly; otherwise, feelings of failure and surrender may result. Conversely, if the patient feels confident about handling the lenses, the feeling of accomplishment improves the motivation to succeed.

The key to successful insertion and removal of both soft and GP lenses is proper manipulation of the lid. For insertion, the fingers are positioned over the lashes, or close to the lid margins while retracting the lids; the lenses can be inserted easily no matter how much resistance is initially present. This is especially important with the older patient who usually has loose lids. If improperly performed, the lids may evert, resulting in insufficient pressure to either insert or remove the contact lens. The customary lid pull "scissors" technique is used

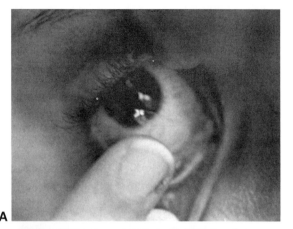

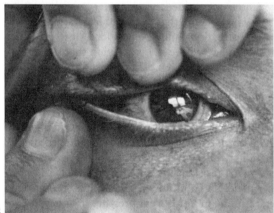

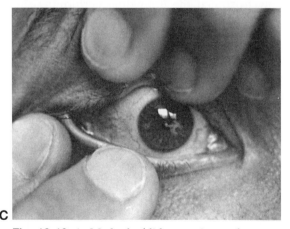

**Fig. 12-13 A,** Method of lid retraction and contact lens insertion best suited for most presbyopic contact lens users. **B,** "Scissors" method of rigid lens removal. **C,** "Squeeze" or ejection method of rigid lens removal.

to remove rigid lenses. Both hands should be used to execute a lens ejection technique. The middle and index fingers of the same hand as the eye are positioned over the lower lid, and the middle and index fingers of the opposite hand hold up the upper lid (Fig. 12-13). The lids are then pulled laterally and, while the patient blinks, the lens is ejected. The lid margins are responsible for the lens ejection. Some patients may experience difficulty in fully opening the lid aperture when inserting a soft lens because of the larger diameter. Once again, both hands should be used to fully retract the lids for soft lens insertion. The middle finger of the opposite hand should be placed underneath the upper lashes; with the lens on the forefinger of the same hand as the eye, the middle finger of this hand is placed over the lower lashes. This should create a sufficient aperture for direct lens placement on the eye. Soft lens removal may be accomplished by the usual decentration and "punching" method or by ejection from pressure of the upper and lower lid margins against the lens edges, pressing into the globe. During the training visit, a minimum of three successful insertions and removals is recommended, although the number depends on the level of the patient's confidence. It may require two or three visits (closely spaced to maximize memorization of the technique and to minimize further anxiety) for the patient to master lens handling. This is occasionally necessary with the patient with presbyopia and hyperopia who is apprehensive and may have difficulty seeing the lens because of the short working distance involved in lens preparation. To assist with this problem, especially with the patient with absolute presbyopia, ordinary reading spectacles can be worn up to the time of lens insertion. In addition, special magnifying lens insertion aids are available, or an illuminated makeup mirror may be useful.

### Educational Methods

Comprehensive education of the presbyopic patient is advised. A four-step process has been recommended.[7] This should include a written manual, verbal education, video education, and re-education.

Instruction manuals for soft and GP lenses are available from all manufacturers and other sources. A patient instruction manual should be

BOX 12-10

**Requirements for Proper Contact Lens Instruction Manuals**

- Benefits of contact lens wear (rigid or soft)
- Insertion and removal
- Cleaning techniques
- Normal and abnormal adaptation symptoms
- Importance of adhering to prescribed wearing schedule
- Causes of reduced wear
- Importance of recommended care regimen
- Spare pairs, spectacles
- Service agreement
- Cosmetic use
- Caring for the lens case

comprehensive and written in layman's language, with print quality that makes it easy to read, understand, and comply with the information presented. This manual should include the information found in Box 12-10.

It also can contain a patient agreement that has the individual office policy on issues such as payment and refund policy, care regimen, and what to do in case of an emergency. This should be signed in duplicate by the patient. This agreement can serve as an informed consent for medicolegal purposes. A special informed consent for monovision patients has been recommended.[43] It should indicate the benefits and possible hazards with monovision in addition to mentioning that alternative forms of vision correction were discussed with the patient. The instruction manuals may be customized by the practitioner and should be printed professionally or by a desktop publishing system. Graphics showing how to handle the lenses are beneficial. These can be provided by a graphic artist or can be obtained from Anadem Publications, Inc. (PO Box 14385, Columbus, OH 43214). The standard educational booklets from Anadem can be customized to the practitioner's satisfaction. Additional useful patient education material is available from manufacturers of presbyopic lenses.

In addition to instructions on handling, the patient needs to be instructed on the functions of the various solutions and how to properly use them. The most important information contained in the manual or patient brochure should be discussed with the patient, and the patient should be encouraged to ask questions.

In fact, the patient should be asked to review how to use the solutions to ensure compliance of cleaning, rinsing, and disinfection steps. Verbal and visual (demonstrated) educational processes are much more important than the written because patients cannot be expected to understand all the information provided and, on occasion, the manual may not be read at all.

A more innovative and effective method of patient education is the use of videotapes on care and handling to supplement the instructional manual and verbal information. A generic rigid lens care and handling videotape is available from the GP Lens Institute/Contact Lens Manufacturers Association (800-344-9060). If any reservations exist pertaining to a patient's ability to handle or care for contact lenses, a videotape reviewed together in the office or for frequent viewing at home would be an excellent supplement to the instruction manual.

Finally, lens care instructions and care compliance should be reinforced at every follow-up visit. For example, patients should be asked to repeat the name and use of the solutions they are currently using, if they have any questions about handling, the condition of their case if available (the optometrist may want to replace the case at regular intervals, such as every 3 months), how they are caring for the lenses, and the wearing schedule. One study showed that if the manufacturer's recommended care instructions are reinforced at every progress visit, only 6% of the solution samples were contaminated; if the care instructions were not reinforced, more than 50% of the samples were contaminated.[96] All these suggestions become more important for the aging patient, who is more likely to forget.

**Care Regimen**

Every product in the care kit provided to a new GP or soft lens patient should be explained because each component is part of a system. Not every patient will carefully read and understand product labels and care instructions. Patients may believe that their wetting/soaking solution also cleans the lenses, or that their cleaning solution is also used for wetting and soaking. If each product is explained and the patient still appears to be confused, the specific care instructions for each care product can be provided in written form. In addition, a large label can be placed on each bottle specifically indicating its function.

The decrease in tear quality and volume that occurs with age, which contributes to lens deposits, makes careful explanation mandatory of the importance of proper and regular cleaning and enzyme use to minimize deposit-related problems. Rewetting drops are frequently prescribed, and their proper application should be reinforced.

### Follow-up Care

Patients with presbyopia who wear contact lenses should be regularly monitored, preferably every 6 months. As a result of their predisposition for dryness-related problems, a careful silt-lamp evaluation with contact lens wear is important. The surface condition and wettability of the worn lens should be carefully evaluated, and aging lenses with deposits must be replaced. If feasible (i.e., with monovision), a 1- to 3-month planned replacement program should be used with soft lens–wearing patients. With lenses off, the cornea should be evaluated with fluorescein dye and the upper eyelids should be everted to rule out papillary changes. In addition, because the bifocal lens designs are often thicker than their single-vision counterparts, the cornea should be evaluated for the presence of corneal edema resulting from possible hypoxia. If striae, central corneal clouding, or another form of edema is present, a thinner design and higher oxygen-transmissible material are indicated. Keratometry and refraction also should be performed during follow-up visits, notably with patients wearing the thicker bifocal designs, in which undesirable curvature and refractive changes may occur.

The presbyopic contact lens market is growing every year. Numerous companies are developing new multifocal lenses in hopes of capturing the baby-boomers, who have, or are reaching, presbyopic age. The cosmetic and sometime functional benefits of contact lenses should therefore be a recommended option for every contact lens–using presbyopic patient and for the many who are becoming aware of multifocal contact lenses. Every patient with presbyopia should not automatically be considered for monovision; in fact, a bifocal diagnostic fitting should be considered as the first option for most presbyopes. Finally, comprehensive education and follow-up care should be performed to ensure patient confidence with care and handling, verify compliance with the care regimen, and minimize the risks associated with contact lens wear.

### THERAPEUTIC (BANDAGE) CONTACT LENS

When a contact lens is applied to heal or protect the eye, as opposed to correct vision or as a cosmetic aid, it is considered a therapeutic, or "bandage," contact lens. This is not a new concept; contact lenses have been used to protect eyes for almost 100 years, beginning with scleral shells[72] and continuing through the early use of hydrogels.[35]

Hydrogel contact lenses in particular have emerged as valuable devices in managing many corneal diseases over the last several decades, with the broad clinical goals listed in Box 12-11.[67]

Most patients who are aided by these bandage hydrogel contact lenses are older. The diseases treated tend to be chronic, use of theses lenses is often on an extended wear basis, and because of this use and the coexistence of other multiple disease processes, both ocular and systemic, these patients are known to be more at risk for corneal infection.[17,26,51]

---

**BOX 12-11**

### Hydrogel Contact Lens Benefits

- Reduction of pain from corneal epithelial defects
- Facilitation and maintenance of corneal epithelial healing
- Protection of the cornea from desiccation (drying)
- Protection of the cornea from mechanical damage from entropion and trichiasis
- Restoration of the anterior chamber after collapse from small corneal perforations
- Drug delivery

---

(Adapted from Mondino BJ, Weissman BA, Manthey R: Therapeutic soft contact lenses. In Stenson SM, editor: *Contact lenses: a guide to selection, fitting and management of complications*, Norwalk, CT, 1987, Appleton & Lange, pp 155-83.)

**TABLE 12-1**

## Parameters of Current FDA-Approved Therapeutic Hydrogel Contact Lenses

| Lens Name & Source | Water Content (%) | Base Curves (mm) | Approximate Center Thickness (mm) | Overall Diameter (mm) |
|---|---|---|---|---|
| **Low Dk** | | | | |
| Softcon (Lombart) | 55 | 8.1/8.4/8.7 | 0.35/0.10 | 14.0/14.5 |
| Plano T/Bausch & Lomb | 39 | Spin cast | 0.17 | 14.5 |
| Permalens/Cooper | 71 | 7.7/8.0/8.3 | 0.10 | 13.5 |
| | | 8.6 | 0.10 | 14.2 |
| CSIT/CIBA | 39 | 8.6/8.9/9.4 | 0.03 | 14.8 |
| | | 8.6/8.9 | 0.03 | 13.8 |
| **High Dk** | | | | |
| Focus Night & Day/CIBA | 24 | 8.4/8.6 | 0.1 | 13.8 |

*FDA*, Food and Drug Administration; *Dk*, oxygen permeability of the lens material.
NOTE: Several previously available therapeutic lens designs have been discontinued by the manufacturers.

## Available Lens Designs

Several hydrogel contact lenses have received specific Food and Drug Administration approval for use in a therapeutic mode (Table 12-1). Lenses are usually prescribed plano (or close to plano) in optical power to provide a parallel-sided uniform thickness shell of hydrophilic plastic to maximize oxygen flux, but some clinicians use optically powered lenses to aid vision as well.[93]

The new silicone hydrogel lenses, because of their limited water content and very high oxygen permeability, may be ideally suited for the bandage lens role.[58] One such lens has received official acceptance in both Europe and the United States (CIBA Focus Night & Day).

Clinicians do not restrict themselves solely to bandage lens designs approved by the Food and Drug Administration, but often use any of the many different types of conventional contact lenses available (especially disposable soft lenses to minimize expense) as custom devices applied in the best interests of their patients' care.

## Therapeutic Hydrogel Contact Lens Fitting Principles

The first principle of therapeutic hydrogel contact lens fitting is that corneal protection demands full corneal coverage. To this end, most hydrogel contact lenses used as bandages will have larger (14.5 to 15.5 mm) rather than smaller (13.0 to 14.0 mm) overall diameters.

Hydrogel and rigid lens thickness should be minimized to maintain oxygenation both for corneal physiology (especially if wear will be extended through one or more sleep cycles) and to promote epithelial healing.[64] The new silicone hydrogels are so permeable to oxygen, however, that this may no longer be a concern.[45]

Lenses should be applied, with the proper selection of base curve and overall diameter, to maintain lens centration and stability. Movement of the lens on the anterior ocular surface should be somewhat less than required of a typical cosmetic application, but not so tight as to totally restrict movement and any potential tear exchange. Minimization of lens movement facilitates patient acceptance by decreasing lid sensation and is helpful in decreasing mechanical trauma to healing epithelial cells. Lenses should not be so steep, however, that indentation of the sclera, conjunctival vascular blanching, central air bubbles, or rippling of the conjunctiva occurs.[66] These may not be serious problems in themselves, but hydrogel lenses, especially if used for extended wear, may steepen with dehydration or changes in pH or aging and then may induce a "tight lens syndrome" in which the eye becomes painful and inflamed, and the epithelium may even slough.[69,86]

Optimum water content is an area of some controversy. Some authors suggest that the higher water content hydrogel lenses are effective in dry eye situations by providing a reservoir of fluid.[88] Others propose that evaporation from the anterior surface of high water content hydrogel lenses draws water from the precorneal tear film and epithelium, perhaps then further dehydrating the anterior surface of the eye.[3] This effect, if it exists, may be helpful in managing bullous keratopathy but can be problematic in cases of dry eye.

In addition, if the patient can manage a therapeutic lens on a daily wear basis, and if the disease being managed allows such use (as opposed to requiring continual overnight wear), such a mode is preferable to reduce the risk of corneal infection and neovascularization and to facilitate the installation of medication. Thinner, lower oxygen transmissibility lenses are ideal for such use. Lens maintenance and cleaning should be with heat (rarely used now), chemical agents, or peroxide as appropriate for the contact lens material and patient situation. Higher oxygen transmissibility (DK/t) lenses should be used when extended wear is elected or necessary. Disposable or frequent replacement silicone hydrogels may be ideal for this use. Cleaning routines as appropriate should be used as frequently as the disease process and the patient's particular situation and removal cycles will allow.

Frequent professional evaluations are essential in the continuing management of therapeutic contact lens patients, especially if the lenses are used under extended wear conditions. The initially fitted patient should be seen 1 to 2 hours after the first lens application to confirm the continued proper mechanical fit of the lens and to observe any acute physiological or physical response. Lens changes are not uncommon at this point to refine the fit. The progress schedule beyond this evaluation varies with the precise situation, but in general patients should be seen the day after application, the day after the first night of lens wear, and at intervals ranging from weekly to monthly or perhaps—when the patient's situation is stable and if the clinician considers risks to be minimal (e.g., the lens is used for daily wear)—at even 3-month intervals. Some situations suggest therapeutic lens management only for short intervals, days or weeks, while healing occurs, and others require maintaining the lens on the eye for months or even years to manage chronic or unresponsive problems. In many such cases patients who are unable to handle their lenses visit the clinician's office periodically for lens cleaning, inspection, and reinsertion. Coordinated comanagement of most of these patients with both a contact lens provider and corneal specialist is considered ideal. Concomitant aggressive medical (e.g., antibiotics, cycloplegics, steroids) and perhaps surgical treatment is often required for best patient care.

### Indications

Box 12-12 lists indications for therapeutic hydrogels.

---

**BOX 12-12**

### Indications for Therapeutic Hydrogels

1. Corneal dystrophies that result in epithelial irregularity and erosion, such as map-dot-fingerprint, Meesman's, Reis-Buckler's, lattice, granular, and macular dystrophies. Hydrogel lenses protect the fragile surface from the rubbing action of the lids to decrease recurrent breakdown of the epithelium, minimizing pain, foreign body sensations, photophobia, and tearing.
2. Other recurrent or chronic epithelial erosions or healing disorders caused by trauma, metaherpetic disease, chemical (especially alkali) burns, or surgery, in which the lens is an alternative to pressure patching the eye to promote reepithelialization of surface defects.
3. Protection from corneal damage from rubbing of inwardly directed eyelashes in entropion with trichiasis or from the inflammation and mechanical abrasion of the large papillae of the upper tarsal conjunctiva in vernal keratoconjunctivitis.
4. Improving patient comfort and healing with Thygeson's superficial punctate keratitis.[34,37]
5. Maintaining comfort for patients with endothelial failure and corneal edema from Fuch's dystrophy or aphakic/pseudophakic bullous keratopathy. Related severe epithelial and stromal edema leads to large epithelial blisters that produce photophobia, foreign body sensation, and pain when they rupture. The presence of a flat hydrogel bandage lens reduces these problems, perhaps by mechanically reinforcing the damaged tissue, reducing the occurrence of ruptures, or covering the otherwise exposed nerve endings from the rubbing action of the lids.
6. Relief of pain associated with superior limbic keratoconjunctivitis.[68]
7. Protecting the cornea in cases of dry eye, with additional artificial tears and ocular lubricants. This use is somewhat controversial and, again, patients are often at greater risk of infection and should be managed conservatively.[25]
8. Bullous diseases of the conjunctiva, such as ocular cicatricial pemphigoid and Stevens-Johnson syndrome, may be partially managed with therapeutic hydrogels.[67] The lenses protect the corneal epithelium from drying and from mechanical damage from eyelid abnormalities such as entropion with trichiasis.

## Indications for Therapeutic Hydrogels

9. Protecting the corneal surface after neurological damage to cranial nerves V or VII to facilitate and maintain the epithelial cells. Because of the very high risk of infection (lesions to cranial nerve V result in anesthesia, and lesions to cranial nerve VII lead to abnormal blinking and secondary hydrogel lens dehydration), this should be considered only after other methods, such as pressure patching, tarsorrhaphy, and conjunctival flap, cannot be considered or have failed.
10. Structural reinforcement and promotion of healing and vascularization of weakened sites in the cornea: reforming the anterior chamber after a small perforation or wound dehiscence[63] in which the contact lens functions as a temporary splint, sometimes concomitant with the use of tissue adhesives, to seal the perforation; or supporting descemetoceles and other stromal thinning disorders (e.g., Mooren's ulcer[2,56]), perhaps to temporize patient care while waiting for definitive surgical treatment.[55]
11. Filamentary keratitis, especially if associated with blinking abnormalities.

### Contraindications

Therapeutic hydrogel contact lenses should not be used in the presence of active microbial infection of the eye. When the contralateral eye is infected, lens wear should be discontinued, if at all possible, until the infection has cleared to preclude the possibility of it spreading to the second eye.

A therapeutic lens should not be used when a patient is unwilling or unable to return for progress evaluations or is unwilling or unable to comply with reasonable care guidelines. Patients should comply with their scheduled visits and be advised to return immediately if they have any pain, injection of the conjunctiva, or reduced vision. The participation of family members in lens handling and follow-up compliance is helpful and should be encouraged.

Additional contraindications include all those that apply to all potential hydrogel lens users: dusty, polluted environments; poor personal hygiene; concomitant lid diseases such as chronic or acute blepharitis; obstructions or infections of the lacrimal drainage system; or filtering blebs, which can serve as a pathway for infection to spread from the surface of the globe to induce endophthalmitis. In general, any actively inflamed eye with lid and conjunctival chemosis is difficult to manage and more likely to develop infectious and inflammatory complications. Most corneal topographies and curvatures, however, can be fitted with today's wide range of available lenses.

### Contact Lens Complications

All the known complications of contact lens wear occur with therapeutic lens use, but they are often both more severe and more prevalent. Of greatest concern is infectious keratitis, which tends to be associated with gram-positive bacteria and fungi in this setting (rather than gram-negative bacteria, as found in cosmetic contact lens wear),[83] and corneal neovascularization. Corneal neovascularization is probably stimulated by both concomitant corneal disease and extended wear; although desirable in some cases to promote the healing process, neovascularization may result in visual loss from corneal opacification in others.[20] The clinician should also be alert for other complications that require clinical management: soiled contact lenses, sterile infiltrates, hypopyon, corneal staining, and giant papillary conjunctivitis.

### Collagen Shields

Contact lens–type devices made from biodegradable porcine collagen were introduced for use in a therapeutic contact lens format. These devices reduce rather than enhance vision and variably dissolve while on the eye over an imprecisely defined period of hours to days. They are currently primarily used in drug delivery (principally antibiotic) rather than as protection, although the lubricant value of the dissolving device in wound healing may be helpful as well.

### Success

Zadnik[100] concludes that therapeutic hydrogel contact lenses are a valuable tool in managing the compromised corneal surface, although they are not universally efficacious. Because these eyes are diseased and their anterior segments compromised before the application of the contact lens, the failure of this device to achieve the therapeutic outcome desired may have been preordained.

## ACKNOWLEDGMENTS

The authors acknowledge the contributions of Bartly J. Mondino, MD, Cheryl Bergin, OD, and Courtney Westrich.

## REFERENCES

1. Ames K: Fitting the presbyope with gas permeable contact lenses, *Contact Lens Spectrum* 16:42-5, 2001.

2. Arentsen JJ, Laibson PR, Cohen EJ: *Management of corneal descemetoceles*, Trans Am Ophthalmol Soc 82:92-105, 1984.

3. Baldone JA, Kaufman HE: Soft contact lenses in clinical disease, *Am J Ophthalmol* 95:851, 1983.

4. Barr JA: Bifocals, multifocals, monovision—what works today, *Contact Lens Spectrum* 18:41-5, 2003.

5. Benjamin WJ, Borish IM: Physiology of aging and its influence on the contact lens prescription, *J Am Optom Assoc* 62:743-52, 1991.

6. Benjamin WJ, Rasmussen MA: Oxygen consumption of the superior cornea following eyelid closure, *Acta Ophthalmol* 66:309-12, 1988.

7. Bennett ES: Lens care and patient education. In Bennett ES, Henry VA: *Clinical manual of contact lenses,* ed 2, Philadelphia, 2000, Lippincott Williams & Wilkins, pp 125-59.

8. Bennett ES, Hansen DW: Presbyopia: gas permeable bifocal fitting and problem-solving. In Bennett ES, Hom MM: *Manual of gas permeable contact lenses,* ed 2, St. Louis, 2004, Elsevier, pp 324-56.

9. Bennett ES, Hansen DW, Baker R: GPs and presbyopes: why today's designs are easier to fit, *Rev Optom* 140:43-6, 2003.

10. Bennett ES, Jurkus JM: Bifocal contact lenses. In Bennett ES, Weissman BA: *Clinical contact lens practice,* ed 2, Philadelphia, Lippincott Williams & Wilkins, pp 531-48.

11. Bennett ES, Jurkus JM, Schwartz CA: Bifocal contact lenses. In Bennett ES, Henry VA: *Clinical manual of contact lenses,* ed 2, Philadelphia, 2000, Lippincott Williams & Wilkins, pp 410-49.

12. Bennett ES, Smythe J, Henry VA, et al: The effect of topical anesthetic use on the initial patient satisfaction and overall success with rigid gas permeable contact lenses, *Optom Vis Sci* 75:800-5, 1998.

13. Benoit DP: Multifocal contact lens update, *Contact Lens Spectrum* 16:26-32, 2001.

14. Bergenske PD: The presbyopic fitting process, *Contact Lens Spectrum* 16:34-41, 2001.

15. Blackwell OM, Blackwell HR: Visual performance data for 156 normal observers of various ages, *J Illum Eng Soc* 1:3-13, 1971.

16. Bridgewater BA, Farkas B, Toscano F: A hydrogel system for the correction of presbyopia, *Contact Lens Spectrum* 14:41-4, 1999.

17. Brown SI, Bloomfield S, Pierce DB, et al: Infections with therapeutic soft contact lenses, *Arch Ophthalmol* 91:274-7, 1974.

18. Byrnes SP, Cannella A: An in-office evaluation of a multifocal RGP lens design, *Contact Lens Spectrum* 14:29-33, 1999.

19. Caffery BA, Josephson J: Rigid bifocal contact lens correction. In Bennett ES, Weissman BA, editors: *Clinical contact lens practice,* Philadelphia, 1991, J.B. Lippincott, pp 42-1 to 42-11.

20. Cogan DG, Kuwabara T: Lipogenesis of cells of the cornea, *Arch Ophthalmol* 59:453-6, 1955.

21. Collins MJ, Brown B, Bowman KJ: Contrast sensitivity with contact lens correction for presbyopia, *Ophthalmic Physiol Opt* 9:133-8, 1989.

22. Collins M, Bruce A, Thompson B: Adaptation to monovision. *Int Contact Lens Clin* 21:218-24, 1994.

23. Collins MJ, Goode A, Brown B: Distance visual acuity and monovision, *Optom Vis Sci* 70:723-8, 1993.

24. Davis R: Pinpoint success with GP multifocal lenses, *Contact Lens Spectrum* 18:25-8, 2003.

25. Dohlman CH, Boruchoff SA, Mobilia EF: Complications in use of soft contact lenses in corneal disease, *Arch Ophthalmol* 90:367, 1973.

26. Donnefeld ED, Cohen EJ, Arentsen JJ, et al: Changing trends in contact lens associated corneal ulcers, *CLAO J* 12:145-9, 1986.

27. Donshik PC, Luistro A: Soft bifocal contact lens fitting with the Alges lens, *CLAO J* 13:174-6, 1987.

28. Du Toit R, Ferreira JT, Nel ZJ: Visual and nonvisual variables implicated in monovision wear, *Optom Vis Sci* 75:119-25, 1988.

29. Du Toit R, Situ P, Simpson T, et al: The effects of six months of contact lens wear on the tear film, ocular surfaces, and symptoms of presbyopes, *Optom Vis Sci* 78:455-62, 2001.

30. Edwards K, Haig-Brown G: An evaluation of bifocal contact lens performance and the design of a new fitting protocol, *Trans BCLA* 30-4, 1987.

31. Erickson P, Schor C: Visual function with presbyopic contact lens correction, *Optom Vis Sci* 67:22-8, 1990.

32. Fisher K, Bauman E, Schwallie J: Evaluation of two new soft contact lenses for correction of presbyopia: the Focus Progressives Multifocal and the Acuvue Bifocal, *Int Contact Lens Clin* 26:92-103, 1999.

33. Fonn D, Dutoit R, Situ P, et al: *Determination of lens prescription for monovision and Acuvue Bifocal contact lenses,* Presented at the Annual Meeting

of the American Academy of Optometry, Orlando, FL, December 2000.

34. Forstot SL, Binder PS: Treatment of Thygeson's superficial punctate keratitis, *Am J Ophthalmol* 88:186, 1979.

35. Gasset AR, Kaufman HE: Therapeutic uses of hydrophilic contact lenses, *Am J Ophthalmol* 69:252, 1970.

36. Ghormley NR: The new Acuvue Bifocal contact lens, *Int Contact Lens Clin* 25:71-2, 1998.

37. Goldberg DB, Schanzlin DJ, Brown SI: Management of Thygeson's superficial punctate keratitis, *Am J Ophthalmol* 89:22, 1980.

38. Gromacki SJ, Nilsen E: Comparison of multifocal lens performance to monovision, *Contact Lens Spectrum* 16:34-8, 2001.

39. Guillon M, Maissa C, Cooper P, et al: Visual performance of a multi-zone bifocal and a progressive multifocal contact lens, *CLAO J* 28: 88-93, 2002.

40. Guth S: Effects of age on visibility, *Am J Optom* 34:463-76, 1957.

41. Hanks A: Contact lenses for presbyopia, *Eye Contact* 9-14, 1984.

42. Hansen DW: Multifocal contact lenses—the next generation, *Contact Lens Spectrum* 17:42-7, 2002.

43. Harris MG, Classe JG: Clinicolegal considerations of monovision, *J Am Optom Assoc* 59:491-5, 1988.

44. Herrin S: How to fit the new bifocal soft lenses, *Rev Optom* 126:57, 1989.

45. Huang P, Zwang-Weissman J, Weissman BA: Is the contact lens "T" still important? *Cont Lens Anterior Eye* 27:9-14, 2004.

46. Iravani N: New multifocal offers best of both worlds, *Contact Lens Spectrum* 17(suppl): 2-5, 2002.

47. Johannsdottir KR, Stelmach LB: Monovision: a review of the scientific literature, *Optom Vis Sci* 78:646-51, 2001.

48. Johnson J, Bennett ES, Henry VA, et al: *MultiVision vs. monovision: a comparative study,* Presented at the Annual Meeting of the Contact Lens Association of Ophthalmologists, Las Vegas, February 2000.

49. Josephson JE, Caffery BE: Hydrogel bifocal lenses. In Bennett ES, Weissman BA, editors: *Clinical contact lens practice,* Philadelphia, 1990, J.B. Lippincott, pp 43-1 to 43-20.

50. Josephson JE, Erickson P, Caffery BE: The monovision controversy. In Bennett ES, Weissman BA, editors: *Clinical contact lens practice,* Philadelphia, 1990, J.B. Lippincott, pp 44-1 to 44-6.

51. Kent HD, Cohen EJ, Laibson B, et al: Microbial keratitis and corneal ulceration associated with therapeutic soft contact lenses, *CLAO J* 16:49-52, 1990.

52. Kirman ST, Kirman GS: Tangent Streak bifocal contact lenses, *Contact Lens Update* 9:65-9, 1990.

53. Kirschen DG, Hung CC, Nakano TR: Comparison of suppression, stereoacuity, and interocular differences in visual acuity in monovision, and Acuvue bifocal contact lenses, *Optom Vis Sci* 76:832-7, 1999.

54. Lee WC: Factors for fitting success, *Contact Lens Spectrum* 14:7a, 1999.

55. Leibowitz HM, Berrospi AR: Initial treatment of descemetocele with hydrophilic contact lenses, *Ann Ophthalmol* 7:1161-6, 1975.

56. Leibowitz HM, Rosenthal P: Hydrophilic contact lenses in corneal disease. I. Superficial sterile, indolent ulcers, *Arch Ophthalmol* 85: 163-6, 1971.

57. Lieblein JS: Finding success with multifocal contact lenses, *Contact Lens Spectrum* 14:50-1, 2000.

58. Lim L, Tan DT, Chan WK: Therapeutic use of Bausch & Lomb PureVision contact lenses, *CLAO J* 27:179-85, 2001.

59. Lloyd M: Fitting a soft disposable bifocal lens, *Optician* 217:18-22, 1999.

60. Loshin DS, Loshin MS, Comer G: Binocular summation with monovision contact lens correction for presbyopia, *Int Contact Lens Clin* 9:161-5, 1982.

61. Mandell RB: A new concept in GP bifocal contact lenses, *Contact Lens Spectrum* 17:34-40, 2002.

62. Mannis MJ, Zadnik K: Contact lenses in the elderly patient, *Geriatr Ophthalmol* 2:23-7, 1986.

63. Mannis MJ, Zadnik K: Hydrophilic contact lenses for wound stabilization in keratoplasty, *CLAO J* 14:199-202, 1988.

64. Mauger TF, Hill RM: Corneal epithelial healing in hypoxic environments, *Invest Ophthalmol Vis Sci* 28(suppl):2, 1987.

65. McGill E, Erickson P: Stereopsis in presbyopes wearing monovision and simultaneous vision bifocal contact lenses, *Am J Optom Physiol Opt* 65:612-26, 1988.

66. Mobilia EF, Yamamoto GK, Dohlman CH: Corneal wrinkling induced by ultrathin soft contact lenses, *Ann Ophthalmol* 12:371, 1980.

67. Mondino BJ, Weissman BA, Manthey R: Therapeutic soft contact lenses. In Stenson SM, editor: *Contact lenses: a guide to selection, fitting and management of complications,* Norwalk, CT, 1987, Appleton & Lange, pp 155-83.

68. Mondino BJ, Zaidman GW, Salamon SW: Use of pressure patching and soft contact lenses in superior limbic keratoconjunctivitis, *Arch Ophthalmol* 100:1932, 1982.

69. Murphy GE: A case of sterile endophthalmitis associated with the extended wear of an aphakic soft contact lens, *Contact Lens Intraoc Lens Med J* 7:5, 1981.

70. Nakagawara VB, Veronneau SJH: Monovision contact lens use in the aviation environment: a report of a contact lens-related aircraft accident, *Optometry* 71:390-5, 2000.

71. Norman CW: Combining simultaneous and alternating vision GP concepts, *Contact Lens Spectrum* 18:21, 2003.

72. Obrig TE: *Contact lenses,* Philadelphia, 1942, Chilton, pp 41-92.

73. Odineal C: Fitting a soft disposable bifocal contact lens, *Contact Lens Spectrum* 16:44-6, 2001.

74. Phillips AJ: Contact lenses and the elderly patient. In Rosenbloom A, Morgan M, editors: *Vision and aging: general and clinical perspectives,* New York, 1986, Professional Press, pp 267-300.

75. Poggio EC, Glynn RJ, Schein OD, et al: The incidence of ulcerative keratitis among users of daily-wear and extended-wear soft contact lenses, *New Engl J Med* 321:779-83, 1989.

76. Quinn TG: Making sense of frequent replacement soft multifocals, *Contact Lens Spectrum* 17: 2002.

77. Quinn TG: The monovision vs. multifocal debate, *Contact Lens Spectrum* 17: 2002.

78. Rajagopalan AS, Bennett ES, Lakshminarayanan V, et al: *Performance of presbyopic contact lenses under mesopic conditions,* Presented at ARVO, Ft. Lauderdale, FL, April 2003.

79. Rajagopalan AS, Bennett ES, Lakshminarayanan V, et al: *Contrast sensitivity with presbyopic contact lenses,* Presented at the American Academy of Optometry annual meeting, Dallas, December 2003.

80. Remba MJ: The Tangent Streak rigid gas permeable bifocal contact lens, *J Am Optom Assoc* 59:212-6, 1988.

81. Rigel LE: What to expect from the Acuvue bifocal, *Optom Today* 6:26-7, 1998.

82. Rigel LE, Castellano CF: How to fit today's soft bifocal contact lenses, *Optom Today* 7(suppl): 45-51, 1999.

83. Schein OD, Ormerod LD, Barraquer E, et al: Microbiology of contact lens-related keratitis, *Cornea* 8:281-5, 1989.

84. Schwartz CA: Portrait of a presbyope in 1999, *Optometry Today* (suppl):5-7, 1999.

85. Shovlin JP: Extended wear for presbyopes? *Rev Optom* 139:55, 2002.

86. Snyder DA, Litinsky SM, Calendar H: Hypopyon iridocyclitis associated with extended wear soft contact lenses, *Am J Ophthalmol* 93:519, 1982.

87. Soni PS, Patel R, Carlson RS: Is binocular contrast sensitivity at distance compromised with multifocal soft contact lenses used to correct presbyopia? *Optom Vis Sci* 80:505-14, 2003.

88. Thoft RA: Therapeutic soft contact lenses. In Smolin G, Thoft RA, editors: *Cornea,* Boston, 1983, Little, Brown, pp 477-87.

89. Vehige JG: Hydron Echelon lens fitting guide. Part III: fitting factors for success. *Contact Lens Spectrum* 7:39-46, 1992.

90. Wan L: Take some frustration out of multifocal fitting, *Contact Lens Spectrum* 18:42-4, 2003.

91. Weale RA: *A biography of the eye: development, age, and growth,* London, 1982, H.K. Lewis.

92. Weinstock FJ, Miday RM: Presbyopic correction with contact lenses, *Ophthalmol Clin North Am* 9:111-6, 1996.

93. Weissman BA: Designing uniform thickness contact lens shells, *Am J Optom Physiol Opt* 59:902, 1982.

94. Westendorf DH, Blake R, Sloane M, et al: Binocular summation occurs during interocular suppressions, *J Exp Psych* 8:81-90, 1982.

95. Wick B, Westin E: Change in refractive anisometropia in presbyopic adults wearing monovision contact lens correction, *Optom Vis Sci* 76:33-9, 1999.

96. Wilson LA, Sawant AO, Simmons RB, et al: Microbial contamination of contact lens storage cases and solutions, *Am J Ophthalmol* 109:193, 1990.

97. Woods C, Ruston D, Hough T, et al: Clinical performance of an innovative back surface multifocal contact lens in correcting presbyopia, *CLAO J* 25:176-81, 1999.

98. Woods JM, Wick K, Shuley V, et al: The effect of monovision contact lens wear on driving performance, *Clin Exp Optom* 81:100-3, 1998.

99. Wooley S: "Doctor, do I have to give up my contact lenses just because I need bifocals?" *Optom Today* 6:40-2, 1998.

100. Zadnik K: Therapeutic soft contact lenses. In Harris MG, editor: *Contact lenses and ocular disease,* Philadelphia, 1990, J.B. Lippincott, pp 632-42.

# CHAPTER 13

# Functional Therapy in the Rehabilitation of Older Adults

**BRUCE C. WICK**

Vision is a complex synkinesis of biochemistry, neural structures, physiology, and learning. The interrelations are often not well understood, but aging causes major changes in visual performance and, as is true in youth, specific deficits frequently do not account for overall performance decrements. The decline of visual abilities with age is a fact of mature life and ranges from severe deterioration to minor reductions in visual function. For most mature adults, the loss of visual sensory and motor abilities influences performance of all perceptual tasks.

Perception of the environment through vision requires that the visual system be able to gather information effectively. Generally, people with otherwise healthy eyes do not experience severe visual acuity impairment with increasing age; however, most have impairment from decreases in oculomotor function.[36] Losses of accommodative ability (presbyopia), field of vision, and eye movement speed and accuracy can cause profound difficulties in binocular information gathering and processing.

These losses often can be remedied by selective rehabilitative techniques. Although perceptual aspects of vision care are important, these aspects are dealt with only partially in this chapter. The primary emphasis of the material in this chapter will be the functional rehabilitation of vision problems, with emphasis on motor aspects of binocular vision for patients with normal static visual acuity.

## OCULOMOTOR FUNCTIONS

A thorough understanding of the basis and development of normal oculomotor function is necessary before any rehabilitation can begin. Equally important is an understanding of the changing normals of age that occur in all individuals. For example, losses in vergence ability and changes in tonic vergence accompany presbyopia and the normal aging process. (Chapter 2 of this text discusses normal changes in visual function with aging.) Rehabilitative techniques should be considered when normal aging changes cause individuals to develop deficits that decrease the required abilities to perform adequately.

## VERGENCE EYE MOVEMENTS

The diagnosis and rehabilitation of oculomotor system dysfunction requires an understanding of pursuit, saccadic, and vergence eye movements.[25] Vergence eye movements generally are considered to consist of four components: tonic, accommodative, disparity (fusional), and proximal.[20] In the diagnosis and treatment of visual motor problems, vergence magnitudes often are related to one another by using various criteria to evaluate whether symptoms are likely to be caused by the findings present.

Components of the total vergence response depend on age and show specific decrements as time passes. There are especially dramatic decreases in accommodative function with a corresponding loss in accommodative vergence and, subsequently, near convergence ability.[14,28,30,40] In light of other decrements in motor and sensory ocular ability with age, disparity vergence ability also decreases with age.

## DIAGNOSIS OF OCULOMOTOR DYSFUNCTIONS

The proper diagnosis of visual problems of older adults is facilitated by taking a thorough, careful history. Patients usually have two or three main visual problems that they want solved. Careful listening by the examiner combined with well-directed questions and a systematic approach to obtaining pertinent information will improve the chances of an accurate history. The value of a complete, accurate history increases with the patient's age because ocular and systemic disease, side effects of medication, and accidental injury all have increased incidence. The history can be conveniently divided into two parts: general and visual.

### General History

A general history should be taken before any examination, and it frequently indicates many tests that should be performed. During examination of older patients, pertinent visual complaints often are obscured by rambling, and sometimes incoherent, details. Often an accompanying member of the family can (or needs to) be consulted because an older patient may overlook key points of illness. In these times, family members can be of great help and keep the patient from becoming frustrated.

### Visual History

Visual history taking should be continued throughout the examination. A fixed sequence of questions can be useful, but information volunteered by the patient during the examination often has the greatest value.[42] Information gathered during the examination may lead to other areas that need to be explored and indicate ancillary tests that will facilitate an accurate diagnosis of the visual problem.

Determining the patient's occupation and hobbies is of the utmost importance for prescriptive purposes. Important issues include working distances, times, lighting conditions, and occupational requirements such as computer use. Older adults are frequently unaware that different types of lenses are needed or are available for various visual tasks or that "computer glasses" that focus the computer screen without an abnormal neck posture can be of great benefit. Thus, in spite of a careful history, many visual requirements may be neglected because the patient is unaware of the visual requirements of specific tasks or the possible solutions that may be available.

Specific questions related to binocular problems should be asked: When do symptoms occur? When do they start? How long do they last? What relieves the symptoms? With what tasks do they occur? Is any diplopia present? When the patient reports newly acquired diplopia, a paretic or restrictive etiologic factor involving oculomotor or systemic pathological condition is usually involved. However, patients frequently confuse double vision with distorted or blurred vision, so true diplopia must be assessed.

Three nonpathological causes of diplopia are possible. With physiological diplopia, many patients are alarmed by a sudden awareness of the condition for objects off the singleness horopter. An anomalous prismatic effect of spectacles can occur with poorly adjusted glasses, errors in spectacle fabrication involving the inclusion of unwanted prism, omission of previously worn prism, or the need for slab-off prism in anisometropia. Strabismus/heterophoria, another cause of diplopia, can be attributed to the following factors:

- *Fusional disturbances.* Intermittent diplopia may be associated with uncompensated heterophoria and comitant heterotropia with inadequate suppression.
- *Postoperative diplopia.* This is a complication of strabismus surgery that may persist for years. It frequently follows cosmetic operations in older patients.
- *Onset of comitant strabismus.* Diplopia is experienced briefly at the onset of a comitant deviation before suppression begins. These patients are typically young children who rarely describe their symptoms accurately.

- *Uncompensated congenital palsy.* In patients with congenital muscle palsies who have maintained single binocular vision by appropriate head posturing and fusional mechanisms, a breakdown in fusional ability may result in sudden diplopia. This occurs particularly with congenital superior oblique palsies in which fusional reserves are weakened (e.g., after a long illness). A review of old photographs will often reveal a head tilt that has been maintained throughout life.
- *Sudden onset of comitant strabismus.* Although almost all comitant strabismus develops insidiously, occasionally a comitant deviation appears suddenly and is accompanied by annoying diplopia. This is most common in patients with high heterophorias who have undergone an artificial interruption of binocular vision for several days (e.g., with unilateral patching or occlusion). When the patch is removed, fusion cannot be maintained and diplopia is constant. Although some cases resolve spontaneously, many require treatment in the form of prisms, lenses, or visual training.
- *A and V patterns.* In these complex forms of horizontal strabismus, the deviation varies with vertical gaze. For example, in A exotropia, the exotropia increases on downgaze. Such patients frequently experience diplopia, especially with reading and other near tasks.
- *Brown's superior oblique tendon sheath syndrome.* This condition involves a congenital superior oblique sheath defect that mechanically limits the affected eye's ability to elevate from an adducted position. Diplopia is noticed on upgaze.

After diplopia has been determined to exist, a routine history is augmented with questions related to (1) the duration of diplopia, (2) its first occurrence, (3) the location of diplopic images, and (4) the frequency and course of their occurrence. For example, diplopia that worsens in the evening is often related to myasthenia and questions should be asked related to muscle weakness, problems with chewing or swallowing, and whether an associated ptosis develops late in the day. Diplopia that worsens in the morning is often related to thyroid eye disease, and questions should be asked related to general thyroid problems, associated swelling or redness of the eyes, and whether a change in the upper eyelid position has developed for one or both eyes (lid retraction).

## TESTS AND MEASUREMENTS
### Comitant Deviations

Once an accurate initial history has been completed, tests are done to evaluate binocular function thoroughly. Ocular health is evaluated (through fundus evaluation, biomicroscope examination, tonometry, visual field testing, the Amsler grid, and testing pupillary reflexes) to be sure that ocular, neurological, or systemic disease is not causing the reported signs or symptoms. The analysis of binocular dysfunction in older adults is described in this section.

A thorough refraction, including tests of binocular and monocular visual acuity, should be performed. Monocular refraction under binocular conditions helps stabilize fusion and visual acuity. American Optical vectographic slides or Turville's distance testing combined with the Borish or other binocular tests for near vision are recommended. Fusional difficulties may cause binocular acuity to be less than the acuity of the better eye.

Obviously, plus additions are needed for older adults to maintain clear vision at near because of loss of accommodative ability. Proper history taking helps determine the best choice for correction, progressive addition lens, bifocal, trifocal, reading, computer lens, or any other. Many tests can determine the addition. Excellent theoretical and test descriptions are available.[4,21] The basic premise is to prescribe the addition so that half of the accommodative amplitude is kept in reserve, or so that the desired working distance is in the central part of the range of clear vision through the near addition.

Heterophoria and binocular vision are evaluated at distance and near. Near evaluations are done through any plus addition indicated by refractive finding. Lateral heterophoria can be measured by various methods: objective and subjective cover tests, Maddox rod (flash and nonflash), and von Graeffe's testing (flash and nonflash).[16] Tests in the natural environment are frequently superior to those made through the phoropter. A properly performed cover test for assessment of phoria magnitude, as well quality of fusional recovery, can be useful.[21,33] The cover test consists of two parts: the unilateral cover test (to detect strabismus) and the alternate cover test (to measure the angle of heterophoria or strabismus). The unilateral cover test is performed as follows:

1. Direct the patient to fixate a small, detailed target.
2. Closely observe one eye (the limbus may be used as a guide) and simultaneously occlude the other eye.
3. Note the direction and estimate the amount of movement required of the eye to fixate the target.
4. Immediately uncover the eye.
5. Repeat if necessary.
6. Bring the occluder beneath the eyes to the opposite side. (Be sure the patient does not alternate fixation.)

If fixation is central for each eye, and no movement of either eye occurs upon covering the opposite eye, heterophoria is present. Strabismus is indicated if movement of one eye occurs upon covering the other. The test should be repeated in different fields of gaze and with right and left head tilt to evaluate noncomitance. For older patients, the near cover test is done through any plus addition required. The alternate cover test is performed as follows:

1. The examiner occludes one eye and directs the patient to fixate a small target with the unoccluded eye.
2. The examiner directs his or her gaze to the cover at a point where the temporal limbus is assumed to be.
3. The examiner quickly moves the occluder to the fixating eye. His or her gaze should not follow the occluder.
4. The direction is noted and the amount of movement required of the uncovered eye to fixate the target is estimated. Movement of the eye with the occluder signifies an exodeviation, and movement opposite to the occluder indicates an esodeviation.
5. The examiner returns the occluder to the original position before the eye.
6. A loose prism (or prisms) of sufficient power is oriented between the occluder and the eye to neutralize the movement just seen.
7. The test is repeated, with the power of the prism or prisms changed until just perceptible movements of opposite direction are observed.
8. The midpoint of this pair of prism values represents the angle of deviation (whether

this deviation was a phoria or tropia is determined by the unilateral cover testing procedure described above).

The test is done in different fields of gaze and with right and left head tilt to analyze noncomitance. Occasionally the alternate cover test will reveal a larger angle than did the unilateral cover test in the presence of strabismus. Such measurements are often evidence of harmonious anomalous correspondence, although for patients with exotropia (especially those with pseudodivergence excess), a properly performed (prolonged) near cover test may reveal more exodeviation than will short, rapid occlusion.

### Lateral Vergence Range and Fixation Disparity Testing

Disparity (fusional) vergence ranges are measured by using loose or rotary prisms in free space and through the phoropter at distance and near. Because loose prisms are presented in discrete steps, they give a good indication of the patient's fusional recovery ability. Measuring vergence ranges by using rotary prisms through the phoropter frequently can be eliminated from the test sequence if forced vergence fixation disparity curves are measured at distance and near.

After determining lateral phorias, forced vergence fixation disparity curves are plotted at distance and near, and prism to reduce fixation disparity to zero is measured in all positions of gaze. Actual fixation disparity is only measured by instruments specifically designed for the task, such as the Sheedy Disparometer and Woolf near card.[26] Most clinical tests (Mallett distance and near fixation disparity tests, as well as Bernell lanterns) measure the prism to reduce fixation disparity to zero—the associated phoria.

Forced vergence fixation disparity curves (Disparometer and Wolff near card) are valuable for the analysis of binocular vision.[29] Figure 13-1 shows typical distance and near forced vergence fixation disparity curves for a symptomatic subject with presbyopia with poor control of a near lateral phoria. Flat curves indicate better compensation for a horizontal phoria (esophoria or exophoria) than do steep curves. For symptomatic patients, prism can be prescribed to approximately center the curve about the y-axis, or the center of symmetry.[24]

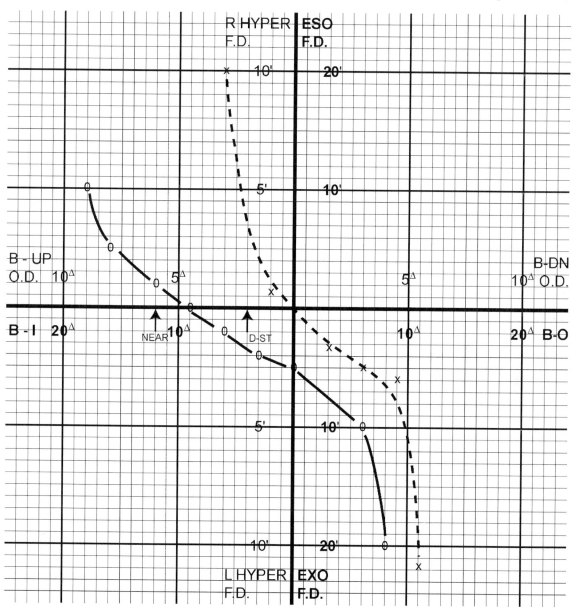

# FIXATION DISPARITY CURVE

NAME **A C**

DATE

DISTANCE X = 4M ; 0 = 40 CM

■ LATERAL ☐ VERTICAL

COMMENTS:

R -0.50    C-0.75 X 94    20/20

L -0.50    C-0.75 X 78    20/20

+2.50

↑ = disoc. phoria

R HYPER  ESO
F.D.     F.D.

10'      20'

5'       10'

B - UP                                         B-DN
O.D. 10△      5△              5△        10△ O.D.

B - I  20△      NEAR 10△    D-ST      10△        20△ B-O

5'       10'

10'      20'

L HYPER  EXO
F.D.     F.D.

**Fig. 13-1** Change in fixation disparity at distance and near is plotted in a graph for various prism powers. The result provides a graphical representation of measurement for the patient with presbyopia with a symptomatic near exophoria. The near exofixation disparity is 5 △ and nearly 10 △ base-in is required to reduce the fixation disparity to zero. (Courtesy James E. Sheedy, University of California, Berkeley, Copyright 1979 Vision Analysis).

The horizontal associated phoria measurement (prism to reduce fixation disparity to zero) generally gives smaller prism prescriptions for symptomatic patients with steep curves than do other criteria for prescribing prisms, and the prescription found usually gives adequate relief of symptoms.[27]

Vision therapy can be prescribed to improve binocularity and modify the curve shape. For older adults, vision therapy progress can be followed by using forced vergence fixation disparity curves. These curves generally flatten with successful therapy, just as do those of younger patients. After therapy, a small fixation disparity generally remains when the actual fixation disparity is measured.[25]

### Vertical Heterophoria and Fixation Disparity Testing

Arriving at the prism prescription for a vertical phoria frequently requires considerable clinical judgment. Various techniques have been recommended for prescription design, including equating vergence ranges, flip prism techniques, and fixation disparity measures. Tests that measure prism to reduce fixation disparities to zero (measured clinically by the American Optical vectographic slides, Turville's infinity balance, the Mallett distance and near unit, and the Borish near card) generally give vertical prism prescriptions that reduce symptoms. Nearly all patients can appreciate a difference of $0.5^\Delta$ on vertical fixation disparity tests.

Vertical heterophoria can be measured at distance and near by Maddox rod assessment, a cover test, or prism dissociation. When a vertical heterophoria is present in an older patient, comitance should be evaluated carefully. Fixation disparity tests probably are the most accurate techniques for prism prescription. Fixation disparity measures have the added advantage that they can be conducted in all fields of gaze under more natural binocular viewing conditions.

When a lateral and a vertical fixation disparity exist simultaneously, the vertical fixation disparity should be corrected first. Then the horizontal fixation disparity curves should be measured. Correcting the vertical fixation disparity will often normalize (flatten) the slope found in horizontal fixation disparity curve measurement.[41]

Vertical prism should be prescribed for vertical fixation disparities but only when it provides improved visual performance (less suppression, increased fusion ranges, and flatter lateral forced vergence fixation disparity curves) and reduced symptoms. Generally, a reduction of vertical misalignment to zero under binocular viewing conditions (prism to reduce fixation disparity to zero) gives the most accurate prism prescriptions. Vertical prism to reduce fixation disparity to zero is generally such a successful correction that a useful clinical rule of thumb is to correct all comitant vertical deviations found on fixation disparity testing. If additional treatment is needed to further relieve symptoms, vision therapy or slab-off prism can be considered after the patient has worn the glasses for a few weeks.

Stereopsis should be measured at distance and near. The stereoscopic threshold is relatively constant up to the ages of 45 to 50 years. After age 50 years, stereopsis declines gradually with increasing age.[23] However, age variations in individuals occur, and "normal" stereopsis may be found even in extremely old persons.

Finally, the near point of convergence should be measured. In youth, the near point of convergence ranges from 1 cm to 4 cm from the spectacle plane.[8] With the onset of presbyopia, a decrease of approximately 1 cm occurs per decade, so by age 70 years the normal convergence near point is 3 cm to 7 cm from the spectacle plane. Debility, systemic medication, and changes in binocular status can cause dramatic individual decrements.

Heterophoria, convergence, and binocular vision should be examined without the patient wearing glasses if the patient does not normally wear them and with glasses (correct or not) if the patient does wear them. For the effects of lens and prism prescriptions to be evaluted, the examination is repeated with the best possible correction and appropriate prescription modification.

### Noncomitant Deviations

Deviations that vary significantly (greater than $5^\Delta$) when the eyes are directed to various fields of gaze are considered noncomitant.[12] These deviations also increase when an eye with one or more paretic muscles fixates; the secondary deviation is larger than the primary. Diagnosis is facilitated by taking a thorough case history and performing tests to measure the amount and extent of diplopia, fusion, and noncomitance. Noncomitant deviations are characterized by one or more of the following:

1. A limitation of monocular motility
2. A change in magnitude of the deviation in various fields of gaze
3. A change in diplopia with various fields of gaze
4. An increase in the angle of deviation when the eye with the paretic muscle fixates

Diagnosis of affected muscles begins with observation. The examiner looks for gross deviations in alignment, signs of lid abnormality, or an unusual head turn or tilt. Patients who have noncomitant deviations often adopt distinctive head positions to compensate for diplopia. Table 13-1 shows head positions adopted in noncomitance and the extraocular muscles affected.

Noncomitance is generally caused by three conditions:

1. Trauma, including head and orbital trauma
2. Neurological disorders (disorders of gaze and muscle palsies caused by dysfunctions of cranial nerves III, IV, and VI)

3. Muscle disorders, including orbital tumors and pseudotumors, that compromise muscle action; thyroid disease; and myasthenia gravis

Tests to detect the affected muscle in noncomitance must take into account that restrictive syndromes (thyroid disease and blow-out fractures) affect eye alignment differently than nerve or muscle dysfunctions (myasthenia gravis and cranial nerve dysfunction cause muscle palsy). In restrictive syndromes diplopia is caused by mechanical resistance to movement of the eye, and diplopia is most noticeable during attempted movements opposite the field of action of the involved muscle or muscles. With nerve dysfunction the deviation increases on attempted gaze into the field of action of the muscle. Recent paretic involvements are characterized by a larger secondary than primary deviation or a sudden onset of symptoms such as diplopia, blurring, and head tilt or turn.

The diagnostic field of action of each extraocular muscle is shown in Table 13-2. To properly diagnose noncomitance, the examiner must evaluate the deviation in the primary position in each of the eight positions of gaze, with right and left head tilt, and with each eye fixating. Evaluation is done monocularly and binocularly to allow determination of the affected muscles. Some tests that can be used for evaluation are the alternate cover test, the Hess-Lancaster screen, and the Maddox rod. A shortcut method to isolate a single cyclovertical muscle in recent noncomitance is the three-step method, which consists of various measurements of ocular alignment.[33] It is not appropriate for lateral muscle palsies or when more than one muscle is affected. The three-step method is conducted by determining which eye has the hyper component in primary position, in which field of gaze the hyper component increases, and whether the hyper component increases on right or left head tilt (Table 13-3).

Two tests are especially helpful for evaluating noncomitance and subsequently monitoring therapy progress.[7] With an arc perimeter or tangent screen, the following should be measured:

1. Monocular field: how far the patient can foveally fixate (follow) a target as it moves along the perimeter surface. This is measured in degrees.

**TABLE 13-1**

### Abnormal Head Posture and Affected Extraocular Muscle

| Turn | Face Position/ Chin Position | Tilt | Muscle Affected |
|------|------------------------------|------|-----------------|
| Right | None | None | RLR |
| Left | None | None | RMR |
| Left | Down | Left | RSO |
| Left | Up | Right | RIO |
| Right | Up | Left | RSR |
| Right | Down | Right | RIR |
| Left | None | None | LLR |
| Right | None | None | LMR |
| Right | | Right | LSO |
| Right | Up | Left | LIO |
| Left | Up | Right | LSR |
| Left | Down | Left | LIR |

*RLR,* right lateral rectus; *RMR,* right medial rectus; *RSO,* right superior oblique; *RIO,* right inferior oblique; *RSR,* right superior rectus; *RIR,* right inferior rectus; *LLR,* left lateral rectus; *LMR,* left medial rectus; *LSO,* left superior oblique; *LIO,* left inferior oblique; *LSR,* left superior rectus; *LIR,* left inferior rectus.

**TABLE 13-2**

### Extraocular Muscles and Their Fields of Action

| Right Eye | | | Left Eye | |
|---|---|---|---|---|
| **Gaze Direction** | **Muscle** | | **Gaze Direction** | **Muscle** |
| Right | RLR | | Left | LLR |
| Left | RMR | | Right | LMR |
| Left, down | RSO | | Right, down | LSO |
| Left, up | RIO | | Right, up | LIO |
| Right, up | RSR | | Left, up | LSR |
| Right, down | RIR | | Left, down | LIR |
| Rotational separation | LIO | | RIO | Rotational separation |
| Vertical separation | LSR / RIO | | RSR / LIO | Vertical separation |
| Patient's left | LLR / RMR | Primary position | RLR / LMR | Patient's right |
| Vertical separation | LIR / RSO | | RIR / LSO | Vertical separation |
| Rotational separation | LSO | | RSO | Rotational separation |

*RLR,* right lateral rectus; *RMR,* right medial rectus; *RSO,* right superior oblique; *RIO,* right inferior oblique; *RSR,* right superior rectus; *RIR,* right inferior rectus; *LLR,* left lateral rectus; *LMR,* left medial rectus; *LSO,* left superior oblique; *LIO,* left inferior oblique; *LSR,* left superior rectus; *LIR,* left inferior rectus.

**TABLE 13-3**

### Three-Step Method for Determining Cyclovertical Muscle

| Paretic Muscle | Hyper Eye in Primary Position | Hyper Greater on Gaze | Hyper Greater on Head Tilt |
|---|---|---|---|
| LIO | Right | Right | Right |
| RIR | Right | Right | Left |
| RSO | Right | Left | Right |
| LSR | Right | Left | Left |
| RSR | Left | Right | Right |
| LSO | Left | Right | Left |
| LIR | Left | Left | Right |
| RIO | Left | Left | Left |

*LIO,* left inferior oblique: *RIR,* right inferior rectus; *RSO,* right superior oblique; *LSR,* left superior rectus; *RSR,* right superior rectus; *LSO,* left superior oblique; *LIR,* left inferior rectus; *RIO,* right inferior oblique.

2. Binocular field: to what extent the patient can bifoveally fixate (follow) a target along the perimeter surface before diplopia or suppression occurs; also measured in degrees.

Anaglyphic or Polaroid techniques help diplopia awareness. An area of suppression or confusion frequently appears before diplopia is noticed. Figure 13-2 shows possible diplopia fields for a right lateral rectus paresis.

During and after optometric rehabilitation, these tests can be used to monitor therapy by checking whether the monocular fixation field has expanded. The extent of the binocular field before diplopia awareness also should increase. This allows objective assessment of therapy progress.

Pupillary and visual field studies should be done when diagnosing any noncomitance. When pupillary function is affected, tumors or aneurysms are suspected. Etiological factors are not determined in every noncomitance, however.

## REHABILITATION OF OCULOMOTOR DYSFUNCTIONS

In geriatrics the objective of treatment has long been recognized to be the restoration of function maximally based on the normal for the age of the patient and the condition present. This may seem obvious to the experienced clinician; however, attempts to restore function beyond normal responses for the age, visual condition, and individual patient will only result in frustration for both practitioner and patient. This may explain the reluctance of many optometrists to engage in the rehabilitation of visual dysfunctions of older patients.

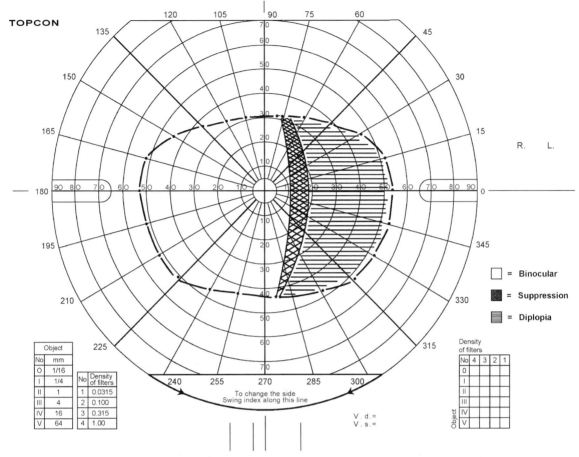

**Fig. 13-2** Representative diplopia fields for a patient with a right lateral rectus paresis.

After an accurate history and diagnosis have been obtained, lens management, prism management, or both are used to improve binocularity maximally. Decisions about lens prescription types (e.g., multifocals including progressive addition, single-vision reading) generally are made based on a case history of working conditions rather than any possible subsequent binocular therapy. The patient is reevaluated after 2 weeks to 1 month. If the patient still shows evidence of decreased binocular function (e.g., macular suppression, decreased amplitude of fusion, fixation disparity, or decreased stereopsis) and symptoms persist, vision therapy is indicated if the patient can be properly motivated. Home vision therapy is generally sufficient for the rehabilitation of older patients' binocular dysfunctions, especially exodeviations. Occasionally the management of esodeviations will need to incorporate office-based therapy along with base-out prism.

### Comitant Deviations

Binocular rehabilitation attempts to develop efficient, comfortable, well-sustained binocular vision by using prisms, lenses, vision therapy, or a combination of these techniques. Motor and peripheral sensory fusion is generally already present. The rehabilitative therapies discussed in this chapter are limited to lateral deviations. Although vertical heterophoria can be treated with vision therapy techniques, the processes needed are somewhat more complicated. Furthermore, experience indicates that vision therapy techniques for vertical deviations are usually less successful in reducing symptoms of older patients than are vertical prism prescriptions.

Vision therapy is designed to enhance stereopsis, version and saccadic ability, and vergence ranges maximally. It is indicated at any age—even into the 90s—when symptoms exist and binocular findings are abnormal. When age-related decreases in monocular skills (pursuit and saccadic ability) are present, a short period of monocular training may be needed (1 week to 2 weeks at most). Rehabilitation for older adults proceeds faster when binocular therapy accompanies monocular therapy and is emphasized exclusively after monocular skills are essentially equal.

Occasionally older patients have problems with even very small heterophorias. Central suppression, reduced vergence ranges, poor version and saccadic ability, and reduced stereopsis influence the extent of these problems. Rehabilitative therapy using appropriate lens and prism corrections is done when these "general skills" problems exist.

## Rehabilitative Management of Exophoria

The overall goals in the rehabilitation of exophoria in older adults are sustained compensation for the exodeviation using increased convergence ability and comfortable binocular vision for needed visual tasks.

Refractive management is usually less successful than vision therapy management for exophoria. Obviously, additional minus lens power at distance is inappropriate for presbyopic patients because of their lack of accommodative ability and base-in prism can actually increase the exodeviation because of prism adaptation.[5,15] Vision therapy is generally sufficient without modification of the refractive correction. However, base-in prism can be useful when vision therapy is not possible.

The following are vision therapy goals for older adults with exophoria:

- Increase voluntary fusional convergence maximally (breakpoints)
- Enhance jump vergences (recovery points)
- Establish central and foveal sensory fusion in free space at the ortho position
- Enhance stereopsis
- Develop reflex vergences

Boxes 13-1 to 13-4 give typical rehabilitative vision therapy procedures for symptomatic near and distance exophoria. Procedures are listed in the order usually prescribed for home therapy, but all procedures are not necessary for every patient. Older patients with symptomatic exophoria at distance and near are managed with rehabilitative vision therapy techniques from all four lists. Therapy for both distance

---

**BOX 13-1**

### Vergence Training for Near Exophoria

- Pencil push-ups. A detailed target is moved from arm's length closer until fusion is lost. This technique is sometimes combined with lights, anaglyphs, or both for antisuppression training.
- Colored circles (Mast/Keystone). These provide a flat fusion convergence demand and can be modified for simultaneous antisuppression training.
- Aperture-rule trainer. With a single aperture, positive fusional vergence training is done using antisuppression and stereoscopic targets. This is often combined with a distance target for jump vergence training.
- Eccentric circles. With these circles used with stereopsis demand, fusion training is done by crossing the eyes to develop convergence ability. This technique can be combined with two targets for jump vergence training.
- Near point chiastopic fusion. This develops convergent fusion by using two ordinary objects (often with antisuppression cues) such as coins, thumbs, or buttons.
- Anaglyphic reading. With a Polaroid or anaglyphic grid of bars and spaces, combined with appropriate glasses, antisuppression training is done. This technique can be combined with lenses or prisms for simultaneous vergence training.[10]
- Mirror stereoscope. A Wheatstone-type stereoscope using two mirrors for dissociation and shaped in the form of a W, using various targets, can train vergence ranges of 40 △ base-in to 50 △ base-out.
- Brock's posture board. With the use of anaglyphs and lights on a Plexiglas board, near antisuppression tests can be done. The technique can be combined with lenses and prisms.
- Three-eye mirror method. A circle is drawn on a mirror. The patient converges and fuses his or her eyes to see one eye fused in the center and two eyes on the outside—all inside the circle. This technique can be combined with a letter on the mirror for jump vergence training.
- Combinations. All these techniques can be combined to increase vergence demand, reduce suppression, and enhance stereopsis.

---

and near exophoria is grouped into two parts: vergence training and antisuppression/stereopsis training. Home therapy is prescribed from each category, and the level of difficulty is increased with improved binocular responses.

When home therapy is appropriate, detailed instruction sheets can ensure patient compliance. Figure 13-3 shows a typical instruction sheet for home therapy that uses push-up convergence. Other sheets can and should be prepared for each rehabilitative technique; examples are given throughout this chapter.

**BOX 13-2**

## Antisuppression/Stereopsis Training for Near Exophoria

- Polachrome Orthoptic Trainer. Vectograms or tranaglyphs and appropriate spectacles are used in antisuppression and convergence therapy.[32]
- Pola-mirror push-ups. The patient looks at his or her eyes in a mirror while wearing Polaroid glasses. Any "blacking out" of one lens (suppression) is noted.[13] The mirror is moved closer and farther away.
- Eccentric circles.
- Anaglyphic reading.
- Brock's posture board.
- Aperture-rule trainer.
- Orthofusor base-out kit. The Polaroid kit is used to improve positive fusional vergence and give antisuppression and stereoacuity training.
- Bar reading (custom-made). A septum is placed between the reading task and the patient to dissociate one eye from the other. Suppression is noted when words are missing. This technique can be combined with lenses and prisms for vergence training.
- Combinations. All these techniques can be combined to increase vergence demand, reduce suppression, and enhance stereopsis.

**BOX 13-3**

## Vergence Training for Distance Exophoria

- Voluntary convergence. During the training of willful crossing of the eyes, visual stimuli are sometimes used. Patients should become aware of the feeling in their eyes as they converge.
- Ductions and versions. Some improvement of saccadic and version ability is often helpful. A swinging Marsden ball can train pursuit movements. Any two targets can be used for saccadic training.
- Pencil pushaways. A detailed fixation target is held close and gradually moved farther away. Sometimes anaglyphs and a light are used.
- Handheld Brewster's stereoscope. This is a refracting stereoscope with a septum. Using any of the hundreds of stereograms available, vergence and antisuppression training are done. Vergence demand is varied by changing the target separation or fixation distance (tromboning).
- Prism demand flippers. With the use of prisms in a lens holder, vergence demand is changed in discrete steps. This technique can be combined with antisuppression exercises (anaglyphs or Polaroid glasses) for powerful training of vergence and fusion ability.
- Chiastopic fusion at far. Two pictures with suppression cues give a fusion demand. Near chiastopic fusion usually must be learned first.
- Risley prism for pursuit. This variable prism, which can be used to increase vergence demand, may need to be combined with antisuppression exercises.
- Polachrome orthoptic trainer. Vectograms or tranaglyphs (Bernell Corporation) and appropriate spectacles are used in antisuppression and convergence therapy.[32]
- Vis-a-vis walkaways. Both examiner and patient wear Polaroid glasses. The patient is to tell of any blacking out of one of the examiner's eyes. This also can be done with a mirror by the patient alone.[12]
- Combinations. All these techniques can be combined to increase vergence demand, reduce suppression, and enhance stereopsis.

As with young patients, the primary therapeutic consideration in treating exophoria in older adults is the patient's ability to compensate for the deviation (an ability that has large individual variations). Because of normal reductions in overall vergence ability in older adults, the magnitude of the deviation is important to the final outcome. Rehabilitative vision therapy alone is generally sufficient for the treatment of exophoria. Frequently a vertical and lateral heterophoria coexist, and deciding whether correcting the vertical phoria is necessary is occasionally difficult. When the vertical phoria is not corrected and initial lateral vergence training is unsuccessful, vertical prism correction is frequently needed to reduce symptoms and ensure the success of lateral therapy.

Some older patients complete all the rehabilitative therapy techniques with little symptomatic relief. These patients require a decrease in overall convergence demand for comfortable, efficient binocularity. Vergence demand can be reduced with base-in prisms or extraocular muscle surgery when the deviation is large enough at all distances. After the deviation has been reduced with prism or surgery, some patients need further vision therapy to eliminate persistent conditions such as foveal sup-

pression and fixation disparity or to develop fine stereopsis.

### Rehabilitative Management of Esophoria

The overall goals in the rehabilitative management of esophoria are to enhance compensation of the esodeviation through increased divergence and provide comfortable binocular vision for needed visual tasks.

Prescription modification is more helpful for esodeviations than for exodeviations and may be successful in relieving symptoms without vision therapy or in minimizing therapy time. Patients with a distance esophoria are frequently

## Antisuppression Stereopsis Training for Distance Exophoria

- Peripheral stereopsis. With the use of large stereoscopic targets (Root rings or Brock's rings), stereopsis responses are elicited peripherally. The patient works to increase the distance from the test so that the test, as well as subsequent stereopsis demand, becomes more central.
- Television trainer. An anaglyphic or Polaroid attachment for the television is available. When appropriate spectacles are worn, suppression is noted when part of the picture turns black. This technique can be combined with prisms or lenses for simultaneous vergence training.
- Brock string techniques. A string is held from a distant target to the nose. The patient sees two strings crossing at the visual axes crossing point. Beads can be put on the string to increase diplopia awareness, and anaglyphs can help eliminate suppression.
- Pola-mirror training with afterimages. A mirror and Polaroid lenses are combined with afterimages. The goal is to see crossed afterimages and both eyes (no suppression).
- Pola-mirror training with two mirrors. This is the same technique as above, but this one uses two mirrors so that fixation distances can be altered to increase or decrease vergence demand and fusion difficulty. It also can be combined with afterimages.
- Chiastopic fusion at far.
- Handheld Brewster's stereoscope.
- Prism bar for saccadic vergences. Prism bars increase vergence demand in discrete, rapid steps. They often are combined with antisuppression exercises. Prism bars can be custom made for each patient to give maximal training.[38]
- Combinations. All these techniques can be combined to increase vergence demand, reduce suppression, and enhance stereopsis.

helped by base-out prism. Vision therapy is then recommended if needed to enhance sensory fusion and give the patient the most comfortable, clear binocular vision possible.

The following are vision therapy goals in the management of esophoria:

- Extend fusional convergence maximally
- Enhance awareness of stereopsis
- Exercise the present ability to achieve sensory fusion (especially peripheral fusion) in as many varied instruments as are available in the office
- Increase fusional divergence (breakpoints) by teaching "relaxation" of the eyes through concentration

- Enhance jump vergence ability (recovery points)
- Establish central and foveal sensory fusion at the angle of deviation by using instruments and then not using instruments
- Develop reflex vergences

Rehabilitative therapy procedures for esophoria attempt to increase disparity (fusional) divergence involuntarily as a response to increased sensory fusion (stereopsis) demands. Sensory fusion is maintained by adding stereopsis to flat fusion skills. Fusional divergence is stimulated reflexively by increased demand. Because of the absence of accommodation caused by presbyopia (compensated by plus additions for clear vision at near), symptomatic near esophoria is rare.

The home rehabilitative therapy sequence for distance esophoria is shown in Box 13-5, Box 13-6, and Figure 13-4.

### Rehabilitative Management of Central Suppression and Fixation Disparity

When older patients have reduced visual skills and binocular instabilities, fixation disparity, foveal and macular suppression, or both are frequently found. Goals in rehabilitation include eliminating central suppression, establishing bifoveal fixation, and developing fine stereoacuity.

Refractive management includes modification of the refractive correction by using prism. Prescriptions are designed with forced vergence fixation disparity curves (see Fig. 13-1). Prism is prescribed to reduced fixation disparity to zero (associated phoria) when steep curves are present. Prism is prescribed to center the flat portion more approximately on the y-axis (center of symmetry) when flat forced vergence fixation disparity curves are measured. Careful refractive management can reduce the need for rehabilitative therapy and enhance therapy success.

Successful rehabilitative therapy of central suppression and fixation disparity requires targets that are small and detailed enough to necessitate bifoveal fixation and enhance central sensory fusion. Using stereoscopic targets rather than flat fusion targets will aid motor processes and thus maintain bifoveal fixation. The techniques are used for "finishing off" procedures for heterophoria with reduced visual skills. Whenever possible, targets should be chosen

These exercises will develop the coordination and focusing ability of your eyes when you are looking at near objects and when you look from far to near objects. You will know you are doing the exercise or exercises correctly when you can fuse the two sets of circles into one circle, with a smaller circle inside that stands out or falls away.

Exercise a total of _____minutes each day. After you can accomplish Procedure 1, add one new procedure each week as you do the exercises. In the beginning you may experience some discomfort such as headaches and eyestrain, so you may have to limit the exercises to a few minutes. As your ability improves, your discomfort will disappear, and the exercise time can be increased. Remember that exercising 15 minutes daily is better than exercising 2 hours once a week! It would be best if you did this exercise at_____,_____, and_____each day. Try to establish a routine so that you always do the exercises at the same time each day.

**Procedure 1:** Hold the two cards together with A's overlapping. Hold a pencil centered between the circles. Look at the top of the lead, and observe the circles on either side without looking directly at them. Slowly move the pencil toward your nose (always looking directly at the lead and keeping it centered) until you see *Four* large circles, or more than two. Continue moving your pencil. Observe the center large circles approaching each other until you see the overlap (superimpose). You then will see *Three* large circles with the center one under the pencil. The center large circle will have a smaller circle inside it that appears to be behind the large circle. If the center circle looks even with the large circle, you are not using one of yours eyes (supression).
*Note:* If you find that only one eye is being used, then in order to use both eyes, do the following:
1. Blink your eyes rapidly.
2. Cover one eye, and then quickly remove the cover.
Next, try to clear the letters. While you continue to maintain the fused circles and depth (one circle behind the other), concentrate on holding the letters clear.

*Correct Response:* When Proceduce 1 is done correctly, you should see three large circles. The center one should be *clear* and composed of two circles –one behind the other.
*Note:* This exercise also can be done with the *B's* overlapping. These are the correct responses:
1. When the *A's* overlap, the center circle should appear behind the larger circle.
2. When the *B's* overlap, the center circle should appear ahead of the larger circle.
If you cannot see the depth or see it as the reverse of the previous description, you are doing the exercise incorrectly and need to try again.

**Procedure 2:** Repeat Procedure 1, but without the aid of the pencil. When you can easily fuse the circle without the pencil, begin moving the cards apart. Keep moving them farther apart until the center circle blurs and then breaks into two. Repeat the exercise_____times, trying to get the cards farther apart each time.

**Procedure 3:** Look to a detailed distant (more than 10 feet away) object, and make it clear. Then look to the cards and fuse the circles, making the center clear and single and noticing the depth. Repeat this until you can easily look from a distant object to the cards and fuse them when they are separated by 12 inches or more. No pencil is to be used in this exercise. Remember to clear the distant object, then look to the cards and fuse and clear the circles. Move the circles farther apart each time.

**Procedure 4:** Place the cards against a wall at a distance of about 5 to 6 feet. The cards should be 5 to 6 inches apart. Fuse them in the same manner you have been using for near. When you can fuse and clear the cards easily at this distance, begin moving them farther apart each time.

**Procedure 5**: When you can fuse the cards (at 5 to 6 feet away) when they are about 2 feet apart, being alternating your fixation from the fused cards at a distance to a detailed near object. Repeat this until you can easily look from the fused cards to the near object, making each clear before you look to the next one.

**Proceduce 6:** Fuse the cards at a distance of 5 to 6 feet with the cards approximately 12 inches apart. Walk toward the cards (keeping them fused) as close as you can until they get blurry or split into two. Repeat this, trying to walk closer each time before the center circle breaks into two. Always try to maintain the correct response: The cards should be clear, and you should see the depth.

**Fig. 13-3** Patient instructions: home vision therapy—free fusion rings (convergence).

that have binocular contours, foveal-sized suppression targets, and fine stereopsis stimulation.

Typical home rehabilitative procedures for fixation disparity and central suppression are shown in Box 13-7, Box 13-8, and Figure 13-5.

A different prism correction is frequently indicated for older patients for distance and near. Bifocals can be prescribed with cement-on or press-on prism segments. Providing bifocals for occasional reading only is often better. For prolonged reading, a single-vision reading correction incorporating the proper near addition and indicated prism correction is frequently the best and most comfortable rehabilitation.

**BOX 13-5**

## Vergence Training for Distance Esophoria

- Ductions and versions. Some improvement of saccadic and version ability is often helpful. A swinging Marsden ball can train pursuit movements. Any two targets can be used for saccadic training.
- Pencil pushaways. A detailed fixation target is held close and gradually moved farther away. Sometimes anaglyphs and a light are used.
- Eccentric circles. With these circles with stereopsis demand, fusion training is done by turning the eyes out to develop divergence ability. This technique can combine with two targets for jump vergence training.
- Prism demand flippers. With prisms in a lens holder, vergence demand is changed in discrete steps. This technique can be combined with antisuppression exercises (anaglyphs or Polaroid glasses) for powerful training of vergence and fusion ability.
- Brock string techniques. A string is held from a distant target to the nose. The patient sees two strings crossing at the visual axes crossing point. Beads can be put on the string to increase diplopia awareness, and anaglyphs can help to eliminate suppression.
- Combinations. All these techniques can be combined to increase vergence demand, reduce suppression, and enhance stereopsis.

**BOX 13-6**

## Antisuppression Stereopsis Training for Distance Esophoria

- Prism demand flippers.
- Hole-in-hand game. The patient looks through a tube with one eye while holding a hand in front of the other eye. The patient strives to see both the hand and an object in the field of view through the "tube hole" in the hand.
- Handheld Brewster's stereoscopes. This is a refracting stereoscope with a septum. With any of the hundreds of stereograms available, vergence and antisuppression training are done. Vergence demand is varied by changing the target separation or fixation distance (tromboning).
- Brock string techniques.
- Polachrome orthoptic trainers. Vectograms or tranaglyphs and appropriate spectacles are used in antisuppression and convergence therapy.[42]
- Flannel board training. Red, green, and yellow pieces are made and put on a piece of black flannel. With anaglyphic glasses, antisuppression exercises can be done. This technique is often combine with tenses and prisms and distance anaglyphic targets.
- Worth dot lights. Four lights—one red, two green, and one white—are arranged in a diamond pattern. They are used with anaglyphs and moved nearer and farther as a good antisuppression technique. This technique can be combined with lenses and prisms for simultaneous vergence training.
- Bagolini's striated lenses. These lenses with fine striations cause a visible streak when the patient looks at a light. Any suppression is noted when one line or part of a line disappears.[43] This technique can be combined with lenses and prisms for vergence training.
- Combinations. All these techniques can be combined to increase vergence demand, reduce suppression, and enhance stereopsis. Figure 13-4 shows a typical home therapy instruction sheet for an esophoria rehabilitation technique.

### Noncomitant Deviations

Management of the noncomitant deviation depends on whether it is of recent onset or is long-standing. Noncomitance of recent onset requires accurate, immediate diagnosis and referral to the appropriate medial practitioner —usually an internist, ophthalmologist, neuro-ophthalmologist, or neurologist. The optometrist plays a significant role in diagnosing, directing the patient to the proper specialist, and judging the urgency of the situation. When the necessary medical care has been completed (and some-times while it continues), functional aspects of the paretic noncomitant deviation are managed by fusion maintenance programs and ocular calisthenics to help prevent secondary contrac-ture. These programs involve careful use of lenses, prisms, occlusion, and vision therapy.

When an extraocular muscle becomes paretic, its antagonist acts unopposed; an eye turn results from weakness of the paretic muscle and subsequent overreaction by the antagonist. Long-standing action by an unopposed muscle can lead to a slow contracture of that muscle. Contracture, which is thought to be caused by

atrophy and hyalinization, frequently occurs over a long period (months or years). When contracture occurs, even when the cause of the noncomitance is muscle paresis, the paresis frequently lessens, the deviation becomes more equal, and a residual deviation remains. This is known as the spread of comitance. Rehabilita-tive intervention can help prevent and relieve the problems of noncomitance (diplopia, spatial localization problems, and contracture).

When diplopia is a significant problem, prism and occlusion often can restore fusion or elimi-nate the diplopic image. Occlusion will always

These exercises will develop good binocular vision while your eyes are diverging (turning outward) as if looking at distant objects. You will know you are using both eyes correctly in each procedure when the pictures viewed are seen as one, they are seen clearly, parts of the targets seen by each eye alone are present simultaneously, and depth is seen in certain cards.

Exercise a total of _____ minutes each day, and increase the number of procedures in each session as you can do them. In the beginning you might experience discomfort such as headaches and eyestrain, so that you may have to limit the exercises to a few minutes. As your ability improves, your discomfort will disappear, and the exercise time can be increased. Remember that exercising 15 minutes daily is better than exercising 2 hours once a week! It would be best if you did this exercise at_____, _____, and _____ each day. Try to establish a routine so that you always do the exercises at the same time each day.

**Procedure 1**: Place the instrument on a table at a comfortable height, with light falling evenly on the target cards. The double-aperture slider is placed at the position marked I or 2 on the front rutler. The target cards should be placed at the 0 position on the back ruler. The AP1 and AP2 cards are the targets for the procedures. To see the targets through the double aperture, place the tip of your nose against the end of the front ruler. If you are wearing a bifocal, tip your head back slightly, and place your lower lip against the ruler. Concentrate and actively try to fuse the targets at all times. Do not be discouraged if you are unsuccessful at first. Repeated efforts at looking at the targets and attempting fusion will lead to success.

Look through the double aperture at card API (later, follow the same procedure with AP2). Close your left eye, and your right eye will see only one box with a black cross. Close your right eye, and your left eye will see only one box with a black ball. The ball is seen only by the left eye, and the cross is seen only by the right eye. If necessary to achieve this, move the aperture slider toward or away from you. Your eyes are now in this position:

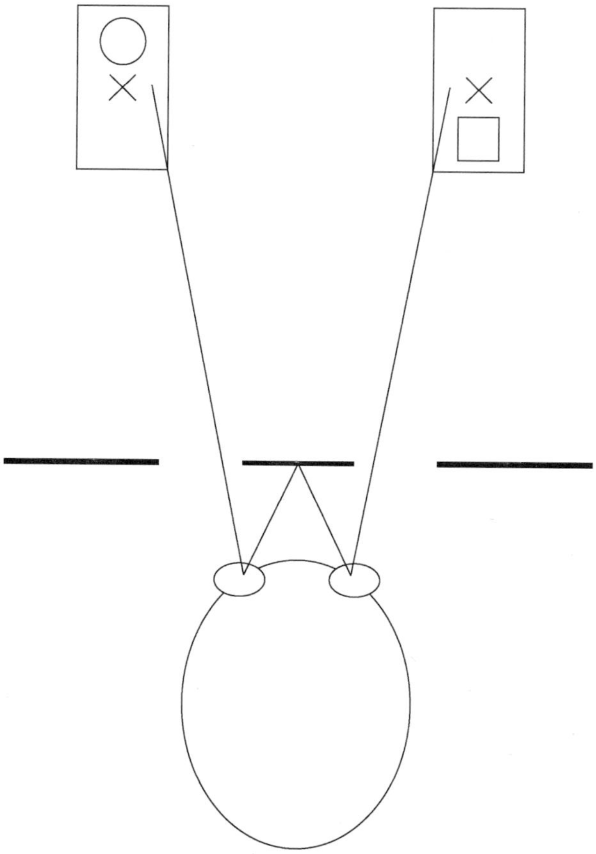

The right eye sees the target on the right side of the card.

The left eye sees the target on the left side of the card.

Look with both eyes, and make the two targets into one target.

**Correct Response:** When you have made the two targets into one (fusion), you will see this:

One box with the cross and ball are seen simultaneously.

**Fig. 13-4** Patient instructions: home vision therapy—double aperture rule trainer.

*Continued*

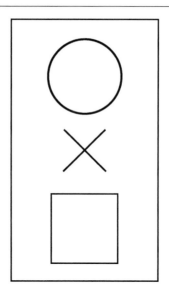

*Note:* If either the cross or the ball is seen alone, it means that although both your eyes are open, the visual information from one of your eyes is not being received (suppression). The result is that of closing one eye. One of your goals in this exercise is to become aware of the information from both eyes and unify it into one visual percept (sensory function). To do so, follow these steps:

1. Cover and uncover one eye, exposing both targets for brief periods while attempting fusion.
2. Blink your eyes rapidly, looking for fusion between blinks.

If you see two boxes instead of one, the visual information is being received, but your eyes are not aimed correctly. Your second goal is to diverge your eyes correctly so that sensory fusion can take place. To do so, look over the aperture slide across the room at a target. You should feel your eyes going outward. As you keep your eyes in an outward position, just notice the targets in the foreground. Now direct your attention to the targets. You should see them as one, and as you concentrate, the fused picture should clear. Repeat this procedure until you can maintain *one fused clear* target.

**Fig. 13-4, cont'd**

eliminate diplopia. However, this technique must be used cautiously because spatial localization is impaired when an eye muscle is paretic. When critical or dangerous tasks are done (e.g., driving, cooking, or dangerous work), the eye with the paretic muscle should be occluded as long as the acuity is sufficiently good so that the patient is safe.

Sector occlusion on a spectacle lens can help prevent diplopia when fusion exists in certain fields of gaze (Fig. 13-6). Alternate occlusion can help provide each eye as much action into the paretic field of gaze as possible.

Occlusion must be done in a manner consistent with attempts to prevent muscle contracture from the paresis. Although it is doubtful whether any method of preventing secondary contracture is fully effective, preventive methods are important to try, and they can only help. The following optical techniques attempt to prevent contracture:

- Conjugate prisms (bases in the same direction) may be worn. Both prisms are placed so that the eyes are forced to look in the direction of the field of the paretic muscle. This stimulates the paretic muscle and relaxes its antagonist.
- A prism can be worn before the eye without the paretic muscle to force that eye into the field of gaze of the paretic muscle. This again attempts to relax the antagonist muscle and stimulate the paretic one.

Nonoptical methods of secondary contracture prevention are also possible. Medical techniques include anesthetic or botulinum injection into the antagonist muscle and early recession surgery of the antagonist before contracture can develop.

Techniques for prevention of secondary contracture are primarily designed to force the paretic eye toward the field of action of the affected muscle. Monocular therapy is designed

---

**BOX 13-7**

### Vergence Training for Central Suppression and Fixation Disparity

- Polachrome orthoptic trainer. Vectograms or tranaglyphs and appropriate spectacles are used in antisuppression and convergence therapy.[32]
- Biopter cards, E series. These are targets with antisuppression cues for use in Brewster-type stereoscopes. They are combined with changeable vergence demand in the stereoscope (tromboning).
- Spache binocular reading. These are targets with antisuppression cues for use in Brewster-type stereoscopes. They are combined with changeable vergence demand in the stereoscope (tromboning).
- MKM binocular reading cards. These are targets with antisuppression cues for use in Brewster-type stereoscopes. They are combined with changeable vergence demand in the stereoscope (tromboning).
- Combinations. All these techniques can be combined to increase vergence demand, reduce suppression, and enhance stereopsis.

---

**BOX 13-8**

### Antisuppression Stereopsis Training for Central Suppression and Fixation Disparity

- Cheiroscopic tracing. With a cheiroscope targets are traced, colored, or filled in. Training can be enhanced by having the patient close his or her or striving to see all lines and colors previously drawn.
- Projectopter. Tranaglyphs or vectograms are projected on a screen for distance antisuppression and vergence training.
- Titmus stereo slides. Slides are used to enhance stereopsis. Vergence ability is altered by using prisms and lenses.
- American Optical vectographic adult slide. A projected polarized slide is used to monitor fixation disparity and suppression as prisms and lenses change vergence demand.
- Mallet distance and near fixation disparity test unit. These fixation disparity tests are used with Polaroid glasses. Lenses and prisms can be used to train vergence while reducing fixation disparity and suppression.
- Combinations. All these techniques can be combined to increase vergence demand, reduce suppression, and enhance stereopsis. A home therapy training sheet is shown in Figure 13-5 for a typical antisuppression training technique.

---

for each eye while the other is occluded. The sound eye exercises in the field of action of the paretic muscle to relax the antagonist muscle and stimulate the paretic one. To exercise the paretic muscle, systematized programs requiring accurate fixations farther and farther into the field of action of the paretic muscle are used.

Boxes 13-9 and 13-10 provide techniques for monocular vision therapy when a muscle paresis is present.

Fusion should be maintained as much as possible in all cases of noncomitance. Prism may be needed to restore fusion in the primary position. Sector prisms in Fresnel form can be used to give increasing fusion ability in the field of the paretic muscle. Prism power is determined empirically, and varying prism power can be used if noncomitance is severe. Prism for fusion does not prevent secondary contracture.

Expansions of motor fusion ranges are indicated in practically all cases of muscle paresis. Motor fusion training is designed to give maximal fusion ability. Sensory fusion was probably present before noncomitance developed, so this type of training may not be needed in all fields of gaze.

Vision therapy goals for patients with muscle paresis include (1) maximally expanding voluntary motor fusion ranges in the field of gaze opposite the paresis, (2) developing reflex vergence in the primary position, and (3) expanding fusional vergence training into the field of action of the paretic muscle.

Rehabilitative therapy is done in the manner indicated for the type of phoria present (see pages 250 and 251). Therapy is similar for recent or long-standing noncomitant deviations. The progress of the therapy should be monitored according to the monocular field of view and binocular diplopia fields, which should increase as fusion and eye movement ability improve.

### PROGNOSIS

Vision therapy is an effective procedure that can improve binocularity in patients with presbyopia. These patients are able to learn therapy procedures easily and often carry them out more faithfully than do younger patients. Thus the tradition of reserving vision therapy primarily for children or young adults is not justified. Problems such as blurred vision, tired eyes, or headaches after reading associated with binocular problems can be helped for most patients of any age.

These exercises will develop simultaneous perception from your two eyes when you are looking at a distance. You will know you are using both eyes when you can see the television clearly through both parts of the therapy device. Remember, your task is to see the whole television picture through both parts of the device at once.

Exercise a total of _____minutes each day, and increase the number of procedures in each session as you can do them. In the beginning, one part of the television may be dark, or you may experience some discomfort; therefore, you may have to limit the exercise to a few minutes. As your ability improves, your discomfort will disappear, and the exercise time can be increased. Remember that exercising 15 minutes daily is better than exercising 2 hours once a week! It would be best if you did this exercise at _____,_____, and _____ each day. Try to establish a routine so that you always do the exercises at the same time each day.

**Procedure 1:** Attach the therapy device to the television set vertically with suction cups.

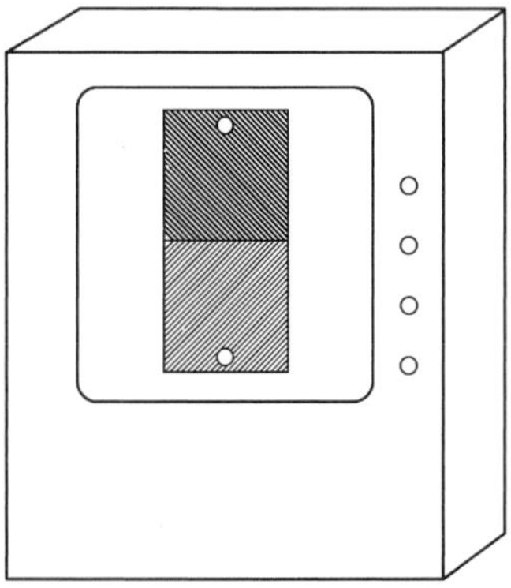

If the device is red and green, put the red part on top. It is very important that the device be vertical; otherwise, the therapy may be ineffective. Put on the special glasses provided by the doctor. If the glasses are red and green, put the red lens over your right eye. If the glasses are not red and green, be very careful to watch the television with your head straight upright. Turn on the television, sit _____feet away from it, and watch it.

*Correct Response:* Looking at the television, you will see the television through both parts of the therapy device at the same time.

*Note:* During this exercise, if one part of the therapy device is black (cannot be seen through), the visual information from one of your eyes is not being received (suppression). The result is like closing one eye. If first one part of the device is black and then the other is black, it is similar to alternately closing one eye and then the other. The visual information is still being received only from one eye at a time. Your goal in these exercises is to become aware of the visual information from both eyes simultaneously.

If you find that only one eye is being used (suppression), do the following to use both eyes:
1. Blink your eyes rapidly, looking for the other eye's image between blinks.
2. Cover one eye; then quickly remove the cover.
3. Turn the room lights down or out.
4. Do any or all of the above in combination.

Ask yourself these questions, and be sure to tell your answers to the doctor evaluating your progress:
1. Does one part of the television therapy device ever go black? If so, when and how often?
2. Does the black part of the therapy device jump from top to bottom and back?
3. If both parts of the device are easy to see through, is the picture on the television clear or blurry?
4. Does this exercise get easier as I do it more often?

**Procedure 2:** Repeat Procedure 1 at a different distance (about _____feet).
Always try to maintain the correct response: clear, easy viewing through both parts of the therapy device at the same time.

**Procedure 3:** As Procedure 2 becomes easy for you, move (closer) (farther) and continue trying to maintain the correct response.

**Fig. 13-5** Patient instructions: home vision therapy—television trainer.

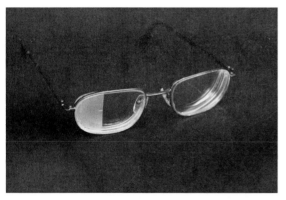

**Fig. 13-6** Temporal occlusion with clear contact paper on the right lens will alleviate diplopia when the patient with a right lateral rectus paresis looks to the right.

**BOX 13-9**

### Sound Eye Fixing (Gaze Direction in Field of Action of Paretic Muscle)

- Watching television or related activity. This is done with the eyes directed in the field of action of the paretic muscle.
- Walking. This is done with the eyes directed toward the field of action of the paretic muscle.
- Balancing exercises. These are done with the eyes directed toward the field of action of the paretic muscle.
- Tracing exercises. Targets are traced toward the field of action of the paretic muscle.
- Prism ductions: large prism changes. Prism vergence is done in large steps toward the field of action of the paretic muscle. The patient tries to maintain fixation farther each time.

**BOX 13-10**

### Paretic Eye Fixing (Gaze Direction Toward Action of Paretic Muscle)

- Tracking a suspended moving ball. The patient attempts to track a Marsden ball farther and farther into the field of action of the paretic muscle.
- Tracing exercises.
- Batting or ringing a moving, suspended ball. The patient attempts to keep a circular ring around a Marsden ball as it swings toward the field of action of the paretic muscle.
- Prism ductions: small prism changes. Prism vergence is done in small steps toward the field of action of the paretic muscle. The patient tries to maintain fixation farther each time.
- Repeating the above exercise while walking.
- Rotating pegboard. The patient tries to put golf tees in a rotating perforated disk. Gradually the disk is moved toward the field of action of the paretic muscle.

For the establishment of the prognosis for success of vision therapy in older adults, records of subjects with presbyopia (n = 161) who had undergone vision therapy for convergence problems (n = 134) or general skills problems (n = 27) were studied.[39] The age range was 45 to 89 years. Patients all had normal acuity for their age. After appropriate refractive management, vision therapy was prescribed as needed. When vision therapy was needed, patients with exophoria generally were successful with 6 weeks of therapy, and patients with esophoria were successful in 6 to 8 weeks. Older patients generally carried out therapy procedures well, and home therapy was satisfactory for most. The conclusion of the study was that for binocular vision problems in older adults who are treated with appropriate prism correction and vision therapy, symptoms are eliminated and test findings are restored to normal for the age and physical condition of the patient 92% (148 of 161) of the time. When the elimination of symptoms was the primary criterion, the success rate for therapy was 97% (156 of 161).

Approximately half of the patients who needed vision therapy remained asymptomatic after therapy was discontinued. In a 3-month follow-up to the study on vision therapy for patients with presbyopia, 47.8% (77 of 161) needed some additional therapy to remain asymptomatic. Generally, patients older than 70 years needed to continue with a maintenance therapy program (68.8%, or 22 of 32). These patients needed to continue minimal home therapy weekly or biweekly, with yearly examinations to assess visual function.[39]

For older patients, just as for younger patients, exophoria responds better than esophoria to vision therapy alone. Vision therapy is generally the only necessary treatment for exodeviations. Esophoria, in contrast, often requires base-out prism management combined with vision therapy. Even when therapy causes symptoms to disappear, the magnitude of the heterophoria usually does not change. Patients more than 20 $^\Delta$ exophoric and 15 $^\Delta$ esophoric may have symptoms remaining after therapy. Extraocular muscle surgery can provide additional relief for selected cases.

Older patients who have noncomitance frequently have partial or complete recovery of paretic muscle function. The recovery of muscle function depends on the nerve innervation, the muscle involved, and the cause of the noncomitance. Overall rates of recovery of paretic muscle function based on the involved cranial nerve are 48.3% for the third nerve, 53.5% for the fourth nerve, and 49.6% for the sixth nerve. When the cause of noncomitance is vascular, the chance of muscle function recovery is approximately 70%. Usually recovery begins within 3 to 6 months. After that time, recovery of paretic muscle function is less likely. When contracture does not occur or can be prevented by functional therapy and muscle function recovers, normal binocularity is restored.

The prognosis for comfortable binocular visual function in noncomitance using the best medical management combined with appropriate optometric intervention (lenses, prisms, patching, and vision therapy) is probably 70% to 80%. Visual function may not be normal, but the patient should be comfortable with minimal diplopia.

## SENSORY ADAPTATION TRAINING
### Monocularity

Older people frequently become monocular because of disease or an accident. They often benefit from advice when adapting to this condition. For example, when monocularity occurs suddenly, depth judgment is lost, particularly for distances within arm's reach. Teaching the patient to touch a plate to the table or a teapot spout to the cup will reduce embarrassment and help prevent accidents. A description of monocular cues to depth (e.g., size constancy, overlap, and perspective) and proper head motion for increased parallax help facilitate safer driving and parking.

### Perceptual Rehabilitation

Declines in visual function with age can be attributed to a reduced ability to gather data (e.g., reduced saccades, version and vergence ability, visual acuity) as well as to a reduced ability to process the data gathered. Optometrists interested in the ability of children to process

data gathered through vision and other senses have worked, through various types of visual/perceptual training, to increase abilities in this area.

Visual processing in older adults significantly decreases when more complex processing tasks are attempted because of age-related slowing of the rate of information processing and different allocation of the resources that control visual function.[9,17,35] Perceptual function in older adults can be evaluated by the following techniques:

- Copy forms (adult variety) and an additional three-dimensional form
- Motor-free visual perception test
- Reading test
- Pegboard test
- Jordan right-left test
- Identification test with objects and pictures

Visual perceptual therapy is used to enhance attention span, form discrimination, and auditory and visual memory in children. Similar procedures can be used to improve visual perceptual function in older adults. A sequenced therapy program that uses sensory-motor interaction enhances basic visual perceptual skills for both older adults and children.

### Aphakic Rehabilitation

Patients with cataracts already have experienced visual function decrease and often are apprehensive about the prospects of life without sight. The optometrist can provide substantial assurance about the outcomes of surgery. Working closely with the ophthalmic surgeon enables the optometrist to advise the patient about what to expect from pseudophakia. A careful explanation of the adaptation to, and correction options in, aphakia and the necessary spectacle correction (at least for near) in pseudophakia will help alleviate patient fear and apprehension. Unfortunately, this necessary assurance sometimes is neglected in referrals back and forth between optometrist and ophthalmologist.

Vision correction after surgery for cataracts presents some unique rehabilitative problems. First, visual acuity must be restored through the use of intraocular lens implants, contact lenses, or aphakic spectacle lenses, and each presents specific problems. Frequently the patient must learn a new way of seeing because of that correction. In addition, convergence demand is increased by the surgery itself, especially for patients who do not have intraocular lens implants.

Aphakic spectacle lenses generally require the most comprehensive rehabilitative techniques. From a purely optical standpoint, an aphakic spectacle lens may cause serious adaptive problems. The lenses magnify what is seen by more than 25%, so objects appear larger and closer than they really are. Aphakic corrections significantly impair initial judgment of depth. The spherical aberration of high plus lenses causes "pin cushion" distortion; that is, lines seem to curve inward, and movement of the eyes behind a fixed spectacle lens causes objects to swim.

The highly magnified central visual field of aphakic spectacle lenses overlaps a portion of the peripheral field and produces a characteristic ring scotoma. The stronger a lens in plus power, the worse the problem is. At intermediate distances (10 to 2 feet), the scotoma causes problems that are not easily overcome. Objects, such as people and chairs, pop in and out of the blind area, and patients see things they cannot turn their eyes to look at, bump into objects, and have trouble negotiating their environment. Visual field limitations of aphakic spectacle lenses are best solved by contact lens correction.

Coordinating hand and eye movements also becomes difficult when aphakic spectacles are first worn, so coordination for near tasks is frequently impaired. Small wooden puzzles, building block figures, and jigsaw puzzles can be used to help patients redevelop the spatial judgment needed for daily tasks. Aphakic adaptation therapy sessions attempt to redevelop the depth judgment and head and eye movements necessary for accurate hand/eye coordination.

### Convergence Requirements

Convergence requirements are altered by cataract surgery. Removal of the lens of the eye shifts the normal visual angle temporally by 2 degrees to 3 degrees per eye. This shift causes an induced exophoria of $10^\Delta$ to $12^\Delta$ for distance and near, which must be overcome by fusional (disparity) vergence reserves. Postsurgically induced exophoria combined with the usually receded near point of convergence in older adults can cause binocular problems that interfere with the

aphakic patient's ability to read comfortably or for very long.

Convergence demands of binocular aphakic spectacle correction are affected by the following:

- Phoria (preexisting phoria combined with altered convergence demands that are caused by the change in the visual angle resulting from lens removal)
- Interpupillary distance
- Spectacle lens vertex distance
- Correcting lens strength (both distance and bifocal additions)

Convergence requirements increase slightly with each diopter of distance lens power increase (provided the vertex adjustment, near additions, and interpupillary distance remain constant). This amounts to approximately $1^\Delta$ of increased convergence demand for each diopter of distance correction. Increasing the bifocal addition causes further dramatic increases in convergence demand.

Near work must be held closer to be clear, and the combined power of the distance lens and the bifocal increases vergence demand still more. Each diopter of increased bifocal addition power increases convergence demand approximately $12^\Delta$. Each 2-mm increase in interpupillary distance increases convergence demands by approximately $1^\Delta$. Greater vertex distances increase convergence demand by approximately $1^\Delta$ per millimeter of increase.

Increased bifocal addition power is the most significant cause of increased vergence demand with aphakic spectacle correction. In general, prescribing the closest spectacle lens vertex distance and the weakest addition possible will minimize problems of increased convergence demand with initial aphakic correction. Patients with aphakia who need strong (+14.00 to +15.50 D) or very strong (greater than +15.50 D) spectacle lens corrections with wide interpupillary distances have large demands on near convergence and are best corrected with contact lenses, especially when strong (greater than +2.50 D) near additions are needed.

Increased convergence demands with the spectacle correction of aphakia are treated with the rehabilitative therapy techniques previously described for near exophoria. These can be combined with puzzle tasks to enhance spatial awareness simultaneously. Rehabilitative therapy is generally successful in developing the convergence ability necessary for near tasks. Occasionally prism segments or near reading corrections with base-in prisms are required for comfortable sustained near vision.

Difficulties in adapting to aphakic spectacle lenses are largely solved by contact lenses or pseudophakic correction. These corrections eliminate many of the size differences and spectacle lens distortions of aphakic spectacle lenses, thus causing significantly fewer adaptive problems. However, increased convergence requirements after cataract surgery are not eliminated by contact lens correction. Convergence therapy is still required for many of these patients to obtain the best binocularity at near. Increased convergence requirements are reduced after intraocular lens implants, and convergence therapy is needed much less frequently.

### Intraocular Lens Implants

Intraocular lens implants are the management of choice after cataract surgery. They solve the problem of spectacle adaptation for patients with cataracts but can cause new problems (aniseikonia and anisometropia) when surgery is initially on only one eye. The problem of aniseikonia also exists when contact lenses are used to correct monocular aphakia. Spectacle lens overcorrections, which are needed for clear vision at near, can be designed to minimize the problems of aniseikonia and anisometropia.

### Aniseikonia and Anisometropia

Aniseikonia is a relative difference in the size, the shape, or both of the ocular images. Clinically significant aniseikonia is aniseikonia greater than 0.75% associated with symptoms related to the use of the eyes (headaches, asthenopia, and spatial distortions) and that is not relieved by accurate refractive or motility correction.[3]

Intraocular lens implants and contact lenses to correct the refractive error after cataract surgery reduce aniseikonia to a minimum in unilateral aphakia. Aniseikonia is usually not considered in spectacle overcorrection of unilateral pseudophakic patients. Lens correction is always needed for clear near vision, even if just a near addition. After a unilateral lens implant, an average ocular image size difference from 1.52% to 2.17% occurs for various anterior chamber lenses.[6,31] The image of the eye without

the implant generally requires magnification. Contact lens correction of unilateral aphakia leaves approximately a 6% image size difference between the two eyes. This 2% to 6% image size difference causes symptoms for many patients.

The rehabilitation of aniseikonia after a unilateral lens implant or monocular contact lens correction of aphakia uses iseikonic lenses. Lens corrections are designed to equalize magnification as much as possible for the two eyes. Lenses are modified by making a thicker, steeper base curve lens for the eye requiring the magnification. If necessary, the opposite lens can be made thinner with a flatter base curve. Complete lens design techniques are available.[37]

Increasing anisometropia during cataract development and after unilateral implants also can lead to binocular vision problems. This rapidly developed anisometropia causes prismatic differences in all fields of gaze, but it especially causes problems on downgaze. Rehabilitation uses lens corrections for reading only or slab-off prism when bifocal lenses are used. The amount of slab-off prism to be prescribed can be measured by using fixation disparity tests. In general, the amount measured by fixation disparity can be prescribed and is almost always less than the amount expected based on calculated prismatic differences between the two lenses. When contact lens corrections are used for unilateral aphakic correction, the contact lens is prescribed so that isometromic (equal) spectacle lens overcorrection is present. In this way, the problem of anisometropia and slab-off prism can be avoided with contact lens correction.

## VISUAL FIELD DEFECTS

Visual field evaluations provide a functional assessment of the location, extent, and quality of the area of best vision.[1] The location, density, size, and number of scotomas are significant in determining the visual care of the patient.[18] Recent field losses may be caused by life- or vision-threatening conditions, and patients with them should be referred to or managed concurrently with appropriate health care practitioners.

When central visual field defects affect visual acuity or patient fixation, the patient is best served by comprehensive low vision evaluation. Some patients have binocular peripheral field loss. Careful analysis with the tangent screen, arc perimeter, and Amsler grid is indicated for optimal evaluation. When complex field loss (multiple scotomas, ring scotomas, peripheral islands of vision, etc.) is present, a low vision evaluation should be done.

Partial monocular field loss is usually not a large problem because the intact field of the other eye compensates adequately. However, when a significant heterophoria is present, partial monocular field loss will occasionally cause fusion difficulty, and the patient will report transient diplopia or confusion. Vergence training or prism corrections are indicated for these patients to give the best possible fusion ability and minimize diplopia.

When binocular congruous field loss is present, techniques such as partial mirrors, mirrors, or prisms can increase the patient's awareness of objects located in the blind area. Bilateral partial conjugate prisms (with bases in the same direction over a portion of the lens) enable the patient to become more aware of objects in the scotomatous area. Although prism does not expand the visual field, without it the patient must make large head or eye movements toward the blind area to detect objects. Prism allows the use of small scanning eye movements to locate objects in the peripheral field. With the prism in place, the apparent position of objects is displaced toward the primary visual direction; objects are then easier for the patient to locate. Usually visual acuity must be essentially normal for prism field enhancement; patients with reduced acuity need appropriate low vision care.

A binocular mirror system also can be used for field defect rehabilitation.[11] Semitransparent mirrors with a 30% reflective coating on the ocular surface are used to allow use of the remaining nasal fields, and temporal fields are seen by reflection. However, the two fields are seen simultaneously, and the mirror device is somewhat cumbersome. Generally prisms are cosmetically superior and probably easier to adapt to.

Monocular mirrors can expand peripheral awareness by blocking out the seeing field of one eye and projecting a superimposed field of the lost area. The mirror allows the user to monitor major changes occurring in the blind field. Images seen in the mirror move rapidly with head movement and are reversed. The patient must learn to suppress the mirror for many tasks and only use it when needed. Large eye movements and hand movements are needed to look at an object in the blind field. The success rate with mirrors is not high because of nausea or disorientation from the moving reversed mirror image.[2]

Prism rehabilitation of visual field defects uses Fresnel prisms put on one sector of each spectacle lens. Prism power is chosen on the basis of the lateral excursion of the patient's habitual eye movements. Larger eye movements allow prisms to be placed farther from the line of sight and lower powers to be used. Prism powers from $10^\Delta$ to $30^\Delta$ can be used depending on the scanning area and patient response. Initial prism power and the location of the prism on the patient's spectacle lens may have to be reduced as the patient's scanning ability improves.

Prisms are placed on the lenses where they will not interfere with primary gaze and normal eye movements. The patient should not be aware of the prisms during normal eye movements and should need only small scanning movements into the prisms to see objects in the blind field. Prisms are usually placed 1 mm or more away from the primary position of gaze.[19,34] They are placed on one lens at a time by occluding one eye and having the patient make eye movements into the blind field with the other eye while the prism is positioned. The leading edge of the prism is moved until the patient is just aware of the prism location. This procedure then is repeated for the other eye, and finally binocular adjustment is done so that both lines of sight simultaneously meet the prism edges. Generally prisms must be used binocularly. When monocular prisms are used, patients may become confused when their gaze first encounters the prism and experience diplopia when looking further into the prism.

The necessity of using prisms is based on the location of the field loss. Right hemianopsias cause reading problems because the patient has difficulty knowing where the next word is and often loses the line. Typoscopes, margin markers in books, and reading slits help the patient improve tracking ability. Occasionally a patient is assisted by learning to read from right to left on an inverted book or by holding the book sideways and reading from the top down, thus avoiding reading in the scotomatous areas. Rehabilitative techniques will assist patients in learning these techniques when necessary.

Left hemianopsias cause fewer problems. Reading ability (right saccades) is generally not impaired, but patients tend to lose their place on returning to the next line. A marker (a finger or other object placed at the start of the next line) usually solves the problem. Superior field losses cause some problems. Because vertical (upward) scanning is difficult, base-up conjugate prism (with bases in the same direction) seems to be superior when prisms are required.[18] Inferior field losses cause mobility problems and reading confusion when the patient tries to find the next line or scan a picture. Prism scanning aids are less successful than improving mobility with head movement and cane travel training.[18]

Careful instruction and training can be valuable in the rehabilitation of visual field defects. Patients must be told that scanning eye movements into the prisms may cause initial confusion and that objects, usually invisible, will appear suddenly in front of them. Images are displaced from their actual position by an amount that depends on the distance of the object seen.

Visual and perceptual rehabilitative therapy can improve judgment of object distance and location. The patient is seated, and objects are brought from the blind field into the seeing field at various distances and speeds (a swinging Marsden ball and ring work well). The patient is trained to judge correct responses by "ringing" the ball as it moves. As improvement is shown, the same and more complex tasks are repeated while the patient stands or walks. When mobility is substantially impaired, referral for mobility training can often greatly benefit the patient.

## PATIENT EDUCATION, MONITORING, AND SELECTION

The availability of the most expert techniques and the finest instrumentation do not ensure the success of therapy. The patient must be educated to understand alternative therapy (lenses, prisms, or vision therapy) along with the scope and magnitude of the problem. Unless the patient can be properly motivated and fully understands the need for, and the technique of, the treatment being used, management will seldom succeed. Literature describing lens corrections, vision therapy, heterophoria, and stroke is valuable in explaining therapy and reinforcing patient cooperation. The following are psychologically sound techniques of greatly increasing patient cooperation with therapy:

- Working well within the patient's limitations is best to give a feeling of success at each session.
- Emphasis on positive results is preferable to a detailed explanation of any dire results that could occur if the therapy is not completed.
- Rehabilitative vision therapy, like any other health routine, must be done regularly. Help the patient set a time of day that ensures compliance. Instructions to do therapy techniques 15 minutes each day at 9 AM, noon, and 6 PM are superior to simple instructions to do these techniques 45 minutes every day.
- Written instructions often are helpful. A daily checklist showing results also can be used in more difficult cases. Routine instruction sheets can be prepared for the patient to reinforce a careful, friendly, personal explanation by the physician. A typical home therapy instruction sheet is shown in Box 13-11.

Monitoring rehabilitative therapy is simplified if the reasons for the therapy are kept in mind. Questioning the patient about any decrease in symptoms, the amount of time spent in therapy, and his or her understanding of techniques is important. Therapy progress can be objectively monitored by repeating appropriate tests. Vergence ranges, the convergence near point, suppression tests, and forced vergence fixation disparity curves can generally be repeated as appropriate. As therapy progresses vergence ranges expand, the near point of convergence improves, and suppression lessens. Force vergence fixation disparity curves are especially helpful for monitoring near binocularity improvement of presbyopic patients. As binocularity improves curves generally flatten, indicating better compensation over a larger range of vergence changes.

Patients should be selected on an individual basis. Nearly all older patients can have some relief of symptoms related to faulty binocular vision when appropriate medical care is com-

**BOX 13-11**

## Functional Therapy in the Rehabilitation of Older Patients

Your specific problems determine the frequency and type of vision therapy (orthoptics) needed to establish a good visual system. Doing orthoptics at the times prescribed is important if learning is to occur, and doing the orthoptics actively and with maximal concentration is equally important if progress is to be made. Remember, your cooperation and efforts at home will largely determine your success.

The following orthoptic program is designed to develop the visual skills needed for comfort and efficiency. When you can do these visual tasks correctly, you will possess visual abilities transferable to your everyday seeing needs.

**Exercise 1**
1. Starting with procedure _____, practice _____ times per day for _____ minutes.
2. When you are able to do all the procedures correctly, limit the exercise to procedure _____ and practice _____ times per ____ for _____ minutes _____.

**Exercise 2**
1. Starting with procedure _____, practice _____ times per day for _____ minutes.
2. When you are able to do all the procedures correctly, limit the exercise to procedure _____ and practice _____ times per ____ for _____ minutes _____.

**Exercise 3**
1. Starting with procedure_____, practice _____ times per day for _____ minutes.
2. When you are able to do all the procedures correctly, limit the exercise to procedure _____, and practice _____ times per ____ for _____ minutes _____.

bined with subsequent rehabilitative therapy. Rehabilitative therapy consists of lenses and prisms combined with vision therapy to improve vergence ranges, eliminate suppression, reduce adverse adaptations after stroke, and improve motility in muscle weakness or restrictive syndromes.

When the patient is mentally capable of understanding instructions, therapy is generally successful in alleviating or reducing symptoms. As with all physical therapy, however, some patients are unwilling or unable to comply. These patients should be managed with lens or prism modification of the spectacle correction to give maximal symptom relief. Patients occa-

sionally have progressive problems that therapy can help only minimally. These patients need continued medical monitoring to be sure the condition is maximally controlled. Rehabilitative therapy can be done concurrently to give the best possible relief of symptoms.

## ACKNOWLEDGMENT

Thanks to my father, Ralph E. Wick, OD, for his help and support in previous versions of this chapter.

## REFERENCES

1. Bailey IL: Visual field measurement in low vision, *Optom Monthly* 69:697-701, 1978.
2. Bailey IL: Mirrors for visual field defects, *Optom Monthly* 73:202-6, 1982.
3. Bannon RE: *Clinical manual on aniseikonia*, Buffalo, NY, 1965, American Optical Co.
4. Benjamin WJ: *Borish's clinical refraction*, Philadelphia, 1998, WB Saunders
5. Carter DB: Fixation disparity and heterophoria following prolonged wearing of prism, *Am J Optom Arch Am Acad Optom* 42:144-52, 1965.
6. Choyce DP: All-acrylic anterior chamber implants in ophthalmic surgery, *Lancet* 2:165-71, 1961.
7. Cohen AH, Soden R: An optometric approach to the rehabilitation of the stroke patient, *J Am Optom Assoc* 52:795-800, 1981.
8. Cooper J, Duckman R: Convergence insufficiency: incidence, diagnosis, and treatment, *J Am Optom Assoc* 49:673-80, 1978.
9. Craik FIM: Age differences in human memory. In Birren JE, Shaie KW, editors: *Handbook of the psychology of aging*, New York, 1977, Van Nostrand.
10. Gibson H: *Textbook of orthoptics*, London, 1955, Hatton.
11. Goodlaw E: Rehabilitating a patient with bitemporal hemianopia, *Am J Optom Physiol Opt* 59:677-9, 1982.
12. Griffin JR: *Binocular anomalies: procedures for vision therapy*, Chicago, 1976, Professional Press.
13. Griffin JR, Lee JM: The Polaroid mirror method, *Optom Weekly* 61:29, 1970.
14. Hamasaki D, Ong J, Marg E: The amplitude of accommodation in presbyopia, *Am J Optom Arch Am Acad Optom* 33:3-14, 1956.
15. Henson DB, North R: Adaptation to prism-induced heterophoria, *Am J Optom Physiol Opt* 57:129-37, 1980.
16. Hirsch MJ, Bing L: The effect of testing method on values obtained for phorias at forty centimeters, *Am J Optom Arch Am Acad Optom* 25:407-16, 1948.
17. Hoyer WJ, Plude DJ: Attentional and perceptual processes in the study of cognitive aging. In Poon LW, editor: *Aging in the 1980s: psychological*

*issues*, Washington, DC, 1980, American Psychological Association.

18. Jose RT, Ferraro J: Functional interpretation of the visual fields of low vision patients, *J Am Optom Assoc* 54:885-93, 1983.

19. Jose RT, Smith AJ: Increasing peripheral field awareness with Fresnel prisms, *Opt J Rev Optom* 113:33-7, 1976.

20. Maddox EE: *The clinical use of prisms and the decentering of lenses*, Bristol, England, 1893, John Wright & Sons.

21. Morgan MW: Accommodative changes in presbyopia and their correction. In Hirsch MJ, Wick RE, editors: *Vision of the aging patient*, Philadelphia, 1960, Chilton, pp 83-112.

22. Parks MM: Isolated cyclovertical muscle palsy, *Arch Ophthalmol* 60:1027-35, 1958.

23. Pitts DG: The effects of aging on selected visual functions: dark adaptation, visual acuity, stereopsis, and brightness contrast. In Sekuler R, Kline D, Dismukes K, editors: *Aging and human visual function*, New York, 1982, Alan R Liss, pp 131-59.

24. Schor C: Analysis of tonic and accommodative vergence disorders of binocular vision, *Am J Optom Physiol Opt* 60:1-14, 1983.

25. Schor C, Ciuffreda KJ: *Vergence eye movements: basic clinical aspects*, Boston, 1983, Butterworth.

26. Schor C, Narayan V: Graphical analysis of prism adaptation, convergence accommodation and accommodative vergence, *Am J Optom Physiol Opt* 59:774-84, 1982.

27. Sheedy JE: Actual measurement of fixation disparity and its use in diagnosis and treatment, *J Am Optom Assoc* 51:1079-84, 1980.

28. Sheedy JE, Saladin JJ: Exophoria at near in presbyopia, *Am J Optom Physiol Opt* 52:474-81, 1975.

29. Sheedy JE, Saladin JJ: Phoria, vergence and fixation disparity in oculomotor problems, *Am J Optom Physiol Opt* 54:474-8, 1977.

30. Sun F, Stark L, Nguyen A, et al: Changes in accommodation with age: static and dynamic, *Am J Optom Physiol Opt* 65:492-8, 1988.

31. Troutman RC: Artiphakia and aniseikonia, *Trans Am Ophthalmol Soc* 60:590-658, 1962.

32. Vodnoy BE: *The practice of orthoptics and related topics*, ed 4, South Bend, IN, 1970, Bernell.

33. von Noorden GK: *Binocular vision and ocular motility*, ed 4, St. Louis, 1990, C.V. Mosby, p 168.

34. Weiss NJ: An application of cemented prisms with severe field loss, *Am J Optom Physiol Opt* 49:261-4, 1972.

35. Welford AT: Experimental psychology in the study of aging, *Br Med Bull* 20:65-9, 1964.

36. Weymouth FW: Effect of age on visual acuity, In Hirsch MJ, Wick RE, editors: *Vision of the aging patient*, Philadelphia, 1960, Chilton, pp 37-62.

37. Wick B: Iseikonic considerations for today's eyewear, *Am J Optom Arch Am Acad Optom* 50:952-67, 1973.

38. Wick B: A Fresnel prism bar for home visual therapy accommodation, *Am J Optom Arch Am Acad Optom* 51:576-8, 1974.

39. Wick B: Vision therapy for presbyopes, *Am J Optom Physiol Opt* 54:244-7, 1977.

40. Wick B: Clinical factors in proximal vergence, *Am J Optom Physiol Opt* 62:1-18, 1985.

41. Wick B, London R: Vertical fixation disparity correction effect on the horizontal forced vergence fixation disparity curve, *Am J Optom Physiol Opt* 64:653-6, 1987.

42. Wick RE: Management of the aging patient in optometric practice, In Hirsch MJ, Wick RE, editors: *Vision of the aging patient*, Philadelphia, 1960, Chilton, pp 214-40.

43. Winter J: Striated lenses and filters in strabismus, *Optom Weekly* 62:531-4, 1971.

## SUGGESTED READINGS

Eskridge JB: Flip prism test for vertical phoria, *Am J Optom Arch Am Acad Optom* 38:415-9, 1961.

Hirsch MJ, Alpern M, Schultz HL: The variation of phoria with age, *Am J Optom Arch Am Acad Optom* 25:535-41, 1948.

Hofstetter HW: A comparison of Duane's and Donder's tables of the amplitude of accommodation, *Am J Optom Arch Am Acad Optom* 21:345-63, 1944.

Hofstetter HW: A longitudinal study of amplitude changes in presbyopia accommodation, *Am J Optom Arch Am Acad Optom* 42:3-8, 1965.

Hugonnier R, Clayette-Hugonnier S: *Strabismus heterophoria, ocular motor paralysis*, St. Louis, 1969, C.V. Mosby.

Morgan MW: The Turville infinity binocular balance test. accommodation, *Am J Optom Arch Am Acad Optom* 26:231-9, 1949.

O'Connor R: Contracture in ocular-muscle paralysis, *Am J Ophthalmol* 26:69, 1943.

Rucker CW: Paralysis of third, fourth, and sixth cranial nerves, *Am J Ophthalmol* 46:787, 1958.

Rush JA, Younge BR: Paralysis of cranial nerves III, IV, and VI: causes and prognosis in 1,000 cases, *Arch Ophthalmol* 99:76-9, 1981.

Rutstein RP, Eskridge JB: Studies in vertical fixation disparity, *Am J Optom Physiol Opt* 63:639-44, 1986.

# CHAPTER 14

# Care of Older Adults Who Are Visually Impaired

**ALFRED A. ROSENBLOOM, JR.**

People are living longer throughout the developed world. Health science break-throughs, health promotion efforts, better nutrition, and other habits of an improved lifestyle have led to a major decline in infant, child, and adult mortality rates in the twentieth century. In 1900 only 4% of the U.S. population was aged 65 years or older. Currently, approximately 13% of the population is at least 65 years old, and more than 70,000 persons are aged 100 years or older. Indeed, a doubling of the population older than 65 years is anticipated to occur during the next 20 years.[53] By some projections, in the year 2030, 20% of the people will be older than 65 years, and by the year 2010 the number of older adults older than 85 years will have doubled to 5.6 million persons.

The burgeoning population of older people also has demographic and psychosocial dimensions. Women and minorities have the highest incidence of severe visual disabilities. Furthermore, approximately two thirds of visually impaired older people have at least one other impairment, such as orthopedic impediments, paralysis, or hearing loss. Older people in the United States are demanding that more attention be paid to the quality and comprehensiveness of their health care. Serving these needs is a continuing challenge.

This chapter considers four aspects of the problem: (1) contemporary aspects of low vision and aging as frames of reference, (2) effective optometric care for older adults, (3) essential clinical skills and understandings, and (4) new directions in the care of older individuals who are visually impaired.

## CONTEMPORARY ASPECTS OF LOW VISION CARE

### Older Adults in Western Society

Providers of vision rehabilitation services are finding that their patient populations are becoming increasingly older and have experienced their visual impairment later in life rather than from congenital causes.[24]

Numerous studies have documented a rapid rise in rates of visual impairment as people age. The Beaver Dam study showed an increase in the prevalence of visual impairment from 0.9% in the 43- to 54-year-old group to 21% in the 75- to 86-year-old group.[28] Other studies have shown similar results.[10,42] Estimates are that worldwide, between 65% and 75% of the population older than 65 years are visually impaired.[3,11]

Contrary to popular opinion, most older people in the United States live independent lives (Box 14-1).[41]

In other developed countries, older adults make up an even larger proportion of the population.

### Leading Causes of Vision Loss in Older Adults

The four major causes of vision loss in persons older than 65 years are age-related macular degeneration, glaucoma, diabetic retinopathy,

---

**BOX 14-1**

### Independent Living Statistics

- Only 5% of individuals older than 65 years are in institutional care (e.g., nursing home).
- Nearly three quarters of those aged 65 to 74 years are homeowners.
- In the 65 to 74 year age group, 62.6% are living with a spouse; 24% live alone, and most of these are women.
- Half of all women older than 75 years live alone.
- Two thirds of all households are headed by people older than 55 years.

---

**BOX 14-2**

### Physical Changes Associated with Normal Aging

- Loss of height and weight
- Loss of muscle mass
- Decreased bone density
- Decline in vision, hearing, smell, and taste
- Decreased reaction time
- Decreased cutaneous and proprioceptive sensation
- Diminished respiratory vital capacity
- Decreased cardiac output
- Decreased glomerular filtration rate
- Decreased hepatic and renal function
- Decreased esophageal peristalsis and sphincter tone
- Loss of brain weight
- Loss of connective tissue elasticity
- Decreased cerebral blood flow
- Diminished immune responses

---

and cataract—all conditions related to the aging process.[3,10] Other causes of visual impairment include optic atrophy, myopic degeneration, retinitis pigmentosa, and corneal dystrophy.

## Aging

Aging describes physiological and related changes in a person's life from maturity to death, including adjustment to the total environment. It is a continuous and highly individualized process, especially in the area of health. Each person adjusts to old age differently.

The impact of vision loss is rarely felt in isolation from the other losses associated with growing older. No two people experience visual loss or the changing self-perceptions associated with aging in the same way. The impact of visual impairment, however, is felt more keenly because of other problems associated with aging (e.g., physical and physiological changes; economic limitations; loss of social independence; and altered roles in the family, workplace, and community).

The social and economic consequences of the aging population are emerging rapidly. Older people have more chronic illnesses and use medical services far more often than younger adults. Persons older than 65 years consume approximately one third of health care expenditures.

Although normal aging is associated with many predictable somatic changes, the timing and severity of these changes is variable. Genetic, environmental, and lifestyle factors affect the rate at which the body ages. Chronological age is a highly imprecise predictor of a person's biological age, psychological age, or state of physical health. Box 14-2 lists some of the more important physical changes associated with normal aging.

The optometrist's role is to understand the effects of aging in dealing with vision rehabilitation. The optometrist should help patients with impaired vision live fulfilling and useful lives and enjoy self-sufficiency, emotional independence, and satisfactory social interactions. Too often the practitioner's goals are aimed at physical well-being; social and psychological aspects are not given the emphasis they deserve.

## EFFECTIVE OPTOMETRIC CARE FOR OLDER ADULTS

The optometrist should adhere to five key principles for geriatric patient care, as shown in Box 14-3, regardless of the nature of the patient's disease, disability, or impairment. Successful aging is facilitated through a process known as life review. In a society that often devalues old age, the older person must develop his or her own unique sense of meaning and purpose; herein lies the creative and growth potential of old age.

Butler[8] proposed the idea that reviewing one's life through reminiscence is a normal, spontaneous, and universal part of the aging process. By reconsidering past life experiences, an individual has the opportunity to work through unresolved conflicts. Past successes and failures can be put in perspective, and a new understanding of the meaning of life is possible. Successful life review can lead to the acceptance of current situations and allows the individual to live more fully in the present.

Effective optometric service involves the art and science of patient care. Patients have become discontented, critical, and hostile as the art of health care gradually becomes separated from the science of health care. Patients have also become increasingly disenchanted with a specialized, high-technology health care system that frequently treats "health problems" rather than human needs.[20,36] To overlook these attitudes diminishes the doctor-patient relationship. The practitioner must view patients as individuals with special needs and abilities.

Because health problems in older adults tend to be complex, effective communication between patient and health provider is essential. Indeed, older adults share with everyone the dual needs for self-importance and social acceptance. Physical limitations often cause older adults to feel isolated. Deficits in hearing and vision may directly interfere with communication. The optometrist should understand the psychological stress that often accompanies aging: loneliness, a sense of uselessness, and anxiety over increasing dependency and impending death.

Low vision plays an enormous role in personal communication. More than half the older population that is visually impaired cannot read standard print, which makes newspapers, magazines, and books—the principal sources of information—of limited use.[39] These people can no longer read personal letters or labels on medicine bottles, instructions, recipes, prices, or signs.

To a great extent, visual impairment also limits a person's ability to relate directly to the environment and causes problems when navigating in unfamiliar environments without assistance.[49] Low vision factors such as restricted field of vision, reduced contrast sensitivity, and lessened visual function correlate to orientation and mobility difficulties such as walking speed and object contrast, resulting in disorientation and mobility incidents.[2]

Visual impairment also appears to be significantly associated with falls and fractures in older persons.[26,32] The risk of death also appears to increase with visual impairment.[27,43]

Vision loss frequently is only one of the conditions impairing the health of older persons. Hearing impairments, decreased stamina, memory loses, respiratory and heart conditions, and arthritis are additional conditions that affect older persons.

The care of the older patient should be effective, humane, and tailored to the limitations and priorities of each individual. In addition to obtaining information essential to a correct diagnosis and treatment plan, the optometrist should assess the cognitive and psychological states of older patients, their ability to carry out activities of daily living, and their socioeconomic needs. This individual must be sensitive to the patient's psychological set; the patient's expressed and perceived needs; the collection of clinical data; and an agreed-on plan of action adapted to the individual's needs, understanding, and motivation.

### Psychological and Functional Effects of Low Vision

Ocular and degenerative disorders tend to increase in incidence and severity among older persons. For a complete discussion of these changes, see Chapters 5 and 6.

Many normal aging changes are exacerbated for the low vision patient.[30] To understand the visual performance characteristics of patients with low vision, differentiation between optical effects and neural effects is necessary.[33] For example, a patient with an optically reduced visual loss resulting from irregularities in the refractive surfaces or media usually has a degradation of the visual image. This deficit results from excessive intraocular scatter, causing lower visual acuity and reduced contrast sensitivity. Patients diagnosed with this deficit have greater difficulty with resolution tasks. As the angular extent of scatter broadens, resolution capacity and performance suffer.

In some patients visual acuity may remain unaffected, but the quality of vision represented by contrast sensitivity of all objects within the visual field is diminished. Marron and Bailey[35] showed that loss of contrast sensitivity and loss of visual field were approximately equally important contributions to impaired mobility because of decreased vision. They also showed that visual acuity was a relatively poor predictor of mobility performance.

Visual acuity, contrast sensitivity, glare sensitivity, color, depth perception, and other functions were compared for 50 older (68 to 87 years) and 20 middle-aged (40 to 60 years) patients by Rumsey.[48] Mean values of each of these visual functions were found to be significantly poorer for the older patients than for the middle-aged patients. Rumsey compared the results of the clinical tests to complaints made by the patients in routine case histories with the following results:

1. A decline in distance vision was reported by 72% of the older group but by only 10% of the middle-aged group.
2. Complaints of diminished driving ability were reported by 45% of the older group and by 25% of the middle-aged group.
3. Problems with glare were reported by 49% of the older group and by 30% of the middle-aged group.
4. Problems with color perception affected 23% of the older group compared with 5% of the middle-aged group.

In discussing these results, Rumsey suggested that when taking case histories, more specific, task-oriented questions might more effectively identify decrements in visual function.

Haegerstrom-Portnoy et al[21] conducted the Smith-Kettlewell Attentional Visual Field Test, making use of a modified Synemed perimeter equipped with a red light-emitting diode (LED) as the fixation point, with peripheral targets in the form of bright-green LEDs. The visual field was first tested in the standard manner, after which the attentional field was tested. During the attentional field test, the examiner briefly turned the red fixation LED off and on at predetermined intervals, and the subject was asked to count silently the number of times the light turned off. The authors noted "whereas standard field extent changes very little with age, attentional field size decreases dramatically, accompanied by enormous increases in variability. Twenty-five percent of the oldest age group have no peripheral fields under conditions of divided attention."

With increased intraocular scatter and absorption of light by the media, higher than normal luminance levels are necessary. Data show an accelerating increase in the effects of glare with age beyond 65 to 70 years. If the individual's environment includes poorly designed light fittings, dimly lit passageways, shadows surrounding objects, and impairments such as disability glare, performance difficulties are increased.

The authors conclude that "standard visual acuity underestimates the degree of visual function loss suffered by many older individuals under the nonoptimal viewing conditions encountered in daily life. All spatial vision functions show a similar rate of decline with age, but the age at which decline begins varies among measures."[21]

Regardless of their causes, losses involving structures within the neural pathway are most commonly expressed as visual field defects. Central field losses typically result in a reduction in visual acuity. These losses may be complicated by metamorphopsia, poor tolerance to variation in luminance, dependence on high luminance levels, lowered contrast sensitivity, and poor mobility despite an intact peripheral visual field. The size and extent of scotomas limit sensitivity of the retina, as only objects of sufficient size, illumination, or contrast will be recognized within these areas. If these scotomas are numerous, the correct localization and subsequent evaluation of visual information may become so difficult that some patients, despite relatively good visual acuity, are unable to read with any efficiency even when using magnification. This effect may be likened to the crowding phenomenon, in which letters can be seen but not interpreted by some patients with amblyopia.

Although not as common as central field losses, peripheral field losses are important within the low vision population. Mobility and the ability to detect environmental hazards are hindered when poor dark adaptation makes patients dependent on high light levels. The fact that older people require higher levels of illumination to meet their visual needs is well established but frequently overlooked.

Because of the effects of aging, older persons require at least twice the amount of illumination required by younger persons. Brilliant[7] notes that nuclear sclerosis produces a yellowing of the lens and a loss of short wavelengths reaching the retina. Incandescent lamps have more energy output in the long wavelengths and less in short wavelengths, which tend to enhance reds, oranges, and yellows and subdue blues and greens. By contrast, fluorescent lighting is usually considered harsh because of its output in the blue portion of the spectrum. Patients complain that fluorescent lighting is disturbing, causing discomfort glare. The use of diffusers and indirect fluorescent lighting tends to minimize these problems. Another light bulb, the neodymium bulb (Chromalux, Lumiram Electric Corp, Mamaroneck, NY) emits 30% less ultraviolet light and blue and 20% to 28% less infrared light than does the incandescent bulb. According to Brilliant, this bulb has shown a significantly improved performance over the standard incandescent bulb for short-term near tasks.

Halogen light has a high intensity and is available in small, portable lamps, but concern surrounds the cost and the high ultraviolet output with the potential for erythemal effects. High-intensity incandescent portable lamps may present a more practical solution to the need for flexible placement of lighting in a cost-effective manner.

### Psychological Set

Psychological factors in aging are influenced by a range of considerations, including physical changes, adaptive mechanisms, and psychopathology. Each older person has a unique psychological profile and social life history. In the absence of disease, character growth and the ability to learn continue throughout life. Losses—of status, physical abilities, loved ones, family support, and income—become more frequent.

Age-related changes in sensation and perception can have a great influence, isolating an individual from the surrounding environment. Diminution of hearing, slowing of intellectual and physical response time, and increasing difficulty primarily with short-term memory may occur.

Many physical and intellectual abilities are retained throughout life, however, and their loss should not be assumed to be a normal aging process. These include the senses of taste and smell, intelligence, and the ability to learn.

Depression is more common in older adults. The signs and symptoms of depression are similar to those seen in younger age groups, although older persons may place greater emphasis on physical symptoms. The role of the optometrist and ophthalmologist is to recognize and refer the patient with depression. In particular, loss of visual function such as moderate or severe visual impairment can precipitate depression. Early recognition may be crucial because older patients are at highest risk for suicide (for men older than 65 years, the risk is five times higher than in the general population.) See Chapter 1 for further discussion of cognitive impairment in older persons.

In addition to physical conditions and aging changes, a patient's performance is influenced by the attitude of the practitioner. Palmore[40] notes that general attitudes of most Americans toward older people and aging tend to be negative. The older years usually are perceived as the worst time in a person's life. Lutsky[34] reports that health care professionals' attitudes towards older people are the same or worse than the those of the general public. Sinick[50] notes that professional personnel in service settings may fail to realize the presence of prejudice despite their commitment to a professional service role. In so doing, they may become condescending, overprotective, and insensitive to the basic needs of older people. Fineman[15] interviewed 42 physicians and nurses and found that they assessed older people to be disengaged, unproductive, and inflexible and to have poor functional and medical status. He notes that geriatric patients tend to be perceived by physicians as "resistant to treatment, rigid in outlook, demanding, and uninteresting."

According to Gilbert[18] and Foley,[16] old age may be equated with inevitable impairment, resulting in less-aggressive treatment or a lower standard of care for older patients. Some health care professionals are uncomfortable providing care for persons the same age as their parents or grandparents. Often older patients remind practitioners of their own unresolved conflicts concerning parental figures.

In caring for older adults, professionals must recognize that an older person's well-being is as important as that of younger individuals. A shortened life span is no basis for making compromises in the scope or quality of health care services. Members of the rehabilitation team must confront their own attitudes toward visually impaired people to render the most effective services.

Barraga and Morris[5] report that many older patients resist attempts at visual rehabilitation because they fear their inability to achieve visual expectations, fear becoming more independent and possibly losing the care and emotional support of family and friends, and lack a desire to invest extra time and effort. Older patients also often do not understand that visual performance may vary from day to day. Mehr[37] notes, "The patient must be ready and eager for help, not seeking restoration of his former vision without limitations. For the patient saying 'yes, but' or preferring dependency to increased visual abilities, a program of masterful inactivity is preferable to an expensive aid." In making a decision about an appropriate therapeutic plan for the low vision patient, the optometrist must consider the psychosocial factors influencing the patient's readiness.

In addition, the visually impaired person may also face inadequacy in all daily activities, such as dressing, grooming, personal hygiene, eating, telling time, and caring for clothes and personal effects—virtually every facet of daily life. He or she may need to relearn many routines. Social insecurities and communication difficulties are experienced; independence may be reduced and self-esteem affected.

Thus the cognitive and psychological states of older patients, their ability to perform daily activities, and their socioeconomic frameworks should be clinically assessed. The services available to assist patients in maintaining their independence should be established. To the extent that practitioners can develop understanding about, and sensitivity to, the realties of being and growing old, they will enhance the quality of the interpersonal relationships with their patients.

## ESSENTIAL CLINICAL SKILLS AND UNDERSTANDING

Access to the eye care practitioner's office ideally should be designed to accommodate geriatric patients (Box 14-4).

Five aspects of providing care for individuals who are visually impaired include the case history interview, low vision examination and functional assessment, therapeutic approaches (appropriate low vision designs and accessory aids), low vision patient management, and patient education and compliance.

### Case History Interview

The success of the rehabilitation process depends on the quality and scope of the case history. The history for older patients should establish their specific needs and desires, their ability to adapt to new situations, their motivation to learn new visual habits, and their understanding of the uses and limitations of the visual aids. If an older patient lives with sighted family members, efforts may be directed toward finding low vision corrections that allow participation in normal family activities (e.g., watching television, card playing, sewing, and playing games). If the patient lives alone, more attention may be focused on functional tasks, such as reading mail and identifying labels on medicine bottles and food packaging.[45] Other important case history information includes ocular and health history, visual capabilities at distance and near, illumination requirements, lifestyle history,

---

**BOX 14-4**

**Various Modifications to Achieve a Geriatric-Friendly Office Environment**

- A safe, well-lit office close to drop-off areas and parking
- Automatic or assisted doors (doorways with pull levers or handles)
- Large-print, legible, and well-placed signs
- Wheelchair-accessible entrances and waiting rooms
- Obstacle-free and well-lit, high-contrast walkways, hallways, and waiting areas (free of rugs, electrical cords, and other hazards)
- Accessible bathrooms with elevated toilet seats, grab bars, and wheelchair-accessible sink

present and previous interests, independent travel abilities, education and reading interests, vocational and avocational activities and goals, and familiarity with rehabilitation services. Brilliant[7] notes that the patient's active participation in the rehabilitation process is critical for success, and nowhere is that participation more important than in the setting of realistic goals and objectives. The patient should prioritize visual goals. A realistic and motivating set of goals greatly enhances the prognosis for success.

The patient should be the primary source of information in gathering the case history; if doubt arises regarding accuracy, other sources such as family or friends should be consulted. For a complete case history to be compiled, multiple sessions may be needed to minimize patient fatigue (Box 14-5).

This information is useful for in-office questioning by the practitioner and in a preexamination interview by telephone or by a low vision assistant in the office.

## Low Vision Examination and Functional Assessment

Michaels[38] notes that the clinical examination of the aging eye does not differ in essentials from that of any other eye, except that it takes more time, more tact, and more patience. "It takes more time because older people frequently have many nonspecific complaints, poorly expressed, and sequentially muddled. Some symptoms may go unreported because of memory loss, fear, or indifference. It takes more tact because, in the nature of things, some senescent diseases are not only chronic but often irreparable. It takes more patience because the aged eye often suffers multiple defects which must be sorted out."

Flexibility and readiness to alter standard procedures are necessary to secure the most accurate and reliable findings. The visual examination must be adapted to the special needs and requirements of the patient. Environmental setting, test distance (usually 10 feet or less), and surrounding illumination are important considerations. Use of the trial frame (including clips for overrefraction), trial lenses, and low vision printed acuity test charts add accuracy, flexibility, and improved patient control. Bailey and Lovie-Kitchin[4] note that the examiner may wish to predict how much change in working distance, dioptric power of an addition, or magnification is required to enable the patient to read a certain size of print. They also recommend using a chart with unrelated words arranged in a logarithmic size progression.

Much of the examination procedure follows a conventional pattern: determination of visual acuities at far and at near; internal and external ocular health examination; retinoscopy; tonometry and slit-lamp biomicroscopy; binocular indirect ophthalmoscopy; ophthalmometry; determination of central and peripheral visual fields, including use of the Amsler grid; and distance and near point subjective testing with low vision and accessory devices suited to the needs and capabilities of the patient. The autorefractor often serves as a valuable auxiliary procedure in determining the refractive state of older patients.

---

**BOX 14-5**

## Key Questions for the Case History Interview

- What is the duration of the visual impairment?
- What is the ophthalmologic diagnosis, treatment, and prognosis?
- What is the state of the patient's general health?
- What drugs or medications are being taken, and for what purposes?
- Do any other health or psychosocial factors affect the patient's lifestyle?
- What is the patient's present level of visual functioning?
- Does the patient see better in bright or dim illumination?
- Does the patient have sensitivity to glare?
- What are the patient's principal vocational, recreational, and daily living activities?
- Are orientation and mobility impaired? Can the patient travel independently and successfully in familiar and unfamiliar surroundings?
- What are the patient's primary visual needs and expectations?
- Is reading an important activity? If so, reading of what type and purpose?
- Can the patient cook, grocery shop, read personal mail or bills?
- Are any low vision devices or appliances being used?
- How does the patient spend a typical day in his or her life? Is the patient living with others or alone?
- Is the patient psychologically ready and motivated for visual rehabilitation?

Functional assessment requires a full understanding of the patient's needs and the complex interaction of factors that influence the perceptual response. These factors include the acuity level required for tasks at various working distances; luminance; figure-ground and contrast differences; and contour interaction relations involving size and style of type, spacing, and print quality. Magnification alone may not improve function in terms of daily activities, orientation, and mobility in the environment. Visual performance is correlated poorly with visual acuity. Accurate refractive technique is of utmost importance, as is the prescription of proper light levels for the patient's various environments. The goal of the low vision practitioner should be to improve function by whatever means to enhance quality of life for the patient.

When possible, previously acquired skills must be reactivated by the practitioner's continuing encouragement, guidance, patience, and empathy. Techniques for achieving accurate clinical findings and their evaluation are described in Chapter 8.

## Therapeutic Approaches (Appropriate Low Vision Designs and Accessory Devices)

Low vision devices that are most valuable to older patients include hand and stand magnifiers, compact telescopic systems for spot checking, high plus reading additions in bifocal or single-vision designs, microscopic types of reading lenses, closed-circuit television systems, and various nonoptical or accessory devices.

A decision on what type of device(s) to prescribe depends on the optometric evaluation derived from the case history and examination findings as well as the evaluation and interpretation of the functional field of vision. According to Faye,[14] the visual field is the single most important factor affecting visual function. Faye identifies three types of field defects that can influence the practitioner's decision on therapeutic correction: no demonstrable field loss, functional field loss involving retinal disease marked by central or paracentral scotomas, and peripheral field loss.

### No Demonstrable Field Loss

Typically, patients with no demonstrable field loss report blurred vision or an image poorly resolved centrally, haze, or a sensation of glare. The evaluation of visual performance depends on the type and size of test objects, contrast, illumination levels, pupil size, and figure-ground interaction.

Therapeutic approaches to a blurred or poorly resolved image include telescopic devices, which help some patients retain their ability to read street, bus, and directional signs and avoid obstacles in travel. For such short-term spotting tasks, hand-held monocular telescopes from 2.5× to 14× are available.

Stand magnifiers often are used by patients with hand tremors, by those with aphakia where added magnification for reading is needed, and as a supplemental correction for the occasional reading of small print.

Most informational display signs can be identified with 20/70 vision under suitable illumination. Patients with diffusely blurred vision need telescopes with good light-gathering properties—often a prism monocular with the largest field. For reading, high addition spectacles, hand or stand magnifiers, or video magnifiers should be prescribed according to near reading acuity.

### Functional Field Loss Involving Retinal Disease Marked by Central or Paracentral Scotomas

Faye[13] notes the common denominators of macular disease: visible pathological condition of ophthalmoscopy, central or paracentral field defects of varying density, decreased central acuity, and central scotoma. Peripheral field functions remain relatively normal. Visual symptoms may vary from lack of clear vision, recognition of faces, and disappearance of parts of words to search difficulties in travel vision.

Brilliant[7] notes that persons with low vision who are myopic or have early-onset vision loss sometimes manifest multiple eccentric fixation points. Because of the possibility of multiple fixation points, distance acuity should not be used to determine magnification needs for near point acuities.

Patients with central scotomas or metamorphopsia typically demonstrate better single-letter visual acuity than continuous text acuity. They may consistently omit letters at the beginning or end of lines and may frequently lose their place and repeat lines already read.

The specific design of the low vision device depends on the patient's level of visual acuity, preference and adaptability, and requirements for daily living. In descending order of frequency, the aids commonly prescribed for older patients are single-vision or bifocal spectacles, hand and stand magnifiers (2× to 9× power), closed-circuit television, handheld and spectacle-mounted telescopes (2.5× to 8×), and telemicroscopic units. Stand magnifiers often are used by patients with hand tremors, by those with aphakia for whom added magnification combined with the bifocal power is needed for reading, and as a supplemental correction for the occasional reading of small print. (See Chapter 15 for further discussion of assistive devices for the older adult who is visually impaired.)

### Peripheral Field Loss

The eye care practitioner must also differentiate between overall contraction of the visual field and sector or hemianopic losses. The most potentially disabling form of functional vision impairment is peripheral field loss. Magnification may not help those with peripheral field loss. Indeed, many patients adopt techniques in traveling and reading that prove more effective than the use of low vision devices.

Patients with irregular scotomatous patterns often have unpredictable near-vision responses. They may identify isolated letters more easily than words, and they may use eccentric viewing and angling of reading materials. An accurate assessment and interpretation of the central and peripheral visual fields should be performed before low vision devices or a rehabilitation program is considered.

In prescribing low vision devices, the practitioner must consider the relative advantages and limitations of various devices. High addition spectacles may be ineffective as low vision devices because of the close distance they impose. Telemicroscopes alleviate the working distance difficulties, but the field of vision becomes small.

Low-powered hand and stand magnifiers can increase the working distance and allow the patient to adapt to a preferred image size. Patients with small central or paracentral fields may prefer closed-circuit television because of the flexible reading distance, the improved ease

and speed in reading, and the illumination and contrast controls.

Accessory devices for mobility and orientation should be considered. Light control is especially important. For patients with sector or hemianopic field defects, trials should be conducted with prisms of varying power and position. Mirrors have been used with some success by patients with homonymous hemianopsias. Prisms also can enhance mobility and scanning, but their success with older adults tends to be limited. On the basis of the author's experience, the success rate with all these techniques is relatively low and depends on patient motivation and adaptability. As a consequence, patients should participate in selecting the best compromise. Frequently the orientation and mobility specialist provides essential adaptive training.

### Accessory or Nonoptical Devices

Accessory or nonoptical devices take many forms. These include large-print materials, matte black cardboard reading slits (typoscopes) and amber acetate sheets to improve contrast, reading stands, adequate illumination, the use of fiber-tipped pens, and visors to control light intensity and glare. Audio or Talking Books should be recommended when limited or unsuccessful trials with optical devices have already been tried; this is especially appropriate if reading is an important part of a patient's lifestyle.

Ogilvie and Johnston (personal communication, 2005) note that high-technology assistive devices continue to play an expanding role in helping ameliorate the disability faced by individuals who are blind or visually impaired. Global positioning systems, cellular telephones, bar code readers, and personal digital assistants are all available in auditory formats designed to meet the personal, social, educational, and vocational mobility, communication, and information management needs of persons who are blind or visually impaired. Video magnification–based reading aids such as closed circuit televisions offer a range of magnification and contrast enhancements unequalled by optical aids. Portable closed-circuit television technology continues to evolve, affording users video-based magnification in a pocket-sized format.

The ever-expanding role the computer plays in our daily lives has led to increased pressure on manufacturers to make their technology accessible to blind and visually impaired persons. Generic accessibility features such as enlargement and color enhancement capabilities are now built into Windows- and Macintosh-based operating systems. Additionally, the availability of feature-rich speech, large-print, and Braille access technology compatible with mainstream software has narrowed the computer functionality gap that still exits between the fully sighted and the blind or visually impaired. Access to the Internet, e-mail, scanning devices, and digital format books has greatly enhanced the visually impaired or blind users' access to information, independence, and communication, countering the effects of reduced mobility and limited print access the disability creates.

Accessory or nonoptical devices should be considered to reduce glare and heighten contrast and illumination. Patients can control outdoor glare by wearing hats with wide brims, visors that attach to the eyeglass frame, and absorptive lenses that reduce ultraviolet and infrared radiation. Tinted lenses may lessen glare but may also reduce reading acuity.

Disability glare presents a special challenge in the diagnosis and management of older adults. Contrast threshold or contrast sensitivity functions of these patients can be essentially normal in low photopic luminance (approximately 30 ft-c), but thresholds for high and medium spatial frequency targets are drastically reduced in the presence of any bright glare source. Because these patients often have 20/20 acuity, their problems can be overlooked by the examiner who does not specifically ask about night vision or glare problems during the case history. These patients can be helped with advice on lighting design to reduce luminance levels and restore contrast. The Brightness Acuity Test (BAT) is useful in measuring the reduction of visual acuity in the presence of glare when a cataract or corneal opacity is present. Glare can be caused by intraocular light scattering; glare testing is likely to be more specific in evaluating anterior segment media opacities. Also, clear antireflective coatings, side and sun shields, and a cardboard reading mask of the appropriate length and width (typoscope) to reduce glare from the surrounding field and improve contrast are generally recommended. Large-print materials, marking pens, heavily lined writing paper, and reading lamps and stands, as well as talking watches and talking calculators, are a few of the many available nonoptical devices.

Contrast and color represent important environmental design considerations. Gradual yellowing of the lens occurs with age and, as a result, blue light is absorbed and scattered selectively. Thus blues become darker and less vivid, and warm tones are perceptually increased. The degree of color bias that occurs with age is quite variable because lens changes vary considerably from individual to individual. A diminished ability to differentiate among similar light tones (pastel colors) or dark shades (blacks, brown, navy) typically occurs with age.[22] Almost any color can be made more visible by improving light intensity, by using full-spectrum light sources, and by using color in a highly contrasting mode. Generally, lighting should be placed on the side of the eye capable of best near vision; it should be direct, close, and adjustable so that the light can be angled to reduce reflected glare.

The eye care professional needs to stress the appropriate use of color contrast as an important factor in managing the environment for older people. For instance, the decoration of homes or facilities for older people should provide color contrast between walls and floor. A knowledgeable use of color also can accent stairways and steps and demarcate other changes in terrain. See Box 14-6 for other important home design safety checks.

The use of nonoptical or accessory devices is especially important because contrast sensitivity is generally lessened in low vision patients. Cullinin[9] identified the importance and effects of poor lighting control: "Among those surveyed who had recently been seen at a specialist's clinic, over 60% apparently saw worse at home than they did at the time of examination." Poor lighting in the home is virtually a universal problem.

A loan system for optical devices that allows a patient to become gradually accustomed to the effects of greater magnification is often desirable. This adaptive process requires reassessment, supervision, and counseling on a continuing basis as frustrations and new needs emerge.

---

**BOX 14-6**

## Interior Safety Checks

**Living area**
Are scatter rugs firmly anchored with rubber backing?
Are electrical cords in good repair, especially on heating pads?
Is adequate night lighting available?
Are stairways continually illuminated?
Is temperature within a comfortable range (70° to 75° F)?
Is the heater vented properly?
Is cross ventilation available?
Is furniture sturdy enough to give support?
Is clutter minimal, allowing enough room for easy mobility as well as lowering the fire hazard?
Are emergency telephone numbers posted in a handy place and easily read, such as for the physician, fire department, ambulance, paramedics, and nearest relative?
If the person has limited vision, does the phone have an enlarged dial?

**Kitchen and bath**
Is the stove free of grease and flammable objects?
Is baking soda conveniently available in case of fire?
Are matches used or does the stove have a pilot light?
Is the refrigerator working properly?
Is the sink draining well?
Is food being stored properly?
Is trash taken out daily?
Is a sturdy stepping stool in evidence?
Are skid-proof mats on the floor?
Are handrails beside the tub and toilet?
Are skid-proof mats in the bathtub and/or shower?
Are electrical outlets a safe distance from the bathtub?

**Outside the home**
Are raised or uneven places on the sidewalks?
Are stairs in good repair?
Are the top and bottom stairs painted white or a bright contrasting color to improve visibility?
Are handrails securely fastened?
Are screens on doors and windows in good repair?
Does the house have an alternate exit?

---

(Adapted from *Hypertext modules in geriatric medicine: computer-based self-instruction modules*, Baylor College of Medicine, 1998.)

---

**BOX 14-7**

## Best Practices in Instruction and Guided Practice with Low Vision Devices

- The development of an individualized vision rehabilitation plan based on clinical and functional assessment for the goals identified by the patient
- Instruction and practice that takes place in a real environment and incorporates teaching the use of vision and devices for the real-world tasks to be performed
- Follow-up by telephone, mail, or home visit that identifies possible vision changes, use and effectiveness of low vision devices, and need for further services

---

care is time consuming, help from an understanding, experienced low vision assistant is desirable. This frees the professional examiner for those procedures necessitating special skills and knowledge.

### Low Vision Patient Management

The management of adaptive problems in the visually impaired individual requires more than the prescription of devices. Proper management frequently requires painstaking instruction and supervised training to create and sustain motivation for visual tasks along with the use of training materials and activities chosen according to the patient's interests (Box 14-7).

Depending on the clinical setting and the needs of the patient, the practitioner should make appropriate referrals. In some cases multidisciplinary care is unnecessary; in others, however, services should be coordinated. Where the services of several specialists are required, one member of the team must take responsibility for identifying needs and coordinating services. Establishing constructive relationships with health care and social service agencies is essential. Because of changing social and family structures, older patients must often seek other support systems. Social service agencies, older adult support groups, and religious and service organizations are available in the community for health care and social support.[25] The practitioner should furnish the patient and the patient's family with a list of resources in the community that could provide needed services. Periodic follow-up increases the patient's compliance and success.

Various patterns of reinforcement or encouragement are needed to keep the patient's enthusiasm and motivation high. Adaptive training should be flexible and emphasize the most effective use of residual vision. Home visits by the assistant or allied professional should be considered. Questions about patient compliance and problems of illumination and contrast in the home often can be resolved by on-site assessment. Because comprehensive low vision

**TABLE 14-1**

**Rehabilitation Services of Most Importance to the Members of the Royal New Zealand Foundation for the Blind, Age 70 Years and Older**

| Service | Members (%) |
| --- | --- |
| Low vision devices and appliances | 97 |
| Vocational rehabilitation | 96 |
| Communication and adult education | 95 |
| Counseling | 94 |
| Recreation and leisure | 93 |
| Orientation and mobility | 91 |
| Advocacy | 89 |
| Techniques of daily living | 88 |
| Network building | 85 |
| Understanding visual impairment | 68 |

Surveys by the Royal New Zealand Foundation for the Blind in 1982 and 1984 identified the greatest rehabilitation needs for those between ages 60 and 69 years: talking books, transportation assistance, information, recreation activities, and advocacy. In 1990 the Foundation asked members 70 years and older to identify the rehabilitation services that were most important to them.[47] Table 14-1 lists the results of the survey.

Orientation and mobility professionals frequently focus their efforts on the home environment but not to the exclusion of other environments significant to their clients. The role of these specialists is to teach how to "utilize the remaining senses in establishing position and relationship to all significant objects in the environment and the subsequent capacity to move independently."[23] The ultimate goal of orientation and mobility training is to enable the individual to enter any environment and travel safely, efficiently, and independently by using a combination of these two skills. Orientation and mobility professionals and rehabilitation teachers frequently work together in providing individualized and comprehensive rehabilitation programs. These programs are most effective when they prevent or defer admission of patients into long-term care facilities. Indeed, independent living training may offer a viable alternative to nursing home placement.

All professionals and paraprofessionals involved in the care of individuals with a visual impairment should assist in the process of reha-

bilitation, which can be thought of as a transition from dependence to independence and finally to interdependence. This transition can be typified by some commonly encountered phrases. The statement, "Of course I can't read; you will have to do it for me," typifies dependence. Independence can be expressed by, "I will try to read this myself," but this also can be a stubborn and self-defeating experience leading to, "This print is just too small. No, you can't help me, I didn't want to read it anyway." Ideally, independence should lead to the ultimate state of interdependence: "I can read this section, but these words are too difficult. Could you help me, please?" This state of rehabilitation recognizes abilities and limitations and graciously requests and accepts assistance. This process requires time, and the patient will fluctuate between stages. The practitioner should seek an understanding of the patient's present state.

The eye care practitioner must be able to look behind the traditional stereotypes and focus on the special needs of each individual. These needs include independence and individuality, physical health and mobility, self-respect, dignity, and privacy. Good health and mobility, in turn, depend on the satisfaction of diverse subsidiary needs such as adequate services to compensate for loss of vision and hearing; a proper nutritional standard; adequate dental care; the maintenance of personal and household standards of cleanliness; and quality, accessible health care.[6]

### Patient Education and Compliance

In contrast to the traditional model of health care, low vision rehabilitation should be oriented to the person rather than to the disease. Such an approach establishes an ongoing, personal relationship with the patient. For older adults unaccustomed to, or overwhelmed by, the diversified maze of the health care system, the optometrist can develop a trusting relationship of support and encouragement. At the same time that this humanistic approach to health care is rightly desirable for the general population, it is critical for older adults and will greatly enhance the patient compliance essential for successful low vision rehabilitation.

Few studies of patient compliance in optometry and medicine specifically concern older adults. Libow and Sherman[31] found that for older patients who had medication prescribed, 50% deviated from the prescribed regimen and 70% did not comprehend the regimen. Noncompliance may result in institutionalization, as shown in a study by Strandberg,[51] who reported that 23% of nursing home admissions were caused primarily by the patient's inability to manage drug therapy at home. Errors in medication and self-medication have accounted for 25% to 95% of the noncompliance problem.[17] Compliance difficulties are increased for older adults for a variety of reasons. Explanations are given too rapidly or poorly, and written instructions are lacking. Environmental hazards such as weather conditions, transportation, or fear of crime deter patients from keeping appointments. Patients have trouble receiving or retaining instructions because of visual and hearing problems or from the loss of short-term memory. They are sometimes unable to open child-resistant medication containers and are confused about regimens with multiple medications.[12]

In a study with experimental and control groups, Talkington[52] found that four factors significantly increased patient compliance (from 53% to 73%):

1. Good rapport and communication between the patient and the health provider
2. Effective interaction in which the patient's concerns were understood and expectations were met
3. Patient understanding of the health problem, causes, treatment regimen, expected outcome of treatment, and the consequences of noncompliance
4. Patient participation in planning the treatment regimen, including the identification, analysis, and solution of problems that might interfere with compliance

## Practitioner's Role in Counseling and Patient Education

Patient education has many facets. The practitioner must realize that every low vision problem is unique and that individual differences increase with age. A slowing of motor functioning is not automatically equated with decreased learning ability; when older adults can pace their own learning, studies show no significant age-related differences in ability. Diversity, rather than homogeneity, is the norm.

The practitioner must pace the instructions according to the learning ability of the patient. The response rate and reaction time of older adults are slower, but not because of lack of motivation. Rushing older adults may result in frustration and reduced motivation. Fear of failure, frustration, and confusion can be reduced by simplifying the environment and the tasks demanded of older adults. Presentation of material in both amount and content should be planned so that the patient's potential for failure is reduced and the opportunity for success is increased.

The practitioner must explain the low vision device(s) (their purpose, use, and limitations); the adaptive training program and its goals; environmental variables, especially lighting; and the importance of continuing follow-up. Informational reinforcement can consist of handouts, demonstrations, discussions, and audiovisual aids; handouts are especially useful as a continuing reminder. Vivian and Robertson[54] (cited in Glazer-Waldman[19]) developed guidelines for patient education that consider word choice, sentence length, and typography to maximize patient comprehension. They also suggest testing the education materials on a sample population before putting them into general use.

To ensure patient participation, the practitioner must provide sufficient opportunity for practice, repetition, and feedback about performance. Adaptive training must emphasize positive reinforcement for correct responses or procedures and retraining for incorrect ones. Evaluation involves assessment of the patient's progress at periodic intervals. An older person's sense of security, control, and orientation to the environment can be heightened with a set schedule of appointments at similar times as well as the use of methods such as telephone inquiries or letter questionnaires. In all cases, rehabilitative success depends on the practitioner's ability to work with the patient to realize attainable goals.

Eye care practitioners working with older individuals with a visual impairment should realize that the primary goals of their work are to develop or maintain self-esteem, self-confidence, and independence. For evaluation of these primary aims, programmed follow-up at periodic intervals should be carried out after the rehabilitation program is complete and the patient has had time to settle into a daily routine. Well-planned rehabilitation programs address the difficulties in communication, travel, personal management, social isolation, recreation, and psychological adjustment related to vision loss and do so in ways that do not place unnecessary demands on the patient.[29]

## NEW DIRECTIONS IN LOW VISION CARE

Today, the findings that are emerging from reliable clinical studies make research in low vision care of older adults an exciting field of inquiry. New technological developments and the broader approach to patient management through involvement of allied health professionals add to the research mandate to expand the boundaries of knowledge about health, disease, and sensory impairment during old age. The ultimate goal is optimal care of visually impaired older persons. This can be achieved by a synthesis of information from studies of normal aging and studies of disease in older adults, yielding a database that allows qualification of, and differentiation among, the effects attributed to age and those attributed to disease.

The focus for the future must be toward research and development. Greater scope and depth in basic and applied research on aging are needed. Relevant topics range from basic biological knowledge to the design of better health care delivery systems, including diagnostic and therapeutic approaches to visual-perceptual problems of older adults.

### Assessment of Visual Performance

Greater research in visual performance is needed. Topics include perceptual problems and adaptations; landmark spotting, and pursuit fixations involving movements of the head, eyes, and body; adaptation to changing environmental conditions; optimal light levels indoors and outdoors; color cues; and figure-ground relationships.

Research should continue in the various conditions that cause loss of vision to allow the development of new procedures for alleviating their effects.

Studies of aging people who maintain normal visual function also are needed. Such studies may identify factors that offer preventive approaches to selected ocular diseases.

New techniques in the assessment of visual performance are needed, with improved correlation between clinical measurements of visual function and visual skills related to a person's lifestyle. This entails new instruments capable of measuring visual functions to understand the visual processes involved in everyday living.

A greater understanding of the activity levels and interests of older adults is needed, as well as the implications for behavior patterns of those with impaired vision. Such knowledge would enable the low vision team to set realistic goals for rehabilitation.

The process by which older patients relearn skills necessary for the successful use of residual vision is poorly understood; consequently, soundly based techniques must be developed for extensive readaptation. This may involve perceptual relearning, the use of eccentric fixation, and methods of expanding the functional field of view.

The outcome of these and related studies may result in the development of a battery of tests used by the practitioner to create a profile of visual function for each visually impaired patient. With the development of this test profile, a multidisciplinary approach would be necessary to consider the patient's overall ability to perform common visually related tasks in everyday life. These data could then be used to implement lifestyle improvements with the use of specific low vision devices.

### Therapeutic Approaches

Epidemiological studies continue to evaluate approaches to preventing, delaying, or ameliorating common ocular diseases that affect the visual function of older adults. The randomized controlled clinical trial approach as used in The Age-Related Eye Disease Study (AREDS) is a promising research design.[1] This study was designed to evaluate the role of antioxidants and minerals in the treatment of age-related macular degeneration and cataract. Thus far, the results of the randomized portion of the study show a significant beneficial effect of treatment with antioxidant vitamins (vitamin C, 500 mg; vitamin E, 440 IU; beta-carotene, 15 mg or 25,000 IU) and minerals (zinc oxide, 80 mg; cupric oxide, 2 mg) for the treatment of age-related macular degeneration. At 5 years of follow-up, the risk of developing advanced age-related macular degeneration was reduced by 25% and the risk of vision loss of 15 or more letters on the logMAR visual acuity chart was reduced by 19% with the combination treatment of vitamins and minerals compared with placebo controls.

New low vision devices must be designed for wider application, versatility, and patient acceptance. The technical challenge is to optimize optical design parameters to combine magnification with distortion-free fields of view.

New accessory devices are required for varied levels of patient disabilities and handicaps. The refinement of these devices may involve microprocessor technology, speech synthesis and recognition, and artificial intelligence. Efforts should continue toward integrating large-character displays with computer and word-processing systems.

Lighting techniques must be examined in relation to intensity, spectral characteristics, heat properties, contrast, and the type of lighting fixture in various environments. Further objective and subjective evaluation is necessary to determine optimal lighting according to a person's near visual acuity, working distance, ocular disease type, and reading position to enhance patient comfort and visual efficiency.

## The Emerging Role of the Health Professional in the Delivery of Low Vision Patient Care

Another major focus must be on the education and preparation of health professionals for the delivery of care to older visually impaired people. A needs assessment study should be undertaken to determine the number and types of professionals needed to adequately serve the growing population of older blind and visually impaired people. Because a positive correlation between knowledge and attitudes exists, professional educators should consider planning strategies to impart knowledge about the aging process and about the health care and social problems of older adults early in school curricula. Training in gerontology should be undertaken at both professional school and the postgraduate levels.[46] A health care professional who understands the social, psychological, and economic aspects of aging can prevent exacer-

bations of illness, achieve patient cooperation with treatment programs, and interact more effectively with patients and their families.

Various alternative models of low vision care delivery should be developed. Such models should delineate the total needs of the patient. The integration of the practitioner into a team is a necessary part of this planning; the nature of the interaction will depend on the health care delivery mode—be it clinic, private or group practice, hospital, or in-home patient care.

Pioneer and current rehabilitation programs for older blind and visually impaired adults should be analyzed and their relative merits evaluated in terms of basic concepts, standards, and principles. Innovative approaches, such as mobile units to provide low vision care for the rural older adult, represent another health care delivery need of increasing significance.

Multidisciplinary teamwork is especially important when caring for older patients. This could be accomplished by the development of one or more comprehensive multidisciplinary centers that encompass patient care, planning, interdisciplinary research, and personnel training. These centers would be responsible for ameliorating the disability (but not necessarily preventing the disease), as well as for diagnosis, treatment, and rehabilitation. They should be staffed by specialists in the basic clinical, social, and public health sciences; bioengineering; and other technical disciplines.

In agency service, a need exists for in-service training of new staff to ensure a comprehensive approach to patient care. The actions of the low vision team must dovetail the programs of care to ensure successful rehabilitation. Feedback from patients is needed to evaluate the quality and adequacy of the services offered because the most important member of any team is the low vision patient.

A delivery system should be developed that is economically viable; disseminates new information and techniques; trains appropriate personnel; and provides grass roots care, specialized assessment, and ongoing support structures. Vision care should be continually evaluated at both the patient and the clinic levels to ensure cost-effective and relevant service delivery. This assumes that goals and objectives have been considered carefully and are realistic given the limits of personnel and money.

Finally, patient care within the community should avoid unnecessary duplication.

Professional services for the visually impaired patient have significantly progressed in the past 50 years since the first low vision clinic in the United States opened its doors. Nevertheless there is still much to be accomplished. New research, advanced technology, and multidisciplinary expertise will be important factors in enhancing our ability to meet human needs.

Equally important is the personal and humane component in rendering effective low vision rehabilitation. Perhaps the practitioner's greatest service lies in encouraging the visually impaired individual to learn new skills and to become independent in every way possible. The extent to which this is achieved depends on the practitioner's ability to foster the patient's aspirations, self-confidence, and potential to realize attainable goals. It is a challenge worthy of the best efforts!

## REFERENCES

1. Age-Related Eye Disease Study Group: Design paper: the age-related eye disease study group (AREDS): design implications. AREDS report no 1, *Control Clin Trials* 20:573-600, 1999.
2. Ambrose GV, Corn AL: Impact of low vision on orientation: an exploratory study, *Review* 29:80-96, 1997.
3. Bailey IL, Hall A: *Visual impairment: an overview,* New York, 1990, American Foundation for the Blind.
4. Bailey I, Lovie-Kitchin J: New design principles for visual acuity letter charts, *Am J Optom Physiol Opt* 53:740, 1976.
5. Barraga N, Morris J: *Program to develop efficiency in visual functioning,* Louisville, KY, 1980, American Printing House for the Blind.
6. Brearley P: Aging and social work. In Hobman D, editor: *The social challenge of aging,* London, 1978, Croom Helm, p 180.
7. Brilliant R: *Essentials of low vision practice,* Boston, 1999, Butterworth-Heinemann, pp 24, 35, 273.
8. Butler RN: The life review: an interpretation of reminiscence in the aged, *Psychiatry* 26:65-76, 1963.
9. Cullinin T: *Low vision in elderly people: light for low vision. Proceedings of a symposium,* London, 1978, University College.
10. Desai M, Pratt LA, Lentzner H, et al: *Trends in vision and hearing among older Americans. Aging trends,* no. 2, Hyattsville, MD, 2001, National Center for Health Statistics.
11. Doubre JH, Boulter E: *Blindness and visual handicaps—the facts,* New York, 1982, Oxford University Press.
12. Ernst N, editor: *Pharmaceutical interventions and the aged,* Dallas, 1981, University of Texas Health Science Center.
13. Faye E: *Clinical low vision,* Boston, 1976, Little, Brown.
14. Faye E: The effect of the eye condition on functional vision. In Faye E, editor: *Clinical low vision,* ed 2, Boston, 1984, Little, Brown, pp 172-89.
15. Fineman N: Health care providers' subjective understandings of old age: implications for threatened status in late life, *J Aging Stud* 8:225-70, 1994.
16. Foley JM: Can dentists find happiness working with elderly patients? Negative attitudes and possibilities for change, *Special Care Dental* 1:197-203, 1981.
17. Gabriel M, Gagnon J, Bryon C: Improving patient compliance through the use of a daily drug reminder chart, *Am J Public Health* 67:968, 1977.
18. Gilbert GH: "Ageism" in dental care delivery, *J Am Dent Assoc* 118:545-8, 1989.
19. Glazer-Waldman H: Patient education. In Ernst N, Glazer-Waldman H, editors: *The aged patient: a sourcebook for the allied health professional,* Chicago, 1983, Year Book Medical.
20. Grayson M, Nugent C, Oken S: A Systematic and comprehensive approach to teaching and evaluating interpersonal skills, *J Med Educ* 52:906-13, 1977.
21. Haegerstrom-Portnoy G, Schneck ME, Brabyn JA: Seeing into old age: vision function beyond acuity, *Optom Vis Sci* 72:141-58, 1999.
22. Hiatt LG: Environmental factors in rehabilitation. In Brody SJ, Pawlson LG, editors: *Aging and rehabilitation II,* New York, 1990, Springer Publishing, pp 151-3.
23. Hill E, Ponder P: *Orientation and mobility techniques: a guide for the practitioner,* New York, 1976, American Foundation for the Blind.
24. Horowitz A, Reinhardt JP: Development of the adaptation to age-related vision loss scale, *J Vis Impair Blind* 92:30-41, 1998.
25. Jacobs P: The older visually impaired person: a vital link in the family and the community, *J Vis Impair Blind* 78:154-62, 1984.
26. Kamel H, Guro-Razuman S, Shareef M: The activities of daily vision scale: a useful tool to assess fall risks in older adults with visual impairment, *J Am Geriatr Soc* 48:1474-7, 2000.
27. Keller BK, Morton JL, Thomas VS, et al: The effect of visual and hearing impairments on functional status, *J Am Geriatr Soc* 47:1319-25, 1999.

28. Klein BEK, Klein R, Lee K: Incidence of age-related cataract: the Beaver Dam study, *Epidemiol Biostat* 116:219-25, 1998.
29. LaGraw SJ: *The rehabilitation of visually impaired people*, Auckland, NZ, 1992, Royal New Zealand Foundation for the Blind.
30. Lederer J: Geriatric optometry, *Aust J Optom* 65:141-3, 1982.
31. Libow L, Sherman F: *The core of geriatric medicine*, St. Louis, 1981, C.V. Mosby.
32. Lord SR, Dayhew J: Visual risk factors for falls in older people, *J Am Geriatr Soc* 49:504-15, 2001.
33. Lubinas J: Understanding the low vision patient, *Aust J Optom* 63:227-31, 1980.
34. Lutsky NS: Attitudes toward old age and elderly persons. In Eisdorfer C, editor: *Annual review of gerontology and geriatrics*, New York, 1980, Springer, pp 286-336.
35. Marron JA, Bailey IL: Visual factors and orientation-mobility performance, *Am J Optom Physiol Opt* 59:413-26, 1982.
36. McKay S: Wholistic health care: challenge to health providers, *J Allied Health* 9:194-201, 1980.
37. Mehr E: Psychological factors in low vision care. In Newman J, editor: *A guide to the care of low vision patients*, St. Louis, 1974, American Optometric Association, p 49.
38. Michaels D: *Visual optics and refraction. A clinical approach*, ed 3, St. Louis, 1985, C.V. Mosby, p 418.
39. Newbold G: *The costs of blindness*, Auckland, NZ, 1987, University of Auckland.
40. Palmore EB: *Ageism. Negative and positive*, ed 2, New York, 1999, Springer.
41. Population Resource Center: *Technology adaptation and the aging*, New York, 1981, Population Resource Center.
42. Reidy A, Minassian DC, Vafidis G, et al: Prevalence of serious eye disease and visual impairment in a north London population: population based, cross sectional study, *BMJ* 316:1643-6, 1998.
43. Reuben DB, Mui S, Damesyn M, et al: The prognostic value of sensory impairment in older persons, *J Am Geriatr Soc* 47:930-5, 1995.
44. Robbins H: Low vision care for the over 80s, *Aust J Optom* 64:243-51, 1981.
45. Rosenbloom A: Care of elderly people with low vision, *J Vis Impair Blind* 76:209-12, 1982.
46. Rosenbloom A: Optometry and gerontology, *Optom Monthly* 73:143-44, 1982.
47. Royal New Zealand Foundation for the Blind: *Focus on rehabilitation: a rehabilitation service delivery plan for people with visual impairment*, Auckland, NZ, 1990, Royal New Zealand Foundation for the Blind.
48. Rumsey KE: Redefining the optometric examination: addressing the vision needs of older adults, *Optom Vis Sci* 70:587-91, 1993.
49. Scott RA: *The making of blind men: a study of adult socialization*, New Brunswick, NJ, 1991, Transaction Publishers.
50. Sinick D: Counseling older persons: career change and retirement, *Vocational Guidance Quarterly* 25:18-24, 1976.
51. Strandberg LR: Drugs as a reason for nursing home admissions, *J Am Health Care Assoc* 4:20-3, 1984.
52. Talkington D: Maximizing patient compliance by shaping attitudes of self-directed health care, *J Fam Pract* 6:591-5, 1978.
53. Taylor HR, Keeffe JE: World blindness: a 21st century perspective, *Br J Ophthalmol* 85:261-6, 2001.
54. Vivian A, Robertson E: Readability of patient education materials, *Clin Ther* 3:129-36, 1980.

## SUGGESTED READINGS

Atchley RC: *Aging: continuity and change*, Belmont, CA, 1983, Wadsworth.
Committee on Vision, National Research Council: *Work, aging, and vision—report of a conference*, Washington, DC, 1987, National Academy Press, p 32.
Conrad KA, Bressler R: *Drug therapy for the elderly*, St. Louis, 1982, C.V. Mosby.
Covington TR, Walker J. *Current geriatric therapy*, Philadelphia, 1984, W.B. Saunders.
Ernst NS, Glazer-Waldman HR: *The aged patient: a sourcebook for the allied health professional*, Chicago, 1983, Year Book Medical.
Grosvenor T: *Primary care optometry*, ed 4, Boston, 2002, Butterworth-Heinemann.
Hobman D, editor: *The social challenge of aging. Aging and social work*, London, 1978, Croom Helm, p 181.
Kirchner C, Peterson R: The latest data on visual disability from NCHS, *J Vis Impair Blind* 74:42-4, 1980.
Kwitko ML: Environmental modifications for the elderly. In Kwitko ML, Weinstock FJ, editors: *Geriatric ophthalmology*, Orlando, FL, 1985, Grune and Stratton, pp 404-10.
Lovie-Kitchin J, Bowman K: *Senile macular degeneration: management and rehabilitation*, Stoneham, MA, 1985, Butterworth.
Lovie-Kitchin JK: Bowman E: Technical note: domestic lighting requirement for the elderly, *Aust J Optom* 66:93-7, 1983.
Mehr EB, Freid AN: *Low vision care*, Chicago, 1975, Professional Press.
O'Hara-Devereaux M, Andrus LH, Scott CD, editors: *Eldercare: a practical guide to clinical geriatrics*, New York, 1981, Grune and Stratton.

Remen N: *The human patient*, New York, 1980, Doubleday.

Rosenbloom AA: Low vision. In Peyman G, Sanders D, Goldberg M, editors: *Principles and practice of ophthalmology*, Philadelphia, 1980, W.B. Saunders, pp 241-77.

Rosenbloom A: Low vision: the next decade [editorial], *J Vis Impair Blind* 86:5, 1992.

Rosenbloom A: A salute to the international year of older persons [editorial], *Optometry* 71:348-50, 2000.

Rosenbloom AA: New aged and old aged: impact of the baby boomer [editorial], *Optometry* 74:211-3, 2003.

Rosenbloom AA: The booming dynamics of aging [editorial], *Optometry* 77:253-5, 2006.

Ross MA: *Fitness for the aging adult with visual impairment: an exercise and resource manual*, New York, 1984, American Foundation for the Blind.

Ryan KM: Rehabilitation services for older people with visual impairments, *Review* 34:31-48, 2002.

Sekuler R, Kline D, Dismukes K: *Aging and human visual function*, New York, 1982, Allan R. Liss.

Simonson W: *Medications and the elderly: a guide for promoting proper use*, Rockville, MD, 1984, Aspen Systems.

Steinberg FU, editor: *Care of the geriatric patient*, ed 6, St. Louis, 1983, C.V. Mosby.

Update on General Medicine, 2003-2004 edition. In *Geriatrics*, San Francisco, 2003, Foundation of the American Academy of Ophthalmology, pp 189-93, 287.

Weale RA: *A biography of the eye: development, growth, age*, London, 1982, H.K. Lewis.

# CHAPTER 15

# Assistive Technologies for the Visually Impaired Older Adult

**GALE WATSON and JOSEPH H. MAINO**

In this chapter, assistive technology is considered as "a broad range of devices, services, strategies and practices that are conceived and applied to ameliorate the problems faced by individuals who have disabilities."[9]

PL 100-407, the Technical Assistance to the States Act, provides the definition of a device:

> Any item, piece of equipment or product system, whether acquired commercially off the shelf, modified, or customized that is used to increase, maintain, or improve the functional capabilities of individuals with disabilities.

Because this definition emphasizes the functional capability of older individuals with disabilities, it is important to our discussion of nonoptical technologies. The successful use of technology in the environment and for the task for which it is intended is the ultimate goal. Functional outcomes are the only important measure of success.

PL 100-407 defines assistive technology service as, "any service that directly assists an individual with a disability in the selection, acquisition, or use of an assistive technology device." The broad spectrum of services that are recognized by this law include (1) evaluating the need for technology; (2) acquiring the technology; (3) selecting, designing, repairing, and fabri-

cating assistive technology systems; (4) coordinating services with other therapies; and (5) training individuals with disabilities and persons working with them to use the technologies effectively.

Technologies may be characterized in a variety of ways that are useful in a discussion of low vision rehabilitation. With the increasing need to look at the service delivery system of low vision as integrated with other forms of physical medicine and rehabilitation in the U.S. health care system, a logical outgrowth of the definitions of technologies and services provided earlier is to characterize low vision technologies in the framework of the technologies that provide improved functional outcomes for other disabilities.

## ASSISTIVE AND REHABILITATIVE OR EDUCATIONAL TECHNOLOGIES

Technologies that help an individual carry out a functional activity are termed assistive. Technology can also serve as a part of the education or rehabilitation process. This technology can be thought of as devices or programs that assist in developing skills for the use of assistive technologies. For example, a flex-armed lamp used to provide illumination for reading is an example of nonoptical assistive technology for enhancing visual ability. Software that assists in enhancing the use of a preferred retinal locus for reading is rehabilitation technology.

## LOW TO HIGH TECHNOLOGIES

Often inexpensive, simple devices that are easy to use may be designated low technology, whereas more complex, more expensive, and more difficult to use devices may be designated as high technology. According to this distinction, typoscopes, canes, and slate and stylus may be thought of as low technology, whereas computer programs, refreshable Braille, and closed-circuit televisions (CCTVs) may be thought of as high technology.

According to Vanderheiden,[26] an appliance is a device that provides benefit independent of an individual's skill level. A tool is a device that requires the development of skill in its use. The distinguishing factor between tools and appliances is the skill level of the user; the benefit a tool provides is directly related to the skill of the user. These concepts can be easily applied with low vision devices. Some devices are intuitive, and their benefit is applied immediately on use, such as lamps and sun lenses. Others cannot be used and benefit cannot be derived unless the user is skilled, such as with computers or CCTVs. The more low vision devices are characterized as tools, the more the need for the appropriate selection of devices and skill acquisition by the user becomes apparent. Some users are able to benefit immediately from a device. Persons whose visual fields are intact are often able to read immediately with spectacle magnifiers with merely a brief demonstration of the focal distance and field of view. Those with central scotoma, however, may require extensive practice and training to identify and use their preferred retinal locus accurately and to develop visual strategies for recognizing words and maintaining comprehension despite slow rates of reading. In this case, the need for practitioners' expertise in prescription and the need for extensive training are related to the attributes of the user as much as the attributes of the tool.

## MINIMAL TO MAXIMAL TECHNOLOGIES

Both persons who are visually impaired and the technology they might require can be considered along a continuum of disability. The dis-

ability related to beginning age-related macular degeneration may require only stronger bifocal or half-eye lenses, protection from glare outdoors, a flex-armed lamp for task lighting, and other minimal technology. A person who has lost vision because of diabetic retinopathy, however, may require maximal technology that includes a computer with speech or Braille output or a long cane or guide dog for safe and efficient travel. These approaches may make use of environmental adaptations such as audible traffic signals, texturized subway guides, and other tools and techniques for independence, safety, and quality of life. Minimal technologies may be those that augment rather than replace function and have been termed orthoses, or orthotic devices. The term prosthetics or prosthetic device is used to describe those devices that replace function. Although these terms were originally developed to describe braces of various types or devices that replace body parts, the terms have been broadened to include all assistive technology devices.

### General Technologies

General technologies are those that are used across a wide range of applications; they are designated as positioning systems, control interfaces, and computers. Although the principles of ergonomics are not widely known or used in low vision service delivery in the United States, they are nonetheless at work in the environments of persons with low vision who are using assistive technologies. When ergonomic positioning is incorrect, persons tire faster and may blame fatigue, headache, or body pains on the low vision device instead of the uncomfortable positioning.

### Commercial to Custom Technology

The continuum in this category includes products commercially available to everyone, to products commercially available to those with low vision, to customization of commercially made products, to a completely customized product. Designers and manufacturers of products that are commercially available to everyone are beginning to use the principles of universal design. These principles have led to products available to the general public that are designed to recognize that enhancing the ability to use vision is important, especially to older persons. Computers are now designed so that universal adaptability includes increasing the print size on the screen. Any kitchen supply store carries measuring cups and spoons with large size markings.

When an older person is no longer able to achieve task function with a commercial universal design technology, then commercial technology designed for persons with low vision can be used. For example, a user with low vision can no longer read the computer screen with the built-in enlarged type. A variety of commercially available devices may assist, such as magnification software (e.g., Zoomtext, Ai Squared, Manchester Center, Vt.) and optical magnifiers.

Ways of categorizing technologies are available to older persons. A few rising tides will carry technology development in this field, including (1) the increasing numbers of older persons who will develop low vision in the coming years, especially baby-boomers; (2) the concept of universal design that will include the demands and requirements of these aging boomers; (3) the increase in miniaturization of computer components; and (4) the increase of "wearable" computer design that will allow access to information with a wide variety of interfaces. As technology is developed at a dizzying pace, many of the design obstacles that have created barriers for the development and deployment of low vision technologies in the past will be removed. Barriers related to optical concepts; the difficulties in designing, developing, and marketing to a low-incidence disability population; and the separation of low vision from other physical medicine and rehabilitation populations are being swept away. As more research is helping define the visual difficulties of normally sighted older persons, the past categorization of low vision is becoming outdated. Many more people have visual difficulties than were previously realized, and they need to understand how to access technologies that will allow them to achieve the independence and quality of life that they expect.

## Visual Function

Visual impairment inhibits gaining sensory information from the environment. The clinical visual functions and descriptions of the types of visual impairments experienced by older persons are described in other chapters. However, in relation to technologies, visual limitations can be characterized in terms of intensity (size), frequency or wavelength (color or contrast), and visual field (central or peripheral or both). Low vision technologies may enhance the visual image by increasing the size, enhancing the contrast, or displacing the visual target in the visual field. But a variety of technologies use other ways of displaying visual information.

## Perceptual Function

The onset of visual impairment creates difficulties with the ability to see targets and interferes with the ability to decode visual information and make sense of what is seen. Factors of visual perception are affected by low vision and the use of assistive technology. In the process of attempting to improve the view of an object by increasing its size, visual perceptual skills may be simultaneously decreased by eliminating cues for perception such as perspective and motion parallax. Perceptual cues related to convergence and binocular disparity are eliminated when monocular devices are used The effective use of assistive technology forces the user to acquire or improve perceptual skills, such as part-to-whole relationships and visual closure, to integrate visual images that will allow effective functioning with a different view of the world.

## Cognitive Function

Cognitive function is important to learning new skills. Individuals who will benefit from technologies must learn to do new things in new ways. The importance of cognitive function has been recognized by Medicare policies that require cognitive testing by some screening, usually the Folstein Mini-Mental State Examination,[7] and that practitioners state how users who score lower than the cutoff will benefit from the service. Cognitive function decreases if the user does not have access to stimulation.[16] Many normally sighted older persons are able to read, watch stimulating television, complete crossword puzzles, and engage in a variety of mentally stimulating tasks that assist them in keeping their cognitive skills. Those techniques are denied, however, to persons with low vision who are not able to access these activities. Low vision devices, training, and daily practice enhance visual function and may also enhance cognitive function and keep the minds of older persons stimulated.

However, even persons who have diminished cognitive function can still benefit from technologies if goals for low vision rehabilitation are switched from independence to reducing caregiver burden. Some low technologies can be used despite decreased cognitive function (such as illumination controls, increased contrast in the environment). Even some high technologies can be useful for individuals with diminished cognitive function if the activity is a familiar one, such as reading materials that are well loved, familiar, and comforting that can still be enjoyed by speech output or on CCTV. Caregivers may get other tasks completed while the person with low vision and reduced cognition is occupied.

## Psychosocial Functioning

Everyone who works in low vision has a story of some individual who has shown great promise of benefit with a low vision device and then did not use it because he or she did not want to be seen using it. Human beings value appearing as much as possible like peer groups and being viewed as strong and capable. Anxiety and depression are common reactions to loss, and age-related visual impairment is complicated by the other losses associated with aging. Older adults may hold many negative stereotypes associated with visual impairment: increased helplessness, inhabiting a world of darkness, increased vulnerability to crime, and the perception that devices mark them as different or to be pitied. Older adults may attempt to pass as fully sighted to avoid having others project these negative stereotypes onto them. But attempting to pass as fully sighted may cause other difficulties. For example, older adults with low vision do not recognize faces well, and the lack of a friendly hello when passing acquaintances may be interpreted as unfriendliness. Failure to use alternative techniques for identifying targets and moving in the environment may lead to falls, burns, incorrect medication dosages, or other safety hazards.

In a study of low vision device use among veterans, most of whom were older men with macular degeneration, family support was the most powerful predictor of continued use of devices up to 2 years after their prescription. Providing information and support to family members who are experiencing the impact of an older relative's vision loss can be powerful. The entire family experiences visual impairment and the caregiving system, not just the older person, and both social and psychological concerns must be addressed. The loss of vision by one family member can disrupt roles in the family, create economic demands, and add stress when tasks previously performed by the older adult must be performed by someone else.

Assisting older adults with low vision in continuing social activities, such as hobbies, crafts, games, and traveling, can help them maintain important contacts with family and peers. Social support and contact were associated with less depression in older adults with low vision.[16] Support groups can assist older adults with low vision in completing and implementing their rehabilitation as well as facilitating adaptation to vision loss.[27] Peer support or mutual aid groups that meet regularly to share concerns may be especially beneficial for older adults. Facilitating assertiveness for older adults is recommended because it is linked to less depression and more social support.[16] Social skills training in assertiveness for older adults with low vision has been shown to be effective in decreasing depression and deriving greater satisfaction in life.[15]

## Motor Control

Manipulating low vision devices is difficult for some older users because of problems with motor control. Hand tremors and arthritis may weaken hands and cause pain. Prospective closed-caption television users may have difficulty manipulating an x-y platform. Low vision devices may cause difficulties with balance and increase the likelihood of falls. According to one study eye position in space was an active, integrated component of standing.[10] Both the oculomotor system and the head motor system in older persons are coordinated to direct gaze and, when necessary, work to suppress the vestibulo-ocular reflex. A breakdown in the gaze control mechanisms in older persons could contribute to the risk of falling and fall-related injuries.

### Ergonomic Positioning

Principles of ergonomics applied to workstations have shown that increased comfort and decreased energy expenditure can increase the work output of persons in a variety of situations.[19] Ergonomics can be defined as "(1) the science of fitting the workplace to the worker, or (2) a biomechanical approach to workplace design."[1] Physiological changes that accompany the aging process include sarcopenia, reduced bone mineral density, reduced maximum oxygen uptake, and reduced muscular strength. Morbidities related to these physiological changes include musculoskeletal instability, osteoporosis, reduced endurance, and a reduction in overall functional ability.[14] If an ergonomically incorrect environment further stresses persons with these known age-related physiological changes, many may experience elevated levels of discomfort.

In a study of ergonomic positioning for older persons who read with devices, reading rate was significantly improved by ergonomic positioning of older readers with low vision, and discomfort while reading was significantly reduced.[28] The study demonstrated that readers who are using low vision devices can benefit from short-term and inexpensive ergonomic interventions that significantly improve reading and may increase the amount of time the reader can spend reading comfortably. Solutions presented by various sources were easily adapted for workstations by readers with low vision in this project.[6,13,20]

### NONOPTICAL DEVICES

#### Devices for Ergonomic Positioning

The clinician should first consider the patient's reading or work environment. The desk or work area should be at an appropriate height for the specific task to be performed. The selection of the chair should be taken seriously. The ABC's of chair selection should be followed (*a*rmrests, *b*ackrests, *c*hair height, and *s*eat). To help the patient select the best chair, a tool such

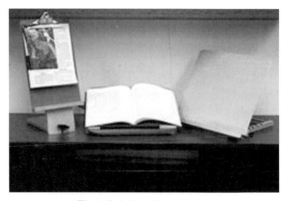

**Fig. 15-1**  Reading stands.

as the Ergonomics Seating Evaluation Form (*http://ergo.human.cornell.edu/ahSEATING.html*) can be used to evaluate the quality of different chairs.

Once the basic ergonomic platform is specified, other tools can be used to position the reading or work material appropriately. In general, the postural and positioning demands are best met with reading stands, easels, copy stands, lapboards, clamps, computer monitor stands, and adjustable tables. Posture and positioning devices are especially important to older adults with arthritis, Parkinson's disease, or other infirmities that affect the ability to hold and manipulate objects.

Tinker[25] showed that reading is improved when the reading material is positioned at a right angle to the patient's line of sight and set 45 degrees down from the vertical. For most applications, simple bookstands or easels provide the best solution to this ergonomic problem. These may include the Eschenbach slanted reading stand and Able Table and Wooden Reading Stand (Able Table Co., Weir Enterprises, Santa Cruz, Calif.) (Fig. 15-1). For reading material on sheets of paper, an inexpensive clamp-on copyholder usually works well. If the reading material is heavy or if it needs to be positioned closer to the patient the Shafer Reading Stand (American Printing House for the Blind, Louisville, Ky.) can be used. When a patient reads in bed, the Posture Rite Lap Desk (Hoyle Products Inc, Glennville, Calif.) has a nonglare, hard surface attached to a fabric cushion (see Fig. 15-1). For computer work, a monitor stand can be used to position the monitor at the best reading distance.

### Relative Size Devices

#### Print

The most commonly used adaptive devices are those that use relative size magnification. These super-sized aids include large print, telephone dials, watches, thermometers, clocks, checks, crossword puzzles, thermostats, calendars, sheet music, and games.

The amount of relative size magnification is the ratio of the size of the original object to that of the enlarged object. For example, if the size of standard print is 1 M and 2.5 M print is used instead, the magnification is 2.5×.*

Other factors leading to improved readability must be considered when using large print. These include print darkness, paper weight and color, letter and line spacing, margin size, and font. In general large print should have clean edges and be of such a size that the lower case *o* is approximately 2.7 mm in height. The paper should be lightweight and have good opacity and high contrast. Line length should be no less than 6 inches, and hyphenation should be kept to a minimum. Finally, periods and commas should be larger than normal.[2]

Large print has both advantages and disadvantages. The advantages include simplicity, ease of use, and acceptance by most people. Large print may also be used in conjunction with low power optical devices as a training tool. Once the individual learns how to use the low power magnifier with the large print, he or she can then more easily progress to higher powered magnifiers with standard-size print.

The primary disadvantage of large print includes the limited amount of magnification, production costs, and limited availability. Few large-print books exceed 18-point type and therefore have only 1.8× magnification. This

low magnification is of little benefit for individuals with visual acuity of 20/400 or less. Production costs soar as print size increases. The number of larger print pages required is governed by the square of the amount of magnification needed. For example, if the size of the print is doubled, four times the number of pages are needed. Other costs such as storage and shipping also increase as print size is enlarged. Although the availability of large-print documents and books has improved over the years, obtaining the latest best seller or most textbooks in large-print versions is still difficult. Several resources for large-print products are available. These include the American Printing House for the Blind and the National Library Service for the Blind and Physically Handicapped. Easily obtainable large-print periodicals and newspapers include *Reader's Digest* and the *New York Times*. Large-print editions of dictionaries, bibles, and cookbooks can be found in most bookstores.

#### Other Devices

Many devices used to accomplish various activities of daily living also come in super-sized formats. The ability to manage finances is an important activity of daily living. Writing checks and balancing a checkbook are key to retaining independence. In addition to check writing guides that can be used with standard-size checks, large-print checks and check registers are available (Fig. 15-2). A large-print check register available from LS&S (Northbrook, Ill.) uses a spiral binding, which allows the register to lay flat. It has seven entries per page and a

---

*In the world of typography, print size is specified according to the point system. One point is approximately $\frac{1}{72}$ of an inch in height. Most print is therefore classified according to point size (e.g., 7-point type). The standard for most print is 10-point type, so an estimate of magnification can be obtained simply by dividing the larger print point size by 10. For example, 18-point type provides approximately 1.8× magnification.

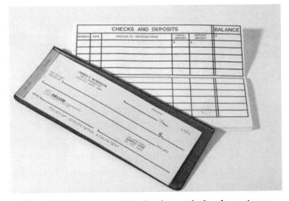

**Fig. 15-2** Large-print checks and check register.

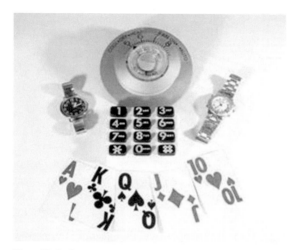

**Fig. 15-3** Large-print watches, phone dial, playing cards, and thermostat.

total of 26 pages. Deluxe Check Printers (Shoreview, Minn.) has a large print check, the Guide-Line, that is available from most banks and comes with a large-print check registry. For older individuals with access to the Internet, online banking and bill paying may make using paper checks obsolete.

Large-print rotary phone dials and large-print push-button overlays or phones can be purchased. Keep in mind that most large-print phones only provide large numbers. The letters are either missing or are still relatively small (Fig. 15-3). For severely vision impaired persons, voice-activated dialing or operator-assisted dialing may provide a better solution.

The ability to tell time is also a necessary activity of daily living. Large-face clocks and watches are obtainable from several distributors. Typically the clock or watch has a white face with large black hands and numbers (see Fig. 15-3). Some large-print watches use light-emitting diodes (LEDs) or liquid crystal displays (LCDs).

All people need to play. Fortunately, many games may be obtained in large-print editions. Various companies have everything from large-print bingo to jumbo-faced playing cards (see Fig. 15-3). Other large-print games include Scrabble, checkers, chess, and Uno. For those who enjoy crafts, spread-eye needles, large-print embroidery designs, large-print tape measures, and other sewing and knitting aids are available.

## Devices for Illumination and Contrast Control

### Illumination

Without light vision is impossible, and without contrast discrimination is impossible. Most eye and vision disorders affect the ability to use available light or reduce the ability to discriminate objects in the environment; consequently, magnification alone is not always enough to improve vision function. Increasing contrast and reducing spatial frequency are typically both used in low vision rehabilitation.

In general, vision performance improves as light increases. So how much light is enough? For normal subjects, performance improves logarithmically, rising rapidly from a low level of illumination until an asymptote is reached.[3,23]

Eye diseases that tend to reduce retinal illumination without light scatter benefit from increased illumination. Individuals who have ocular disorders that both reduce illumination and scatter light may not benefit from more light. As a matter of fact, increased light may actually reduce vision and vision function. This phenomenon is seen when doing a glare test on an individual with cataracts. Acuity under dim room light is typically better than when the room lights are turned on. On the whole, individuals with macular disease do better with increased illumination, whereas those with cataract may do worse. Individuals with glaucoma do approximately the same as normals (more light equals better performance).[11,18,24] Other eye diseases associated with glare and photophobia include aniridia, achromatopsia, albinism, clinically significant diabetic maculopathy, retinitis pigmentosa, and various cone dystrophies. Many treatments for ocular disease can also affect the need for illumination. For example, laser photocoagulation may increase glare and reduce the ability to adapt to changing levels of illumination, whereas the use of miotics to treat glaucoma, which also constricts pupil size, results in the need for increased illumination.

Higher levels of illumination can result in glare, which in turn can reduce visual performance or even result in visual discomfort. When glare causes discomfort or pain (photophobia) it is called *discomfort glare*. When it interferes with vision performance, it is referred to as *disability glare*. There are several ways to control glare. The type, size, brightness, and position of the source can be changed, the contrast between the light source and the surroundings can be changed, or filters that change the quality or quantity of light entering the eye can be used.

The eye care professional can help the patient select the appropriate light for a given task. Fortunately, numerous types of lights (fluorescent, incandescent, neodymium, halogen) are commercially available. The least expensive but most difficult to control is natural sunlight. Although many people with vision impairment prefer sunlight, it can produce discomfort and reduce the individual's ability to adapt quickly to changing light conditions. Sunlight is most often controlled by the use of light filters, visors, and clip-on side shields or by using hats with brims.

Many older persons do not function well with fluorescent light. Standard fluorescent illumination is harsh; provides little contrast; and accentuates blues, greens, and yellows. Because it contains a higher percentage of ultraviolet light, it can make the eye's lens fluoresce, resulting in glare or haze. Newer fluorescent lights are now available with a range of color temperatures that mimic incandescent light. Because fluorescent lights "burn" cooler than most other types of lights, they may be useful in situations in which the person must be close to the light source.

Incandescent illumination puts out light of longer wavelengths and is considered a "warm" light, appearing more yellow than blue. An incandescent light source tends to be pinpoint and directional and produces more contrast and shadows than fluorescent fixtures. Incandescent lights require the use of diffusers and shades to reduce glare. Because the longer wavelength of incandescent light is not scattered as much as the longer wavelength of fluorescent lights, it is usually preferred by individuals with cataracts, corneal edema, or other media opacities that tend to scatter light. Many older persons prefer small, movable, adjustable incandescent light sources when reading or performing other tasks.

The Chromalux (Lighting Manufacturers & Distributors, Inc., Barrington, Ill.) bulb (neodymium light source) produces illumina-

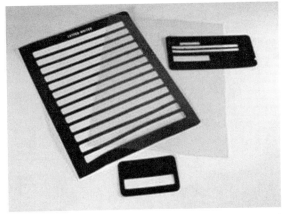

**Fig. 15-4** Typoscopes, yellow acetate filter, and writing guides.

tion that is similar to sunlight. Available in 60- and 100-W frosted bulbs, use of a neodymium light source may increase short-term task performance.[8]

Halogen light, although bright, produces a great deal of heat and ultraviolet rays. Although some low vision devices incorporate halogen lights with a rheostat, the typical halogen light fixture is not useful for most people with vision impairment.

Light position is important to control glare and intensity. The ideal light source should be movable, be adjustable, and have a rheostat to control output. It should be placed on the side of the better-seeing eye and positioned to avoid glare. If the light does not contain a rheostat, moving the light closer to or further from the material being viewed can control intensity. Keep in mind the intensity varies by the square of the distance from the source—moving the light twice as close makes the illumination four times as bright.

The typoscope, invented by Charles Prentice in 1897, effectively reduces stray light and glare from surrounding text and acts as a line guide when reading (Fig. 15-4).[22] When the typoscope is combined with a yellow acetate filter, contrast also increases.[4]

Pinhole glasses, stenopaic slits, and controlled-pupil contact lenses have also been used as a diagnostic tool to determine if glare and photophobia are contributing factors to the patient's complaint.

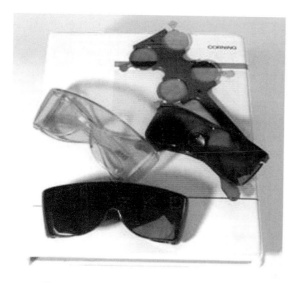

**Fig. 15-5** NoIR and corning light filters.

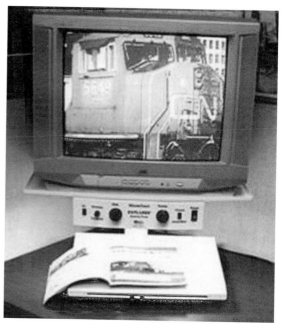

**Fig. 15-6** CCTV.

### Light Filters

Clinicians prescribe light filters to reduce glare and photophobia, improve residual visual function, reduce adaptation time, and improve orientation and mobility. Unfortunately, little objective evidence supports clinically significant improvement in visual performance with light filter use.[12] A literature review by Eperjesi et al[12] regarding the impact of light filters on visual acuity, contrast sensitivity, and visual field did provide some insight into what type of light filter may be best for a specific ocular condition. So why are light filters prescribed? For many individuals, tints do seem to improve vision function and occasionally even improve the level of vision impairment (better acuity or improved contrast sensitivity).

### Available Filters

NoIR Medical Technologies (South Lyon, Mich.) manufactures two types of light filters: the NoIR and UVShield. According to the company, the UVShield provides visible light and 100% ultraviolet light protection and the NoIR blocks near infrared and 100% ultraviolet and offers visible light protection. Currently NoIR offers more than 25 UVShield and 18 NoIR filters. These polycarbonate filters retain their shape and have several different form factors, including large and standard fit-overs, clip-ons, and standard sunglass styles. Fit-overs also

have polycarbonate side shields that are the same color as the front; consequently, they are ideal for blocking stray light that comes in from the side or above most standard light filters (Fig. 15-5). Children and infant versions are also available (*http://www.noir-medical.com/*). (See Chapter 11 for information on available glass photochromic lenses.)

## ELECTRONIC MAGNIFICATION

### Closed-Circuit Television

The CCTV is an effective low vision rehabilitation device that provides electronic magnification and, in some cases, image enhancement to allow vision-impaired persons to perform such tasks as reading and writing. The basic CCTV consists of a monitor; camera; various controls for magnification, contrast, and polarity; and an x-y table (a reading platform that moves vertically and horizontally so the material can be viewed) (Fig. 15-6). This device typically provides up to 60× magnification and allows the user to control image size, brightness, contrast, and image polarity (black letters on a white background can be reversed to white letters on a black background). Individuals can also view the monitor binocularly, write and read at a comfortable distance and change viewing distance and magnification to maximize the linear

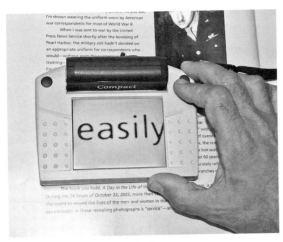

**Fig. 15-7** Compact.

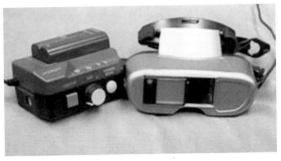

**Fig. 15-8** Jordy.

functional field of view by changing the working distance from the CCTV monitor.

When prescribing a CCTV, keep in mind that ergonomics are important. The CCTV workstation should include a comfortable, adjustable chair and have the CCTV controls and monitor at the correct height. Older persons may also require a pair of glasses that focus the monitor for the intended viewing distance.

Many improvements in CCTVs have occurred over the years. Modern systems may have high-resolution color or black-and-white monitors, liquid crystal display color and black-and-white monitors, multiple cameras (to produce split screens), and CCTV/computer combination devices. Handheld CCTV cameras, pocket-size electronic magnifiers, and head-mounted CCTVs are also available. The handheld/stand CCTV camera system (e.g., Flipper, Enhanced Vision Systems, Huntington Beach, Calif.) can use the patient's own home TV as a monitor. Various pocket-size electronic magnifiers, such as the Compact (Optelec, Tieman Group; Chelmsford, Mass.), are also available. This palm-size, handheld device offers up to 8× magnification, a battery life of 2 hours, and five viewing modes (Fig. 15-7). The Jordy (Enhanced Vision Systems) is a small, lightweight, battery-operated device that can be worn like a pair of glasses or used as a desktop video magnifier when placed on its docking stand (Fig. 15-8). Finally, Eschenbach (Ridgefield, Conn.) has incorporated a computerized scanner into their latest electronic reading system, the myReader

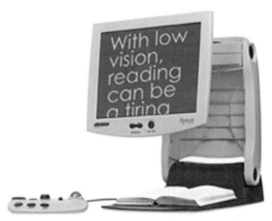

**Fig. 15-9** myReader.

(Fig. 15-9). This new device scans a page of text and then allows the individual to play it back as a wrapped paragraph, a continuous line, or one word at a time.

As devices become more complex, providing the individual with appropriate training becomes more important. CCTV training involves familiarization with the equipment, determination of the best device parameters to optimize visual performance, demonstration and use of the x-y table, and eccentric viewing therapy. Additionally, the individual may also be taught how to scan documents for salient information to get an overview of the material, write, and read.[20]

## Computers

For many vision-impaired computer users, free or relatively inexpensive solutions may be possible. For example, current versions of Windows and the Macintosh operating system have built-in low vision accessibility options. In Windows XP, go to Start → Accessories → Accessibility → Magnifier. The Windows XP built-in magnifier is a screen enlarger that enlarges a portion of the display, making the screen easier to read. The Windows XP accessibility option can enlarge the screen up to nine times and can also increase contrast. The Apple Macintosh operating system includes a program called CloseView. The built-in program is also a screen enlarger. It magnifies all screen images (text, graphics, menu bar, and the mouse cursor) up to 16 times. Additionally, CloseView can inverse the Macintosh display (so that text appears white on a black background instead of vice versa; see *http://www.apple.com/disability/vision/easyaccess.html*). Although the Windows magnifier and CloseView are not intended as replacements for a full-featured screen-enlargement utility, they may be all that is required for individuals with mild or moderate vision loss.

A larger monitor may help other computer users. For example, increasing the monitor size from 15 inches to 22 inches increases the magnification by almost 1.5 times. Other choices include using a monitor stand or arm so the user can move the monitor closer to take advantage of relative distance magnification. If the individual moves the monitor from a working distance of 40 cm to 10 cm, magnification is increased by a factor of four. Other inexpensive options include snap-on screen magnifiers and screen polarizers. For older computer users with poor typing skills, the computer's keyboard characters can be enlarged by using key tops with large-print characters or by using press-on large-print characters.[21]

Although this chapter primarily describes nonoptical devices that assist vision-impaired older adults, remember that in some instances telemicroscopes may also be used to read the computer screen. One device that allows the individual to look at the computer monitor and keyboard, across the room, and at reference material all without having to manually re-focus is the Ocutech (Chapel Hill, N.C.) autofocus telescope (Fig. 15-10).

Older individuals with visual acuity of 20/200 or less may also benefit from the use of stand-alone large-print computer programs. The number of large-print access computer programs continues to increase every year. A

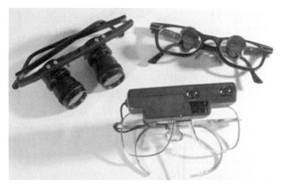

**Fig. 15-10** Eschenbach near telescope, designs for vision near telescope, and the Ocutech autofocus telescope.

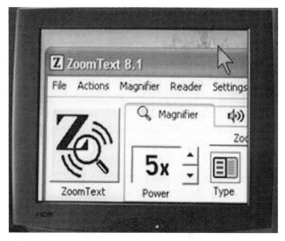

**Fig. 15-11** ZoomText computer screen magnifier.

review of all these programs is beyond the scope of this chapter, but a few well-established programs that provide most of the functionality vision-impaired computer users need are described.

Two of the most commonly used programs for Windows include ZoomText and MAGic (Freedom Scientific Inc., St. Petersburg, Fla.; Fig. 15-11). Both programs come in several versions and offer up to 16× magnification, mouse pointer enhancements, flexible color contrast and, depending on the version, speech output. (See *http://www.aisquared.com* and *http://www.freedomscientific.com*.) Free trial versions of the software are available before purchase.

Nonvisual computer access is required when screen-magnifying software fails to meet the needs of the vision-impaired person. Fortunately numerous options are available. For Windows, two of the most used programs include Window-EYES (GW Micro, Fort Wayne, Ind.) and JAWS (Freedom Scientific). Braille access solutions also exist. Obviously, when a profoundly visually impaired person is evaluated, working with the state Agency for the Blind or other local or regional aging resources is important. These rehabilitation agencies may have assistive technology specialists to determine the most appropriate nonvisual computer access technology for the person.

## HEARING AIDS AND ASSISTIVE LISTENING DEVICES

Among adults aged 70 years or older, 18.1% report vision impairment, 33.2% note a hearing loss, and 8.6% have both a vision and a hearing loss.[5] Several kinds of hearing aids are available. The primary types include behind the ear (BTE), in the canal (ITC), and completely in the canal (CIC) (Fig. 15-12). A BTE hearing aid fits behind the ear and has a small ear hook that extends over the top of the auricle into the ear canal. The ITC is small enough to fit into the ear canal and looks like a large ear plug. The CIC is the smallest device and is almost completely inserted into the canal, thereby making it nearly invisible (see Fig. 15-12).

Assistive listening devices (ALDs) are typically much larger than hearing aids and usually consist of a headphone and microphone (Fig. 15-13). Use of an ALD can be advantageous, especially when background noise exists. Unlike most traditional hearing aids that amplify all

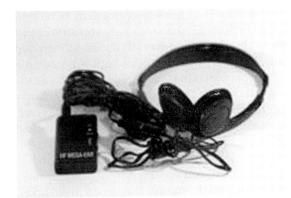

**Fig. 15-13** External assistive listening device.

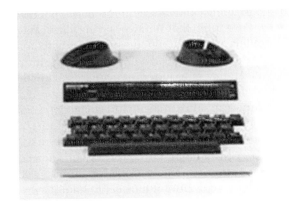

**Fig. 15-14** Telecommunication device for the deaf.

sounds equally, ALDs amplify the primary signal, not the competing noise. ALDs that use an FM sound system are found at movie theaters, concert halls, and churches. Infrared sound systems are available for home TVs and various telephone amplifiers, and telecommunication devices for the deaf are also available to help the hearing-impaired older person (Fig. 15-14). (See Chapter 9 for a more complete discussion of age-related auditory impairment.)

Helen Keller, who was both blind and deaf, noted that she would prefer to have her hearing back instead of her vision because she believed that although blind people were cut off from things, deafness cut her off from people.[19] Therefore the optometrist and the ophthalmologist should consider the need for hearing aids or assistive listening devices when working with older persons.

The performance of activities of daily living is improved with the use of assistive devices.

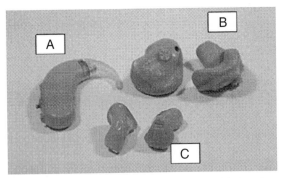

**Fig. 15-12** BTE (**A**), ITC (**B**), and CIC (**C**) hearing aids.

Unfortunately, many eye care practitioners tend to underestimate the usefulness of these aids. Additionally, most vision-impaired patients are unaware of the multitude of available assistive devices; consequently, the eye care practitioner should provide information and make recommendations to help patients select the best devices for a given task.

## REFERENCES

1. Anshel MH, Freedson P, Hamill J, et al: *Dictionary of the sport and exercise sciences*, Champaign, IL, 1991, Human Kinetics.
2. Arditi A: Typography, print legibility and low vision. In Cole RG, Rosenthal BP, editors: *Remediation and management of low vision*, St. Louis, 1996, Mosby, pp 237-48.
3. Bailey I, Clear R, Berman S: Size as a determinant of reading speed, *J Illum Engin Soc* 22:102-17, 1993.
4. Bailey I, Kelty K, Pittler G, et al: Typoscopes and yellow filters for cataract patients, *Low Vision Abstr* 4:2-6, 1978.
5. Campbell VA, Crews JE, Moriarty DG, et al: Surveillance for the sensory impairment, activity limitations and health-related quality of life among older adults—United States. 1993-1997, *MMWR* 48:131-56, 1999.
6. Carter K: Assessment of lighting. In Randall J, editor: *Understanding low vision*, New York, 1983, American Foundation for the Blind, pp 403-14.
7. Cockrell JR, Folstein MF: Mini Mental State Examination (MMSE), *Psychopharmacology* 24: 689-92, 1988.
8. Cohen JM, Rosenthal BP: An evaluation of an incandescent neodymium light source on near point performance of a low vision population, *J Vision Rehab* 2:15-21, 1988.
9. Cook AM, Hussey S: *Assistive technologies: principles and practice*, Mosby, 2002, Philadelphia.
10. De Fabio RP, Paul S, Emasithi A, et al: Evaluating the eye-body coordination during unrestrained functional activity in older persons, *J Gertontol A Biol Sci Med Sci* 56:571-4, 2001.
11. Eldred KB: Optimal illumination for reading in patients with age-related maculopathy, *Optom Vis Sci* 69:46-50, 1992.
12. Eperjesi F, Fowler CW, Evans B: Do tinted lenses or filters improve visual performance in low vision? A review of the literature, *Ophthalmic Physiol Optics* 22:68-78, 2002.
13. *Ergonomic guidelines for arranging a computer workstation: 10 steps for users*, CUErgo, Cornell University Department of Design and Environmental Analysis, http://ergo.human.cornell.edu/ergoguide.html, accessed May 2001.
14. Guyton AC: *Human physiology and mechanisms of disease*, Philadelphia, 1982, W.B. Saunders.
15. Harrell RL, Strass F: Approaches to assertive behavior and communication skills in blind and visually impaired persons, *J Vis Imp Blind* 80: 794-8, 1986.
16. Hersen M, Kabacoff RI, Van Hasselt VB, et al: Assertiveness, depression and social support in older visually impaired adults, *J Vis Imp Blind* 89:524-30, 1995.
17. Holmes A: Sensory aids: hearing assistive listening aids and signaling devices for the hearing impaired. In DeRuyter O, editor: *Clinicians guide to assistive technology*, St. Louis, 2002, Mosby, pp 199-206.
18. Julian WG: The use of light to improve the visual performance of people with low vision, *Proceedings of the 20th Session of the CIE*, D116:1-4, 1983.
19. Leat S, North RV, Bryson H: Do long wavelength pass filters improve low vision performance? *Ophthalmol Physiol Opt* 10:219-24, 1990.
20. Lund R, Watson GR: *The CCTV book: habilitation and rehabilitation with closed circuit television systems*, Froland, Norway, 1997, Synsforum Ang.
21. Musick J: Clinical strategies for the visually impaired computer user. In Cole R, Rosenthal B, editors: *Remediation and management of low vision*, St. Louis, 1996, Mosby, pp 219-20.
22. Prentice CF: *The typoscope*, Philadelphia, 1897, Keystone.
23. Rea MS, Ouellette MJ: Relative visual performance: a basis for application, *Lighting Research & Technology* 23:135-44, 1991.
24. Sloan LL, Habel A, Feiock K: High illumination as an auxiliary reading aid in diseases of the macula, *Am J Ophthalmol* 76:745, 1973.
25. Tinker MA: Effect of sloped text upon the readability of print, *Am J Optom Arch Am Acad Optom* 33:189-95, 1956.
26. Vanderheiden GC: Service delivery mechanisms in rehabilitation technology, *Am J Occup Ther* 41:703-10, 1987.
27. Van Zandt PL, Van Zandt SL, Wang A: The role of support groups in adjusting to visual impairment in old age, *J Vis Imp Blind* 88:244-52, 1994.
28. Watson GR, De l'Aune WR, Stelmack J, et al: A national survey of veterans' use of low vision devices, *Optom Vis Sci* 74:249-59, 1997.

## SUGGESTED READINGS

Gormezano S, Stelmack J: Efficient, effective clinical protocols for the prescription of selective absorption filters. In Stuen A, Arditi A, Horowitz MA et al, editors: *Vision '99: vision rehabilitation: assessment, intervention and outcomes*, New York, 1999, Swets & Zeitlinger, pp 206-7.

Leguire LE, Suh S: Effect of light filters on contrast sensitivity function in normal and retinal degeneration subjects, *Ophthalmol Physiol Optom* 13:124-8, 1993.

National Institute for Occupational Safety and Health: *Musculoskeletal disorders and workplace factors: a critical review of epidemiological evidence for work-related musculoskeletal disorders of the neck, upper extremity and low back*, Cincinnati, 1997, NIOSH.

North Carolina State University: *Principles of universal design*, Raleigh, NC, 2001, The Center for Universal Design.

Such GV, Whittaker SG: Computer assistive technology for the low vision patient. In Brilliant R, editor: *Essentials of low vision practice*, Boston, 1999, Butterworth-Heinemann, p 298.

Tupper B, Miller D, Miller R: The effect of a 550 nm cut off filter on the vision of cataract patients, *Ann Ophthalmol* 17:67-72, 1985.

Van den Berg TJTP: Red glasses and visual function in retinitis pigmentosa, *Doc Ophthalmol* 73:255-74, 1990.

Watson GR, Ramsey V, De l'Aune WR, et al: Effect of ergonomic enhancement on reading with low vision, *J Vis Impair Blind* 98:228-40, 2004.

Zigman S: Vision enhancement using a short wavelength light-absorbing filter, *Optom Vis Sci* 67:100-4, 1990.

Zigman S: Light filters to improve vision, *Optom Vis Sci* 69:325-8, 1992.

# CHAPTER 16

# Older Drivers

MELVIN D. SHIPP

A lthough they are ubiquitous today, roughly 100 years ago no one had an automobile in the United States. Now almost everyone aged 16 years and older has a driver license and access to an automobile. This sea change in personal transportation has resulted in both intended and unintended consequences.

As a society, we are much more mobile and independent but are more likely to die in a traffic crash than any other accidental cause of death (e.g., airplane crash, drowning, gunshot). Previously, unintentional fatalities and injuries were viewed as either accidental (random, unpredictable, and unavoidable occurrences) or the result of individual carelessness. The current view is that injuries arise from multiple causes, most of which are amenable to intervention through public policy.[33] Consistent with this view, the term crash will be used in lieu of accident because the latter term suggests the absence of viable control measures.

Death from unintentional injuries is among the top 10 causes of death in America. Importantly, motor vehicle crashes are the leading cause of unintentional injury deaths in the United States.

## U.S. TRAFFIC CRASH TRENDS

Annual traffic fatality rates per 100,000 population rose rapidly from 1961 to 1966, dipped in the early 1970s, and exhibited minor increases through 1973. In 1974 these rates dropped, presumably because of the combined effect of the fuel crisis and the adoption of a national 55-mph speed limit.

In general, from the mid-1970s through the early 1980s, annual traffic fatality rates per 100,000 population remained relatively stable. Since the late 1980s, annual traffic fatality rates have declined. This decline has been attributed to changes in automobile design, highway design, seat belt laws, development of air bags, improvement in rescue operations and medical practice, and other developments.* However, the effect is variable with age. Although most driver age groups have experienced a decline in crash fatality rates, the rate for older drivers has not declined as rapidly as other age cohorts.

In spite of recent declines, traffic-related injuries and fatalities represent a continuing public health concern. Older drivers are the most rapidly growing segment of the driving population in the United States, and, although they drive fewer miles, older drivers have the highest rate of crashes per mile driven.[9,17,245]

Older adults are at higher risk for reduced vision function because of normal aging and age-related conditions, which may be associated with higher risk for crash involvement. The extent to which licensure policies and practices accurately identify and remove visually

---

*References 69, 108, 228, 248, 251, 259.

at-risk older drivers from U.S. roadways has not been fully investigated. Because inappropriate licensure policies may inappropriately deny driving privileges—particularly for older individuals—pursuing valid and uniform policies and practice is important.

## FINANCIAL IMPACT

Although the annual rate of fatal motor vehicle crashes in the United States is declining, motor vehicle crashes remain significant at the individual and societal level. In 1990 the economic impact of motor-vehicle crashes was roughly 2.5% of America's gross national product: an estimated $137.5 billion.[22] These cost estimates include both direct (medical care, property damage, etc.) and indirect (loss of income, lost productivity, etc.) costs. Costs related to traffic fatalities were estimated as $702,000 per event, nearly 80% of which is related to lost workplace and household productivity.[22] The costs of nonfatal injuries were estimated at $589,000 per event. Almost 30% of the first-year medical costs of persons hospitalized for traffic-related injuries were paid for by government sources such as Medicaid and Medicare.[82] These costs continue to increase in conjunction with other national economic indicators.

Traffic crashes result in both health and economic consequences. Health consequences include injury, disability, and death. Economic consequences include the direct and indirect costs associated with (1) providing treatment, (2) the loss of productivity and earnings, and (3) the loss of property. Often motor vehicle crashes produce multiple injuries, which generate even higher social costs. Costs vary with the intensity and duration of medical treatment, survival, and the duration of work-related disability.[83,191,260] Treatment costs include goods and services expended in emergency services, hospitalization and outpatient care, drugs, medical supplies and equipment, and rehabilitative services.

The loss of productivity and loss of earnings represent indirect costs.[191,260] For older victims, the indirect costs to society for lost years of life and productivity are low because of retirement from work and a shortened life expectancy, so the direct costs for treatment for older crash victims predominate.[48]

In 1980 the present-value direct and indirect costs associated with motor vehicle injuries ($14.4 billion) was second only to cancer ($23.1 billion).[83,191] Coronary heart disease and stroke, although preceding unintentional injuries as leading causes of death, trail in economic importance at $13.7 billion and $6.5 billion, respectively. Clearly the health and economic consequences of traffic crashes are not trivial. Raffle[182] reported that if the fatalities and casualties from crashes in the United Kingdom were caused by an infectious disease, there would be an outcry of concern from the public and press.

In a 3-year study of the use of hospital and intensive care unit resources in treating injured older adults in North Carolina trauma centers, 21,214 cases were reviewed.[39] After controlling for severity of injury, the researchers found that older adults had longer mean lengths of stay than younger adults or children. Although 22% of older adult injuries were transportation related, these injuries generated 38% of hospital charges ($14 million). The authors concluded that a 10% reduction in both transportation and fall-related injuries among older adults could save $3.5 million over 3 years in North Carolina.

During calendar year 1992, the Centers for Disease Control and Prevention (CDC) estimated there were 89.8 million visits to hospital emergency departments (EDs) in the United States. Of this total, 34.0 million (37.8%) were injury related: an average of 13.5 injury-related ED visits per 100 persons.[29] Accidental falls and motor vehicle crashes accounted for 41% of these ED visits. The total lifetime costs of losses of motor vehicle crashes exceed costs associated with falls, despite of the higher incidence of falls.

The CDC estimated that more than $9.2 billion was spent on injury-related ED visits in 1992. A study by the Federal Highway Administration (FHA) and the National Highway Traffic Safety Administration (NHTSA) reported that in 1990 the medical costs (e.g., medical, emergency services, rehabilitation) resulting from motor vehicle crashes was $13.9 billion.[22] In 1985 motor vehicle injuries accounted for 9% of total injuries but 31% of total economic costs.[191] These findings suggest that unintentional injuries are associated with significant morbidity and economic costs.

## DEMOGRAPHICS AND TRAFFIC SAFETY

Age, sex, race, and socioeconomic status may be important factors in the consequences of traffic crash injuries. The same severity crash is more likely to be fatal to an older driver than to a younger driver.[53,146] Older adults are more frail and therefore more susceptible to life-threatening injuries and severe outcomes subsequent to trauma. For both sexes, the fatality risk at age 70 years is roughly three times that at age 20 years.

In an analysis of U.S. Department of Transportation statistics from 1980 and 1989, Barr[17] observed that although total driver fatalities fell by 8.4%, among drivers 65 years and older fatalities increased 43%. Although older adults comprise roughly 12% of the U.S. population, they disproportionately accounted for 28% of injury-related fatalities.[48] Using data from the Fatal Accident Reporting System (FARS), for 1975 to 1983, Evans[54] observed that fatality risks were roughly 25% higher for females than for males in the 15- to 45-year cohort, whereas for younger and older age cohorts, males were more at risk.

A study of an older inner-city population suggests possible differences in traffic injury-related morbidity and mortality rates by race and socioeconomic status (SES), with minority individuals of lower SES having lower traffic-related mortality and morbidity rates.[72] This difference may be associated with motor vehicle ownership. Neither regression nor time series models using specific economic indicators (e.g., rates of employment, unemployment and non-labor forces) provide improved forecasting models for motor vehicle fatalities, suicides, and homicides.[187]

Age-specific traffic fatality rates per 100,000 licensed drivers have consistently remained highest for the youngest and oldest drivers.[53,251] In general, older drivers appear more hazardous than their younger counterparts; the crash rate (per licensed driver) per mile driven is lowest for drivers in their late 20s and highest in drivers older than 60 years.[9,30,68,192,251]

Driver performance is often stereotyped on the basis of age; younger drivers are perceived as having high-risk behaviors and older drivers as having diminished capacity.[157,158] Older drivers are in fact a heterogeneous group. Individual variations in information processing efficiency, depth judgment, decision-making ability, and speed of reaction are extreme.[38]

Rigdon[192] reports that older adults are more apt to be involved in fatal crashes because of failure to yield the right of way, not obeying traffic signs or officers, and inattentiveness. Traffic crashes involving older drivers are more likely to be multivehicle collisions that result in more serious injuries than those involving younger drivers.[188] In addition to being more at risk while driving, older drivers are more likely to be responsible for the crashes in which they are involved.[38]

A 1986 study of 8210 drivers aged 36 to 50 years old and 5853 drivers older than 55 year old in British Columbia reported that although older drivers had fewer crashes, their safety record relative to kilometers driven was poorer and they were more often at fault in a multi-vehicle crash.[38] Weather was a significant factor differentiating 36- to 50-year-old drivers from drivers aged 65 years and older; middle-age drivers have more weather-related crashes than drivers aged 65 years and older. The authors attributed this difference to the tendency of older drivers to avoid difficult driving situations. The relative risk of crash responsibility increased dramatically for drivers older than 65 years.

Driving is a complex dynamic activity, requiring rapid and continuous integration of cognitive, sensory, and motor skills.[37,127,232] Age-related decrements in driving competency are likely to have important implications for traffic safety.[43] Older drivers may possibly make more errors in perception, judgment, decision making, and reacting.

According to Marottoli,[139] most older drivers are aware of their diminished capacity and adjust their driving habits accordingly by driving fewer miles and shorter distances, driving during optimal lighting and weather conditions, and driving on familiar roads. In spite of evidence that some visually impaired drivers voluntarily restrict their driving activities, traffic fatality trends for older drivers suggest that self-imposed restrictions or compensations for diminished functional ability are inadequate.[14] Effective means of preventing motor vehicle crashes represent an opportunity to reduce untimely deaths, disability, and health care costs associated with unintentional injury. If genuine opportunities exist to control this age-specific rise in traffic fatalities, these options should be implemented.

## Personal Demographics and Experience

The automobile is the dominant mode of travel for older Americans. The proportion of older individuals with driver licenses is increasing, particularly among women.[57,227] Women tend to outlive their husbands. Many older women rely on their husbands to drive.[227] When their husbands die, some widows obtain a license for the first time or drive more regularly than they did when their husbands were alive.

A study of the impact of age, sex, and race on North Carolina motor vehicle crashes during even-numbered years (1974 to 1988) reported that although the proportion of older drivers increased during the study period, their crash rates per licensed driver were lower than other age cohorts.[214] The crash rates for older drivers (55 years or older) declined more than those of younger drivers in terms of crashes per driver and crashes per estimated miles traveled. A factor associated with this decline in crash rate for older drivers was a decrease in weekend and nighttime driving. The authors concluded that older drivers limit their driving to situations they feel capable of handling, and only better older drivers expose themselves to higher risk driving situations. Unlike younger drivers, older drivers were less likely to combine their driving with alcohol use, speeding, and other behaviors known to increase crash risk. The greatest declines were for drivers 65 years and older, particularly in minority populations. Men had a higher crash rate per miles driven than women, but this difference declined with increasing age. Crash-related variables evaluated in this study included information on the driver (e.g., age, sex, level of injury, seat belt use, culpability), the vehicle (e.g., vehicle type, damage severity), and crash characteristics (e.g., location, time of day, day of the week, crash type, number of vehicles involved). This study supports the notion that personal demographic variables may have a differential effect on crash risk and crash involvement.

A 1995 study replicated a 1990 investigation of variations in driving errors and violations between male and female drivers. In the initial study, young drivers reported that they committed more dangerous errors and dangerous violations than older drivers.[23,185] Also, although driving frequency did not differ, male drivers admitted to more dangerous violations and crash involvement than female drivers. The initial and subsequent study corresponded. According to Blockley and Hartley,[23] this supported the premise that driving errors stem from different psychological mechanisms with differences in sex, socioeconomic status (SES), and culture. Blockley and Hartley concluded that their observed age and sex differences in violation-prone driver behavior might imply the need for targeted remediation strategies.

Hakamies-Blomqvist[78] observed in a study of 2315 fatal crashes in Finland (from 1984 to 1990) that both sexes manifested age-related changes in accident characteristics (e.g., increasing frequency with aging), but that female drivers were affected at an earlier age and to a higher degree. The female drivers in this study were less experienced than male drivers. The authors concluded that although the proportion of older Finnish female drivers will grow, future cohorts of female drivers will be more experienced and more skilled because of changing societal norms. This increase in female drivers could result in improved traffic safety.

A gender-related cohort effect may therefore currently exist. Older women having less driving experience than either older male drivers or their younger female counterparts because of societal norms and role expectations may drive less and have fewer crashes. Alternatively, older female drivers may be more risk averse, less likely to drive in hazardous conditions, and more compliant than other age-sex driver cohorts. Spousal survival rates for women are higher than those for men. Surviving female spouses may be more apt to obtain alternate transportation or stay at home than their male counterparts. Clearly, gender variations among licensing jurisdictions could mask or confound the effect of vision-related licensing policies.

A study of 350 older California drivers observed that older drivers tended to self-restrict more than younger drivers, primarily by avoiding driving at night, sunrise, and sunset.[86] However, the reported level of self-restriction was highly variable regarding vision function loss and age. Vision test scores and age accounted for less than 10% of the variation in the investigated types of self-restriction (e.g., night driving frequency, avoidance of rain or fog, avoidance of sunrise or sunset, avoidance of driving alone, avoidance of left turns, and avoidance of heavy traffic). This suggests that the presence of other influential variables was not accounted for in this study.

A population-based study of 629 community-dwelling older drivers reported a relation between vision-related driving self-restriction and poorer performance on nonstandard measures of acuity—namely, depth perception and spatial vision function.[249] Importantly, poor visual attention, an important risk factor for crashes, was not recognized by at-risk drivers.

## American Drivers

U.S. life expectancy is expected to increase, and older adults will likely represent an ever-increasing percentage of the population.[8] In concert with the "graying of America," older drivers are increasing in number.[17,69] By the year 2020, the number of older drivers is expected to increase by almost 50%.[154]

The average American driver is becoming older. From 1979 to 1989, drivers aged 70 years and older increased by 56.5% while the number of drivers aged 19 years of age and younger decreased by 18.5%. In 1990, 9.8 million American drivers were aged 19 years or younger, and 13.5 million were aged 70 years and older.[234] Roughly 88% of older Americans rely on private automobiles for their transportation needs.[94] Most older persons live in very-low-density communities where alternative transportation to the privately owned automobile is rare.[196] Most older adults drive their own cars, and almost 100% will have driven by the turn of the century.[197]

A 10-year prospective study of community-dwelling older drivers observed that a substantial proportion continue to rely on their automobiles and drive in their ninth decade of life.[102] The anticipated increase in the average age of older drivers may result in further increases in age-specific crash and fatality rates.

### Aging and Driving

The proportion of older drivers is likely to increase, and these drivers will have an accompanying increased likelihood of vision impairments and risk for vision-related crashes. These projections underscore the importance of effective policies for accurately identifying high-risk drivers and enhancing traffic safety.

The normal aging process is accompanied by declining vision performance and function.* Persons older than 65 years are at higher risk for decreased vision performance.[26,122,137,142,250] Often, individuals with age-related vision impairments are only slightly aware of moderate to severe changes in their ability to see, primarily because these vision losses progress very slowly.

### Aging and Traffic Crashes

The U.S. Department of Transportation estimates that approximately 50% of all motor vehicle crashes are related to poor vision.[237] Yet, despite the assumed importance of vision in driving, the relation between vision performance and crash risk—particularly among older adults—has not been empirically established.[165,245] On the other hand, some research findings suggest the potential for identifying drivers at risk for vision-related crashes.[104,256]

## VISION AND AGING

As a group, older drivers have a higher incidence and prevalence of functionally impaired vision because of age-related ocular conditions and diseases than do younger drivers. These visual impairments are likely associated with the overrepresentation of older drivers in motor vehicle crashes per mile driven.

Until relatively recently, ocular disease-free older adults—those free from identifiable eye disease—were commonly thought to also be free from functional vision problems. This view has changed.[165] Several discrete anatomical and physiological changes are associated with aging in the human eye and a concurrent loss of vision function.†

A fine line exists between normal and a diseased state. Differentiating between declining

---

*References 120, 151, 155, 165, 217-219, 228, 245.
†References 9, 32, 105, 108, 119, 165, 217-219, 254.

visual performance characteristic of normal aging and pathological age-related disease is challenging for clinicians and scientists.[70] Some minor, age-related ocular changes are considered normal changes, but in more advanced stages they are classified as diseased.[165] These changes are invariably accompanied by changes in visual performance manifested as a loss of central or peripheral vision. As a result of normal aging processes within the eye, older persons (aged 65 years and older) tend to have poorer visual acuity, reduced night vision, and a higher prevalence of sight-compromising eye diseases (see Chapter 2 for a discussion of normal age-related vision changes).[155,165,213,217-219]

Elliott et al[52] report that a decline in visual acuity in normal, healthy eyes may begin at approximately age 30 years, much earlier than the age of 50 years cited in commonly used references.[173,247] They also observed that normal visual acuity in healthy eyes is much better than 20/20 (6/6), and in young patients is at least 20/10 (6/3) under optimal testing conditions. Nevertheless, visual acuity function varies significantly with age. Survey data from the U.S. Department of Health Education and Welfare estimated that in 1977, whereas 1.5% of the 18- to 24-year age group had visual acuity worse than 20/20, for the 65- to 74-year age group, 68.0% would have visual acuities worse than 20/20.[10]

An investigation of the impact of aging on visual search performance with 24 young adults (mean age, 21.5 years) and 24 older adults (mean age, 66.17 years) found a slowing of visual processing speed with age.[135] The researchers concluded that older adults experience a declining efficiency in accumulating, processing, and responding to selective attention tasks. Population-based epidemiological studies have reported declines in visual acuity with aging, even in the absence of ocular disease. The visual acuity declines were attributed to increased light scattering by ocular media, miotic pupils, decreased retinal illumination, and decreased neural function.* These changes were associated with self-reported visual problems of older drivers.[126]

The prevalence of sight-threatening eye conditions among persons aged 65 to 74 years exceeds 85%.[107] Investigators estimate that approximately 10% of persons older than 65 years have undetected eye disease or visual impairment and that the prevalence of undetected eye disease increases with age.[19,142] In a study of 1000 Danish citizens, Vinding[240] found the following increases in prevalence of age related maculopathy (ARM): 2.3% for ages 60 to 64 years, 5.9% for ages 65 to 69 years, 12.1% for ages 70 to 74 years, and 27.3% for ages 75 to 80 years. These increases were comparable for men and women.

The prevalence of vision impairment in the United States is expected to increase in coming decades. Crews[42] has projected that the number of older persons experiencing vision impairments will more than double within the next 30 years. These persons will also experience other age- and disease-related changes.[193] These impairments—losses or abnormalities of psychological, physiological, or anatomical structure or function at the organ level—may result in disabilities or handicaps that affect mobility and quality of life for older persons.[257]

Importantly, individuals with either normal age-related vision changes or progressive vision losses caused by sight-threatening diseases and conditions are only slightly aware of moderate to severe changes in their ability to see. The prevalence of both cataracts and ARM increase as a function of age. In fact, no personal demographic variable is more strongly associated with these conditions than age.[114,115,117,217-219] Both conditions involve degenerative changes that are considered part of the normal aging process. Although ARM specifically affects central vision, cataracts may impair both central and peripheral vision. A more detailed discussion of these conditions follows.

### Crystalline Lens Changes

The most common age-related changes in the human eye occur in the crystalline lens. With age, this structure becomes more dense and loses its elasticity. Functionally, at approximately age 40 years, these changes result in a condition known as presbyopia—a decrease in the ability of the eye to accommodate or change focus. This normal aging change is more noticeable when performing near tasks. Regarding driving, a reduction in accommodative function could interfere with visualizing an instrument

---

*References 92, 104, 116, 123, 226, 238, 250, 261.

panel or impede the ability to quickly change focus from distance objects to the instrument panel, or vice versa.

A more insidious and profound age-related change in the crystalline lens is that it becomes less transparent, most notably in persons aged 60 years and older. This loss of transparency can result in a significant loss in visual function (loss of visual acuity, altered color vision, altered contrast sensitivity). Typically, when this loss of transparency is accompanied by a loss of visual acuity, the opacified lens is labeled as a cataract.[9,218] Studies have shown that these changes can be directly related to traffic crash involvement.[169]

The prevalence of cataracts increases rapidly after age 60 to 65 years.[2,106,141,221,222] Cataracts are found more frequently among black Americans, persons with diabetes, rural dwellers, and persons with high exposure to ultraviolet B light and are inversely related to the number of years spent in school.[87,93,179,258] Cataract treatment involves the surgical removal of the opaque lens and replacement with a compensatory corrective lens—spectacle, contact, or intraocular lens.

In a prospective study of 293 older patients, cataract surgery with intraocular lens implantation was associated with improved visual acuity, mental status scores, manual performance, and subjective function. These improvements were maintained at 1-year follow-up.[7] A similar study of 1021 patients with cataracts found improved quality of life function—nighttime driving, daytime driving, community activities, mental health, and life satisfaction—with cataract surgery and treatment of other chronic ocular disorders, including refractive services.[26] Substantial differences in anisometropia accompany the aging process and gender is an important marker for changes in refractive error.[77]

A case-control study of patients undergoing cataract surgery and those without cataracts reported that improvements in vision performance as measured by visual acuity, contrast sensitivity, and disability glare were independently linked to improvements in activities of daily living scales.[147] These findings suggest a concordance between improved vision performance and quality of life among patients undergoing cataract surgery. In a prospective study of 174 patients undergoing cataract surgery with intraocular lens implantation, the investigators observed a positive impact on traffic safety for the subjects, with reduced crash involvement compared with 103 control (no surgery) patients.[167]

A random sample of Medicare beneficiaries suggests that cataract complication rates for retinal detachment and endophthalmitis have remained low or have improved.[101] However, evidence suggests that the rigor of the research methods in these studies varies considerably, and the quality of outcome studies on the safety and effectiveness of contemporary cataract surgery needs to be improved.[180]

**Retinal Changes**

A common age-related retinal change involves the macula. The macula is the region of the retina responsible for central vision. It has the highest concentration of cones—the photoreceptors responsible for detailed color vision. Normal aging may result in mild histological changes in the macula, with or without clinical signs or symptoms. When these changes produce clinically significant reductions in visual performance, they are diagnostically classified as ARM (age-related maculopathy).[9,96,217]

Functionally, patients with advanced ARM experience visual distortions, altered color perception, and a profound loss of central vision. A study comparing crash involvement of 20 patients with central vision impairment caused by Stargardt disease or cone-rod dystrophy with 29 control subjects found a higher rate (per licensed driver) of nighttime crashes for the impaired drivers.[215]

ARM is a leading cause of vision loss in the United States, England, and other industrialized countries.[58,220,222] The prevalence of ARM increases with age, with more than a quarter of individuals older than 75 years experiencing this condition.[123,152] ARM is a disease of unknown etiology, but studies suggest that prolonged exposure to high levels of blue and visible light may be important in its occurrence.[220,222] A study of 4926 persons aged 43 to 83 years residing in Beaver Dam, Wisconsin, found that exposure to sunlight was associated with ARM frequency.[44]

Changes in the function of the peripheral retina are also associated with aging. With normal aging sensitivity declines throughout the visual field.[27] These functional changes do not necessarily result from morphological changes. Notably, one case study suggests that in the absence of a significant pathological condition, the alignment of photoreceptors does not deteriorate with aging.[198]

A comparative study of 15 younger subjects (22.9 ± 1.3 years) and 13 older subjects (66.6 ± 4.5 years), found a significant age-related deterioration in visual sensitivity to motion, which was more pronounced in central than peripheral vision.[254] The simulated restriction of young (24 to 35 years old) drivers' binocular visual fields resulted in impaired identification of road signs, prolonged reaction time, and inaccurate speed estimation.[256]

A survey of 126 patients with ARM observed that the loss of vision function associated with this condition was directly related to a reduction or avoidance of driving under certain environmental conditions.[46] These situations included driving when visibility was reduced (e.g., rain, nighttime) or in complex traffic conditions (e.g., highway, rush-hour traffic).

## Glaucoma

Glaucoma, one of the nation's leading causes of preventable blindness, is manifested by a gradual, and frequently asymptomatic, loss of peripheral or side vision.[104] According to the National Society to Prevent Blindness, more than 2 million Americans have glaucoma and more than half are unaware of it.

Because it manifests itself with few or no symptoms, glaucoma usually remains undetected until vision is lost.[155] Groups at high risk for glaucoma include black Americans older than 40 years, those with a family history of glaucoma, and all individuals older than 60 years.[152] Given the increasing prevalence of glaucoma with advancing age, several authors stress the importance of assessing peripheral vision in older drivers.*

## Diabetic Retinopathy

Diabetes is a relatively common systemic condition that results in sight-threatening complications: cataracts, glaucoma, and retinopathy. Over time, diabetes produces characteristic changes in ocular tissues independent of the level of therapeutic control. Although the ocular

manifestations may progress more rapidly and more severely than for persons without diabetes, changes in visual performance may not be fully appreciated. Laser treatment (e.g., panretinal photocoagulation) may be used to arrest the progression of diabetic retinopathy. Unfortunately, panretinal photocoagulation, the mainstay treatment for retinal disease related to diabetes, has been associated with failure to pass visual field tests for driver license renewal.[95]

## Retinitis Pigmentosa

Retinitis pigmentosa (RP) is a group of inherited diseases characterized by night blindness and constricted peripheral vision.[109] Despite the progressive loss of peripheral vision, 25% of patients with RP maintain good central visual acuity throughout life. However, by age 50 years, at least half of patients with RP experience some loss of central vision in addition to peripheral vision loss. A study comparing crash data on 21 drivers with RP and 31 normally sighted control subjects found that the degree of visual field loss of drivers with RP was a significant predictor of crash involvement.[216]

## Ocular Melanoma

The loss of an eye in the treatment of cancer (malignant choroidal melanoma) results in a reduction of peripheral vision on the affected side. Edwards and Schachat[50] observed that 7 of 56 patients who had lost an eye from this condition voluntarily discontinued driving within a 15-year period because of a subjective decrease in visual function. The remaining patients continued to drive with extra side-view or wide-angle rear view mirrors.

## VISION FUNCTION AND CRASHES

Vision is estimated to account for 90% of the information drivers use when operating a vehicle.[9,205] To date, empirical evidence is lacking of a significant predictive relation between changes in vision function and automobile crashes.[203] Although suggestive, efforts to determine the role of vision in driving have not been useful in identifying at-risk older drivers.[9,13,137]

Although the association between reduced vision function and poor driving is strong for older persons, this does not infer a causal relation. Importantly, a variety of age-related factors may be more important in crashes.

---

*References 61, 104, 141, 219, 233, 245.

In a pioneering investigation involving more than 17,500 California drivers, Burg[28] found only weak correlations between aspects of vision function and driving performance. For persons older than 54 years, both dynamic and static visual acuity was weakly correlated with traffic crash rates; dynamic visual acuity was more strongly related to crashes. Burg also found weak relations between traffic crashes and other vision functions, specifically, the extent of the visual field and disability glare. Glare recovery time is significantly longer for older people, explaining at least in part their reported difficulty with night driving. For persons aged 54 years or less, no meaningful relations between visual function and crashes were found.

Currently, only static visual acuity is routinely assessed by standard vision screening for driver licensing. A small but consistent correlation exists between static acuity and accident involvement, particularly for older drivers.[45]

Early studies of visual field limitations (i.e., loss of peripheral vision) did not find consistent relations between this measure of vision performance and traffic crashes.[28,204] A limitation of early studies was the use of crude screening devices rather than more sophisticated clinical testing.[205] In a study involving the screening of 10,000 volunteers with clinical visual field testing, Johnson and Keltner[104] found a 13% incidence of binocular visual field loss for persons older than 65 years compared with 3.0% to 3.5% for persons aged 16 to 60 years. Importantly, more than half of the persons with a visual field loss in this study were unaware of any eye problems before testing. The investigators observed that drivers with severe binocular vision field loss had crash and conviction rates twice those of drivers with normal visual fields. Currently, only a small percentage of U.S. licensing jurisdictions requires testing of peripheral vision as a condition of licensure.

The useful field of view (UFOV), or attention window, is the size of the visual field in which useful information can be acquired in a single glance. Unlike standard binocular visual field testing, UFOV measures the effective field of view. UFOV combines assessments of peripheral vision and cognitive function and measures the visual field in terms of the ability to detect and identify visual stimuli. In other words, a person with a normal binocular visual field may have a restricted UFOV, a relatively common situation among older adults. In the most extreme cases of UFOV restriction, individuals are sensitive to distraction and are unable to divide their attention effectively between central and peripheral viewing tasks.[13]

A study by Ball et al[15] stressed the importance of the UFOV in driving safety. In their study of 294 drivers aged 55 years and older, they observed that the 126 subjects with a 40% or greater reduction in UFOV were six times more likely to *have* been involved in crashes than subjects with little or no UFOV reduction. Older adults experienced more difficulty than younger individuals with visual search, peripheral vision, and cluttered visual scenes, which the authors hypothesize to be related to UFOV.

A study by Wood and Troutbeck[256] investigated the effect of simulated visual impairment on the driving performance of 10 older subjects (60 to 74 years of age). Goggles were altered to simulate the visual effects of cataracts, visual field restriction, and monocularity (i.e., one eye). Driving performance was evaluated on a test track with no other vehicles, and visual performance was assessed with a clinical visual field testing device (Humphrey Field Analyzer), a visual acuity testing instrument (Pelli-Robson Chart), and the UFOV. Wood and Troutbeck reported that driving performance was significantly reduced, although the subjects met minimal vision standards for driver licensing. The investigators observed significant correlations between the driving performance and both the UFOV and the Pelli-Robson Chart.

Some investigators of driving performance and traffic safety have concluded that future research in vision and crashes should focus on higher-order vision-related functions: visual search, effective visual field, and divided attention among visual and other tasks.* Future studies may demonstrate whether these factors are better able to predict poor driving performance than contemporary vision screening or clinical tests.[205]

## NONVISION FUNCTION AND CRASHES

In addition to changes in vision function, a variety of health conditions specific to older adults may influence driving performance. An extensive literature suggests age-related declines

---

*References 9, 12, 15, 162, 166, 202.

in sensory, mental, and motor function; presbycusis (hearing loss); sleep apnea; depression; dementia; decreased strength; diminished dexterity; and sudden death behind the wheel as covariates in traffic violations and crashes.*

In addition to requiring a high degree of physical coordination and mental alertness, driving is a visually complex task. Typically, individuals experience a slow and steady decline in some perceptual, cognitive, and motor skills in their 40s.[144,150]

## Health Status

Among the noninstitutionalized older men and women in the Framingham Study cohort, stroke, depressive symptoms, hip fracture, knee osteoarthritis, and heart disease accounted for more physical disability than any other diseases.[73] Of these conditions, stroke was the leading cause of functional limitation.[59] A study of 283 community-living persons aged 72 years and older found that as the number of physical and sensory impairments increased, risk for motor vehicle crash involvement, moving violations, or being stopped by the police increased commensurately.[140]

Although older drivers with sensory and motor impairments may reduce their driving appropriately, those with cognitive impairment may not recognize their limitations.[188] A retrospective review of driving records of 249 outpatients in a dementia clinic in British Columbia reinforces the need to better identify high-risk drivers.[230] The traffic crash rate per licensed driver was 2.5 times higher for 165 patients with dementia relative to an age-, sex-, and residentially matched sample of randomly selected drivers within the province. However, a 2.2 times higher traffic crash rate was also observed for 84 patients without dementia relative to their matched control sample. Tuokko et al[230] observed that other neurological, medical, and psychiatric conditions were present in the drivers without dementia, which could have affected their driving performance. Crashes caused by older drivers may be caused by age-related dementing disease or the psychogenic

side effects of medications for chronic health conditions.[15,103,232] In a study of the impact of hearing loss on the function of older adults, Bess et al[21] observed that progressive hearing loss is a common chronic condition associated with progressive physical and psychosocial dysfunction. Yet a review of investigations and experimental studies by Booher[24] found little evidence to suggest that hearing-impaired individuals did not drive as safely as the general population. Booher allowed that further study was needed to establish minimal requirements for impaired individuals. The consequence of hearing loss in driving may not be important because according to investigators the ambient noise inside automobiles traveling in excess of 35 mph provides a masking similar to a very severe hearing loss.[227]

## Mental Health Status

Accurately estimating the proportion of older individuals with memory deficits or psychological impairment is difficult. Barakat and Mulinazzi[16] observe that only 2% to 3% of persons aged 65 years and older are institutionalized for psychiatric illness but suggest that the prevalence is closer to 10%.

In addition to compromises in memory, other Alzheimer disease (AD) symptoms include selective attention, divided attention, hearing impairment, diminished sustained attention and comprehension, and visual dysfunction.[62,171,231] In some AD cases, visual impairment is the initial or dominant manifestation, although not typically a reduction in visual acuity.

Studies have reported that patients with AD were generally inferior to control subjects in color perception, contrast sensitivity (low-frequency stimulus), stereoacuity (depth perception), perceptual organization, face and object recognition, and spatial reasoning.[43,200,203] A study of 77 subjects with AD and 111 healthy control subjects observed that visual dysfunction was a common sign of AD.[149] A related study of 72 subjects with AD found that fundamental visual processing abilities such as contrast sensitivity were related to cognitive dysfunction in object recognition.[81,97]

## Socioeconomic Status and Behavioral Factors

Driving errors resulting in traffic crashes do not occur at random.[175] Risk factors for crash

---

*References 5, 16, 20, 32, 36, 40, 41, 49, 60, 62, 63, 81, 85, 107, 110, 121, 126, 127, 131, 134, 136, 139, 159, 160, 164, 168, 171, 181, 183, 184, 188, 189, 201, 208, 209, 232, 241-244, 252.

involvement also include social and behavioral factors (e.g., elevated blood alcohol level, not wearing seat belts, driving without a driver license), associations that are not unique to the United States.[212]

A study assessing the ability to predict motor vehicle fatalities in the United States or within various subpopulations found that information about employment status did not improve forecasting.[187] The logic of this study was that with higher economic activity, the level of motor vehicle travel would be higher, as would the risk of fatal crash involvement. The authors were unable to improve on prediction estimations based simply on prior crash fatalities and concluded that other economic variables (e.g., disposable personal income) might be more useful in making such predictions.

A study of population traffic fatality rates within the 48 contiguous states (1979 through 1981) reported that death was inversely related with per capita income.[11] Baker et al[11] observed that a variety of factors might underlie the strong inverse correlation between traffic death rates and population density or income. Per capita income was higher in metropolitan areas. According to Baker et al, the correlation between traffic fatality rates and income may have been partly attributable to an interaction with population density, which was not controlled for in this study. The author observed that seat belt use varied dramatically with median property value—higher income was associated with higher rates of seat belt use. Very old vehicles, more common in rural areas, were less likely to have seat belts. Seat belt use was considered a significant causal factor in the inverse relation between the traffic death rate and income.

In a Swedish study of 396 multiple-vehicle and 201 single-vehicle fatal passenger crash fatalities from 1980 through 1989, single-vehicle victims were more often less restrained, younger, inebriated men.[161] In a survey of 1800 southern California motorists, Hemenway and Solnick[84] reported that southern California drivers with more than a high school education were more likely to both speed and be involved in a crash. Holding other factors constant (age, sex, and miles driven), Hemenway and Solnick observed that those who attended college were more likely to have been involved in a crash during the prior year. By contrast, other studies have found that less well-educated individuals have more accidents.[84]

Motor vehicle crashes are the largest single cause of death from unintentional injuries in most developing countries.[212] Crash fatality rates for men are up to five times higher in those countries. In a longitudinal analysis of male and female drivers (1975 to 1990), Evans[55] observed that beyond the age of 65 years, U.S. car-driver fatalities for men increased dramatically, whereas the rates for women did not. The higher representation of men in these studies may represent a sex-based difference in traffic policy compliance. A state-level survey by Hemenway and Solnick[84] determined that male respondents were more likely than female respondents to engage in high-risk driving behaviors—speeding, running red lights, and drinking and driving—and to be involved in crashes; however, after controlling for mileage, no significant difference in crash involvement was found.

## NONDRIVER CRASH-RELATED FACTORS
### Environmental Conditions, Traffic Conditions, and Legal Issues

Within the United States an increasing percentage of older persons live in suburban and rural areas, whereas younger persons tend to reside in metropolitan areas.[227] This difference in residence affects the mobility options available to older and younger Americans.

Public transportation accounts for a small amount of suburban travel because the population density in the suburbs is generally too low to justify public transit systems. Aggregate data from a survey of transportation behavior between 1977 and 1983 found that persons older than 65 years used private automobiles more frequently, as drivers and as passengers, and public transit less frequently relative to younger age groups. Reliance on private automobiles by older individuals was highest in rural areas, where travel options were limited.

Fatal traffic crashes may result from factors not intrinsic to the driver. A Swedish study analyzing relations between traffic fatalities that involve older persons and the environment provides some important insights about nonvision factors and traffic safety.[211] Autopsy and police reports were used to investigate 379 fatal traffic crashes of older (60 years or older) drivers between 1977 and 1986. In most cases, the fatally injured older drivers were responsible for the collision. Most older-adult traffic fatalities involved vehicle-vehicle crashes and occurred on straight roads, during daylight hours, and at intersections (rather than nonintersections). Ice or snow was the major precrash factor for roughly one third of the crashes. The fatality rate of male drivers was twice that of female drivers. Only 4% of the fatally injured drivers were driving under the influence of alcohol.

The findings in the preceding study mirror those of an investigation of older driver multi-vehicle crashes in the United States from 1975 to 1986.[239] Most crashes in this investigation occurred during daylight, on dry roads, and without alcohol involvement. According to this study, 88% of the crashes occurred at intersections and were caused by driving error or traffic violation by an older adult driver. Icy or wet roads were an important injury risk factor for older drivers.

Investigators have reported an association between traffic fatalities and natural illumination. Variations in illumination and climate may differentially affect older and younger drivers, with older drivers being more susceptible than younger drivers to crashes in poor visibility conditions. Although older drivers tend to avoid difficult driving situations, inclement weather, such as icy or wet roads, is an important crash risk factor for older drivers.[38]

A Finnish study found that older drivers (65 years and older) were better able to compensate for difficult driving conditions than younger and middle-aged drivers (aged 26 to 40 years).[79] Relatively fewer crashes occurred at nighttime and under bad weather and poor road surface conditions. Older drivers had more crashes in sunny weather (76.4% compared with 34.9% for the comparison group). According to the authors the older drivers were less often in a hurry, alcohol intoxicated, or distracted by non-driving activities.

Since the 1980s a continuing tendency for reductions in traffic fatalities has occurred. These reductions have followed identifiable geographic trends; the north-central region having the largest reduction, followed by east and west coastal regions, with the smallest reduction in the southwest states.[30] Also, the reduction in fatalities was greater in urban areas than in rural areas, particularly for multivehicle crashes.

Variations in the mileage between and among states and differing driving patterns of older and younger drivers could possibly introduce variability in the magnitude of fatal collisions. Janke[99] observes that mileage alone may be an inaccurate measure of crash exposure. According to Janke, high-mileage drivers accumulate distances on highways or limited-access roads, whereas low-mileage drivers tend to be nonhighway drivers. High-mileage drivers are more often middle-aged drivers, whereas low-mileage drivers tend to be older drivers. After negotiating the entrance to highway traffic and becoming part of the one-way flow of traffic, highway driving is less risky than nonhighway driving. Hence nonhighway drivers frequently encounter more challenging driving conditions: intersections and multidirectional traffic flows.

Relative to road classification, the interstate system had the smallest reduction. Cerrelli[30] reported that the reduction in fatalities for passenger car occupants was not uniform. Intermediate and larger cars experienced a 29% reduction compared with a 2% reduction for compacts and smaller cars. The reduction in fatalities was very similar among the major vehicle classifications: passenger cars (–15%), motorcycles (–16%), and trucks (–16%). This trend has been attributed to improvements in automobile design, highway design, seat belt laws, air bags, and emergency treatment.*

Regarding car mass compared with size in two-car crashes, mass (i.e., weight per unit volume) is the dominant factor in fatality risk.[56] A reduction in car mass increases occupant fatality risk. According to Evans,[54] car mass and car model are functions of preferences influenced by driver age and sex. This age-related difference in automobile preference may influence the likelihood of a fatal outcome in equivalent crash situations.

In a retrospective Swedish study of 396 multiple-vehicle and 201 single-vehicle fatal passenger crash fatalities, single-vehicle victims were more often less-restrained, younger, inebriated men whose crashes occurred during the weekend between 9:00 PM and 6:00 AM on dry road surfaces.[161] In a similar retrospective study of older drivers, most vehicle occupants were killed in head-on vehicle-vehicle crashes, during daylight hours, and at intersections or

---

*References 69, 108, 228, 248, 251, 259.

on straight roads. In 31% of those crashes, ice or snow was a major precrash factor.[211] These studies suggest that non–driver-related factors may affect older drivers differently than younger drivers.

In a study of population traffic fatality rates in the 48 contiguous states, poor roads and high speeds were associated with higher death rates.[11] Poor roads were considered an important factor in higher traffic fatality rates in areas of low population density. This relation was not associated with age. Speed of travel was an important determinant of traffic crash fatalities, especially in rural areas. The use of seat belts was less common in rural areas and varied dramatically with median property value.

The practice of licensing drivers has changed little since the mid-1950s.[229] Performance standards are set by individual states but are fairly consistent. Licensing and relicensing practices are based primarily on age. However, age is not a good predictor of an older driver's functional ability.

States with the largest older populations seem to be the most lax regarding license renewal requirements.[192,236,259] This is likely related to political factors. Florida, the state with the largest proportion of older drivers, allows drivers to renew by mail for up to 6 years. Pennsylvania, with the third-highest percentage of older drivers, allows mail renewal unless drivers are reported to the relicensing board by their physicians as not meeting minimal physical or mental standards or are chosen for in-person renewal by lottery. Only eight states require knowledge testing for all renewal applicants.[229,236] The impact of this variation in policy and practice on traffic safety has not been fully investigated.[229]

### Traffic Fatalities and Natural Illumination

Most traffic fatalities occur at night. Researchers have determined that reduced visibility (i.e., low conspicuity) is an important contributor to some types of traffic crashes.[4,210] At dusk and dawn the eye is less sensitive to perceiving contrasts, and when driving at night the eyes never become fully dark adapted because of intermittent exposure to intense light sources (e.g., headlights of oncoming cars).[37]

An important research finding by Mortimer and Fell[151] was that the rate of crash involvement in darkness (per 100 million vehicle miles driven) for drivers aged 65 years or more was greater than for drivers aged 25 to 64 years. In 1991 the nighttime traffic fatality rate was 3.7 times that of the daytime rate: 4.4 per 100 million miles compared with 1.2 per 100 million miles.[154]

Using FARS data for an 11-year period (1980 to 1990), Owens et al[163] analyzed 104,235 crashes that occurred during morning and evening time periods—often called the "twilight zones." Most of the fatal crashes occurred in the evening (70.3%) and in clear atmospheric conditions (85.7%). They found 12.1% more fatalities during these time periods than would be predicted by chance alone. For the fatal crashes occurring during the darker portions of these periods no significant relation to time of day (e.g., rush hour, non–rush hour), the day of the week, or alcohol consumption by the driver was found. Under conditions of reduced illumination with good atmospheric conditions, the proportion of fatal crashes was 9.8% greater than expected by chance alone; under degraded atmospheric conditions this proportion was 25.6% greater than chance.

Researchers have reported that poor visibility from reduced illumination and poor atmospheric conditions was a major factor in fatal crashes with less-conspicuous hazards (e.g., pedestrians, joggers, and bicyclists). However, this does not appear to play a major role in the incidence of other classes of fatal crashes (e.g., automobile to automobile).

### Traffic Fatalities and Population Density

Differences in population density may reflect the degree of exposure to other vehicles, driving conditions, or alternative means of transportation. For example, sparsely populated areas provide fewer opportunities to interact with other drivers, and the risk of a vehicle-vehicle crash is lower than in more populated areas; rural areas have fewer total crashes but more fatal crashes. Alternatively, less-congested areas may permit higher speeds, which in turn could be related to an increased risk of fatal crashes; in highly populated areas average speeds may be lower because of traffic congestion.

In some densely populated areas, mass transit (e.g., rail, bus) may provide an alternative means of transportation and may reduce the risk of fatal crash involvement. In less-populated regions, public transportation alternatives are less common. Differences in the availability of alternative means of transportation could alter the effect of policy differences among licensing jurisdictions.

## THE LAW AND PUBLIC HEALTH

The U.S. Constitution is the supreme law of the land; any federal or state law in conflict with the U.S. Constitution is invalid. Similarly, any state statute in conflict with that state's constitution is invalid. Both the Ninth and Tenth Amendments to the U.S. Constitution suggest that people have inherent individual rights. These individual rights are broadly interpreted by the courts and constrained only to the extent that they interfere with the explicit powers granted to the federal government (or prohibited to the states) by the Constitution or the individual rights of other citizens.[253]

In contrast to the federal government's explicit powers, state governments have extremely broad inherent powers to act. These powers are not limited to the exercise of those explicitly defined by the state or federal constitution. The state's power to govern—generally known as police powers—include reasonable laws necessary to preserve the public order, health, safety, welfare, and morals.

In conflicts between the state exercising its police powers and a claim that individual constitutional rights are being violated by that exercise of power, the courts weigh the relative merits of the state action against the abridgment of individual rights. If the court finds that the state's action is unnecessarily broad and that the state's purpose can be carried out by less-dramatic means, the courts can invalidate the law or regulation. The courts have almost always upheld a state's exercise of police powers as long as they protect the public's health, safety, welfare, or morals.

### 1990 Americans with Disabilities Act

The issue of equity is important in regulations for driver licensure and relicensure. As a group, older adults have higher rates of vision impairment and are more likely to be denied driver licenses as a result of failing vision-screening examinations. The Americans with Disabilities Act (ADA) of 1990 prohibits discrimination against persons with disabilities.

Although advanced age is not considered an impairment under this statute, age-related functional deficits are considered impairments. Thus vision-related changes would be considered disabilities under this law.

The state legislature, through its police powers, has the authority to control and regulate the use of highways, and the courts have usually found in favor of reasonable laws necessary to preserve the public health, safety, and welfare. Under the equal protection clause, the government is required to treat similarly circumstanced individuals in a like manner.[138] The only requirements are that legislative action must not abridge a constitutional right or freedom and that it be rationally related to legitimate governmental interests.[253] Importantly, the ADA emphasizes reasonableness but does not require that others be placed at risk in the process of creating opportunities for persons with disabilities.[172] From this perspective, a license to drive could be considered a privilege, not a constitutional right. Therefore, if licensing requirements are applied in a uniform and nondiscriminatory manner, and individuals are afforded an equal opportunity to obtain a license, the spirit of this clause will be satisfied, provided that the criteria for eligibility are not prejudicial.[253] But, given the present lack of empirical evidence of a predictive relation between vision testing and traffic safety, current vision testing criteria could be challenged as being discriminatory against older adults.

According to Reese,[186] the notion that driving is a privilege and not a right should be discounted because of the profound effects on mobility associated with the denial of a driver license. He maintains that the ability to use roadways should not be tested by the privilege notion, but by the standards of due process of law. In the case of driver licensing, license suspensions and revocations are always for cause and are designed to fit or correct deficiencies. For example, to address the increasing problem of drunk driving, many states have adopted per se laws to facilitate the suspension and revocation of driving privileges of offenders. In some licensing jurisdictions, the law provides for immediate action, whereas in others, action is delayed until a record of conviction is received by the licensing agency.[223] The latter approach is presumably designed to protect individual rights by ensuring due process. However, in the process of complying with the spirit of the Ninth and Tenth Amendments, this approach may indirectly increase public risk.

For the legal system to work effectively, laws must clearly define specific relationships between individuals and institutions. Also, they must be enforceable. In general, the law is imperfectly enforced, not only because of undetected violations, but also because of conflicting ethical and societal concerns. Some rights are enforced and defined not by the legal system but by the force of prevailing ethics. This is particularly true in the health care delivery system. Ethics are principles of conduct recognized and enforced by associates or professional peers; in many cases ethics are not enforced in any pragmatic sense. Conversely, ethics can be vigorously enforced and, particularly with regard to health care providers, the sanctions available to professional associates can have serious personal or economic impact.[253] The conundrums associated with the professional and ethical activities and responsibilities of health care providers relative to the duty to warn are significant. Within the realm of traffic safety, this imperfect enforcement may have direct personal and economic effects.

In the United States, a driver's license is intrinsically tied to mobility, independence, and quality of life. Retirees, widows, and the lifelong poor are the groups most likely to have economic difficulties, and the very old are also apt to find their retirement incomes inadequate because cost-of-living adjustments in private pensions do not keep pace with inflation.[8] Lowered incomes may force older persons to give up their private automobiles or use them less often. Yet older people still need access to health care services, markets, and social groups to give meaning to their lives. Often this can only be accomplished at someone else's inconvenience. These factors are relevant to the psychology of aging and control-related constructs of perceived control, self-efficacy, and learned helplessness.[125] Given a choice, most people prefer staying active, innovative, and independent. The extent to which these control-related constructs influence visually impaired older drivers' decisions to drive will affect policy enforcement.

At the state level, traffic safety involves a delicate balance between the protection of individual rights and the public's health and safety. Those involved in protecting the public from incompetent drivers must effectively and fairly balance those competing interests. Nondiscriminatory, objective standards are clearly needed to guide those involved in legislating, regulating, and enforcing policies that protect the interests of both the individual and the public.

### Legal and Ethical Issues

Inappropriate or overly restrictive vision standards for licensing might intrude unnecessarily on the mobility and personal liberties of older adults. A long-term trend away from public transportation has occurred in the United States.[8] The lack of alternative means of transportation could seriously affect the quality of life of older Americans. These factors emphasize the importance of effective and fair policies that balance the individual needs of older Americans with societal interests.

Some have argued that the ability to use roadways should not be tested by the privilege notion but by the standards of due process of law. The ADA (Americans with Disabilities Act) emphasizes reasonableness; it does not require that others be placed at risk in creating opportunities for persons with disabilities.[172] From the ADA perspective, a license to drive would be considered a privilege, not a constitutional right. The requisite requirements under the ADA are that eligibility criteria are not prejudicial and that licensing requirements are applied in a uniform and nondiscriminatory manner. As such, objective, nondiscriminatory standards are requisite to allow states to meet their dual responsibilities of enforcing policies that protect the interest of both the individual and society.

Mandatory reporting requirements place health providers in a potentially duplicitous position, serving as both the agent of individual patients and as the agent of society at large. With mandatory reporting requirements, health providers would be vulnerable to claims of negligence by victims of visually impaired drivers under the concept of proximate causation. Mandatory reporting requirements by health providers prompt several ethical questions. Should individuals who voluntarily seek professional services—perhaps for signs and symptoms unrelated to driving—be reported if they do not meet minimal vision standards for driving privileges? Do mandatory reporting requirements conflict with patient confidentiality? Does professional responsibility to society outweigh responsibility to the patient? Can practitioners afford to be identified with patients losing their driver licenses? What are the legal ramifications of not enforcing standards or not reporting drivers with impaired vision?

Qualified privilege requires that disclosure of confidential information be done in good faith, be accurate, be limited to necessary information, and be provided only to individuals who should receive the information. Thus a good faith report to an agency, addressing legitimate interests of a patient, does not breach the duty of confidentiality. Several states have physician reporting statutes permitting the reporting of patients who, in the physician's professional opinion, are unable to drive safely. These statutes protect physicians who properly notify appropriate authorities about functionally disabled patients without incurring a breach of duty regarding confidentiality. Without such statutory reporting provisions, health care providers would probably not voluntarily report adverse patient information.

Because individuals are frequently unaware of vision impairments, these statutes may play a role in enhancing traffic safety. To provide optimal public protection from vision-related crashes, this reporting authority should be broadened to include optometrists—a profession representing nearly two thirds of U.S. eye care professionals.

## THE PUBLIC'S HEALTH

Most of the risk factors associated with the three leading causes of death—heart disease, cancer, and cerebrovascular disease—are irreversible or difficult to change. Additionally, the risk of death from these chronic conditions is specific to a given individual. In contrast, most risk factors associated with the fourth leading cause of death in the United States—unintentional injury fatalities—are amenable to change. Furthermore, in the case of unintentional injury the risk of injury or death may extend to others. Thus fatalities arising from unintentional injuries should be more responsive to effective preventive measures than heart disease, cancer,

and cerebrovascular disease, and preventive interventions should provide both individual and societal benefits.

Public policy emphasizing preventive measures has the potential to play a significant role in determining the nation's health and reducing avoidable costs. The promotion and adoption of effective safety legislation at the national and state levels should help reduce deaths, injuries, and economic costs associated with avoidable traffic crashes. With a better understanding of the sequence of events and the types of factors involved, developing effective systems to prevent injury and death from motor vehicle crashes is possible.[75]

### Vision Function, Traffic Safety, and the Law
#### Duty to Warn

All health providers are required to conform to standards of conduct prescribed by the law in treating their patients. Physicians are in a unique position to counsel older drivers about adjusting their driving habits in concert with functional changes and limitations, but they often have little knowledge of their patients' driving habits or their mobility needs.[143] Importantly, empirical evidence suggests that educational intervention in high-risk drivers can statistically reduce crash involvement.[170]

In general, health care practitioners often evaluate patients with severely reduced physical and mental function, thereby incurring a clinical and legal duty to warn those patients of their increased risk of injury. The courts have upheld this duty when the proximate cause of an injury to a patient is deemed to be associated with a failure to warn by the doctor.[224] Several cases have broadened the provider's responsibility to include third parties injured by patients whose judgment was impaired by medication. This increased risk of provider culpability gives rise to important ethical and legal considerations.

A loss in vision function may be dangerous to others as well as the patient. A physician caring for individuals with significantly impaired vision has a responsibility to inform these patients of their impairment or be subject to a suit by a third party injured by such individuals. For example, a person injured by a driver with vision performance below the state standards for licensure could conceivably seek recourse for damages from both the driver and the driver's eye care professional.

Eye care professionals assume two important traffic safety roles: evaluating and treating patients who fail vision screening evaluations and informing patients when their vision status is below state standards for driving.[233] These roles prompt a variety of professional, ethical, and legal questions (see Chapter 20 for a discussion of ethical issues in the care of the older adult).

The success of preventive and curative treatment depends in part on the patient's willingness to adopt and maintain recommended behaviors. Unfortunately, public participation in preventive health efforts and individual adherence to prescribed treatments and recommended behavior changes are less than optimal.[18] Adherence requires that individual patients have both knowledge and understanding to fully cooperate with recommended treatment and behavior modification. Jette and Branch[102] suggest that a considerable amount of nonadherence by patients may be unintentional because of inaccurate patient-provider communication. In traffic safety, the quality of patient-provider communication may have individual, societal, and legal consequences.

The theory of reasoned action posits that an individual's intention to perform a particular behavior can be accounted for by a combination of factors.[3] This model suggests that individual beliefs are influenced by outside groups and subjective norms (what others thinks she or he should or should not do). Family members may reinforce or undermine health providers' attempts to alter high-risk behaviors.

Thus in addition to the health provider, other social factors play an important role in an individual's adherence to specific health regimens and behavioral changes. Regarding traffic safety, compliance with legal constraints or functional driving ability could be positively or negatively influenced by these factors.

## Privileged Communications

The concepts of privileged communications and confidentiality are based on the notion that information entrusted to a health provider by a patient will not be divulged to a third party without the consent of the patient. In fact, health providers can be held liable for disclosing confidential information about patients, even though such disclosures may be true and accurate.[35] The unauthorized publication of patient information, broadly categorized as invasion of privacy, can constitute a civil offense. Also, the public disclosure of information that places a patient in a false light could also result in legal action against a physician for which damages may be awarded.

In some instances health professionals need to communicate important health information to others for the sake of the patient or society at large. Examples include reports to spouses and agencies, as in the case of communicable diseases, or in the case of driving, reporting those patients who do not meet minimal vision standards for driving privileges.

Legal cases have established the qualified privilege of physicians to divulge confidential information about a patient when the patient's life is in danger or in the case of "necessity"—when necessity implies the presence of an imminent desperate, serious, or threatening condition.[91] Qualified privilege extends to situations in which the author and recipient of a written report have a common interest and a moral or social duty to act in the public interest on matters of public concern.[35] Qualified privilege requires that disclosure of confidential information be done in good faith, be accurate, be limited to necessary information, and be provided only to individuals who should receive the information. Therefore a good faith report to an agency, addressing legitimate interests of a patient, does not breach the duty of confidentiality.

Several states have adopted physician reporting statutes that require or permit the reporting of patients who, in the physician's professional opinion, are unable to drive safely.[59] These statutes are designed to protect the physician who notifies appropriate authorities of a patient with compromised vision function without incurring a breach of duty regarding confidentiality. Only Connecticut specifically includes vision disorders within the category of reportable conditions.

Importantly, optometrists, although representing nearly two thirds of all eye care professionals, do not have a duty to report patients whose vision does not meet legal standards for driver licensure in any state.[34] In fact, optometrists who voluntarily report such patients risk legal action. Obviously a lack of legal protection for this large professional group could negatively affect public safety.

A patient whose vision function does not meet legal vision standards should be warned not to drive. However, as previously discussed, a warning does not ensure that visually impaired patients will actually refrain from driving. Ideally, health providers should be protected from legal action when accurately reporting persons not meeting minimal vision standards for driver licensure.

Most states have established medical advisory boards that have the function of providing professional opinions on the degree to which various medical conditions or impairments interfere with safe driving.[67,80] When persons with medical impairments are identified during the license renewal process and are referred for evaluation, the medical advisory board evaluates the medical records of these individuals and determines whether the applicant's medical condition would interfere with safe driving. The ultimate decision for relicensure, however, rests with the licensing bureau. In a 1986 study of the effectiveness of this process in Texas, Gober[67] found a 46% reduction of violations and a 53% reduction in collisions for the study group, with significant declines in collisions caused by blackouts, general debility, neurological impairments, and vision impairments.

Some states have instituted policies for restricted driver licenses, allowing for operation of a vehicle within a limited range of a person's home.[69] Other jurisdictions have made changes in roadway signage to enhance visibility.[118] Several states have modified relicensing policies that require more frequent driver examinations, often including knowledge and road tests for older motorists. These alternatives seek to satisfy the mutual goals of public safety and independence. The effectiveness of these alternatives has not been empirically established.

## Public Policy and Traffic Safety

The primary purpose of public policy requiring vision testing for driver license renewal is to identify and, when necessary, restrict drivers with functional vision impairments as a means of enhancing traffic safety. These policies are predicated on the notion that poor vision is causally related to poor driving and crashes. Some states require vision testing for driver license renewal; others do not. Among those states requiring vision testing, the frequency and types of vision tests performed vary considerably.

When shaping public policy, lawmakers and regulators must carefully balance societal needs and individual rights. Often legal, behavioral, and ethical forces interact in ways that undermine the intent of statutes designed to protect the public. At issue in the case of relicensing policies is whether the combination of these forces and contemporary vision standards protect the public health and safety to a greater extent than they reduce the quality of life of older Americans.

For effective evaluation of the need, or the appropriateness of, existing vision-related relicensing policies effectively, the magnitude of traffic fatalities in the United States and the impact of traffic fatalities on the public's health must be understood.

In 1903, Massachusetts and Missouri became the first states to enact driver license laws.[223] Since that time, all states and the District of Columbia have adopted comprehensive systems to test and license drivers with the goal of ensuring public safety. Driver licenses are granted or denied on the basis of an applicant's ability to satisfy prescribed standards of knowledge of state laws and practices; demonstrate driving proficiency; and, in varying degrees, demonstrate adequate visual, mental, and health function. All licensing agencies have the legal responsibility and authority to monitor, restrict, or revoke the driver licenses of individuals who represent an unwarranted risk to themselves or others.[177] Several states have instituted systems to penalize traffic violators through administrative action.

Traffic safety statues also have been legislated at the national level. The Beamer Resolution (P.L. 85-684) authorized states to enter into driver license compacts and enabled joint action among states in enhancing traffic safety. Specifically, this federal law provided an exchange of information among the states on violation-prone drivers to permit the identification of violations in jurisdictions other than the state in which the license originated. This law supported the one license concept in which the owner of a valid driver license is considered a legal operator in all other jurisdictions. In 1986 the U.S. Commercial Motor Vehicle Safety Act was passed. Among other things, this law imposed federal requirements on drivers of vehicles involved in foreign and interstate commerce.[223]

Three guiding principles have been suggested in selecting injury prevention strategies: (1) a mixed strategy that focuses differentially on the preinjury, injury, and postinjury phases; (2) emphasis on passive measures that do not require action by the individuals being protected; and (3) measures that will most effectively reduce injury losses. The Institute of Medicine/National Research Council concluded that "the second strategy—providing automatic protection—will generally be more effective than the first, and that the third—providing automatic protection—will be the most effective."[33,157] Consistent with these observations, societal interventions involving changing vehicles or environments have been used to reduce the number of motor vehicle crashes.[191]

Most legislative efforts involve a fault-based approach to prevent injury, namely, restricting high-risk behaviors and identifying and removing individuals at high risk for injury. Examples include mandatory seat belt laws, mandatory motorcycle helmet protection, and vision screening.

Three major arguments are used to oppose injury-prevention laws: (1) they do not work—statutes, ordinances, and government regulations are not effective ways of reducing injury; (2) even if they do work, the restriction of individual liberty is too great to justify such an intrusive approach; and (3) the economic cost involved in making them work is too great to justify such approaches. Supporters of such laws find all three of these challenges unconvincing and argue that injury prevention holds the prospect of saving thousands of American lives per year.[33,148,225] In the area of traffic safety, strong proponents are found on both sides of the prevention argument.

The preceding illustrates the challenges federal and state lawmakers face in balancing individual rights and the needs of society relative to traffic safety. Despite near universal agreement that vision plays a preeminent role in driving performance, that vision performance deteriorates with age, and that older adults disproportionately have more crashes, a limited empirical basis is available for current state vision screening policies.

As America becomes progressively older, determining the impact of age-related changes in vision function on driving performance, the effectiveness of contemporary vision screening tests in identifying high-risk drivers, and the impact of vision-related driver license renewal policies and practices on older adults and society will all become more important.

## VISION SCREENING

The purpose of vision screening at driver license renewal is to identify drivers with vision impairments and correct the problems or, if necessary, restrict the drivers. All states require some level of vision screening for initial licensing; however, not all state some level of vision screening as a condition for license renewal. The practice of licensing drivers has changed little since the 1950s.[229] The existence of state-level vision standards for driver licensing suggests a shared assumption among states that vision plays an important role in driving performance.

Vision screening tests are designed to identify individuals with impaired vision function. All U.S. jurisdictions require vision screening for initial licensing. However, vision testing requirements and procedures for driver licensing are not uniform among states.[233] At present U.S. jurisdictions vary considerably in the frequency, types of tests, and pass/fail criteria.

Most people commonly assume that the strict application of vision standards will decrease traffic fatalities, yet there is a lack of empirical evidence that vision screening tests are predictive of traffic crash involvement.[166] Older drivers may effectively compensate for their loss of vision function and not experience vision-related traffic crashes more frequently than other age groups.[205]

Furthermore, some have argued that older drivers, cognizant of their impaired functional capacity, may voluntarily adjust their driving behaviors by driving less frequently, more slowly, during daylight hours, and so forth.[141]

Thus older drivers may be at risk for a restriction or loss of driving privileges because of age-related vision impairments even though those impairments may not increase their level of traffic crash involvement.[1,20]

The loss of a driver license has significant implications for both older individuals and society.[141,245] Currently, many states do not have the capacity to provide alternative means of transportation for those at risk for losing driving privileges.[245] Although vision testing for license renewal represents an appropriate use of police power and is carried out for society's benefit, this requirement could adversely affect the social, health, and economic well-being of many older Americans. The mere existence of a vision-testing requirement for license renewal may have a chilling effect on older drivers and may lead to unnecessary self-restriction. Obviously, stringent vision testing for driver license renewal or age-related vision testing should reduce the magnitude of automobile crashes; otherwise the risk of inappropriately denying driving privileges to older drivers would be high. These factors emphasize the importance of effective and fair policies that balance the individual needs of older Americans against those of society.[207]

As has been previously discussed, older persons are susceptible to a loss of visual acuity, altered color vision, diminished light sensitivity, increased susceptibility to glare, and reduced peripheral vision. The prevalence of each of these impairments increases with age. Regarding driving, these impairments result in difficulty visualizing other vehicles, pedestrians, or traffic signals, especially when driving at night.*

The United States has considerable variation in the frequency, types of testing, and pass/fail criteria among jurisdictions for driver license renewal. Also, a wide variation in visual standards, testing methods, and test frequency is found among different counties despite efforts for uniformity.[31,45,194]

A study of vision screening results of driver license renewal applicants in Oregon provides some important insights to vision testing.[190] Investigators reported that one of five drivers renewing their licenses did not meet the vision screening standards, but their license did not

include necessary restrictions. These persons tended to be older than the average driver.

## Uneven Application of Driver License Policies?

A number of important questions exist about contemporary vision testing for license renewal What is the appropriate renewal period? What are the appropriate test procedure(s)? Are vision screening tests valid and reliable? Are vision standards uniformly enforced?

Because most vision testing procedures are semiautomated, human error during test administration is possible. For example, in a lax testing environment, examinees might cheat by memorizing eye charts. Alternatively, examiners in certain jurisdictions may be tougher in administering tests and applying standards.

Differences between policy and practice between and within licensing jurisdictions are likely in the enforcement of reporting and law enforcement because licensing authorities are authorized to exercise discretion in the administration of licensing and relicensing policies. Also, some individuals drive despite license revocation and suspension; in 1995, 28% of the fatal crashes in Alabama were associated with unlicensed, uninsured drivers.

## Renewal Periods

With progressive aging, a time will come when a person's vision is too poor to permit safe driving. Currently, which performance criteria best defines this point is not clear. A visual standard for safe driving is obviously needed. Also, because the likelihood of vision impairment increases with advancing age, increased frequency of vision assessment with advancing age may be appropriate. At present, the appropriate tests, test procedures, and test frequencies have not been determined.

Among those states requiring mandatory vision screening for renewal, the intervals range from 3 to 6 years.[236] However, in states with renewal by mail policies, the time between in-person vision screenings can exceed 7 years. Some states have age-related requirements that require more frequent license renewal by older drivers, satisfactory road test performance, or the submission of medical reports.[235]

In general, state-level vision testing requirements are not consistent with anticipated age-

---

*References 16, 116, 118, 120, 165, 232.

related vision changes because the incidence and prevalence of ocular diseases, the use of corrective lenses, and functional losses in central vision and peripheral vision function increase dramatically beyond age 65 years.* If age-related vision changes and crash rates are causally related, perhaps the frequency of vision testing should vary with age. On the basis of an investigation of the relation between reduced visual fields and traffic crashes, Keltner and Johnson[113] recommend that the visual acuity and visual fields of drivers older than 65 years be evaluated every 1 to 2 years.

## Tests Administration and Types of Vision Tests

According to Graham,[69] vision testing for relicensure may not be cost effective, even when targeted specifically at older drivers. In a 4-year state-level study comparing in-person driver license renewal (i.e., with written tests and vision screening) to a renewal by mail program (i.e., mail-in extensions for clean record drivers), no significant differences were found in subsequent rates of crashes or convictions for the two groups.[98,100,111,112] The authors concluded that the omission of renewal testing made essentially no difference in the subsequent crash experiences of clean-record drivers and suggested as a possible explanation that visually impaired individuals took compensatory or corrective action on their own.[100,112] An alternative explanation may be that the test was not appropriately administered or evaluated.

Generally, non–eye care professional staff administer vision screening tests with semiautomated testing devices.[202] The vision testing options include static visual acuity (distance and near), color vision, depth perception, lateral and vertical phoria, and horizontal visual field.

In a comparison of two popular vision screening devices—Orthorater and Keystone—different failure rates were observed under both normal and reduced illumination.[246] The Keystone vision tester was consistently more stringent than the Orthorater. The test-retest reliability for the Keystone machine was assessed for a subset of 100 employees for within-machine and between- and within-group varia-

tion. Mann-Whitney and Wilcoxon tests showed no significant differences for the comparisons. Spearman correlations of the vision testing options ranged from 0.57 to 0.96. Because of inconsistencies, the Keystone vision tester was not recommended for measuring peripheral vision. Waller et al[246] does not recommend testing visual acuity under reduced illumination conditions because no significant relations were found between performance on this test and poorer driving records.

Despite differences in optotype and testing procedures, the Orthorater and Keystone vision screening devices are comparable, with small, but clinically insignificant, systematic differences. Test-retest reliability and interrater reliability for these semiautomated devices are good to high ($r > 0.70$).[202] An experienced examiner has been estimated to be able to administer a full range of tests in less than 3 minutes.[233]

### Static Visual Acuity

All states require visual acuity testing as a common component of vision screening.[9] Static visual acuity tests measure the ability to discriminate stationary high-contrast targets (i.e., black on white). The minimal standards for best-corrected static visual acuity range from 20/40 to 20/70 for binocular drivers. For persons with one blind eye, the minimal acuity ranges from 20/25 to 20/70.[9,232,236] These standards were derived at by consensus.

According to a 1990 report, on the basis human factor assumptions on road sign design, drivers should have static visual acuity that allows the identification of 1-inch letters for every 35 feet of distance from a roadway sign. This is roughly equivalent to 20/23.[124] Bailey and Sheedy[10] estimate that 96.5% of the adult population would meet the 20/40 standard, but 13% would not meet the 20/23 standard—roughly 50% of whom would be in the older than 70 years age group. The Snellen visual chart is the most commonly used vision test to assess static visual acuity; however, newer technologies (e.g., Flow S-chart, Bailey-Lovie chart) have higher reliability.

From 5% to 10% of drivers from 60 to 65 years of age have corrected visual acuity worse than 20/40, the minimal acuity level for an unrestricted license in a majority of the 51 U.S. licensing jurisdictions.[9,116,235] In a study of 13,786

---

*References 9, 104, 106, 115, 116, 128, 129, 132, 152, 164, 165, 240, 245.

drivers, Hofstetter[89,90] observed that drivers with poor acuity had significantly more crashes and repeated crashes during a 12-month period than those with good acuity. Hills and Burg[88] found that drivers older than 54 years showed consistent relations between static visual acuity and dynamic visual acuity but that the predictive values were low.

A study of 900 individuals between the ages of 58 and 102 years were assessed on a variety of psychophysical tests to determine the impact of aging on visual performance.[76] The investigators found that high-contrast acuity is reasonably maintained, even into very old ages. However, the authors caution that high-contrast acuity underestimates the degree of functional vision loss suffered by older individuals. Contrast sensitivity assessment provided a better indication of functional vision status.

### Depth Perception

Depth perception judgments may be binocular (i.e., using both eyes) or monocular (i.e., using one eye only). Stereopsis—binocular depth perception—results from disparate lateral imaging of an object on the retinas of both eyes.[199] A monocular appreciation of depth can occur from visual size comparisons, shadow casting, variations in color and brightness, movement parallax, and stereoscopic cues. While driving, most depth perception cues are monocular rather than binocular.

In driver vision testing, depth perception is assessed by stereoscopic vision test. A variety of stereoscopic optotypes are used in modern testing, most of which do not fully evaluate threshold capabilities.[199] Although dynamic stereoacuity may be related to traffic safety, definitive work has yet to be done.

The depth perception used while driving and current vision testing procedures have an obvious disconnect. Perhaps the absence of a relation between traffic safety is attributable to weak construct validity between testing and functional requirements.

### Peripheral Vision

Glaucoma, one of the leading causes of blindness in older adults, restricts peripheral vision but does not affect central vision. Hence a person may have visual acuities that satisfy minimal driver license requirements but be legally blind because of restricted peripheral vision.

The visual field is the total area visualized with both eyes while looking straight ahead at a constant fixation point. The Transportation Research Board of the National Research Council recommends that drivers with a field of view limited to a range of 45 to 70 degrees to either side of fixation should be required to install special mirrors to compensate for restricted visual field.[237]

Peripheral vision impairments may adversely affect driver performance and traffic safety.[104,105] In 1990 only 12 licensing jurisdictions had a statutory requirement for peripheral vision testing as a condition for relicensure.[235] The additional time to assess visual fields (2 minutes per eye) of one fourth of the 162 million drivers in 1988 was estimated at $45 million per year.

### Vision Screening and Traffic Safety

Although static visual acuity testing is the most frequently used measure of visual function, studies have shown that central vision alone is not effective in predicting adequate visual performance for driving-related tasks or future crash involvement.[6,9,12] In a Canadian study of crash involvement of 70-year-old drivers, visual acuity alone was not a significant risk for crash involvement. The risks of crashes in those with minimal visual acuity and lack of binocularity was only moderately higher (odds ratio, 1.23; 95% confidence interval, 0.88-1.72) than among other drivers.[71] A study of 1000 British drivers' crash histories and their performance on a vision screening instrument (Keystone Telebinocular) revealed significant positive associations between vehicle crashes and visual acuity.[45] This association was strongest for older drivers.

Decina and Staplin[47] performed unannounced visual testing (visual acuity, horizontal visual field, and contrast sensitivity) on 12,400 Pennsylvania drivers at the time of license renewal. After controlling for self-reported mileage, no significant relations were found between visual acuity or horizontal visual fields and crash data extracted from Pennsylvania Department of Transportation crash records for all drivers (January 1986 through August 1989). However, for drivers aged 66 years and older the combination of visual acuity, horizontal visual fields, and contrast sensitivity was significantly related to increasing crash involvement.

## Alternative Vision Screening Tests

### Dynamic Visual Acuity

Dynamic visual acuity testing involves the recognition of a letter or detail on a moving target. Dynamic visual acuity decreases with age and is related to traffic crashes.[9,202,204] Unfortunately, dynamic visual acuity testing is time consuming and difficult to administer. Driver age and dynamic visual acuity interact in a complex manner with traffic safety.[9]

For example, Schieber[202] found that both young drivers with the best dynamic visual acuity and drivers older than 54 years with the poorest dynamic visual acuity had higher frequencies of traffic crashes and convictions. This most likely resulted from the influence of uncontrolled factors that differentially affect crash rates for these age cohorts.

### Contrast Sensitivity

Tests of contrast sensitivity determine how much contrast an individual requires to detect different size bar grating patterns.[25,164,168,255] The standard test pattern consists of bar gratings with different spatial frequencies; low spatial frequencies are large-sized patterns, whereas high spatial frequencies are smaller-sized patterns. When the results are plotted as log contrast sensitivity versus log spatial frequency, the data are well described by a parabolic curve, even for low vision observers.[174]

Contrast sensitivity measures the ability to distinguish targets against low-contrast backgrounds (e.g., dark gray on light gray). Contrast sensitivity assessment is thought to be more relevant to the visual requirements of driving than static visual acuity is because the test simulates vision challenges associated with adverse driving conditions (e.g., dusk, rain, fog).[164,206] Investigations of functional vision loss have shown that static visual acuity testing is less reliable than testing with low-contrast targets.[64-66,164,165,202]

Under daylight conditions, older adults demonstrate a loss of sensitivity for patterns with intermediate and higher spatial frequencies compared with younger adults, with older adults requiring roughly three times more contrast to discriminate the same patterns.[261] This loss in sensitivity is primarily caused by optical rather than neurological changes. In a study of within-session and between-session reliability with certain contrast sensitivity charts (Vistech VCTS 6500) reliability was found to be low.[187] A study by Rohaly and Owsley[195] suggests that the contrast-sensitivity functions of older adults cannot be described by a single parabolic curve and that the Pelli-Robson chart does not adequately predict peak contrast sensitivities for this age group.

Importantly, older individuals may have adequate acuity for high-contrast targets but inadequate acuity with low-contrast targets. Therefore current vision screening methods may not adequately identify drivers with functionally impaired vision. Clinically, contrast sensitivity measurements appear to be useful in explaining symptoms of poor vision in a patient with good visual acuity.[51] Several investigators suggest the use of contrast sensitivity testing (i.e., testing with low-contrast targets) to identify mild changes in visual performance in drivers.[164,165,202]

Preliminary research suggests that the Pelli-Robson charts provide the same information as contrast sensitivity assessments. Several researchers suggest that the Pelli-Robson contrast sensitivity chart as a screening device provides both visual acuity and contrast sensitivity assessments without additional costs and inconveniences associated with Snellen acuity testing combined with contrast sensitivity testing.[173,205] The Pelli-Robson chart consists of 16 triplets of 4.9-cm letters. Each triplet of letters has the same contrast. The contrast of successive triplets decreases by a factor of 0.15 log units. Several case studies have shown that patients with glaucoma, diabetic retinopathy, macular degeneration, and cataract exhibit defects in contrast sensitivity testing.

### Useful Field of View

Older individuals with normal visual fields often have reduced attention windows or UFOV. One research team found that the relation between UFOV and crashes in older drivers is stronger than correlations between the more commonly used visual sensory tests (e.g., visual acuity, peripheral vision) and crashes.[15] This suggests that an age-specific requirement for UFOV testing would enhance traffic safety. Unfortunately, UFOV testing is considered costly and time intensive.[36] To date, none of the jurisdictions requires an assessment of UFOV for license renewal.[223]

Hennessy[86] observed that voluntary avoidance of driving at sunrise and sunset by 350 older drivers was associated with reduced vision function as measured by the Pelli-Robson low-contrast acuity test and the UFOV test. Self-restriction (e.g., reduced night driving, avoidance of rain and fog, driving during twilight conditions, driving alone, and performing left turns) was most strongly associated with low UFOV performance.

According to Shinar and Schieber,[205] of the visual functions (dynamic visual acuity, motion perception, visual field, contrast sensitivity, and higher order perceptual functions), corrected static visual acuity—with glasses or contact lenses—is most resistant to deterioration from aging. Therefore an assessment of static visual acuity alone would not reflect other visual and higher order age-related changes in vision function related to traffic safety.

## POLICY-RELATED STUDIES

Traffic safety is an important public health issue that, given our aging society, will become increasingly problematic in the future. State governments have the right and responsibility to protect the public health, yet in the area of traffic safety ineffective policies may adversely affect the mobility and quality of life of older adults. The proper design and exercise of the law in traffic safety are important in balancing individual rights and societal needs.

By using state-specific fatal crash records from 1986 through 1988, Nelson et al[156] compared fatal motor vehicle crash ratios of younger and older drivers licensed in states requiring vision testing for license renewal with states that did not. Specifically, fatal crash ratios of nine states without vision testing for license renewal were compared to the fatal crash ratios of 11 contiguous states with vision testing requirements. The investigators found significantly lower fatal crash involvement in states requiring testing than states without testing and concluded that vision testing as a condition for relicensure appeared warranted for individuals aged 65 years and older. These findings

suggest that, although specific aspects of vision function and specific vision tests have not been unequivocally related to traffic crashes, the combined effect of relicensing policies and practices may enhance traffic safety.

A 4-year (1985 to 1989) nationwide study investigated the relation between driver license renewal policies and fatal crash rates of drivers older than 69 years.[130] The investigators evaluated the effect of vision tests, knowledge tests, and road tests on older driver fatal crash rates while accounting for differences among states in factors likely to influence older motor vehicle crashes. The investigators observed that tests of visual acuity, adjusted for renewal period, were associated with lower fatal crash risk for older drivers. Knowledge tests provided a nonsignificant further reduction, whereas road tests had no effect.

Another nationwide study reported that state-level vision-related licensure renewal policies were associated with lower older driver–related traffic fatality rates and lower crash-related costs.[206] Shipp[206] estimated that if mandatory vision testing policies had existed in all licensing jurisdictions, an estimated 222 (12.2%) fewer vehicle occupant fatalities associated with older drivers would have occurred between 1989 and 1991. Conservatively, these excess deaths represented $31 million in non-workplace and nonhousehold productivity-related economic costs.

In the Shipp study, although the presence of a vision testing requirement was associated with lower fatal crash involvement, no differential impact was found with different types of vision test(s) or combinations thereof. In part, this may have been attributable to wide variations among the licensing jurisdictions on what constitutes minimal standards, variations in testing procedures, and frequency of testing. Because visual acuity testing was common to all test batteries, perhaps acuity testing alone may adequately identify drivers with functional vision impairments. Alternatively, this may signal a need for revised or stricter screening standards or a need for testing procedures with higher predictive value.

Before these studies no empirical evidence had been published to support the effectiveness of vision testing policy in preventing fatal traffic crashes. The results of these investigations suggest that vision-related relicensing policies may prove helpful in enhancing traffic safety and reducing crash-related costs in states without such policies.

Several researchers have reported that older drivers frequently are aware of their functional limitations and voluntarily adjust their driving behaviors. Other researchers submit that older drivers effectively compensate for their loss of vision function, thereby reducing their vision-related traffic crashes. The findings of these current studies indicate that such adjustments by older drivers are inadequate and suggest the need for state-level policy changes in jurisdictions without vision-related relicensing policies to protect the public's health.

## Policy Implementation Challenges

The adoption of vision testing renewal policies by jurisdictions without such policies generates a variety of concerns, most of which are related to the costs associated with changing facilities, staffing, and equipment. The new requirements would likely increase license processing time, and alterations or expansions of existing facilities might be required. Similarly, staffing changes might become necessary, requiring the hiring of new staff or upgrading of existing staff to assume expanded responsibilities. Lastly, costs would be associated with the purchase and maintenance of vision testing devices. The key concern in implementing a new vision testing policy is cost effectiveness; specifically, would the costs of adopting a new vision testing policy for relicensure be less than the costs of avoidable traffic crashes?

A Pennsylvania-based pilot vision screening program in three licensing centers from February to August 1989, provides some insight on the cost effectiveness of vision-related relicensing policies in a jurisdiction without such requirements.[47] At the time of the study, Pennsylvania did not have a requirement for vision testing for license renewal. One component of this program used the pass/fail requirements of the minimal vision standards for initial licensure. Of the 12,710 motorists who voluntarily participated in the screening, 424 (3.3%) failed to meet the minimal visual standards; among operators aged 65 years and older, 9.5% did not meet the minimal standards. Of those not meeting the minimal vision standards, 54.2% were unaware

of their vision problems before testing. Of those participants who were aware that they had a vision problem before the screening, 48.2% had not changed their driving behaviors. The second component of this program involved binocular contrast acuity assessment with sign grating targets. From 1.2% to 8.3% of the participants failed the eight levels of the contrast sensitivity testing. An analysis of vision status and traffic violations suggested that periodic screening of drivers by existing vision standards alone would not be cost effective, but the addition of contrast sensitivity testing would be cost effective under certain conditions (e.g., testing of middle- and high-range frequency and follow-up examination by an eye care professional).

This study provides only qualified support for the efficacy of vision-related relicensing policies in improving traffic safety. The results of this study and ongoing research on UFOV, contrast sensitivity, and other screening tests suggest that certain alternative vision screening tests may have higher predictive values and may more accurately identify high-risk drivers than current practices. An important concern is the cost effectiveness of these new vision-testing options relative to existing procedures.

The primary purpose of population-based screening is to diagnose and treat diseases and conditions in asymptomatic, apparently healthy individuals.[145] Because screenings are designed for large groups of people, the tests should be innocuous, efficient, and inexpensive. Nonprofessionals should be able to administer the screening tests. Ideally, the tests should have high sensitivity, specificity, and reliability, and the treatment for positively identified individuals should be acceptable and available. According to Shinar and Schieber,[205] introducing new tests may be impractical because "(1) there is insufficient agreement on which visual skills are most critical, (2) for all but photopic (i.e., daylight) acuity, there are no pass/fail criteria that can be scientifically defended, and (3) the complex visual skills that seem to more relevant to driving are susceptible to practice effects."

Because the prevalence of sight-compromising diseases and conditions in the United States is low for persons younger than 50 years, vision testing for individuals in this age group would have a very low yield. Age-specific vision testing for relicensing would seem to be more cost effective than a universal requirement for all drivers. Importantly, because the prevalence of reduced vision function increases significantly with age, at some age the prevalence will be so high that simply requiring a comprehensive eye examination by an eye care professional as a condition of relicensing would be more cost effective.

## SUMMARY

Vision performance declines with age. Frequently, because of the slow rate of progression, individuals with age-related vision changes do not fully appreciate the extent of their visual impairments. In most cases, with early detection these impairments may be easily corrected with a complete or near-complete restoration of functional performance.

Research on contemporary vision tests and testing procedures have not established a strong relation between test performance and older driving. Nevertheless, the crashes in which older drivers are overrepresented indicate the presence of visual difficulties.[13] Driving is a visually complex task. Functional vision status is only one of many factors affecting the driving performance of older Americans. A variety of factors influence traffic crashes. Fatal crashes may result from the independent effect of any of driver or non–driver-related factors. Fatal crashes could also arise from interactions between one or more driver and non–driver-related factors.

The current view is that fatal and nonfatal injuries result from multiple controllable causes, implying that the adoption and enforcement of effective safety legislation should help reduce deaths, injuries, and economic costs associated with avoidable injuries. Purportedly, the most effective preventive strategies involve passive measures that do not require action by those being protected.

Although traffic fatalities as a whole have been decreasing during the past 2 decades, since 1980 the fatality rates of older drivers have increased relative to other age cohorts and in terms of miles driven. In light of these traffic safety trends and projected demographic changes in the U.S. population, empirical information about effective and efficacious strategies to enhance traffic safety is urgently needed to provide a rational basis for designing and implementing effective prevention strategies.

An important cautionary note for policy makers is that new and evolving traffic safety policies must carefully balance individual rights and societal needs. Although the results of recent policy studies suggest a beneficial effect on traffic safety by vision-related license renewal policies, evaluating the possibility that these policies may cause unnecessary driving cessation by otherwise competent individuals is important. The implementation of new licensing policies must be weighed against the potential benefits of improved traffic safety as well as the potential adverse impact on the mobility and quality of life of older Americans and their families.

Eye and vision care professionals have an important role to play in this emerging public health challenge. In addition to bringing this issue to the attention of policy makers, these experts must also address the individual needs of older Americans and their families and public safety of society at large.

## REFERENCES

1. Adams JM, Hoffman L: Implications of issues in typographical design for readability and reading satisfaction in an aging population, *Exp Aging Res* 20:61-9, 1994.
2. Agency for Health Care Policy Research: *Clinical practice guideline:number 4. Cataracts in adults: management of functional vision impairment*, Rockville, MD, 1993, U.S. Dept. of Health and Human Services, Public Health Service, Agency for Health Care Policy and Research.
3. Ajzen I, Fishbein M: *Understanding attitudes and predicting social behavior*, Englewood Cliffs, NJ, 1980, Prentiss-Hall.
4. Allen MJ: *Vision and highway safety*, New York, 1970, Chilton.
5. Antecol DH, Roberts WC: Sudden death behind the wheel: natural disease in drivers of four-wheeled motorized vehicles, *Am J Cardiol* 66:1329-35, 1990.
6. Appel SD, Brilliant RL, et al: Driving with visual impairment: facts and issues, *J Vision Rehab* 4:19-31, 1990.
7. Applegate WB, Miller ST, et al: Impact of cataract surgery with lens implantation on vision and physical function in elderly patients, *JAMA* 257:1064-6, 1987.
8. Atchley RC: *Social forces and aging*, Belmont, CA, 1985, Wadsworth.

9. Bailey H, Sheedy JE: Vision screening and driver licensure. In *Transportation in an aging society: improving mobility and safety for older persons. TRB special report 218*, Washington, DC, 1988, Transportation Research Board, pp 294-324.

10. Bailey IL, Sheedy JE: Vision and the aging driver. In London R, editor: *Problems in optometry*, Philadelphia, 1992, J.B. Lippincott.

11. Baker SP, Whitfield RA, et al: Geographic variations in mortality from motor vehicle crashes, *N Engl J Med* 316:1384-7, 1987.

12. Ball K, Owsley C: Identifying correlates of accident involvement for the older driver, *Hum Factors* 33:583-95, 1991.

13. Ball K, Owsley C: The useful field of view test: a new technique for evaluating age-related declines in visual function, *J Am Optom Assoc* 63:71-9, 1992.

14. Ball K, Owsley C, et al: Driving avoidance and functional impairment in drivers, *Accident Analysis and Prevention* 30:313-22, 1988.

15. Ball K, Owsley C, et al: Visual attention problems as a predictor of vehicle crashes in older drivers, *Invest Ophthalmol Vis Sci* 34:3110-23, 1993.

16. Barakat SJ, Mulinazzi TE: Elderly drivers: problems and needs for research, *Transportation Quarterly* 41:189-206, 1987.

17. Barr RA: Recent changes in driving among older adults, *Hum Factors* 33:597-600, 1991.

18. Becker MH, editor: *Theoretical models of adherence and strategies for improving adherence. The handbook of health behavior change*, New York, 1990, Springer.

19. Beers MH, Fink A, et al: Screening recommendations for the elderly. *Am J Public Health* 81:1131-40, 1991.

20. Berkman LF, Berkman CS, et al: Depressive symptoms in relation to the physical health and functioning in the elderly, *Am J Epidemiol* 124:372-88, 1986.

21. Bess FH, Lichtenstein MJ, et al: Hearing impairment as a determinant of function in the elderly, *J Am Geriatr Soc* 37:123-8, 1989.

22. Blincoe LJ, Faigin BM: *The economic cost of motor vehicle crashes, 1990,* Washington, DC, 1992, U.S. Department of Transportation.

23. Blockey PN, Hartley LR: Aberrant driving behaviour: errors and violations, *Ergonomics* 38:1759-71, 1995.

24. Booher HR: Effects of visual and auditory impairment in driving performance, *Hum Factors* 20:307-20, 1978.

25. Bosse JC: An argument for the inclusion of contrast sensitivity testing into the routine optometric regimen, *N Engl J Optom* 42:6-10, 1998.

26. Brenner MH, Curbow B, et al: Vision change and quality of life in the elderly: response to cataract surgery and treatment of other chronic ocular conditions, *Arch Ophthalmol* 111:680-5, 1993.

27. Brenton RS, Phelps CD: The normal visual field on the Humphrey Field Analyzer, *Ophthalmologia* 193:56-74, 1986.

28. Burg A: Vision and driving: a report on research, *Hum Factors* 13:79-87, 1971.

29. Burt CW, Fingerhut LA: Injury visits to hospital emergency departments: United States, 1992-1995, *Vital Health Stat 13* 9:1-76, 1998.

30. Cerelli EC: *The 1983 traffic fatalities early assessment*, Washington, DC, 1984, National Highway Traffic Safety Administration.

31. Charman WN: Visual standards for driving. *Ophthal Physiol Opt* 5:211-20, 1985.

32. Charness N, Bosman EA: Age-related changes in perceptual and psychomotor performance: implications for engineering design, *Exp Aging Res* 20:45-59, 1994.

33. Christoffel T: The role of law in reducing injury, *Law, Medicine & Health Care* 17:7-16, 1989.

34. Classé JG: Optometrist's duty to warn of vision impairment, *South J Optom* 4:66-9, 1985.

35. Classé JG: *Legal aspects of optometry*, Stoneham, MA, 1989, Butterworth.

36. Colsher P, Wallace RB: Geriatric assessment and driver functioning, *Clin Geriatr Med* 9:365-75, 1993.

37. Connolly PL: Vision, man, vehicle and highway. In Selzer ML, Gikas PW, Huelke DF, editors: *The prevention of highway injury*, Ann Arbor, MI, 1967, Highway Safety Research Institute, pp 122-49.

38. Cooper PJ: Differences in accident characteristics among elderly drivers and between elderly and middle-aged drivers, *Accident Analysis and Prevention* 22:499-508, 1990.

39. Cornoni-Huntley J, Ostfeld AM, et al: Established populations for epidemiologic studies of the elderly: study design and methodology, *Aging Clin Exp Res* 5:27-37, 1993.

40. Crancer A Jr, McMurray L: Accident and violation rates of Washington's medically restricted drivers, *JAMA* 205:74-8, 1968.

41. Crancer A, O'Neall PA: A record analysis of Washington drivers with license restrictions for heart disease, *Northwest Med* 69:409-16, 1970.

42. Crews JE: The demographic, social, and conceptual context of aging and vision loss, *J Am Optom Assoc* 65:63-8, 1994.

43. Cronin-Golomb A, Corkin S, et al: Visual dysfunction in Alzheimer's disease: relation to normal aging, *Ann Neurol* 29:41-52, 1991.

44. Cruickshanks KJ, Klein R, et al: Sunlight and age related macular degeneration—the Beaver Dam Eye Study, *Arch Ophthalmol* 111:514-8, 1993.

45. Davison PA: Inter-relationships between British drivers' visual abilities, age and road accidents histories, *Ophthal Physiol Opt* 5:195-204, 1985.

46. DeCarlo DK, Scilley K, et al: Driving habits and health-related quality of life in patients with age-related maculopathy, *Optom Vis Sci* 80: 207-13, 2003.

47. Decina LE, Staplin L: Retrospective evaluation of alternative vision screening criteria for older and younger drivers, *Accident Analysis and Prevention* 25:267-75, 1993.

48. DeMaria EJ: Evaluation and treatment of the elderly trauma victim, *Clin Geriatr Med* 9: 461-71, 1993.

49. Dubinsky RM, Williamson A, et al: Driving in Alzheimer's disease, *J Am Geriatr Soc* 40:1112-6, 1992.

50. Edwards MG, Schachat AP: Impact of enucleation for choroidal melanoma on the performance of vision-dependent activities, *Arch Ophthalmol* 109:519-21, 1991.

51. Elliott DB, Whitaker D: How useful are contrast sensitivity charts in optometric practice? *Optom Vis Sci* 69:378-85, 1992.

52. Elliott DB, Yang KCH, et al: Visual acuity changes throughout adulthood in normal, healthy eyes: seeing beyond 6/6. *Optom Vis Sci* 72:186-91, 1992.

53. Evans L: Older driver involvement in fatal and severe traffic crashes, *J Gerontol Soc Sci* 43: S186-93, 1988.

54. Evans L: Risk of fatality from physical trauma versus sex and age, *J Trauma* 28:368-78, 1988.

55. Evans L: How safe were today's older drivers when they were younger? *Am J Epidemiol* 137:769-75, 1993.

56. Evans L, Frick MC: Car size or car mass: which has greater influence on fatality risk? *Am J Public Health* 82:1105-12, 1992.

57. Federal Highway Administration: *1990 National personal transportation: summary of travel trends,* Washington, DC, 1992, United States Department of Transportation.

58. Ferris F III: Senile macular degeneration: review of epidemiologic features, *Am J Epidemiol* 118:132-51, 1983.

59. Fisk GD, Owsley C, et al: Vision attention and self-reported driving behaviors in community-dwelling stroke survivors, *Arch Phys Med Rehab* 83:469-77, 2002.

60. Foley DJ, Wallace RB, et al: Risk factors for motor vehicle crashes among older drivers in a rural community, *J Am Geriatr Soc* 43:776-81, 1995.

61. Freeman PB: Visual requirements for driving, *J Rehab Optom* Summer:6-7, 1984.

62. Friedland RP, Koss E, et al: Motor vehicle crashes in dementia of the Alzheimer type, *Ann Neurol* 24:782-6, 1988.

63. Gilley DW, Wilson RS, et al: Cessation of driving and unsafe motor vehicle operation by dementia patients, *Arch Intern Med* 151:941-6, 1991.

64. Ginsburg AP: Contrast sensitivity, drivers' visibility, and vision standards. In *Visibility for highway guidance and hazard detection, transportation research record 1149,* Washington, DC, 1987, Transportation Research Board, National Research Council, pp 32-9.

65. Ginsburg AP: Next generation contrast sensitivity testing. In Rosenthal B, Cole R, editors: *Functional assessment of low vision,* St. Louis, 1996, Mosby–Year Book, pp 77-88.

66. Ginsburg AP, Evans DW, et al: Large-sample norms for contrast sensitivity, *Am J Optom Physiol Opt* 61:80-4, 1984.

67. Gober G: Initial medical advisory board review of medical impairment: effect on driver performance and traffic safety, *J Texas Med* 86:64-8, 1990.

68. Graca JL: Driving and aging, *Clin Geriatr Med* 2:577-89, 1986.

69. Graham JD: Injuries from traffic crashes: meeting the challenge, *Ann Rev Public Health* 14:515-43, 1993.

70. Gray LS, Heron G, et al: Comparison of age-related changes in short-wavelength-sensitive cone thresholds between normals and patients with primary open-angle glaucoma, *Optom Vis Sci* 72:205-9, 1995.

71. Gresset JA, Meyer FM: Risk of accidents among elderly care drivers with visual acuity equal to 6/12 or 6/15 and lack of binocular vision, *Ophthalmol Physiol Opt* 14:33-7, 1994.

72. Grisso JA, Schwarz DF, et al: Injuries in an elderly inner-city population, *J Am Geriatr Soc* 38:1326-31, 1990.

73. Guccione AA, Felson DT, et al: The effects of specific medical conditions on the functional limitations of elders in the Framingham study, *Am J Public Health* 84:351-8, 1994.

74. Gunby P: As nation grows older, traffic safety officials confront questions of who should drive, *JAMA* 268:307-8, 1992.

75. Haddon W Jr: Keynote address: options for the prevention of motor vehicle crash injury, *Israel J Med Sci* 16:45-65, 1980.

76. Haegerstrom-Portnoy G, Schneck ME, Brabyn JA: Seeing into old age: vision function beyond acuity, *Optom Vis Sci* 76:141-58, 1999.

77. Haegerstrom-Portnoy G, Schneck ME, et al: Development of refractive errors into old age, *Optom Vis Sci* 79:643-9, 2002.

78. Hakamies-Blomqvist L: Aging and fatal accidents in male and female drivers, *J Gerontol Soc Sci* 49:S286-90, 1994.

79. Hakamies-Blomqvist L: Compensation in older drivers as reflected in their fatal accidents, *Accident Analysis and Prevention* 26:107-12, 1994.

80. Hales RH: Functional ability profiles for driver licensing, *Arch Ophthalmol* 100:1780-3, 1982.

81. Hansotia P, Broste SK: The effect of epilepsy or diabetes mellitus on the risk of automobile accidents, *N Engl J Med* 324:22-6, 1991.

82. Harris JS: Source of payment for the medical cost of motor vehicle injuries in the United States, 1990, Washington, DC, 1992, National Highway Traffic Safety Administration.

83. Hartunian NS, Smart CN, et al: The incidence and economic costs of cancer, motor vehicle injuries, coronary hearth disease, and stroke: a comparative analysis, *Am J Public Health* 70:1249-60, 1980.

84. Hemenway D, Solnick SJ: Fuzzy dice, dream cars, and indecent gestures: correlates of driver behavior? *Accident Analysis and Prevention* 25: 161-70, 1993.

85. Henderson R, Burg A: *Vision and audition in driving*, Washington, DC, 1974, Department of Transportation.

86. Hennessy D: *Vision testing of renewal applicants: crashes predicted when compensation for impairment is inadequate*, Sacramento, CA, 1995, California Department of Motor Vehicles.

87. Hiller R, Sperduto RD, et al: Epidemiologic associations with cataract in the 1971-1972 National Health and Nutrition Examination Survey, *Am J Epidemiol* 118:238-49, 1983.

88. Hills BL, Burg A: *A reanalysis of California driver vision data: general findings*, Los Angeles, 1977, Transport and Road Research Laboratory.

89. Hofstetter HW: Visual acuity and highway accidents, *J Am Optom Assoc* 47:887-93, 1976.

90. Hofstetter HW: The correlation of traffic accidents with visual acuity, *Optom Monthly* 69: 161-6, 1978.

91. Holder AR: Disclosure of confidential information, *JAMA* 216:385-6, 1971.

92. Hoyer WJ, Plude DJ: Aging and the allocation of attentional resources in visual information-processing. In Sekuler R, Kline D, Dismukes K, editors: *Aging and human visual function*, New York, 1982, Alan R Liss.

93. Hu H: Effects of ultraviolet radiation, *Med Clin North Am* 74:509-14, 1990.

94. Hu PS, Young JR, Lu A: *Highway crash rates and age-related driver limitations: literature review and evaluation of databases*, Oak Ridge, TN, 1994, Oak Ridge National Laboratory.

95. Hulburt MFG, Vernon SA: Passing the DVLC field regulations following bilateral pan-retinal photocoagulation in diabetics, *Eye* 6:456-60, 1992.

96. Hyman LG, Lilienfeld AM, et al: Senile macular degeneration: a case-control study, *Am J Epidemiol* 118:213-27, 1983.

97. Jackson GR, Owsley C: Visual dysfunction, neurodegenerative diseases, and aging, *Neurol Clin* 21:709-28, 2003.

98. Janke MK: Safety effects of relaxing California's clean-record requirement for driver license renewal by mail, *Accident Analysis and Prevention* 22:335-49, 1990.

99. Janke MK: Accidents, mileage and the exaggeration of risk, *Accident Analysis and Prevention* 23:183-8, 1991.

100. Janke MK: Assessing medically impaired older drivers in a licensing-agency setting, *Accident Analysis and Prevention* 23:183-8, 1991.

101. Javitt JC, Street DA, et al: National outcomes of cataract extraction, *Ophthalmology* 101:100-6, 1994.

102. Jette AM, Branch LG: A ten-year follow-up of driving patterns among the community-dwelling elderly, *Hum Factors* 34:25-31, 1992.

103. Jick H, Hunter JR, et al: Sedating drugs and automobile accidents leading to hospitalization, *Am J Public Health* 71:1399-400, 1981.

104. Johnson CA, Keltner JL: Incidence of visual field loss in 20,000 eyes and its relationship to driving performance, *Arch Ophthalmol* 101: 371-5, 1983.

105. Johnson CA, Marshall D Jr: Aging effects for opponent mechanisms in the central visual fields, *Optom Vis Sci* 72:75-82, 1995.

106. Kahn HA, Leibowitz HM, et al: The Framingham Eye Study. I. Outline and major prevalence findings, *Am J Epidemiol* 106:17-32, 1997.

107. Kane RL, Kane RA, et al: Prevention and the elderly: risk factors. *Health Services Research* 19:945-1006, 1985.

108. Kanouse DE: Improving safety for older motorists by means of information and market forces. In *Transportation in an aging society, vol 2*, Washington, DC, 1988, Transportation Research Board.

109. Kanski JJ: *Clinical ophthalmology*, London, 1989, Butterworth-Heinemann.

110. Katz RT, Golden RS, et al: Driving safety after brain damage: follow-up of twenty-two patients with matched controls, *Arch Phys Med Rehabil* 71:133-7, 1990.

111. Kelsey SL, Janke MK: Driver license renewal by mail in California, *J Safety Res* 14:65-82, 1983.

112. Kelsey SL, Janke MK, Peck RC, et al: License extensions for clean-record drivers: a 4-year follow-up, *J Safety Res* 16:1491-67, 1985.

113. Keltner JL, Johnson CA: Visual function, driving safety, and the elderly, *Ophthalmology* 94:1180-8, 1987.

114. Kini MM, Leibowitz HM, et al: Prevalence of senile cataract, diabetic retinopathy, senile macular degeneration and open-angle glaucoma in the Framingham Eye Study, *Am J Ophthalmol* 85:28-34, 1978.

115. Klein BE, Klein R: Cataracts and macular degeneration in older Americans, *Arch Ophthalmol* 100:571-3, 1982.

116. Klein R: Age-related eye disease, visual impairment, and driving in the elderly, *Hum Factors* 33:521-5, 1991.

117. Klein R, Klein BEK, et al: Prevalence of age-related maculopathy: the Beaver Dam Eye Study, *Ophthalmology* 99:933-43, 1992.

118. Kline DW: Visual aging and the visibility of highway signs, *Exp Aging Res* 17:80-1, 1991.

119. Kline DW: Optimizing the visibility of displays for older observers, *Exp Aging Res* 20:11-23, 1994.

120. Kline DW, Kline TJB, et al: Vision, aging, and driving: the problems of older drivers, *J Gerontol Psychol Sci* 47:27-34, 1992.

121. Koepsell TD, Wolf ME, et al: Medical conditions and motor vehicle collision injuries in older adults, *J Am Geriatr Soc* 42:695-700, 1994.

122. Kosnik WD, Sekuler R, et al: Self-reported visual problems of older drivers, *Hum Factors* 32:597-608, 1990.

123. Kosnik W, Winslow L, et al: Visual changes in daily life throughout adulthood, *J Gerontol Psychol Sci* 43:P63-70, 1988.

124. Krause RA, Shelley MC II, Horton G, et al: *Positive guidance: new visions for safer highways: the report of the National Advisory Task Force on Positive Guidance,* Lexington, KY, 1990, The Council of State Governments, Center for Transportation.

125. Kuhl J: Aging and models of control: the hidden costs of wisdom. In Baltes MM, Baltes PB, editors: *The psychology of control and aging,* Hillsdale, NJ, 1986, Lawrence Erlbaum, pp 1-33.

126. Legh-Smith J, Wade DT, et al: Driving after a stroke, *J Royal Soc Med* 79:200-3, 1986.

127. Lerner N: Giving the older driver enough perception-reaction time, *Exp Aging Res* 20: 25-33, 1994.

128. Leske MC: The epidemiology of open-angle glaucoma: a review, *Am J Epidemiol* 118:166-91, 1983.

129. Leske MC, Sperduto RD: The epidemiology of senile cataracts: a review, *Am J Epidemiol* 118:152-165, 1983.

130. Levy DT, Vernick JS, et al: Relationship between driver's license renewal policies and fatal crashes involving drivers 70 years or older, *JAMA* 274:1026-30, 1995.

131. Lings S, Dupont E: Driving with Parkinson's disease, *Acta Neurol Scand* 86:33-9, 1992.

132. Liu IY, White L, et al: The association of age-related macular degeneration and lens opacities in the aged, *Am J Public Health* 79:765-9, 1989.

133. Lovie-Kitchin JE: Validity and reliability of visual acuity measurements, *Ophthalmol Physiol Optics* 8:363-70, 1988.

134. Lucas-Blaustein MJ, Filipp CL, et al: Driving in patients with dementia, *J Am Geriatr Soc* 36:1087-91, 1988.

135. Madden DJ, Allen PA: Aging and the speed/accuracy relation in visual search: evidence for an accumulator model, *Optom Vis Sci* 72:210-6, 1995.

136. Mader S: Hearing impairment in elderly persons, *J Am Geriatr Soc* 32:548-53, 1984.

137. Mangione CM, Phillips RS, et al: Development of the "activities of daily vision" scale, *Med Care* 30:1111-26, 1992.

138. Mariner WK: Access to health care and equal protection of the law: the need for a new heightened scrutiny, *Am J Law Med* 12:345-80, 1986.

139. Marottoli RA: Driving safety in elderly individuals, *Connecticut Medicine* 57:277-80, 1993.

140. Marottoli RA, Cooney LM, et al: Predictors of automobile crashes and moving violations among elderly drivers, *Ann Intern Med* 121: 842-6, 1994.

141. Marottoli RA, Ostfeld AM, et al: Driving cessation and changes in mileage driven among elderly individuals, *J Gerontol Soc Sci* 48:S255-60, 1993.

142. Martinez GS, Campbell AJ, et al: Prevalence of ocular disease in a population of study subjects 65 years old and older, *Am J Ophthalmol* 94: 181-9, 1982.

143. Martinez R: Older drivers and physicians, *JAMA* 274:1060, 1995.

144. Mattis S: Mental status examination for organic mental syndrome in the elderly patient. In Bellak L, Karasu TB, editors: *Geriatric psychiatry,* New York, 1976, Grune & Stratton.

145. Mausner JS, Kramer S: *Mausner & Bahn: epidemiology—an introductory text,* Philadelphia, 1985, W.B. Saunders.

146. McCoy GF, Johnstone RA, et al: Injury to the elderly in road traffic accidents, *J Trauma* 29: 494-7, 1989.

147. McGwin G Jr, Scilley K, et al: Impact of cataract surgery on self-reported visual difficulties: comparison with a no-surgery reference group, *J Cataract Refract Surg* 29:941-8, 2003.

148. McKinlay JB, McKinlay SM, et al: A review of the evidence concerning the impact of medical measures on recent mortality and morbidity in the United States, *Int J Health Services* 19: 181-208, 1989.

149. Mendola JD, Cronin-Golomb A, et al: Prevalence of visual deficits in Alzheimer's disease, *Optom Vis Sci* 72:155-67, 1995.

150. Mor V, Murphy J, et al: Risk of functional decline among well elders, *J Clin Epidemiol* 42:895-904, 1989.

151. Mortimer RG, Fell JC: Older drivers: their night fatal crash involvement and risk, *Accident Analysis & Prevention* 21:273-82, 1989.

152. National Advisory Eye Council: *Vision research: a national plan: 1994-1998*, Bethesda, MD, 1993, National Institutes of Health.

153. National Research Council and Institute of Medicine: *Injury in America: a continuing health problem*, Washington, DC, 1985, National Academy Press.

154. National Safety Council: *Crash facts 1992*, Chicago, 1992.

155. National Society to Prevent Blindness: *Vision problems in the United States—1980: data analysis*, New York, 1980, National Society to Prevent Blindness.

156. Nelson DE, Sacks JF, et al: Required vision testing for older drivers, *N Engl J Med* 326:1784-5, 1992.

157. Nelson TM, Evelyn B: Experimental intercomparisons of younger driver perceptions, *Int J Aging Hum Dev* 36:239-53, 1993.

158. Ng SH: Information-seeking triggered by age, *Int J Aging Hum Dev* 33:269-77, 1991.

159. Odenheimer GL, Beaudet M, et al: Performance-based driving evaluation of the elderly driver: safety, reliability, and validity, *J Gerontol Med Sci* 49:M153-9, 1994.

160. O'Hanlon JF: Discussion of medications and the safety of the older driver by Ray et al, *Hum Factors* 34:49-51, 1992.

161. Ostrom M, Eriksson A: Single-vehicle crashes and alcohol: a retrospective study of passenger car crashes in northern Sweden, *Accident Analysis and Prevention* 25:171-176, 1993.

162. Overley ET: *Prospective follow-up of older drivers: relationship between vision and future vehicle crashes*, Birmingham, AL, 1994, University of Alabama.

163. Owens DA, Helmers G, Sivak M: Intelligent vehicle highway systems: a call for user-centered design, *Ergonomics* 36:363-9, 1993.

164. Owsley C, Ball K: Assessing visual function in the older driver, *Clin Geriatr Med* 9:389-401, 1993.

165. Owsley C, Burton KB: *Aging and spatial contrast sensitivity: underlying mechanisms and implications for everyday life*, New York, 1991, Plenum Press.

166. Owsley C, Ball K, et al: Visual/cognitive correlates of vehicle accidents in older drivers, *Psychol Aging* 6:403-15, 1991.

167. Owsley C, McGwin G Jr, et al: Impact of cataract surgery on motor vehicle crash involvement by older adults, *JAMA* 288:841-9, 2002.

168. Owsley C, Sekuler R, et al: Contrast sensitivity throughout adulthood, *Vis Res* 23:689-99, 1983.

169. Owsley C, Stalvey BT, et al: Visual risk factors for crash involvement in older drivers with cataracts, *Arch Ophthalmol* 119:881-7, 2001.

170. Oswley C, Stalvey BT, et al: The efficacy of an educational intervention in promoting self-regulation among high risk older drivers, *Accident Analysis and Prevention* 35:393-400, 2003.

171. Parasuraman R: Attention and driving skills in aging and Alzheimer's disease, *Hum Factors* 33:539-57, 1991.

172. Parmet WE: Discrimination and disability: the challenges of the ADA, *Law, Medicine and Health Care* 24:274-81, 1991.

173. Pelli DG, Robson JG, et al: The design of a new letter chart for measuring contrast sensitivity, *Clin Vis Sci* 2:187-99, 1988.

174. Pelli DG, Rubin GS, et al: Predicting the contrast sensitivity of low vision observers, *J Opt Soc Am* 3:P56, 1986.

175. Perneger T, Smith GS: The driver's role in fatal two-car crashes: a paired case-control study, *Am J Epidemiol* 134:1138-45, 1991.

176. Peters HB: Vision screening with a Snellen chart, *Am J Optom Arch Am Acad Optom* 38: 487-505, 1961.

177. Petrucelli E, Malinowski M: *Status of medical review in driver licensing: policies, programs and standards*. Springfield, VA, 1992, National Highway Traffic Safety Administration, p 1.

178. Pitts DG: The effects of aging on selected visual functions: dark adaptation, visual acuity, stereopsis, and brightness contrast. In Sekuler R, Kline D, Dismukes K, editors: *Aging and human visual function*, New York, 1982, Alan R. Liss.

179. Pitts DG, Cullen AP, et al: Ocular effects of ultraviolet radiation from 295 to 365 nm, *Invest Ophthalmol Vis Sci* 16:932-9, 1977.

180. Powe NR, Tielsch JM, et al: Rigor of research methods in studies of the effectiveness and safety of cataract extraction with intraocular lens implantation, *Arch Ophthalmol* 112:228-38, 1994.

181. Radloff LS: The CES-D scale: a self-report depression scale for research in the general population, *Appl Psychol Meas* 1:385-401, 1977.

182. Raffle PAB: The cost of casualties to the community, *J Royal Soc Med* 84:390-3, 1991.

183. Ray WA: Medication and the safety of the older driver: is there a basis for concern? *Hum Factors* 34:33-47, 1992.

184. Ray WA, Fought RL, et al: Psychoactive drugs and the risk of injurious motor vehicle crashes in elderly drivers, *Am J Epidemiol* 136:873-83, 1992.

185. Reason J, Manstead A, et al: Errors and violations on the roads: a real distinction? *Ergonomics* 33:1315-32, 1990.

186. Reese JH: *The legal nature of a driver's license*, Washington, DC, 1965, Automotive Safety Foundation.

187. Reinfurt DW, Stewart JR, et al: The economy as a factor in motor vehicle fatalities, suicides, and homicides, *Accident Analysis and Prevention* 23:453-62, 1991.

188. Retchin SM, Anapolle J: An overview of the older driver, *Clin Geriatr Med* 9:279-96, 1993.

189. Reuben DB: Dementia and driving, *J Am Geriatr Soc* 39:1137-8, 1991.

190. Rice D, Jones B: *Vision screening of driver's license renewal applicants*, Salem, OR, 1984, Department of Transportation.

191. Rice DP, Mackenzie EJ, et al: *Cost of injury in the United States: a report to Congress*, San Francisco, CA, 1989, Institute for Health & Aging, University of California and Injury Prevention Center, The Johns Hopkins University.

192. Rigdon JE: Car trouble: older drivers pose growing risk on roads as their numbers rise, *The Wall Street Journal* p A1, Oct. 29, 1993.

193. Ritchie K: The screening of cognitive impairment in the elderly: a critical review of current methods, *J Clin Epidemiol* 41:635-43, 1988.

194. Roberts HJ: *The causes, ecology and prevention of traffic accidents*, Springfield, IL, 1971, Charles C Thomas.

195. Rohaly AM, Owsley C: Modeling the contrast sensitivity functions of older adults, *J Optom Soc Am* 10:1591-9, 1993.

196. Rosenbloom S: The mobility needs of the elderly. In *Transportation Research Board: transportation in an aging society*, Washington, DC, 1988, National Research Council.

197. Rosenbloom S: Transportation needs of the elderly population, *Clin Geriatr Med* 9:297-310, 1993.

198. Rynders MC, Grosvenor T, et al: Stability of the Stile-Crawford function in a unilateral amblyopic subject over a 38-year period: a case study, *Optom Vis Sci* 72:177-85, 1995.

199. Sachsenweger M, Sachsenweger U: Stereoscopic acuity in ocular pursuit of moving objects, *Documenta Ophthalmologica* 78:1-133, 1991.

200. Sadun AA, Borchert M, et al: Assessment of visual impairment in patients with Alzheimer's disease, *Am J Ophthalmol* 104:113-20, 1987.

201. Scherr PA, Albert MD, et al: Correlates of cognitive function in an elderly community population, *Am J Epidemiol* 128:1084-101, 1988.

202. Schieber F: High-priority research and development needs for maintaining the safety and mobility of older drivers, *Exp Aging Res* 20: 35-43, 1994.

203. Schlotterer G, Moscovitch M, et al: Visual processing deficits as assessed by spatial frequency and backward masking in normal aging and Alzheimer's disease, *Brain* 107:309-25, 1983.

204. Shinar D: *Driver vision and accident involvement: new findings with new vision tests. Proceedings of the American Association for Automotive Medicine 22nd Conference and the International Association for Accident and Traffic Medicine VII Conference*, Ann Arbor, MI, 1978, American Association for Automotive Medicine.

205. Shinar D, Schieber F: Visual requirements for safety and mobility of older drivers, *Hum Factors* 33:507-19, 1991.

206. Shipp M: Potential human and economic cost-savings attributable to vision testing policies for driver license renewal, *Optom Vis Sci* 75:103-18, 1998.

207. Shipp MD, Penchansky R: Vision testing and the elderly driver: is there a problem meriting policy change? *J Am Optom Assoc* 66:343-51, 1995.

208. Shute RH, Woodhouse JM: Visual fitness to drive after stroke or head injury, *Ophthalmol Physiol Optics* 10:327-32, 1990.

209. Sims RV, McGwin G Jr, et al: Exploratory study of incident vehicle crashes among older drivers, *J Gerontol A Biol Sci Med Sci* 55:M22-7, 2000.

210. Sivak M: A review of literature on nighttime conspicuity and effects of retroreflectorization, *HSRI Research Review* 10:9-17, 1979.

211. Sjögren H, Björnstig U, et al: Elderly in the traffic environment: analysis of fatal crashes in northern Sweden, *Accident Analysis and Prevention* 25:177-88, 1993.

212. Smith GS, Barss P: Unintentional injuries in developing countries: the epidemiology of a neglected problem, *Epidemiol Rev* 13:228-66, 1991.

213. Sommer A: Eye care for the elderly: looking better! seeing better! *Ophthalmology* 94:1178-9, 1987.

214. Stutts JC, Martell C: Older driver population and crash involvement trends, 1974-1988, *Accident Analysis and Prevention* 24:317-27, 1992.

215. Szlyk JP, Alexander KR, et al: Assessment of driving performance in patients with retinitis pigmentosa, *Arch Ophthalmol* 110:1709-13, 1992.

216. Szlyk JP, Fishman GA, et al: Evaluation of driving performance in patients with juvenile macular dystrophies, *Arch Ophthalmol* 111: 207-12, 1993.

217. Tasman W, Jaeger EA, editors: Acquired macular disease. In *Duane's clinical ophthalmology,* Philadelphia, 1989, J. B. Lippincott.

218. Tasman W, Jaeger EA, editors: Clinical types of cataracts. In *Duane's clinical ophthalmology,* Philadelphia, 1989, J. B. Lippincott.

219. Tasman W, Jaeger EA, editors: Glaucoma: general concepts. In *Duane's clinical ophthalmology,* Philadelphia, 1989, J. B. Lippincott.

220. Taylor HR, Muñoz B, et al: Visible light and risk of age-related macular degeneration, *Trans Am Ophthalmol Soc* 88:163-77, 1990.

221. Taylor HR, West SK, et al: Effect of ultraviolet radiation on cataract formation, *N Engl J Med* 319:1429-33, 1988.

222. Taylor HR, West SK, et al: The long term effects of visible light on the eye, *Arch Ophthalmol* 110:99-104, 1992.

223. Teets MK, editor: *Highway Statistics 1994,* Washington, DC, 1994, Federal Highway Administration.

224. Tennehouse DJ: The physician's duty to warn: a new twist, *Survey Ophthalmol* 28:317-8, 1984.

225. Teret SP, Jacobs M: Prevention and torts: the role of litigation in injury control, *Law, Medicine & Health Care* 17:17-22, 1989.

226. Tobimatsu S: Aging and pattern visual evoked potentials, *Optom Vis Sci* 72:192-7, 1995.

227. Transportation Research Board: *Transportation in an aging society: improving mobility and safety for older persons,* Washington, DC, 1988, National Research Council.

228. Transportation Research Board: *Committee on the safety and mobility of older drivers,* Washington, DC, 1993, National Research Council.

229. Transportation Research Board-National Research Council: *Vision screening for driver licensure,* Washington, DC, 1988, National Research Council.

230. Tuokko H, Tallman K, et al: An examination of driving records in a dementia clinic., *J Gerontol Soc Sci* 50B:S173-81, 1995.

231. Uhlmann RF, Larson EB, et al: Relationship of hearing impairment to dementia and cognitive dysfunction in older adults, *JAMA* 261:1916-9, 1989.

232. Underwood M: The older driver—clinical assessment and injury prevention, *Arch Internal Med* 152:735-40, 1992.

233. Ungar PE: Standardizing and regularizing driver vision test. In Gale AG, editor: *Vision in vehicles,* New York, 1986, Elsevier Science.

234. U.S. Department of Commerce, Economics, and Statistics Administration, Bureau of the Census: *1990 census of population: social and economic characteristics—United States,* Washington, DC, 1993, U.S. Government Printing Office.

235. U.S. Department of Transportation: Guidelines for motor vehicle administrators. In *State and provincial licensing systems: comparative data 1990,* Washington, DC, 1990, National Highway Traffic Safety Administration.

236. U.S. Department of Transportation: *State and provincial licensing systems: comparative data 1990,* Washington, DC, 1990, National Highway Traffic Safety Administration.

237. U.S. Department of Transportation: *Addressing the safety issues related to younger and older drivers,* Washington, DC, 1993, National Highway Traffic Safety Administration.

238. van den Berg TJ: Analysis of intraocular straylight, especially in relation to age, *Optom Vis Sci* 72:52-9, 1995.

239. Viano DC, Culver CC, et al: Involvement of older drivers in multivehicle side-impact crashes, *Accident Analysis and Prevention* 22: 177-88, 1990.

240. Vinding T: Age-related macular degeneration—macular changes, prevalence and sex ratio, *Acta Opthalmologica* 67:609-16, 1989.

241. Wallace RB, Retchin SM: A geriatric and gerontologic perspective on the effects of medical conditions on older drivers: discussion of Waller, *Hum Factors* 34:17-24, 1992.

242. Waller JA: Chronic medical conditions and traffic safety: review of the California experience, *N Engl J Med* 273:1413-20, 1965.

243. Waller JA: Cardiovascular disease, aging and traffic accidents, *J Chronic Dis* 20:615-20, 1967.

244. Waller JA: Research and other issues concerning effects of medical conditions on elderly drivers, *Hum Factors* 34:3-15, 1992.

245. Waller PF: The older driver, *Hum Factors* 33: 499-505, 1991.

246. Waller P, Gilbert E, Li K: *An Evaluation of the Keystone Vision Tester with recommendations for driver's licensing programs,* Raleigh, NC, 1980, North Carolina Department of Transportation.

247. Weale RA: Senile ocular changes, cell death, and vision. In Sekuler R, Kline D, Dismukes K, editors: *Aging and human visual function,* New York, 1982, Alan R. Liss.

248. Wells JK, Williams AF, et al: Coverage gaps in seat belt use laws, *Am J Public Health* 79:332-33, 1989.

249. West CG, Gildengorin G, et al: Vision and driving self-restriction in older adults, *J Am Geriatr Soc* 51:1348-55, 2003.

250. Weymouth FW: Effect of age on visual acuity. In Hirsch MJ, Wick RE, editors: *Vision of the aging patient*, Philadelphia, 1960, Chilton, pp 37-62.

251. Williams AF, Carsten O: Driver age and crash involvement, *Am J Public Health* 79:326-7, 1989.

252. Wilson T, Smith T: Driving after stroke, *Int Rehabil Med* 5:170-7, 1983.

253. Wing KR: *The law and the public's health,* Ann Arbor, MI, 1990, Health Administration Press.

254. Wojciechowski R, Trick GL, et al: Topography of the age-related decline in motion sensitivity, *Optom Vis Sci* 72:67-74, 1995.

255. Wood JM, Lovie-Kitchin JE: Evaluation of the efficacy of contrast sensitivity measures for the detection of early primary open-angle glaucoma, *Optom Vis Sci* 69:175-81, 1992.

256. Wood JM, Troutbeck R: Effect of restriction of the binocular visual field on driving performance, *Ophthalmol Physiol Optics* 12:291-8, 1992.

257. World Health Organization: *International classification of impairments, disabilities, and handicaps: a manual of classification relating to consequences of disease,* Geneva, 1980, World Health Organization.

258. Young RW: The family of sunlight-related eye diseases, *Optom Vis Sci* 71:125-44, 1994.

259. Zador PL, Ciccone MA: Automobile driver fatalities in frontal impacts: air bags compared with manual belts, *Am J Public Health* 83:661-6, 1993.

260. Zeidler F, Pletschen B, et al: Development of a new injury cost scale, *Accident Analysis and Prevention* 25:675-87, 1993.

261. Zhang L: Aging, background luminance, and threshold-duration functions for detection of low spatial frequency sinusoidal gratings, *Optom Vis Sci* 72:198-204, 1995.

# CHAPTER 17

# Nutrition and Older Adults

**BARBARA CAFFERY**

**B**y the year 2030, 57 million Americans will be aged 65 years or older. The increasing number of older adults presents the health care community with significant challenges. Health care providers are increasingly looking for ways to prevent the disease processes that occur with age. The regulation of nutritional status is one of the forefronts in this area.

One of the most devastating occurrences in later life is loss of vision. The Blue Mountain Study assessed the impact of visual impairment on health-related quality of life and determined that noncorrectable vision impairment was associated with reduced functional status and well-being, with a magnitude comparable to major medical conditions.[13] Thankfully, particularly in eye care, nutrition is playing a greater role in the prevention of vision loss. Macular degeneration stands out as the most important recent example in which the treatment of the dry form of this devastating disease includes taking vitamin supplements. Clearly, understanding the role of malnutrition, both undernutrition and obesity, in older adults on age-related disease, including ocular diseases, is important for all health care providers.

Age-related vision loss is most commonly seen with cataract, macular degeneration, glaucoma, retinal vascular disease, and diabetic retinopathy. Research suggests that nutrition has a role to play in all these conditions except glaucoma, a condition in which the relations are not yet clear. The interaction of nutrition and these diseases is complex. Inadequate antioxidant intake can lead to excess free radical formation that has a direct impact on cataracts and macular degeneration. Free radicals also play a role in the formation of arterial plaques and therefore contribute to vascular causes of vision loss, such as retinal vein and arterial occlusions, and may also influence the course of macular degeneration. Excess fat intake can cause increased blockage of arteries that may cause retinal and vein vascular occlusions. Poor nutritional intake that exacerbates age-related suppression of the immune system allows inflammatory processes such as those that occur in Bruch's membrane in the macula to progress. Obesity is a risk factor for diabetes and the complications of retinopathy. Thus the overall health and nutritional status of older patients must be of concern to promote the maintenance of good vision.

Older adults are particularly prone to nutritional problems because of the frequency of poverty, loneliness, neglect, and mental disabilities. In fact, the magnitude of the problem of malnutrition cannot be overestimated. Ryan et al,[57] in a study of older adults in the United States, determined that "poor nutrition is a major problem in the nation's elderly." Thirty-seven percent to 40% of the population of community-dwelling individuals older than 65 years have inadequate nutritional intake.

Of equal importance is the problem of obesity. The percentage of older people with obesity will likely continue to grow as the problem of excess weight occurs in younger and younger people. Eighty-seven percent of older Americans have diabetes, hypertension, dyslipidemia, or a combination of these diseases. All these diseases can contribute to vision loss and are controlled in part by diet and exercise. The new epidemic of type 2 diabetes in North America has obesity as one of its major risk factors. The Third National Health and Nutrition Examination Survey (NHANES III, 1988 to 1994) indicated that 34% of women and 44% of men are considered overweight in the United States, and an additional 27% of women and 34% of men are considered obese. Older black American women and poor women have the higher rates of obesity. An added risk factor in older adults is that fat tends to distribute around the central areas of the body. This increases the risk for diabetes, hypertension, and lipid abnormalities.[59] Certainly nutrition plays a large role in the treatment of these conditions, as much of the morbidity associated with these diseases can be reduced by diet and weight loss.[55]

Recognizing that not all the available research indicates that obesity is a risk factor for all diseases in older adults is important. For example, some research suggests that increased weight is a protective factor for hip fracture.[26] This type of information highlights the fact that, especially in the geriatric population, each case must be considered on an individual basis. Generally, however, for the purposes of this chapter the ideas of normal weight and a healthy diet are stressed as important to long-term ocular health.

This chapter begins with some terms and definitions, followed by a rationale for understanding the importance of nutrition in older adults when providing primary health care to this population. The review of the physiology of aging emphasizes free radical formation and immunosenescence because of their impact on vision loss. The influence of nutrition on these processes is discussed. Finally, a clinical approach to understanding the risk factors for malnutrition in older adults and for and formulating a history that will screen for malnutrition is presented.

## DEFINITIONS AND TERMS

The following terms and their meanings are used throughout this chapter:

Nutrition: A function of living plants and animals that consists of taking in and assimilating, through chemical changes (metabolism), material by which tissue is built up and energy liberated; its successive stages are known as digestion, absorption, assimilation, and secretion.

Malnutrition: Faulty nutrition resulting from malassimilation, poor diet, or overeating.

Undernutrition: A form of malnutrition resulting from a reduced supply of food or from inability to digest, assimilate, and use the necessary elements.

Obesity: Fatness, corpulence, general adiposity, or an abnormal increase of fat in the subcutaneous connective tissue. A body mass index of 25 to 29.9 is considered overweight, and a body mass index of 30 or greater is considered obese.[43,45]

Weight loss (clinically important): More than 10 pounds in 6 months or 4% to 5% of body weight in 1 year.

Body mass index (BMI): The ratio of weight in kilograms to height (in meters squared)

Low BMI: A BMI of less than 17 is definitive for protein-energy undernutrition (PEU) and for being consistent with but not diagnostic of PEU if between 17 and 20.

Sarcopenia: Age-related loss of muscle mass.

Cachexia: Body cell mass is diminished as a function of illness, injury, or disease; an active cytokine-mediated disease.

Wasting: Loss of body cell mass without increased cytokine production.

Protein-energy undernutrition (PEU): Insufficient intake of foods with evidence of physical wasting and biochemical markers such as reduced albumin.

## AGING EFFECTS ON NUTRITIONAL REQUIREMENTS

A decline in organ function accompanies the aging process. Those occurring in the gastrointestinal system influence the nutritional needs of older adults.

Several studies have shown that older patients do not require as many calories per day to maintain their weight. The Baltimore Longitudinal Study of Aging showed a decrease in energy intake in older adults that was a result of both reduced physical activity and decreased basal metabolism.[42] The recommended energy intake from the Recommended Dietary Allowance (RDA) is 2300 kcal for the reference 77-kg older man and 1900 kcal for the reference 65-kg woman aged 51 years or older.[23]

High-protein diets are often less well digested and absorbed in older adults.[69] A daily intake of 1 g/kg appears to meet the needs of the older population.[65] Carbohydrate absorption is also slightly impaired with aging.[21] The digestion and absorption of fat is equivalent to that of young adults when measured at normal consumption levels of 100 g. At higher dietary levels of more than 120 g/day, older adults show less fat absorption than young adults; institutionalized older persons may absorb even less.[51,58] The RDA has no recommendations for fat, but a prudent diet is widely believed to have 30% or fewer calories from fat.

Inadequate vitamin status is a common finding in older adults that relates to either poor food choices or inadequate dietary intake.[63] Table 17-1 describes the recommended intake of various vitamins and an assessment of whether the recommendation is appropriate for older

adults. Mineral intake has also been assessed, and Table 17-2 shows the standards and how they apply to older adults.

Nutritional intake in older adults is obviously a complex subject. As with all assessments in this population, individual lifestyles must be considered when analyzing and recommending dietary advice.

## DOES MANIPULATION OF DIET WORK IN OLDER ADULTS?

As clinicians consider the addition of nutritional counseling to the routine care of patients, understanding the rationale behind this type of advice is important. If, after a certain stage of life, does all the hard work involved in modifying food intake mean anything to the patient's well-being? The important question is whether manipulation of the diet in older persons has beneficial effects. This issue has been addressed in the general medical literature, especially in the area of nutrition and mortality rate. Research also shows that a healthy diet and weight control do affect the morbidity associated with

**TABLE 17-1**

### Estimate of Adequacy of RDA for Vitamins in Older Adults

| Vitamin | Current RDA for Age ≥51* | Adequacy of RDA for Older Adults | Physiological Reason for Change |
|---|---|---|---|
| Vitamin A | 800-1000 µg | May be too high | Change in unstirred water layer may lead to increased absorption in older adults; decreased uptake by the liver of newly absorbed vitamin A |
| Vitamin D | 5 µg | Is too low | Lack of sun exposure, decreased number of intestinal vitamin D receptors, reduced vitamin D absorption, reduced vitamin $D_3$ synthesis in skin, and impaired renal 1-$\alpha$ hydroxylation suggest that the dietary requirement might be higher |
| Vitamin E | 8-10 mg | I/C data† | — |
| Vitamin K | 65-80 µg‡ | I/C data† | — |
| Thiamin | 1-1.2 mg | Adequate | — |
| Riboflavin | 1.2-1.4 mg | Adequate | — |
| Niacin | 13-15 mg | I/C data† | — |
| Vitamin $B_6$ | 1.6-2.0 mg | Is too low | Serum homocysteine levels rise when dietary vitamin $B_6$ is <2.0 mg/day, and poor response to $B_6$ supplements in normal range suggests altered absorption or metabolism |
| Folate | 180-200 µg | May be too low | |
| Vitamin $B_{12}$ | 2.0 µg | May be too low | |
| Ascorbate | 60 mg | Adequate | — |
| Biotin | 30-100 µg | I/C data† | — |
| Pantothenate | 4-7 mg‡ | I/C data† | — |

Amounts are from 1989 RDA guidelines.
*RDA for both men and women.
†Insufficient or conflicting data.
‡Estimated safe and adequate daily dietary intake.

**TABLE 17-2**

### Estimate of Adequacy of RDA for Minerals in Older Adults

| Mineral | Current RDA for Age ≥51* | Adequacy of RDA for Older Adults | Physiological Reason for Change |
|---|---|---|---|
| Calcium | 800 mg | Too low | |
| Iron | 10 mg | Adequate | |
| Zinc | 12-15 mg | Adequate | |
| Copper | 1.5-3.0 mg† | Adequate | |
| Selenium | 55-70 µg | Adequate | |
| Magnesium | 280-350 mg | Too high | |
| Chromium | 50-250 µg† | Too high | |

From Russell RM, Suter PM: Vitamin requirements in elderly people: an update, *Am J Clin Nutr* 58:4-14, 1993.
*RDA for both men and women.
†Estimated safe and adequate daily dietary intake.
Amounts are from 1989 RDA guidelines.

diabetes in older adults and other populations. This more directly relates to the issue of vision loss and diabetic retinopathy. Finally, the use of antioxidant supplements is considered standard of care in macular degeneration.

Some of the most convincing work comes from the literature on undernutrition and mortality rate. Older patients have been observed for the markers of undernutrition that include weight loss, morphometric changes, poor nutritional intake, and biochemical measures of malnutrition such as albumin, transferrin, and retinal binding protein. The syndromes of undernutrition include body composition changes with aging or sarcopenia, cachexia, wasting, protein-energy malnutrition, and failure to thrive.

In the outpatient setting, commonly used definitions of undernutrition include loss of more than 10 pounds in 6 months, loss of 4% to 5% of body weight in 1 year, or loss of 7.5% of body weight in 6 months. This sudden drop in weight has a clinical importance, as demonstrated by a study of veterans. A 4-year cohort study determined that the annual incidence of involuntary weight loss among veterans monitored in an outpatient setting was 13.1%. In a 2-year follow-up period, those with involuntary weight loss had an increased risk of death that was 28% among those who lost weight versus 11% among those who did not.[68] Clearly, nutrition does indeed have a large impact on the well-being of older patients.

The morbidity research in diet and diabetes is another good example of the importance of nutritional status in older adults. Certainly the length of time that the disease has been present

contributes to the morbidity rate of diabetes. Older patients who have had diabetes for a longer time are therefore at higher risk for diabetic retinopathy. The impact of nutrition on the complications of diabetes is clear. The Diabetes Control and Complications Trial (DCCT) demonstrated that strict regulation of blood sugar with the frequent use of injections and proper diet dramatically reduces the complication rate.[1] This means that fewer patients will lose vision from diabetic retinopathy if they maintain a normal weight and a healthy diet.

The Age Related Eye Disease Study (AREDS) stated that "patients of any age who demonstrate extensive intermediate size drusen or who have advanced macular degeneration in one eye should consider taking a supplement."[29] The following antioxidants were recommended: 500 mg vitamin C, 400 IU vitamin E, 15 mg beta-carotene, 80 mg zinc, and 2 mg copper. The results show that in these populations, the supplements decreased the risk of advanced macular degeneration in 25% of the group.

Therefore, as research continues to suggest that healthy nutritional status in older patients is important for their general well-being and longevity as well as their continued good visual health, eye care practitioners will inevitably be more involved in their patients' nutritional status.

## THEORIES OF AGING AND THE NUTRITIONAL IMPACT

The importance of nutrition in the aging process can best be understood by observing the physiology of aging.

The process of aging that occurs in the body is complex and still only mildly understood. The process is slow and varied in individuals. It appears that our genes control the development and growth of our bodies until a certain age, at which point a new set of aging messages occur within cells and the body simply ages. The control of this time clock within our bodies is only beginning to be understood. With time, our bodies experience the loss of the viability of individual cells that then affect the function of the organ or tissue in which they are found. On a systemic level this can be seen as tumor formation in the lungs with the inhalation of pollutants such as cigarette smoke as the ability to control free radical oxidation deteriorates, or the incurable pneumonia that occurs when immune systems falter. At the ocular level the most visible example is cataract formation that occurs when the proteins are oxidized over time. Of greater concern is the macular degeneration that occurs because of a breakdown in free radical containment, vascular supply, and immune function.

The many theories of aging include inappropriate cellular proliferation, reduced basal metabolic rate, reduced rate of DNA repair, reduced rate of protein synthesis, increased catabolism, reduced immune response, and free radical damage. Although all these theories likely interrelate, the latter two theories of free radical damage and immunocompetency are the most important for this chapter in the understanding of age-related vision loss and the influence of nutrition.

Free radical formation and oxidative stress are part of both cataract and macular degeneration. Free radical formation also damages blood vessel walls and leads to cardiovascular disease, which in turn can affect the vascular supply to the retina and add to the problems of macular degeneration. This pathological condition may also induce retinal vascular diseases and contribute to the damage that occurs in diabetic retinopathy. Understanding the pathophysiological factors of these theories will help explain how nutrition can slow or prevent the end-stage pathologic condition.

## FREE RADICALS AND OXIDATIVE STRESS

Free radical formation and the subsequent oxidative stress have been implicated in human disease and the process of aging. Aging bodies have reduced defenses against such activity, and this explains in part why certain diseases are more prevalent in older adults.

Oxidative stress is a process in which molecules that are missing an electron take electrons from other molecules, resulting in a breakdown in cellular metabolism and function. The cells may completely malfunction and die, or their DNA may be altered to produce malfunctioning cells. The latter effect of oxidation can produce cancer cells that then replicate without control.

An atom that contains one or more orbital electrons with unpaired spin states defines the free radical species. The radical may be a very small molecule such as oxygen or nitric oxide, or may be part of a larger molecule such as a protein, carbohydrate, lipid, or nucleic acid. Some of the common free radicals are derived from oxygen (superoxide anion, hydroxy radical, peroxide radicals, singlet oxygen), hydrogen peroxide, carbon, nitrogen, and sulfur.

Free radical formation is a normal outcome of functioning cells within our bodies. For example, most cells produce superoxide anions with the necessary intracellular activities of microsomal and mitochondrial electron transport systems. Myeloid cells such as neutrophils and macrophages are especially prone to producing superoxide anions because, as they kill bacteria, their plasma membrane-bound electron transfer complex (reduced nicotinamide adenine dinucleotide phosphate oxidase) interacts with oxygen to produce this radical.

Although the body does form endogenous free radicals from within normally functioning cells, many exogenous sources of these destructive molecules exist over which more control can be exerted. These include cigarette smoke, smog, and sun-related ultraviolet radiation.

The natural occurrence of free radicals within the body is controlled by the natural antioxidants that are produced. The breakdown of this balance that occurs with aging allows disease processes to flourish.

### Various Sources of Free Radicals
#### Oxygen Species

The very act of breathing can create free radicals. Atmospheric oxygen is a radical, but it is unusual in that it is not particularly reactive with biological molecules. Its lack of aggressiveness is a result of the fact that the two orbital electrons participating in oxidation reactions have the same spin state. When atmospheric oxygen molecules do react, however, they produce a very reactive state called a superoxide anion. This superoxide anion can combine with other reactive species such as nitric acid, which is produced by macrophages, to yield even more reactive species.

Superoxide anion is quickly turned into hydrogen peroxide by superoxide dismutase, which is found universally in both the cytoplasm and the mitochondria of cells. Hydrogen peroxide can then diffuse over considerable distances and can pass membranes in the process. Hydrogen peroxide and superoxide anions can occur in extracellular space and in blood plasma as a result of the membrane-associated reaction in myeloid cells such as neutrophils and macrophages. Hydrogen peroxide is lethal to cells when the concentration is too high.

Hydroxyl radicals react with many biological macromolecules. The rate of reaction of the hydroxyl molecule is diffusion controlled, and therefore it reacts very closely to its site of production and is site specific.

Peroxyl radicals occur during the oxidation of lipids and are associated with the action of prostaglandin H synthetase in prostaglandin synthesis. The peroxyl radical species can diffuse large distances.

Singlet oxygen is formed by the oxidation of other partially reduced oxygen species, resulting in an oxygen molecule with paired electrons in the reactive orbit.[8]

Metals play a role in the modulation of free radical activity. In the presence of iron or copper, superoxide anion can give rise to a highly reactive hydroxyl radical species. Some forms of bound iron participate in this process readily, whereas other complexes of iron prevent it from occurring.

### Nitrogen Species

Nitric oxide is an abundant free radical that is an important biological signal in such physiological processes as smooth muscle relaxation and immune regulation.[4] The nitric oxide synthetase enzyme produces this species by an oxidative reaction that uses arginine as its substrate.

Nitric oxide is particularly active in macrophages and neutrophils. Cells that pro-

duce both superoxide anion and nitric oxide cause a great deal of activity when they are gathered in an inflammatory response. At these times, nitric oxide and superoxide anion may react together to produce the highly active peroxynitrate that attacks both protein cysteine and methionine.

The complexity of the oxidative stress reactions is a function of the number of radical species, the site of production, the action of enzymes, and the availability of transition metals.

### Effect of Free Radicals on Molecules

#### Carbohydrates

Hydroxyl radicals react with carbohydrates by randomly abstracting a hydrogen atom from one of the carbon atoms.[67] This leads to chain breaks in important molecules such as hyaluronic acid. This activity is documented in joints, where inflammation involving neutrophils produces large amounts of oxyradicals and an ensuing reduction in synovial fluid.

#### Nucleic Acids

Nucleic acids undergo reactions with hydroxyl radicals that produce breaks in the molecule. The base portion of the polymer may also be affected and is likely responsible for the genetic defects produced by oxidative stress. In fact, 8-hydroxyguanosine is often used as a marker for genetic defects in human beings. This molecule is a product of hydroxy radical attacks on DNA.

#### Proteins

Three main measurable events occur when proteins are damaged by free radical activity. First, aggressive radicals such as hydroxyl radicals can fragment proteins in plasma, and these can be identified and measured. This most often occurs with proline and histidine.[17] Second, proteins may contain metal binding sites that make them particularly prone to oxidative damage at those sites. When this occurs, the signal sequences that result can be recognized by specific cellular proteases.[15,61] Finally, many intracellular proteins have reactive sulfhydryl groups on specific cysteine residues that can be oxidized to specific disulfide forms that can be reduced again. Also, some proteins have a reactive methionine that can undergo reversible modification to methionine sulfoxide.[6]

*Lipids*

Lipid peroxidation of polyunsaturated lipids is a facile process. This oxidation affects materials present in dietary constituents and greatly affects the flavor of food. Lipids are important constituents of cellular membranes. Oxidation of membrane lipids seriously affects membrane function.[24]

Most peroxidized membrane lipids result from oxidative stress within an intact cell. However, some dietary material can incorporate into the cell structure.[71] The oxidation of membrane lipids sets up a chain reaction within the cell membrane that creates a profound effect on cell function.

The products of lipid peroxidation are easily detected in blood plasma and are often used as an estimate of total oxidative stress. Malondialdehyde is the most commonly measured product.

## How The Body Protects Itself From Free Radical Oxidation

Because the body naturally creates free radicals, nature allows numerous built-in mechanisms for protecting human cells from their devastating effects. In fact, the loss of balance between the creation and the scavenging of free radicals is what leads to disease. The many reasons for this loss of balance include all behaviors that promote free radical formation. These include cigarette smoke, exposure to ultraviolet radiation, and polluted air. The imbalance can also occur if the diet lacks sufficient antioxidants. The most common cause of this imbalance is the simple process of aging. Over time, the body may not be able to keep up with the destructive efforts of free radicals.

The built-in mechanisms of destruction of free radicals differ depending on the location of the stress and which molecules are involved. For example, cell membrane damage is caused by both exogenous and intracellular free radical stresses. Think of ultraviolet sunlight exposure and the effect on facial skin. Tocopherols (e.g., vitamin E) are the best at preventing this cell wall damage because they react with both peroxyl and hydroxyl free radicals to reduce their destructive potency. Vitamin E breaks the oxidative destructive chain of events because it closely associates with the polyunsaturated components of the cell membrane.[50]

Another example of our body's ability to fight free radical damage occurs in the plasma. When oxidative events begin in plasma, a variety of antioxidant mechanisms are set into motion. Bilirubin and uric acid are waste products in plasma that are good scavengers of oxyradicals. The most important antioxidant proteins of plasma include ceruloplasmin, albumin, transferrin, haptoglobin, and hemopexin. Along with vitamin E, they must work actively to reduce the formation of atheromas on the vessel walls as low-density lipoproteins become oxidized and promote such formations.[62]

Within and around cells, the effects of hydrogen peroxide are mitigated by catalase. This heme protein breaks down the lethal hydrogen peroxide ($H_2O_2$) into water ($H_2O$) and oxygen ($O_2$). This particular reaction is well known to contact lens practitioners because this activity can be observed in the In-A-Wink system (Ciba Vision, Atlanta, Ga.) of contact lens care.

When free radicals begin to act within the cell cytoplasm, glutathione comes to the rescue. Glutathione is a low-molecular-weight thiol that participates in cellular antioxidant systems to slow or eliminate the destructive events of the oxidative process within cells. Its importance in the protection of cellular function is evidenced by its abundance in cytoplasm, nuclei, and mitochondria.[44]

## Nutritional Manipulation of the Defense of Free Radicals

More and more research is establishing the role of nutrition in the defense of the body against free radicals. For example, low blood vitamin C concentrations in the older British population were found to be strongly predictive of death.[22]

Nowhere is the issue of antioxidants and function more clearly viewed than in the formation of cataracts. This common age-related condition can serve as a model of how nutrition can affect oxidatively induced disease. The research also suggests the complexity of the problem of studying nutritional effects on tissue function because not all studies show the expected results.

The pathophysiological factors of age-related cataract include the breakdown of proteins within the intraocular lens. New cells are formed throughout life within the lens, but older cells are not lost. Instead, they are compressed into the nucleus of the lens. The lens itself also slowly dehydrates. Thus the proteins of the intraocular lens are subject, throughout their lives, to the stresses of exposure to light and other high-energy radiation and oxygen. Many of these insults cause oxidative damage to these proteins and lead to cataractogenesis.[33] If those stresses are increased by adding extra ultraviolet exposure (as a result of geography or profession) and smoking, the accelerated aging that occurs in this structure can be seen.

Many epidemiological studies show associations between elevated risk of various forms of cataract and exposure to higher intensities of ultraviolet light.[14,37,38] Increasing intensity of light increases the amount of free radical activity. The continuous generation of oxygen and its derivatives is well described in the chemistry literature. Thus even a small amount of photo sensitizer in the lens or aqueous can lead to continuous generation of oxygen. With age the ability to scavenge these molecules is reduced, and the oxidative effects on the lens proteins is increased.[65]

Further studies demonstrate that increased free radical production from such sources as smoking increase the risk for cataract. Both smoking and chewing tobacco produce stresses that result in diminished levels of antioxidants, ascorbate, and carotenoids and enhanced cataract at younger ages.[31,70]

The high oxygen levels of hyperbaric chambers also increase the risk for cataract.[48] One study also noted reductions in glutathione and increases in glutathione disulfide, which are changes normally seen in aging. Thus the protective aspects of antioxidation are reduced in these patients. In a sense these cataracts have aged very quickly.

Reasonable clinical belief exists in the benefits of antioxidant intake in the prevention of cataract. The results, however, are complex and not as straightforward as desired. Ascorbate is one of the more aggressive antioxidants found in the lens. Several studies have found correlations between vitamin C supplement use and risk for cataract. Jacques et al[34] studied 165 women with high vitamin C intake (mean, 294 mg/day) and 136 women with low intake (mean, 77 mg/day). Those with higher intakes for more than 10 years had a 70% lower prevalence of early opacities and greater than 80%

lower risk of moderate opacities compared with those who did not take supplements. Hankinson et al[30] helped corroborate these findings by using cataract surgery as the end point. However, after controlling for confounders such as age, diabetes, smoking status, and energy intake, they did not observe an association between total vitamin C intake and rate of cataract surgery.

Some studies are less clear. Mares-Perlman et al[41] reported that past use of supplements containing vitamin C was associated with a reduced rate of nuclear cataract but an increased prevalence of cortical cataract. This study highlights the fact that not all cataracts are the same and the protective nature of some antioxidants affect nuclear, cortical, and posterior subcapsular cataracts differently.

Consumption of vitamin E supplements proved protective of cataract formation in a study by Robertson et al.[54] They found that the prevalence of advanced cataract was 56% lower in persons who consumed more than 400 IU of vitamin E than in those not consuming supplements. However, Mares-Perlman et al[41] showed only weak associations between vitamin E supplements and nuclear and cortical cataract.

An excellent summary of the literature by Taylor[64] states that the literature suggests some benefit to antioxidant intake regarding diminished risk for cataract but that not all the studies clearly show the benefits.[64]

Free radical oxidation is more prevalent in older adults and has an effect on systemic systems and ocular function. Older patients must consume sufficient antioxidants to control as much as possible the breakdowns that occur as a function of this chemical process. The simplest way to provide this protection is by taking vitamin supplements.

## IMMUNOCOMPETENCE THEORY OF AGING

Many of the common disorders of old age, including infection, cancer, autoimmune disorders, immune complex diseases, and degenerative vascular diseases, are in part a result of declining immunological competence.

The interactions among dietary intake, immunocompetence, and health are now recognized. Epidemiological studies of young children in developing countries have documented a steep rise in mortality rate with progressive worsening of nutritional status. A striking similarity between impaired immunity and the high burden of disease has been observed in older adults, young infants, and immunosuppressed adults.[11]

Immunological studies have confirmed that protein energy malnutrition and deficiencies of several nutrients result in impaired immune responses. Many individuals older than 65 years have obvious or subclinical deficiencies. The belief is that malnutrition contributes to immunological senescence in ways that are not well understood, and that the correction of nutritional deficits and imbalances can help reverse the impairment of cell-mediated immunity commonly observed in older adults.[10,11]

Older adults need to maximize their immune systems to avoid infection, the inappropriate inflammation of cardiovascular disease, and the breakdowns that occur in autoimmune disease. Interest in the immune system among eye care providers is clear. They are particularly sensitive to the anterior segment processes of episcleritis, scleritis, and dry eye that occur in autoimmune disease and to the inflammation that is part of macular degeneration.

Studies have shown that the provision of protein energy supplements and the correction of deficiencies in iron, zinc, and vitamins C, E, and B complex are associated with improved immune response.[12] This improved nutritional status may enhance immunocompetence and reduce the burden of illness experienced by older adults.

## AGE-RELATED CHANGES IN IMMUNE FUNCTION

The most extensive changes seen with age are in cell-mediated immunity and T-cell function. Most of the research in this area has been done on laboratory animals.

### Stem Cells

Stem cells with the ability to colonize peripheral lymphoid organs such as the spleen and develop immunocompetent cells decrease in number with age in many strains of mice. This may reflect the clinical reality of the aging patient with sepsis who often cannot produce leukocytes. This failure may reflect low bone marrow reserves as well as the fact that under stress of infection and cell destruction, older individuals may not be able to increase cell production.

### T Cells

Cell-mediated immunity, which is responsible for delayed hypersensitivity reactions, killing of tumor cells, lysis of infected viral cells, and transplantation rejection depends on the integrity of T cells. Individuals older than 65 years show delayed cutaneous hypersensitivity responses to recall antigens derived from bacterial and fungal products as well as strong chemical agents. The response is reduced in frequency and size. This impaired response may be caused by changes in T-cell number and function, decreased lymphokine production, or poor inflammatory response. Research has also shown that functional alterations—including reduced proliferation response to mitogens and antigens, decreased production of lymphokines such as macrophage migration inhibition factor, and impairment of autologous mixed lymphocyte reaction—of synthesis of interleukin-2 or T-cell growth factor and of natural killer cell activity are common in older adults.[25,27,28,32,40]

### B Cells

The number of B cells is generally comparable in younger and older adults.

### Phagocytosis

Little investigation of phagocytosis in old age has been attempted. Some researchers suggest that polymorphonuclear leukocytes obtained from older adults have reduced migration ability. The uptake of particles and microorganisms is unchanged, and the ability to kill ingested bacteria remains intact.[49] The antigen-processing ability of macrophages may be compromised with age. This may cause an inability to localize antigen effectively in the lymphoid follicles of regional lymph nodes. If this occurs in relation to tumor cells as well, it may explain the gap in immune surveillance against cancer cells in old age.

## NUTRITIONAL MODULATION OF IMMUNE RESPONSE

Nutritional status is a critical determinant of immunocompetence. When called on, the immune system must synthesize protein in the form of antibodies and complement and cause the proliferation of T and B lymphocytes. Missing nutrients will slow the process, allowing disease to take control.

Most of the research in this area has been done in young children. However, these principles likely apply to older adults as well. In young children with protein-energy malnutrition, cell-mediated immunity is impaired.[2,9,12,36] The ability to respond in delayed hypersensitivity reactions is reduced, the number of rosette-forming T cells is decreased, and their response to mitogens is greatly reduced. The maturation of T-cell precursors is impaired because of a decrease in thymic inductive factors.

Several nutrients are particularly responsible for these changes. Zinc is essential for immunocompetence. Zinc deficiency results in marked impairment of cell-mediated immunity. Vitamin $B_6$ deficiency also directly interferes with the immune response. The effects of iron deficiency are more controversial, but lymphocytic and granulocyte functions are compromised in iron deficiency.

In an early study, Chandra[11] looked at the nutritional and immunological status of a group of older people who showed no evidence of underlying systemic disease. Among those with clinical hematological and biochemical evidence of nutritional deficiency, cutaneous hypersensitivity response, T-cell number, and response to mitogens were all delayed. Nutritional advice with supplementation resulted in improved functions in all immune areas tested.[44]

Zinc and vitamin C supplementation have also been studied. With only 1 month of supplementation in a population of adults older than 70 years, circulating T cells and serum immunoglobulin G antibodies both increased in number.

The prevalence of nutritional deficiencies in older adults is considerably higher than in young adults.[7,53] Older adults experience a higher frequency of illness than young adults. The common causes of morbidity in older adults suggest that they have a compromised immune response; this conclusion has been verified by many studies. The frequent occurrence of nutritional deficiencies and changes in body composition has also been noted in older adults. Because nutritional status has much to do with immune competence, and restoration of nutritional well-being is associated with improved immune response in this population, the subject of nutrition in older adults should be addressed by all health care practitioners.

Improved nutrition in older adults is expected to reduce the burden of illness in old age.

## WHY EYE CARE PROFESSIONALS SHOULD ASSESS NUTRITIONAL STATUS IN OLDER ADULTS

The importance of the nutritional status of older patients to eye care professionals is now clearly related to maintaining useful and clear vision throughout life. Vigilance that was once kept for patients who smoked may now be matched by the necessary vigilance for nutritional factors such as obesity and undernutrition, especially in older adults.

Problems do occur in attempting to obtain the nutritional status of older adults. They are a far less uniform group of people than are younger patients. Children have normal weights, heights, and energy levels and are generally well. Older adults vary in many ways. They often have diseases that may have changed their health status immensely, take medications that can complicate their dietary intake and absorption, and are greatly influenced by their social status and living arrangements. Their cognitive and emotional well-being may also influence their ability to eat properly.

Over the past few decades several attempts have been made to develop a screening tool that would identify older patients who are at risk for malnutrition and who would benefit from further nutritional counseling.[52] The assessments fall into the following three main types:

1. A brief self-reported screening instrument such as the Nutritional Screening Initiative's DETERMINE checklist or the Mini-Nutritional Assessment
2. A clinician-determined brief screening instrument such as the Subjective Global Assessment
3. Multiple-method techniques such as the Prognostic Nutritional Index or Hospital Prognostic Index

The Nutritional Screening Initiative is a partnership of many American health professionals who believe in a tiered approach to screening. The first approach is a simple checklist that can be completed by the patient or caregiver. It consists of 10 questions scored from 0 (lowest risk) to 21 (highest risk); those with higher risk are then referred for further screening.

The second tier of tests has both level I and level II testing. The level I testing includes height and weight measurements and the calculated basal metabolic index (BMI) as well as questions about weight loss or gain within 6 months, eating habits, living environment, and functional status. Level II includes much more in-depth analysis, including anthropomorphic measurements, serum albumin and cholesterol levels, and cognitive and affected status.

Eye care professionals who have older patients should have some ability to screen their patients for nutritional status. All the quick devices have pitfalls that are difficult to overcome. A recall of food intake during the past 24 hours may not represent normal behavior. A longer recall may be impossible for the patient to remember. The most effective method appears to be an interview that asks the patient to recall food intake for as long as memory allows. Simple questions such as "what did you eat for breakfast yesterday and today?" can help to determine whether the patient has traditional eating habits. Specific question about how many fruits and vegetables were eaten yesterday can help determine the risk for malnutrition. The interviewer can then construct an average daily intake from the bits of information.

## RISK FACTORS FOR MALNUTRITION

Because getting concrete answers may be difficult, knowing the risk factors for malnutrition can help raise the index of suspicion. Risk factors become particularly important when clinical appearance may be misleading in this population. Clinically, low dietary intakes and abnormal biochemical findings are rarely found to be associated with the disturbances of form and function that indicates clinical malnutrition. Low nutritional status may thus be present in the absence of overt disease. Also, malnutrition refers to the absence of sufficient caloric intake as well as obesity that comes with the excess intake of calories.

Because clinical assessment of older adults is difficult to perform and often yields poor findings, the risk factors for malnutrition are important to know. In England, a study found that older people living alone eat fewer foods that require preparation than married couples and therefore might be considered a group at risk.[3]

In 1972, Exton-Smith[20] found housebound older people to be at risk; another study found that widowers older than 80 years were the highest risk group.[5]

American studies have also addressed the issues of risk factors for malnutrition in older adults. These include depression, poverty, women living alone, obesity, underweight, mental disorders, dehydration,[39,46,60] lack of sunlight,[47] reduced taste,[35] and drug therapy.[66]

## INTERACTION OF SOCIAL, ENVIRONMENTAL, AND MEDICAL RISK FACTORS

Primary and secondary causes of malnutrition can be defined in older adults.[19] Research distinguishes between social or environmental causes that call for public health measures and physical or mental disorders that call for appropriate medical treatment. In 1979 the Department of Health and Social Services in Great Britain reported on risk factors for older men and women (Box 17-1).[18]

Many risk factors are related. The Gerontology Nutrition Unit at London University suggested the risk factors shown in Box 17-2 can be explored by any medical or nonmedical personnel.[16]

Any health examination of older adults should include a history that addresses the issue of nutritional status and dietary intake. Knowing the risk factors for malnutrition can help determine the extent of the nutritional analysis.

---

**BOX 17-1**

### Risk Factors

**Social**
    Living alone
    Housebound lifestyle
    No regular cooked meals
    Poverty bracket
    Social class
    Low mental test score
    Depression

**Medical**
    Chronic bronchitis
    Emphysema
    Gastrectomy
    Poor dentition
    Difficulty swallowing
    Smoking
    Alcoholism

## SUMMARY

As the North American population ages, age-related diseases will be a part of all primary health care practices. The goal of health care providers is to prevent these diseases from occurring or slow their progress and reduce their morbidity. Nutritional counseling is a part of the treatment that should be available to these patients.

Common age-related ocular diseases include cataract, macular degeneration, diabetic retinopathy, and vascular retinal occlusions and hemorrhages (Box 17-3). These diseases are in part associated with the normal physiological changes of aging that include free radical oxidation and immunosenescence. Nutritional factors such as the intake of antioxidants, undernutrition, obesity, and balanced meals influence the course of these diseases. All primary health care providers should routinely establish a screening history for nutritional status and take the time to educate patients about the role of nutrition in maintaining good visual health throughout life (Box 17-4).

## REFERENCES

1. Anderson EJ, Richardson M, Castle G, et al: Nutrition interventions for intensive therapy in the Diabetes Control and Complications Trial. The DCCT Research Group, *J Am Diet Assoc* 93:1104, 1993.
2. Beisel WR: Single nutrients and immunity, *Am J Clin Nutr* 35:417-68, 1968.
3. Bransby ER, Osborne B: A social and food survey of the elderly living alone or as married couples, *Br J Nutr* 7:160-80, 1953.
4. Bredt DS, Snyder SH: Nitric oxide: a physiologic messenger molecule, *Ann Rev Biochem* 63:175-95, 1994.
5. Brockington CF, Lempert SM. In *The social needs of the over eighties. The Stockport survey of the aged*, Manchester, England, 1966, Manchester University.
6. Brot N, Weisbach H: Biochemistry and physiological role of methionine sulfoxide residues in proteins, *Arch Biochem Biophys* 223:271-81, 1983.
7. Burr ML: The nutritional state of the elderly. Demographic and epidemiological considerations. In Chandra RK, editor: *Nutrition, immunity and illness in the elderly*, New York, 1985, Pergamon Press, pp 5-18.

8. Cadenas E: Biochemistry of oxygen toxicity, *Ann Rev Biochem* 1989;58:79-110, 1989.

9. Chandra RK: Nutritional deficiency and susceptibility to infection, *Bull World Health Organ* 57:167-76, 1979.

10. Chandra RK: Nutrition, immunity and infection: present knowledge and future directions, *Lancet* I:688-91, 1983.

11. Chandra RK: Nutritional regulation of immune function at the extremes of life, in infants and in the elderly. In *Malnutrition: determinants and consequences*, New York, 1984, Alan R. Liss, pp 254-61.

12. Chandra RK, Dayton D: Trace element regulation of immunity and infection, Nutr Res 2:721-33, 1982.

13. Chia E, Wang JJ, Rochtchina E, et al: Impact of bilateral visual impairment on health-related quality of life: the Blue Mountain Eye Study. *Invest Ophthalmol Vis Sci* 45:71-6, 2004.

14. Cruickshank KJ, Klein BE, Klein R: Ultraviolet light exposure and lens opacities: the Beaver Dam Study, *Am J Public Health* 82:1658-62, 1992.

15. Davies KJ: Protein damage and degradation by oxygen radicals. I. General aspects, *Biol Chem* 262:9895-901, 1987.

16. Davies L: *Three score years...and then?* London, 1981, William Heineman Medical Books.

17. Dean RT, Wolff SP, McElligott MA: Histidine and proline are important sites of free radical damage to proteins, *Free Radic Res Commun* 7:97-103, 1989.

18. Department of Health and Social Services in British Isles: *Nutrition and health in old age. Report on health and social subjects*, London, 1979, Department of Health and Social Security.

19. Exton-Smith AN: Nutrition of the elderly, *Br J Hosp Med* 5:639-45, 1971.

20. Exton-Smith AN: *Nutrition of household bound people*, London, 1972, King's Fund.

21. Feibusch JM, Holt PR: Impaired absorptive capacity for carbohydrate in the aging human, *Dig Dis Sci* 27:1095-100, 1982.

22. Fletcher AE, Breeze E, Shetty PS: Antioxidant vitamins and mortality in older persons: findings from the nutrition add-on study to the Medical Research Council Trial of Assessment and Management of Older People on the Community, *Am J Clin Nutr* 78:999-1010, 2003.

23. Food and Nutrition Board, National Research Council: *Recommended dietary allowances*, ed 10, Washington, DC, 1989, National Academy Press.

24. Gardner HW: Oxygen radical chemistry of polyunsaturated fatty acids, *Free Radic Biol Med* 7:65-86, 1989.

25. Girard JP, Paychere M, Cuevas M, et al: Cell-mediated immunity in an aging population, *Clin Exp Immunol* 27:85-91, 1977.

26. Greenspan SL, Myers ER, Maitland LA, et al: Fall severity and bone mineral density as risk factors for hip fracture in ambulatory elderly, *JAMA* 271:128-33, 1994.

27. Gupta S, Good RA: Subpopulations of human T lymphocytes. X. Alterations in T, B, third population cells and T cells with receptors for immunoglobin M(tu) or G(Ty) in aging humans, *J Immunol* 111:1101-7, 1979.

28. Hallgren HM, Buckley CE, Gilbertsen VA, et al: Lymphocyte phytohaemagglutin responsiveness, immunoglobins and autoantibodies in aging humans, *J Immunol* 111:1101-7, 1973.

29. Hammond BR Jr, Johnson MA: The age-related eye disease study (AREDS), *Nutr Rev* 60:283-8, 2002.

30. Hankinson SE, Stampfer MJ, Seddon JM, et al: Intake and cataract extraction in women: a prospective study, *Br Med J.*305:335-9, 1992.

31. Hankinson SE, Willett WC, Colditz GA, et al: A prospective study of cigarette smoking and risk for cataract surgery in women, *JAMA* 268:994-8, 1992.

32. Hijmans W, Radl J, Bottazzo GF, et al: Autoantibodies in highly aged humans, *Mech Ageing Dev* 26:83-9, 1984.

33. Jacques PF, Taylor A: Micronutrients and age-related cataracts. In Bendich A, Butterworth CE, editors: *Micronutrients in health and in disease prevention*, New York, 1991, Marcel Dekker, pp 359-79.

34. Jacques PF, Taylor A, Hankinson SE, et al: Long-term vitamin C supplement use and prevalence of early age-related lens opacities, *Am J Clin Nutr* 66:911-6, 1977.

35. Kamath SK: Taste acuity and aging, *Am J Clin Nutr* 36:766-75, 1982.

36. Keusch GT: Nutrition, host defenses and the immune system. In Gallin JI, Fauci AS, editors: *Advances in host defense mechanisms, vol 2*, New York, 1982, Raven Press, pp 275-357.

37. Klein BE, Cruickshank KJ, Klein R: Leisure time, sunlight exposure and cataracts, *Documenta Ophthalmol* 88:295-305, 1994.

38. Klein BEK, Klein R, Linton KLP: Prevalence of age related lens opacities in a population: the Beaver Dam Eye Study, *Ophthalmology* 99:546-52, 1992.

39. Kohrs MB: A rational diet for the elderly, *Am J Clin Nutr* 36:796-802, 1982.

40. Lokhorst HM, van der Lindon JA, Schuurman HJ, et al: Immune function during ageing in man: relation between serological abnormalities and cellular immune status, *Eur J Clin Invest* 13: 209-14, 1983.

41. Mares-Perlman JA, Klein BEK, Klein R, et al: Relationship between lens opacities and vitamin

and mineral supplement use, *Ophthalmology* 101:315-55, 1994.

42. McGandy RB, Barrows CH, Spanias A, et al: Nutrient intakes and energy expenditure in men of different ages, *J Gerontol* 21:581-7, 1996.

43. Meisler JG, St. Jeor S: Summary and recommendations from the American Health Foundation's Expert Panel on Healthy Weight, *Am J Clin Nutr* 63:474S-7S, 1996.

44. Meister AI: Glutathione metabolism and its selective modification, *J Biol Chem* 263:17205-8, 1988.

45. Mokdad AH, Serdula MD, Dietz WH, et al: The spread of the obesity epidemic in the United States, 1991-1998, *JAMA* 282:1519-22, 1999.

46. Nordstrom JW: Trace mineral nutrition in the elderly, *Am J Clin Nutr* 36:819-22, 1982.

47. Omdahl JL, Garry PJ, Hunsake LA, et al: Nutritional status in a healthy elderly population: vitamin D, *Am J Clin Nutr* 36:1225-33, 1982.

48. Palmquist BM, Phillipson B, Barr PO: Nuclear cataract and myopia during hyperbaric oxygen therapy, *Br J Ophthalmol* 60:113-7, 1984.

49. Pamblad J, Jaak A: Ageing does not change blood granulocyte bacteriacidal capacity and levels of complement 3 and 4, *Gerontology* 24:381-5, 1978.

50. Pascoe GA, Reed DJ: Cell calcium, vitamin E and the thiol redox system in toxicity, *Free Radic Biol Med* 6:209-24, 1989.

51. Pelz KS, Gottfried SP, Sooes E: Intestinal absorption studies in the aged, *Geriatrics* 23:149-53, 1968.

52. Reuben DB, Greendale GA, Harrison GG: Nutrition screening in older persons, *J Am Geriatr Soc* 43:415-25, 1995.

53. Rivlin RS, Young EA, editors: Symposium on the evidence relating selected vitamins and minerals to health and disease in the elderly population in the United States, *Am J Clin Nutr* 36:977-1086, 1982.

54. Robertson J McD, Donner AP, Trevithick JR: Vitamin E intake and risk for cataracts in humans, *Ann NY Acad Sci* 570;372-82, 1989.

55. *The role of nutrition in maintaining health in the nation's elderly: evaluating coverage of nutrition services for the Medicare population,* Washington, DC, 2000, Institute of Medicine, National Academy Press.

56. Russell RM, Suter PM: Vitamin requirements in elderly people: an update, *Am J Clin Nutr* 58:4-14, 1993.

57. Ryan AS, Craig LD, Finn SC: Nutrition intakes and dietary patterns of older Americans: a national study, *J Gerontol* 47:M145-50, 1992.

58. Sawaya AL, Saltzman E, Fuss P, et al: Dietary energy requirements of young and older women determined by using the doubly labeled water method, *Am J Clin Nutr* 62:338-44, 1995.

59. Schwartz RS: Obesity in the elderly. In Bray GA, Bouchard C, James WPT, editors: *Handbook of obesity.* New York, 1997, Marcell Dekker, pp 103-14.

60. Siegel JS: Some demographic aspects of aging in the United States. In Ostfeld AM, Gibson DG, editors: *Epidemiology of aging,* Bethesda, MD, 1975, National Institute of Health, pp 17-82.

61. Stadtman ER: Metal ion-catalyzed oxidation of proteins: biochemical mechanism and biological consequences, *Free Radic Biol Med* 19:315-25, 1990.

62. Steinbrecher UP, Zhang H, Loughheed M: Role of oxidatively modified LDL in atherosclerosis, *Free Radic Biol Med* 9:155-68, 1990.

63. Suter PM, Russell RM: Vitamin requirements of the elderly, *Am J Clin Nutr* 45:501-12, 1987.

64. Taylor A: Nutritional and environmental influences on risk for cataract. In Taylor A, editor: *Nutritional and environmental influences on the eye,* Boca Raton, FL, 1999, CRC Press, pp 53-94.

65. Taylor A, Jaques PF: Relationship between aging, antioxidant status and cataract, *Am J Clinical Nutr* 62:1439S-47S, 1995.

66. Vestal RE: Drug use in the elderly: a review of problems and special considerations, *Drugs* 16:258-82, 1978.

67. von Sonntag C: The chemistry of free-radical-mediated damage, *Basic Life Sci* 58:287-317, 1991.

68. Wallace JI, Schwartz RS, La Croix AZ, et al: Involuntary weight loss in older outpatients: incidence and clinical significance, *J Am Geriatr Soc* 43:329-37, 1995.

69. Werner I, Hambraeus L: The digestive capacity of elderly people, In Carlson LA, editor: *Nutrition in old age,* Uppsala, Sweden, 1972, Almquist and Wiksell, pp 55-60.

70. West SK, Munoz B, Emmett EA, et al: Cigarette smoking and risk of nuclear cataracts, *Arch Ophthalmol* 107:1166-9, 1989.

71. Wills ED: The role of dietary components in oxidative stress in tissues. In Sies H, editor: *Oxidative stress,* Orlando, FL, 1989, Academic Press, pp 197-220.

# CHAPTER 18

# Delivery of Vision Care in Nontraditional Settings

GARY L. MANCIL and SUZANNE M. HAGAN

With current demographic trends of independence maintained over a longer number of years, older adults are generally able to continue with well-established, lifelong health care patterns in private practice settings. Optometric care traditionally has been provided in the private-practice setting, but more recently optometrists have been expanding their sphere of services beyond their offices into institutional and other out-of-office settings. The growing mobile service delivery system in the United States (encompassing everything from health care to car repair) suggests that the convenience factor appeals to many segments of the population. For instance, relatively independent older adults residing in retirement communities may prefer to receive vision care on site rather than travel to an office.

Older adults who are physically fit to travel to a traditional office setting for vision care should be encouraged to do so. A growing number of older adults, however, find that continuing to receive vision care in the private-practice setting is difficult. This change comes with the onset of frailty, most often seen in the population of adults aged 85 years and older. With advancing age, patients are more likely to experience a variety of health problems that may result in loss of independence and restrictions in their mobility. More than 40% of those older than 65 years become institutionalized at some point in their lives, with an average stay of approximately 2.5 years.[44] Furthermore,

reduced vision is associated with self-reported disability.[41,47] This larger number of frail older adults who remain in the community but require significant assistance is growing much faster than the nursing home population.

Loss of independence is most often the result of age-related physical or mental health disorders such as atherosclerotic vascular disease (including cerebral vascular accident and congestive heart disease), adult-onset diabetes mellitus, chronic obstructive pulmonary disease, age-related dementias (including organic brain syndrome, Alzheimer's disease, and Parkinson's disease), and degenerative joint disease.

Alzheimer's disease is associated with visual symptoms such as reading difficulty, blurred or "poor" vision, difficulty navigating spaces or recognizing faces, visual hallucinations, and visual agnosia. Biological analysis reveals optic nerve degeneration and loss of retinal cells among patients with Alzheimer's disease.[17]

Several conditions that increase with age—cardiovascular, musculoskeletal, and respiratory conditions as well as sensory impairments—contribute to immobility and disability among older persons.[20] A 9-year study of those aged 65 years and older showed that nearly half develop at least one of three chronic eye diseases as they grow older: diabetic retinopathy, glaucoma, or age-related macular degeneration.[23] Another study showed that the rates of eye examinations for these eye diseases fell far below the frequencies recommended.[24] For many of these patients, transportation to an eye care practitioner's office is lacking or available only through assistance from family, friends, or community resources (which are infrequently found) or through considerable personal expense.

Fear of blindness is second only to fear of cancer among our nation's older adults, according recent testimony before Congress.[39] Vision and eye health problems are the second most prevalent chronic health care problem in the United States. In older adults, untreated vision problems can hasten the loss of independence and result in increased incidence of falls and hip fractures.[19,26,38,48]

With decreasing personal independence, older adults are likely to be forced into new living arrangements, and the variety of settings in which they may choose to reside are sometimes described as the "housing continuum." For example, older adults could theoretically move along this continuum through various options ranging from a fully independent private home (sometimes receiving support from community resources) to a situation of total dependency. Along the continuum, they might use an assisted living private residence (incorporating regular assistive services such as homemaker/chore assistance and supportive medical services), congregate care or supported living arrangement with full-time caretakers, or a so-called life care or continuing care community (combining independent living arrangements with the availability of extensive medical and supportive services). Adult day care/day hospital services provide a form of respite care (see later) for an older person's usual caregiver or short-term rehabilitation. Hospice care provides for the needs of dying patients and their families. Respite care provides temporary support to relieve stress of caring for frail older persons. Older adults recovering from an acute illness who are discharged from the hospital but are not well enough to return to the community may enter a convalescent unit or nursing facility. In this instance, the treatment goal is to facilitate the expected return to the community. With the onset of greater dependency, a nursing home providing skilled and intermediate care may encompass the greatest degree of supportive living. Skilled nursing facilities provide the highest level of supportive care outside hospitals.

Such options in patterns of elder living are reflected by changes in how optometry schools are training students and in how optometrists practice. One study reports that clinical rotation through a nursing home internship was considered by students to be a valuable part of their clinical training.[13] According to a recent survey by the American Optometric Association, nearly 20% of all optometrists in the United States currently see patients who live in the long-term care environment and report that they visit three to four facilities on a regular basis.[32] Several studies show that fewer than half of nursing home residents received regular eye examinations, and that this population has a high prevalence of remediable visual impairment.[21,42] In studies in France and Australia, the actual rate of visual impairment among institutionalized older persons is higher than predicted and higher than that of their noninstitutionalized counterparts.[45,46]

## ESTABLISHING VISION CARE PROGRAMS IN NONTRADITIONAL SETTINGS

The initial steps in establishing a vision care program as an outreach of an existing private practice require an analysis of the practice itself. Providing care on site necessitates that the specialist, staff, or both be away from the office, so this must be an appropriate decision for the practice. Reimbursement expected to the practice through the program is also a consideration. Because many patients encountered in nontraditional settings rely on Medicare or Medicaid as their insurance, issues of accepting assignment and level of reimbursement often are determined by the insurance carrier. Obtaining information from the carrier in advance of implementing any new program, as well as evaluating the availability of practice time to devote to this activity, enables better decisions to be made regarding the frequency and length of time the eye care practitioner is able to devote to out-of-office care. On the basis of this analysis, practices adding an associate or experiencing reduced growth may benefit to the greatest degree from establishing outreach programs. The optometrist proposing a vision care program of this nature must determine the fees for on-site care (which are likely to be considerably higher than in-office fees for similar levels of care). Although under review, current regulations by the Centers for Medicare and Medicaid Services (CMS) at this writing do not permit two fee schedules for the same set of services.[30] Therefore the optometrist contemplating outreach services in addition to ordinary services at a traditional office may want to establish a second business entity for that area of the practice so that appropriate fee schedules can be established.

A second decision to be made is which opportunities are optimal for providing care in nontraditional settings. Settings geographically convenient to the existing practice should be given preference because of decreased travel time. Additional questions to consider include how many potential patients may be accessed in a particular setting and what, if any, existing arrangements for vision care are in place.

## Key Staff Interactions

The decisions of how to initiate contact and whom to approach on the facility staff of the out-of-office setting have the potential to set the tone for the entire vision care program. A letter of introduction should be sent to the administrator and other key staff (e.g., nursing director and social worker). The letter should state the optometrist's interest in serving the patients' visual needs, professional qualifications and expertise, and the intention to follow the letter with a phone call requesting an appointment. Whenever possible, the letter should be addressed to specific individuals rather than simply unnamed positions or titles, and the follow-up phone call should take place soon after the letter is sent.

The key staff contact person may vary, but the social worker or other community services contact staff person is often the individual most aware of residents' visual needs. In fact, one of the social worker's major responsibilities is to ensure that the appropriate resources (including those from the community) are called on to meet patient needs. In some settings, the nursing staff serves this role and may represent the primary contact. The program administrator is an important contact and should be included in the early discussions, although usually other staff will determine the details of a new program for vision care. However, regular communication with, and support from, the top administrator can overcome ambivalence from other key staff.

One important issue is to what degree the facility staff will need to be involved. Supervisors and administrators may need to be assured that bringing a vision care program into their facility will not be time intensive to their staff. Nursing staff, for instance, may be accustomed to physicians expecting an assistant to accompany them during their rounds. This degree of staff support is typically not required in a vision care program. Nevertheless, a minimal degree of support is needed from the staff.

Their involvement typically includes educating patients and their sponsors (typically a family member or significant other with medical power of attorney) about the availability of vision care services on site; making available medical records for the patients; in some settings (e.g., nursing homes) facilitating an order from the attending physician requesting vision care; directing or transporting patients to a central site for evaluation; filing reports in the patients' charts; and following up on or initiating treatment or referral as recommended by the optometrist (in some settings in conjunction with the patients' attending physicians).

Other issues of concern to the agency or institution staff are fees charged for on-site vision care and the need for careful communication regarding this to the patient (and in most settings, the patient's sponsor). In many agency and institutional settings, patients are insured by a combination of Medicare and Medicaid, necessitating that the optometrist accept assignment. A fee schedule will likely be requested and shared with patients and/or sponsors. This fee schedule should be as clear and complete as possible.

A formal agreement or contract should be drafted to clarify and document what each party expects of the other. This allows the optometrist to negotiate important issues such as exclusivity of care and to specify other aspects of the on-site visits, such as availability of patient charts, level of staff assistance, and minimal number of patients to be scheduled. The contract may stipulate whether the optometrist serves on an "on-call," case-by-case basis or schedules regular, periodic visits. While scheduled visits for a predetermined, minimal number of voluntary patients is often preferred, provisions also need to be made for providing additional services as needed (such as urgent or emergency care).[11] Furthermore, the contract may specify exclusivity of the optometrist's services and provide recommendations regarding primary referral sources. Conformance to Health Insurance Portability and Accountability Act and CMS regulations regarding patient confidentiality and availability of patient eye examination records for purposes of audit may also need to be documented. Conditions and terms for eyeglasses provision may be specified in the contract, such as when eyeglasses need to be paid for in advance and how and when they are to be delivered.

In turn, the agency or institution may wish to document in the contract the availability of the optometrist, the responsibility of patients or their insurers to pay fees involved for professional services, the responsibility of the optometrist to carry adequate insurance coverage, and the expected conduct of both parties.

## Instrumentation, Equipment, and Locale

Providing vision care on site in a nontraditional setting (such as an agency or institution) can be accomplished with a minimal amount of ophthalmic equipment. However, at present, portable versions of in-office instrumentation allow a level of on-site evaluation that formerly was not possible (Figs. 18-1 to 18-8).

Of special note are portable versions of lensometers (Fig. 18-1), applanation tonometers (Fig. 18-4), biomicroscopes (Fig. 18-5), keratometers or autorefractors (Fig. 18-6), interferometers (Fig. 18-1), and fundus cameras. This equipment also has uses in the traditional office, especially for wheelchair-bound or other physically challenged patients who cannot easily adapt to traditional office instruments. Box 18-1 lists essential and recommended equipment for use in providing vision care on site in a nontraditional setting. Figures 18-1 to 18-3 show how equipment is packed in individual cases that are loaded onto a platform cart for transport.

Scheduling of appointments should be based on considerations for maximizing patient performance as well as minimizing extraneous dis-

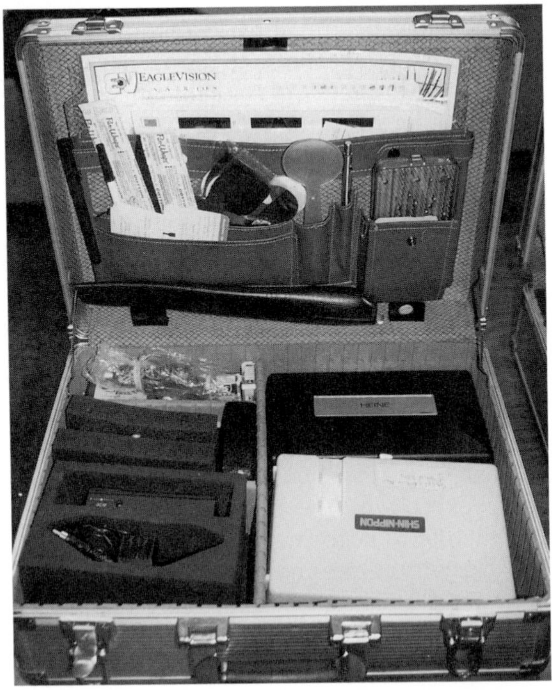

**Fig. 18-1** Case packed with examination equipment, including a portable lensometer, a diagnostic kit, spectacle-mounted BIO, interferometer, foreign body removal kit, occluders, and miscellaneous items.

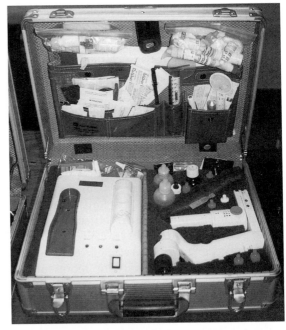

**Fig. 18-2** Case with disassembled portable slit lamp and its base, tonometer, diagnostic and therapeutic drugs, and miscellaneous items.

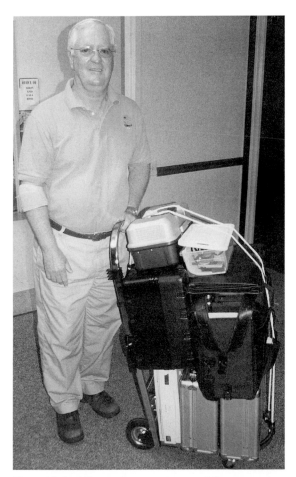

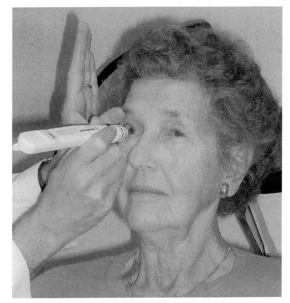

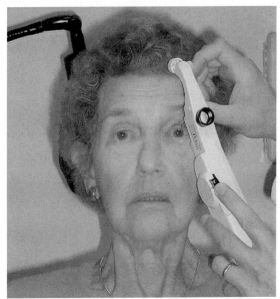

**Fig. 18-3** All equipment for mobile eye care, including a portable photocopier, loaded onto a platform cart.

**Fig. 18-4** Portable equipment such as a handheld tonometer enable sophisticated testing to be performed in any environment.

tractions during the examination. As a rule, older adults may prefer mid-morning appointments. Other considerations include medication schedules (some medications cause drowsiness), social activities (many older adults prefer not to miss a favorite crafts class or television show), the desire of family members to be present during the examination (and hence the need to consider their schedules), naps, and staff shift changes.

In the initial phases of proposing and implementing any new program, an appropriate locale should be selected. This may include treatment rooms, conference rooms, classrooms, private offices, or empty patient rooms. Access to an area that can be closed off from noise and activity, in which lighting can be controlled, and from which a sink is easily reached is a desirable feature.

**Before the Examination**

An example of an Advanced History Form is show in Figure 18-9. A signed permission or consent form from either the patient or the sponsor is necessary before conducting an examination (Fig. 18-10). A written order from

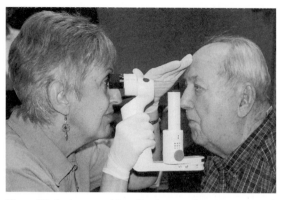

**Fig. 18-5** A portable slit lamp (biomicroscope) affords a good view of the anterior structures of the eye, even in a wheelchair-bound patient, and can be used with a condensing lens to evaluate disc, macula, and posterior pole.

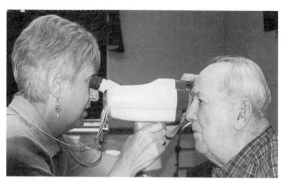

**Fig. 18-6** When patients in a long-term care environment need to be referred for cataract extraction, a portable autorefractor/keratometer enables corneal curvatures or K readings to be relayed to the ophthalmologist.

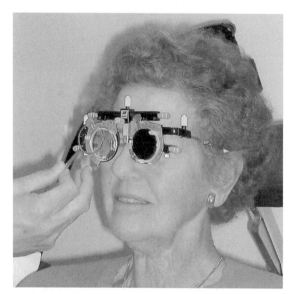

**Fig. 18-7** Trial frame refraction using loose lenses and the handheld Jackson Crossed Cylinder is effective in out-of-office examinations.

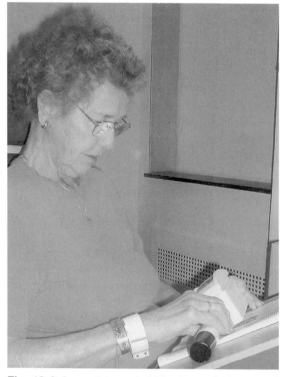

**Fig. 18-8** Low vision rehabilitation techniques and devices can be evaluated and prescribed in any nontraditional office setting.

---

*ADVANCE HISTORY FORM*

Patient Name _____

Address _____

_____

Phone _____ Contact Person _____

Who will be present during the exam? _____

Relationship _____

Directions: _____

_____

_____

_____

Primary Physician _____ Phone _____

Last Seen _____ For what purpose? _____

_____

Pharmacy Name _____ Phone _____

Previous Eye Doctor's Name _____ Last seen _____

*Nature of Current Vision Problems/Complaint*

_____

_____

_____

---

**Fig. 18-9** Advance history form.

the patient's primary care physician is also adequate. Obtaining both pieces of documentation is even better. A "blanket" authorization to examine all patients in a long-term care facility is considered insufficient reason for an eye examination, according to CMS, and lack of proper documentation may jeopardize payments or cause CMS to demand repayment, often with fines or interest, after an audit. However, when allowed, the optometrist can assist the facility staff in prioritizing which residents would benefit from an eye examination by conducting a chart audit of all residents and providing a written summary of the findings (within HIPAA guidelines).

A check of the patient's insurance coverage, usually found on the face sheet just inside the front cover of the patient chart, will help ensure that the optometrist is a provider on the patient's plan. Many Medicare health mainte-

nance organizations require prior authorization before they will pay for an eye examination. The optometrist's liaison at the facility should provide a copy of the face sheet for the optometrist's records and can point out or flag who may need prior authorization for an eye examination and obtain this authorization before the eye examination.

The optometrist should carefully review the patient's medical chart for medical conditions and current medications, including any topical eye medications. Table 18-1 lists commonly encountered abbreviations in patients' medical charts that may be unfamiliar to optometrists coming from a traditional office setting.

**Recommended Examination Sequence**

As is the case when examining an older adult in any setting, clear and accurate communication skills must occur throughout the process.

**Eye Care Services Consent Form**

*(Optometric practice)* will provide eye examinations and optical services to any resident or client of this facility. Such services will take place on a regular basis.

Residents of long-term care facilities or clients of custodial care services often have unmet eye care needs. Vision impairment is a common chronic condition. Many such persons may suffer from undetected glaucoma, cataracts, retinal disease, or untreated eye infections. Others may slowly lose usable vision because their glasses prescriptions have not been regularly checked or updated. Still others may be unable to read or perform other close work because they are not provided with special low vision aids.

Services provided by *(Optometric practice)* include: *Comprehensive Eye Examinations* including eye health and vision testing; *Diagnosis and treatment of eye diseases* including glaucoma and infections; *Surgical Co-Management; Complete spectacle service* (orders/adjustments/minor repairs); Regularly scheduled visits and urgent care; *Low vision services*

Medicare, Medicaid, private insurance, and private payment cover the professional fees for these services. We are Medicare participating providers and we accept assignment. This means that we will always accept the amount that Medicare approves for an eye examination. Please sign and return the form below if you are interested in eye care services. If you have questions about these services, please contact the social services director at your facility or our office.

**Lifetime Consent Agreement**

The patient, legal guardian or health care surrogate authorizes *(Doctor and/or optometric practice) to* examine the eyes and treat, if necessary, the patient listed below. This consent may be withdrawn at any time.

Medicare Authorization — Signature on File

HICN_____

I request that payment of authorized Medicare benefits be made on my behalf to *(Doctor and/or optometric practice)* for any services furnished me by that provider. I authorize any holder of medical information about me to release to the Centers for Medicare and Medicaid Services (CMS) and its agents any information needed to determine these benefits or the benefits payable for related services. I understand my signature requests that payment be made and authorizes release of medical information necessary to pay the claim.

**Supplemental Insurance Authorization**

Policy Number_____

If other health insurance is indicated in Item 9 of the CMS 1500 form or elsewhere, my signature authorizes release of the information to that insurer or agency. *(Optometric practice)* accepts the charge determination of the Medicare carrier as the full charge. I understand that I am responsible only for the deductible, co-insurance and noncovered services. Co-insurance and deductible are based upon the charge determination of the Medicare Carrier.

**Release of Information to other Health Care Providers**

I understand that in the course of providing optometric services, *(Optometric practice)* may advise referral to other specialists for treatment including surgery.Should referral occur, I authorize release of examination results, which may be transmitted electronically, to other health care providers.

Notice of Privacy Practices for the Health Insurance Portability and Accountability Act of 1996 (HIPAA)

I understand that this facility or agency has a copy of the Notice of Privacy Practices for *(Optometric practice)*. I also understand that I may obtain a copy of this document by request from *(Optometric practice)*.

_____

Patient Name

Date

_____

Printed Name of responsible party/Signature
Name of Facility

**Fig. 18-10** Sample consent form useful for optometric practice outside a traditional office.

**BOX 18-1**

## Equipment Useful in Out-of-Office Examinations

**Essential Equipment**
Diagnostic kit
Occluder
BIO
20 D lens
Trial lens set
Halberg/Janelli clips
Handheld Jackson Crossed Cylinder (JCC)
Trial frames
Acuity charts
    Distance: 10-ft Snellen, Feinbloom
    Low vision, near: reduced Snellen, Lighthouse
    near vision card, or Duke reading card
Frames (traditional styles with adjustable nosepads)
Ophthalmic materials (tools, screws, hinges, temples)
Tonometer (e.g., Perkins, Tonopen*)
Ophthalmic drugs (diagnostics and therapeutics)
Slit lamp (biomicroscope)
Amsler grid

**Optional Equipment**
Gonioscopy lenses
Portable lensometer
Fundus camera (portable)
Interferometer (portable)
Low vision devices
Assistive listening devices (e.g., "hardwire")
Portable autorefractor/keratometer
Forceps, punctal dilators
Portable pachymeter
Bailey-Lovie low-contrast visual field test
Portable, automated tangent screen
Damator or Oculus "visual field tests"
Optokinetic nystagmus drum
Teller card preferential looking "visual acuity test"
Five-hole punch
Two-way radios
Platform cart/carrier
Carrying cases
Portable photocopier

**Miscellaneous Equipment**
Tape
Extension cords
Three-pronged adaptors
Portable lighting
Measuring tape
Rx pads
PD ruler
Penlight
Extra bulbs and batteries
Engraving tool
Gloves*
Alcohol wipes†
Tissues*

---

*Medtronic Solan, Jacksonville, Fla.
†Often provided by the facility.

**TABLE 18-1**

## Medical Abbreviations and Definitions

| Abbreviation | Definition |
|---|---|
| AF | Atrial fibrillation |
| ASHD | Arteriosclerotic heart disease |
| BKA | Below-the-knee amputation |
| BPH | Benign prostatic hypertrophy |
| CAD | Coronary artery disease |
| CHF | Congestive heart failure |
| COPD | Chronic obstructive pulmonary disease |
| CRI | Chronic renal insufficiency |
| CVA | Cardiovascular accident (stroke) |
| DJD | Degenerative joint disease |
| DVT | Deep vein thrombosis |
| ESRD | End-stage renal disease |
| GERD | Gastroesophageal reflex disease |
| MI | Myocardial infarction |
| MRSA | Methicillin-resistant *Staphylococcus aureus* |
| N/V | Nausea and vomiting |
| OA | Osteoarthritis |
| OBS | Organic brain syndrome |
| OCD | Obsessive-compulsive disorder |
| PUD | Peptic ulcer disease |
| PVD | Peripheral vascular disease |
| RA | Rheumatoid arthritis |
| SDAT | Senile dementia, Alzheimer's type |
| SOB | Shortness of breath |
| SVT | Supraventricular tachycardia |
| URI | Upper respiratory infection |
| UTI | Urinary tract infection |

Furthermore, the chief complaint must always match the assessment. If the patient cannot articulate a symptom, that is, the examination is being conducted because of physician request or family/sponsor wishes, the optometrist should document that as the chief complaint. A sample examination form is shown in Figure 18-11.

In testing visual acuities, the clinician working in a nontraditional setting may need auxiliary lighting. Clip-on spot lighting is commercially available to address this need. Portable visual acuity test charts (traditional Snellen and others) are appropriate, as are low vision test charts. A lightbox with a variety of charts using different optotypes is extremely helpful (Fig. 18-12). In noncommunicative patients, techniques such as an optokinetic nystagmus drum and preferential viewing are appropriate.[14,29] A 10-foot test distance (or less) may be used, depending on the room characteristics where the examinations take place. In

Name_____Date_____

Facility_____DOB_____Age_____

Medical & Ocular History _____provided by patient _____obtained from chart_____

(dated)

Allergies/sensitivities to medications _____ none _____

Current meds *see chart* _____

Current eye meds *none* _____

     ROS with major dysfunctions/ surgeries/ injuries noted

      *Normal*

____*Constitutional* fever weight loss/gain cancer MRSA_____

____*Sensory* presbycusis peripheral neuropathy

____*CV* angina HTN CVA MI TIA CHF ASHD AF CAD PVD DVT_____

____*Derm* rash decubitus rosacea cellulitis _____

____*Endocrine* hypothyroid IDDM NIDDM _____

____*ENT* asthma SOB COPD CHF pneumonia _____

____*GI* constip diar PUD hepatitis GERD obesity appendectomy_____

____*GU* neurogenic bladder ESRD BPH hysterect incontinence UTI_____

____*Lymphatic/hematologic* anemia hyperchol dehydration _____

____*Musculoskeletal* RA OA DJD osteoporosis fx amputee _____

____*Psych* SDAT Parkinson's depress anx OBS psychosis schizo_____

*OCULAR*

blepharitis

blindness / reduced VA

cataract / extraction

conjunctivitis

corneal dystrophy / degen / PK

dry eye / SPK

glaucoma suspect / PI / I trab

mac degen exud nonexud h/o

laser

Date of last H & P _____by Dr_____GNP_____

Pertinent Clinical Findings

*Affect* (calm/ agitated/ alert/ weeping/ confused/ sleepy/ withdrawn)

*Oriented* (time place person)

*Date of LEE*_____pt unable to provide by Dr_____

H/o spectacle wear(y,n) if y, age of present spectacles _____ condition good fair poor

    ___no current SRx

      *Cc*_____exam requested by patient/ family/ physician_____

*HPI* (Sx loc qual severity duration timing context modifiers unable 2° to pt mental status)

_____

PERRLA___APD  NPC ___cm CT< Motility____FROM Confr. Fields___FTFC___FTFM

_____unable

D 20< ph        D 20<        Ks          VAsc

                VAcc

N 20<         N 20<

Current SRx<               Ret<   MR<

                   add

Today's SRx<

PD:                 seg ht:

type:              frame:

T$_A$ / @ _____I gtt P F / OU Dil ____ gtt OD____gtt OS

    Paremyd T 0.5/1%P 2.5%          C 1/ 2%

*SLE*

    *Internal* 90D 20D direct

nml     *OD*        *OS*     *OD*        *OS*

L/L     _____ *collarettes meib*    ONH *D/F/P PPA*

Tear_*poor debris*              C/D

Lac Sys_*open*              PVD

Con_____ *ping concret inj*        ves *tort*

Scler____ *hyaline*           mac *FR*

Corn_____ *arcus NaFl stain*               *scarring*

AC _____X        X         bkgd *drusen RPF*

*changes*

Iris *rube PI surgpup*           vitr *floater*

Lens *NS PSC cort pseud (ACIOL PCIOL) fibrosis aphake*  periph *intact / not*

    *seen*

(Drawings of external structures)       (Drawings of fundus)

Assessment                   Plan

*Signature*

F/U_____days/mos/yr

**Fig. 18-11** Sample examination form.

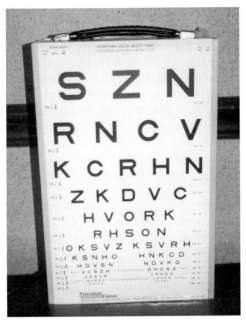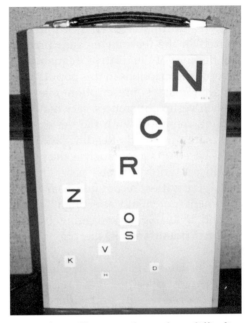

**Fig. 18-12** Because low light levels often make use of a wall-mounted eye chart difficult, a lightbox with a variety of charts may be advisable. This lightbox, shown with a Snellen-type chart *(left)*, can be made more practical by a practitioner-made overlay that occludes all but one letter on each line *(right)*.

testing near visual acuity, use good lighting and a test chart that features a wide range of letter sizes or numerals.

A Feinbloom low vision chart or other source that uses numeric optotypes is invaluable, not only for patients who are visually impaired, but also for the evaluation of patients with conditions such as cerebrovascular accident or Alzheimer's disease, which may involve cognitive deficits. Because of aphasia or visual agnosia, many such patients can appreciate and verbalize numerals or symbols but cannot do the same for an alpha optotype subtending the same or even larger visual angle.[16]

Pupillary testing, gross observation of the eyes and adnexa, and evaluation of ocular motility and binocularity are appropriate tests to administer next. Confrontation visual field testing should be attempted on every patient because a visual field test is required for complete examination and because significant field loss may accompany stroke or other systemic insults. Portable tangent screen fields, the Damato portable visual field test, Amsler grid charts, and automated portable visual field instruments are available.

Refraction should proceed with trial frame or Halburg/Janelli clip methods while giving appropriate consideration to increased difference thresholds expected in this population. Retinoscopy is of considerable value in many patients and should be used routinely, although some patients have pupillary miosis or media opacities that reduce the usefulness of this test. Radical retinoscopy may serve as a means of overcoming these problems, or it may be done after dilation.

Subjective refraction is best conducted with Halberg/Janelli clips over the patient's habitual correction when possible (otherwise trial frame methods suffice). The habitual correction can be neutralized with a portable lensometer or through hand lens neutralization techniques. Trial lenses and handheld Jackson Cross Cylinders provide a means for accurate cylinder action in any setting. The availability of both ±0.50 and ±1.00 cross cylinders provides for most needs. Trial frame refraction can be used successfully with this population as well (see Fig. 18-7). When refraction is done at the patient's habitual spectacle plane (with Halberg or Janelli clips), the combination of lenses (habitual spectacle lenses with spheres and cylinders added during the overrefraction) can be neutralized in the lensometer and directly prescribed. Because of the relative frequency of high hyperopic prescriptions in this population, adjustments in glasses prescription may be required when vertex differences vary between the trial frame compared with the vertex distance of the frames fitted. Reading addition prescribed is based on factors such as the possibility of reduced vision (thereby necessitating higher adds), the patient's common near tasks and environment (potentially affecting working distance), and available task lighting (which takes on added importance in the presence of cataract).

Evaluation of the lids, adnexa, and anterior segment of the eye typically follows refraction. High-quality, portable slit lamps (biomicroscopes) are available and have applications both in the private office setting and the out-of-office setting (see Fig. 18-5). In the absence of handheld, portable slit lamps, a diagnostic kit or other illumination source used in conjunction with a magnification system (condensing lens or magnifier) provides additional information beyond that obtained from gross observation only. A simple cobalt blue filter attached to the end of a transilluminator or penlight, with the use of fluorescein dye, helps assess tear quality or detect gross corneal staining.

Binocular indirect ophthalmoscopy should be performed after dilation of each patient (except where dilation is contraindicated because of the risk of angle closure or the presence of iris fixated intraocular lenses, or is not needed because of large surgical pupils). The handheld slit lamp in combination with condensing lenses (e.g., 60 D, 78 D or 90 D) can be used to evaluate the optic nerve, macula, and posterior pole. Information gained from these procedures is invaluable and not otherwise obtainable by any other test means. In addition, medicolegal precedents dictate that examination through dilated pupils be used routinely in optometric evaluations.[3]

Optometrists who provide care regularly in these settings may also wish to provide certain special procedures and services on site. These may include pachymetry, contrast sensitivity testing, glare disability testing, interferometry, ocular photography, and low vision care.

Providing care in a nontraditional setting also creates an opportunity for input (formally or informally) on uses of environmental design from the optometrist's background and expertise. In any setting, the optometrist can assess use of lighting, color, and contrast and make recommendations to improve the visual environment for older adults.

For this population, obtaining glasses may be just as difficult or impossible as obtaining vision care in the community. Therefore any on-site optometric evaluation must include services for the repair and ordering of glasses. In many instances, simply reconditioning, repairing, or modifying existing glasses will fulfill the patient's needs. However, any examination in a nontraditional setting should offer selection and ordering of glasses. Ophthalmic lens type prescribed must be appropriate for the common spectacle corrections and visual demands of older adults.

In addition, the frames should be engraved with the patient's name or initials to increase the chances that misplaced spectacles and their owners will be reunited.[11,16] Whenever eyeglasses are dispensed in an environment where a medical chart for the patient is available, document under the progress notes the date that eyeglasses were dispensed and adjusted, and sign the entry. Thus, if the eyeglasses are misplaced, a record that they were dispensed is available.

Eyeglasses are covered by Medicare when co-managing or caring for patients after cataract surgery. Medicare requires a signed and dated proof of delivery from the patient. Again, document in the chart when eyeglasses are dispensed to a resident of a long-term care environment. When filing the claim, the place of service code must be the patient's home (box 12 on the claim).[4]

### Reporting and Follow-up

Because of the high incidence of eye health problems in this population, following up with patients regularly on subsequent visits is important. This is facilitated in an arrangement for regularly scheduled visits to an agency or institution as opposed to on an "on-call" basis.[11]

Patients examined in nontraditional, out-of-office settings are likely to present special challenges in the area of follow-up and compliance.

The following verbiage can be formulated on an adhesive strip to be affixed to the Progress Notes section of each patient's medical chart
___F/U eye exam/ consult for (condition/complaint)_____
___Complete eye exam/ consult at request of (patient /family/ physician) for (condition/complaint)_____
Copy of the eye examination is in (Progress Notes/ Consults)
New orders: ___Yes ___No
F/U:____Days____Weeks_____ Months___Year____prn
Name of practice_____
Name of optometrist_____
Optometrist's telephone number_____

**Fig. 18-13** Sample progress note.

Therefore the clinician must provide documentation to all concerned parties, patients, staff at the agency or institution, other health care providers, and family or sponsors. Forms can be designed that facilitate reporting with minimal time required from the clinician. In particular, a three-part, carbon-copy form (one copy for the patient or the family/sponsor, one for the agency or institution, and one for the clinician) conveniently meets this need in most instances. Alternatively, a portable copy machine may be brought along if one is not available at the facility. Sample examinations are shown in Figures 18-9 and 18-11, and a sample progress note is shown in Figure 18-13. A brief cover letter with a copy of the report can be provided to other health care providers to augment general information contained in the examination report or when referral is desired.

Document every patient encounter in the progress notes or consults section of the chart with a brief note that records any order change or referral request. If a copy of the eye examination is filed in the chart—a practice that is highly recommended—the note should state such.

Keeping carbon copies or photocopies of every written order, whether for medications or for ophthalmological referral, ensures completeness of the optometrist's record and will help ensure positive results from any audit.

## Coding

Table 18-2 lists applicable codes for the examination and place of service. Do not use nursing home assessment codes 99301-3 because these are for primary care physicians only.[5,12]

**TABLE 18-2**

### Coding for the Eye Examination and Place of Service

| Type of Service | CPT Codes | Place of Service | Code |
|---|---|---|---|
| Comprehensive examination | 92004 (new patient) | Home | 12 |
| | 92014 (existing patient) | Assisted living | 13 |
| Intermediate examination | 92002 (new patient) | Nursing facility | 32 |
| | 92012 (existing patient) | Skilled nursing facility* | 31 |
| Nursing facility services (for disease-focused examinations ranging in complexity from limited to extensive) | 99311-13 | — | — |
| Refraction | 92015 | | |

Adapted from Hagan S: Reach out to patients in long-term care facilities, *Primary Care Optometry* 8:40-2, 2003.
*To be used when patient is in a skilled facility in a bed that is funded by Medicare Part A.

## VISION CARE NEEDS IN NONTRADITIONAL SETTINGS

### The Long-Term Care Setting

Nursing home residents have a high incidence of vision disorders and eye health problems that worsen over time. Data from the Beaver Dam Eye Study document vision decline and visual field loss, which are worse for nursing home residents and group home residents compared with the general population.[22] As previously mentioned, the more common ocular disorders in those aged 65 years and older are age-related cataracts, age-related macular degeneration, open-angle glaucoma, and diabetic retinopathy.[23] Visual handicaps are known to influence quality of life in a negative fashion, yet vision needs go largely unmet.[24,49] Vision impairment has been targeted as a condition affecting vulnerable older adults in need of improvement because of its prevalence among nursing home residents.[43] In another study, 51 (almost 25%) of 238 residents were identified as being in need of low vision evaluation.[33] In short, the optometrist's role in providing care in the nursing home setting is significant.[10,15,27]

A report on the results of the vision evaluation must be added to the patient's chart in the nursing home. This can be done by simply adding notes in SOAP format (subjective, objective, assessment, plan) to the consultants section of the chart or by using the wording shown in Figure 18-13 when a copy of the eye examination form is also left in the chart. Originals of the evaluation, records of telephone calls, and copies of any orders will need to be maintained by the optometrist, as will copies of the face sheet and the signed consent form and physician order for the eye examination.

## The Hospital Setting

Routine vision care is not often requested for patients undergoing hospitalization for acute illnesses. Rehabilitation centers, sometimes referred to as convalescent hospitals, provide a moderately intense level of care over an extended period. In such cases the goal is to facilitate transition back to independence in the community. In rehabilitation centers, optometric services ranging from eye health evaluation and management to replacing lost glasses to vision rehabilitation services can support the goal of return to independence in the community.

Optometrists commonly have clinical privileges in hospitals operated by the Department of Veterans Affairs, the Public Health Service, and the various branches of the military. In other hospitals, optometrists in the community may establish hospital privileges and therefore may be called on for a variety of needs. The American Optometric Association offers guidelines to optometrists who are interested in obtaining hospital privileges.[36]

## Community Service Agency Setting

A variety of programs sponsored by government agencies, various religious groups, and private agencies exist to provide community assistance for older adults. Older adults served in these settings are candidates for on-site eye care. Examples include senior centers or nutrition centers, senior clubs, day hospitals, adult day care centers, and rehabilitation centers. In settings in which older adults are highly independent, the optometrist's role is more likely to provide health education to reduce the gap in knowledge and provide knowledge, skills, and resources that enable them to meet their own health care goals and objectives.[25,31] In other settings, however, vision screening or even comprehensive on-site optometric services may be more appropriate.[28]

In each setting, an appropriate contact person must be identified in an effort to access older adults who can benefit from optometric care. This individual's title may be center director, program administrator, or ombudsman. Meeting with the director of the local Area Agency on Aging generally can provide all the information and contacts needed to instigate a new program. Contact may be initiated through an introductory letter followed by a phone call. In many instances, administrators in these settings are most interested in having a presentation or vision screening provided by the optometrist. Some settings will be appropriate for providing more comprehensive care on site.

## The Private Home Setting

Most older Americans reside in private homes. However, with advancing age the chances of an older adult who resides in a private home requiring assistance with activities of daily living increase dramatically. Although only 6% of the population aged 65 to 69 years requires such assistance, almost 32% of the population older than 85 years requires assistance. Nearly 71% of the long-term care population resides in the community.[9] Special housing needs are concentrated among the population of those aged 75 years and older, a reflection of the high incidence of physical disability in this population.[35] Furthermore, 30% of noninstitutionalized older adults reside alone.[8]

Community-based or home care has been shown to be an alternative to inappropriate or premature institutionalization.[18] Furthermore, this alternative for caring for frail, older people is more cost effective than institutionalization and, in fact, is preferred by potential program beneficiaries.[34] The success of the home care option in the future depends on a number of factors, including commitment on the part of health policy makers and the availability of health care professionals with interest and expertise in this area of health care.[2,7] Leaving the private office setting to travel to a home to provide a single examination is not cost effective. In some instances this practice may be more practical, such as when an established patient of a private practice becomes homebound, a close relative of an active family of patients is involved, or when conditions in a practice leave an optometrist with unfilled office time. Whenever possible, making provisions to examine the patient in the office setting improves the range of services offered as well as efficiency.

However, examination of the patient in the home environment gives the optometrist the opportunity to provide a complete eye examination and make practical suggestions regarding placement of lighting, adjustment of seating, and other environmental modifications to help the patient achieve visual goals.

The provision of optometric care in the home setting incorporates many of the considerations previously discussed. In seeking to access these patients, caregivers must be made aware of the availability of the service through communication or marketing. In an existing private practice, patients who receive care in the practice can become a source of referrals. In addition, other optometric and ophthalmological offices that do not offer the service, as well as social workers and all members of the network of resources for older adults, must be informed. Brochures, press releases, and newspaper articles also can be prepared to inform the local aging network and the community at large of the service. In some areas, brokers who market health care services to nursing homes can assist in placing optometrists in these settings.

Interaction with caregivers and family members is a major aspect of providing home care. Without family caregivers, many frail older adults who live at home would require nursing home care, and by some estimates 80% of the care provided to frail older adults is provided by families.[6,40] These individuals represent a major source for information before an examination through the use of advance forms or phone calls, and they are also likely to be the on-site support persons during the examination. A caregiver's presence in the examination is not always desired. In some instances the patient will perform better and be more at ease if a caregiver is not present. Once the practitioner is made aware of an adverse relationship, steps should be taken to remove the distraction from the examination. In extreme cases of adverse relationships, such as when elder abuse is suspected, states may have mandatory reporting requirements that apply to all professionals (including optometrists) who provide care to an older adult. In arranging for the appointment, it is helpful to know who will be present, their relationship to the patient, and their goals for the examination (as well as the patient's goals). Consideration for optimal time of day, equipment needed, examination sequence, environmental vision assessment, and reporting parallel those factors previously discussed.

### The Mobile Clinic Setting

Another means of providing vision care in nontraditional settings is through the use of a mobile eye clinic. Optometrists who emphasize on-site care as an aspect of their practices may operate mobile clinics. Indeed, the mobile vision clinic adds a dimension of versatility in that it can serve patients in any of the settings previously described. Additionally, some optometrists practice full-time optometry in so-called nontraditional settings, thus eliminating the physical confines (and overhead expenses) of a traditional office.

The mobile clinic method of health care delivery can take place in a number of ways. In one scenario, the clinic is designed for bringing patients on board and providing care within the mobile unit itself.[37] In another, the necessary equipment simply is transported in an ordinary vehicle to the site where the care will be deliv-

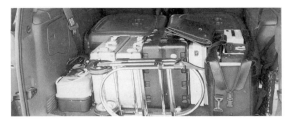

**Fig. 18-14** All cases of ophthalmic equipment, supplies, and a platform cart can be stowed in the back of a van or other motor vehicle or in the trunk of a car for transport to any site.

ered (Fig. 18-14). This latter method is perhaps best suited for accessing bedridden patients in nursing homes, private homes, and rehabilitation facilities.

## FUTURE TRENDS IN NONTRADITIONAL SETTINGS

Given emerging trends that have rapidly shifted population demographics, the need for providing vision care in nontraditional settings may be expected to increase. The development of on-site services for home care, nursing home care, and other settings can be instrumental in reaching a large and growing underserved population. However, as stated by Berkowitz et al[1] more than 20 years ago, "As governments and organizations pursue cost avoidance strategies, individuals will get squeezed into 'solutions' that do not fit their real needs."

The current trends in health policy place the major emphasis on cost containment, but the high health care costs generated during the time older adults spend in a state of disability and dependence at the end of life also need to be considered. Maintaining independence in the community (including through improving access to a variety of community-based services) can be more cost effective than providing for years of dependence and institutionalization. Policy, then, is perhaps the greatest obstacle to the provision of vision care in nontraditional settings. Despite this paradox, optometrists are better prepared educationally, better equipped technically, and better dispersed geographically to meet this growing need than ever before in history.

## REFERENCES

1. Berkowitz M, Horning M, McDonnell S, et al: An economic evaluation of the beneficiary rehabilitation program. In Rubin J, editor: *Alternative in rehabilitating the handicapped,* New York, 1982, Human Sciences Press.
2. Bernstein LH, Hankwitz PE, Portnow J: Home care of the elderly diabetic patient, *Clin Geriatr Med* 6: 943-57, 1990.
3. Classe JG: A review of 50 malpractice claims, *J Am Optom Assoc* 60:694-706, 1989.
4. Corcoran S: Post cataract surgery glasses, *Optom Manage* 38:57, 2003.
5. Corcoran S: A whole new world: documentation rules and CPT codes for services to nursing home patients, *Optom Manage* 38:86, 2003.
6. Covinsky KE, Eng C, Lui LY, et al: Reduced employment in caregivers of frail elders: impact of ethnicity, patient clinical characteristics, and caregiver characteristics, *J Gerontol A Biol Sci Med Sci* 56: M707-13, 2001.
7. Cummings JE: Innovations in homecare, *Generations* 12:61-4, 1987.
8. DeSylvia DA: The older patient: part I, *High Performance Optometry* 4:1-5, 1990.
9. DeSylvia DA, Williams AK: Health and housing continuum. In *Optometric gerontology: a resource manual for educators,* Rockville, MD, 1989, Association of Schools and Colleges of Optometry, pp 5.1-5.13.
10. Durkin JR, Newcomb RD: Optometry in nursing homes, *J Am Optom Assoc* 63:102-5, 1992.
11. Eger N: Taking a closer look at nursing homes, *Optom Manage* 34:38-44, 1999.
12. Eisenberg J: Billing for nursing home visits, *Rev Optom* 135:8, 1998.
13. Elam J: Optometry students' attitudes about nursing home rotations, *Optom Educ* 28:137-9, 2003.
14. Friedman D, Munoz B, Massof R, et al: Grating visual acuity using the preferential-looking method in elderly nursing home residents, *Invest Ophthalmol Vis Sci* 43:2572-8, 2002.
15. Gorman NS: Nursing home practice, *Optom Econ* 1:18-21, 1991.
16. Hagan S: Reach out to patients in long-term care facilities, *Primary Care Optom* 8:40-2, 2003.
17. Holroyd S, Shepherd M: Alzheimer's disease: a review for the ophthalmologist, *Surv Ophthalmol* 45:516-24, 2001.
18. Holt SW: The role of home care in long term care, *Generations* 11:9-12, 1986.
19. Ivers R, Norton R, Cumming R, et al: Visual impairment and risk of hip fracture, *Am J Epidemiol* 152:633-9, 2000.
20. Janicki MP, Davidson PW, Henderson CM, et al: Health characteristics and health services utiliza-

tion in older adults with intellectual disability living in community residences, *J Intellect Disabil Res* 46:287-98, 2002.

21. Keller B, Hejkal T, Potter J: Barriers to vision care for nursing home residents, *J Am Med Dir Assoc* 2:15-21, 2001.

22. Klein R, Klein B, Lee K, et al: Changes in visual acuity in a population over a 10-year period: the Beaver Dam Eye Study, *Ophthalmology* 108:1757-66, 2001.

23. Lee P, Feldman Z, Osterman J, et al: Longitudinal prevalence of major eye diseases, *Arch Ophthalmol* 121:1303-10, 2003.

24. Lee P, Feldman Z, Ostermann J, et al: Longitudinal rates of annual eye examinations of persons with diabetes and chronic eye diseases, *Ophthalmology* 110:1952-9, 2003.

25. Livingston PM, McCarty CA, Taylor HR: Knowledge, attitudes, and self care practices associated with age related eye disease in Australia, *Br J Ophthalmol* 82:780-5, 1998.

26. Lord S, Dayhew J: Visual risk factors for falls in older people, *J Am Geriatr Soc* 49:508-15, 2001.

27. Mancil GL: Delivery of optometric care in non-traditional settings: the long-term care facility (symposium). *Optom Vis Sci* 66: 9-11, 1989.

28. Mancil GL: Eye care delivery in nontraditional settings. In Aston SJ, DeSylvia DA, Mancil GL, editors: *Optometric gerontology: a resource manual for educators*, Rockville, MD, 1989, Association of Schools and Colleges of Optometry, pp 16.1-16.12.

29. Marx MS, Werner P, Cohen-Mansfield J, et al: Visual acuity estimates in noncommunicative elderly persons, *Invest Ophthalmol Vis Sci* 31:593-6, 1990.

30. Medicare plans to specifically exempt physician fees from "excessive charge" rule, *American Optometric Association News*, vol 42, November 3, 2003.

31. Minkler M, Pasick RJ: Health promotion and the elderly: a critical perspective on the past and future. In Dychtwald K, editor: *Wellness and health promotion for the elderly*, Rockville, MD, 1986, Aspen Publications.

32. More optometrists seeing nursing facility patients, *American Optometric Association News*, vol 39, April 23, 2001.

33. Morse AR, O'Connell WO, Joseph J, et al: Assessing vision in nursing home residents, *J Vis Rehabil* 2:5-14, 1988.

34. Nassif JZ: There's still no place like home, *Generations* 11:5-8, 1986.

35. Newman SJ: The shape of things to come, *Generations* 9:14-7, 1985.

36. *Optometric hospital privileges*, American Optometric Association St. Louis, Mo.

37. Optometry on the road, *J Am Optom Assoc* 72:333-4, 2001.

38. Palmer R: Falls in elderly patients: predictable and preventable, *Cleve Clin J Med* 68:303-6, 2001.

39. Researcher makes case for doubling federal eye research budget, *American Optometric Association News*, vol 41, June 2, 2003.

40. Rubin RJ: Private versus public responsibilities for long-term care. In Dunlap BD, editor: *New federalism and long-term care of the elderly*, Millwood, VA, 1985, Center for Health Affairs.

41. Rubin GS, Roche KB, Prasada-Rao P, et al: Visual impairment and disability in older adults, *Optom Vis Sci* 71:750-60, 1994.

42. Scilley K, Owsley C: Vision specific health related quality of life: content areas for nursing home residents, *Qual Life Res* 11:449-62, 2002.

43. Sloss EM, Solomon DH, Shekelle PG, et al: Selecting target conditions for quality of care improvement in vulnerable older adults, *J Am Geriatr Soc* 48:363-9, 2000.

44. Spillman B, Lubita J: New estimates of lifetime nursing home use: have patterns of use changed? *Medical Care* 40:28, 2002.

45. Taiel-Sartral M, Nounou P, Rea C, et al: Acuite visuelle et pathologie oculaire chez le sujet age residants en maison de retraite: etude orleanaise sur 219 personnes, *J Fr Ophthalmol* 22:431-7, 1999.

46. Van Newkirk M, Weih L, McCarty C, et al. Visual impairment and eye diseases in elderly institutionalized Australians, *Ophthalmology* 107:2203-8, 2000.

47. Wallhagen MI, Strawbridge WJ, Shema SJ, et al: Comparative impact of hearing and vision impairment on subsequent functioning, *J Am Geriatr Soc* 49:1086-92, 2001.

48. Wang J, Mitchell P, Cumming R, et al: Visual impairment and nursing home placement in older Australians: the Blue Mountains Eye Study, *Ophthalmic Epidemiol* 10:3-13, 2003.

49. Williams RA, Brody BL, Thomas RG, et al: The psychosocial impact of macular degeneration, *Arch Ophthalmol* 116:514-20, 1998.

# CHAPTER 19

# *Public Health Aspects of Older Adult Patient Care*

## NORMA K. BOWYER

The demographic shift toward an aging population poses major challenges for public health programs and practices in the twenty-first century. This chapter defines public health, primary care, and their interrelated functions and also reviews trends in aging demographics and sets forth the nation's public health vision and eye health goals and objectives for all Americans. Also, this chapter examines public health and primary care and highlights important health-related topics relevant to older populations and their implications for public health. It discusses the influence of aging on current public health program priorities. The chapter concludes exploring potential public health strategies the nation has set forth in the *Healthy People* series to address the future direction of public health for vision and aging issues as the population ages.

## WHAT IS PUBLIC HEALTH?

Public health is what society does together to ensure the conditions in which people can be healthy.[14] Just as a person's health is greater than the health care he or she receives, public health is more than services, programs, education, and activities provided by governmental health agencies. It also collectively encompasses the resultant impact of individual personal choices and environmental influences.

## Role of Government in Public Health

In 1988, the Institute of Medicine (IOM) published *The Future of Public Health,* which provided guidance to the public health community by setting the foundation of public health through delineating the core functions of public health agencies at all levels of government. These functions are (1) assessment: systematic collection and analysis of information on the health of the community; (2) assurance: services provided to achieve population health goals; and (3) policy development: direction of operations and resource allocation for the health system.[14] These basic functions were descriptively refined through identifying public health competencies and articulating the public health Vision, Mission and Essential Public Health Services (Box 19-1 and Fig. 19-1).[21,22] The public health agenda for the nation, *Healthy People 2010,* through assessment, that is, systematic collection and analysis of vision and eye health data, set forth 10 national public health vision objectives. All but two of these objectives directly address needs of aging America. Furthermore, assurance, quantifying and examining the needs of the nation, especially with awareness for specialty populations, brought about changes in policy development through resource allocation and operation guidance, most notably in the areas of glaucoma and diabetes.

## Role of the Individual in Public Health

In the section "Shared Responsibilities," the 2000 public health agenda for the nation *Healthy People 2000* challenges that "Each of us whether acting as an individual, an employee or employer, a member of a family, community group, professional organization, or government agency, has both an opportunity and an obligation to contribute to the effort to improve the Nation's health profile."[25] Public health includes more than the governmental actions of local, county, state, or federal health agencies. Public health activities, although very important to the health and well-being of a community, are more than restaurant and sanitation inspections. Public health is more than indigent care for the needy

or less fortunate. Public health is more than annual influenza immunizations or vision screenings before reissuance of driver's licenses. Public health is what individuals do on a day-to-day basis. Public health ultimately includes the collective actions chosen by the individual; for example, the decision whether to smoke cigarettes. These are individual choices or actions of self-responsibility that an individual makes in his or her daily life, creating a more or less healthy lifestyle. In concert with controllable and uncontrollable factors (such as genetics and personal health status of the individual), when examined collectively, these choices contribute to the health status of the nation.

### Is Aging a Public Health Concern?

Three essential characteristics of a public health issue include disease burden, change in incidence (suggesting preventability), and concern about risk.[27] High disease burden means that the disease is sufficiently common enough that many people feel that it might happen to them. A high disease burden can be magnified by a second, related element, that is, the burden was previously low and increased at a high enough rate as to make the change obvious. Public concern is the third element in societal acceptance of a health condition as a public health issue. With the rapidly increasing number of individuals attaining older age and having greater needs in such areas as low vision resources and services, the public begins to call for societal, community, and governmental intervention to help support individuals and families by sharing a greater portion of the high disease burden so that aging Americans can maintain their quality of life and independent lifestyles.

### Public Health and Primary Care

In 1996 the IOM produced another landmark report, *Primary Care: America's Health in a New Era*, which updates the definition of primary care in the United States.[15]

  In previous reports and IOM documents the essence of primary care was defined as accessible, comprehensive, coordinated, and continual care delivered by accountable providers of personal health services. The older definition has been widely used and was helpful as a beginning point for redefining and updating the new definition of primary care (Box 19-2).[15]

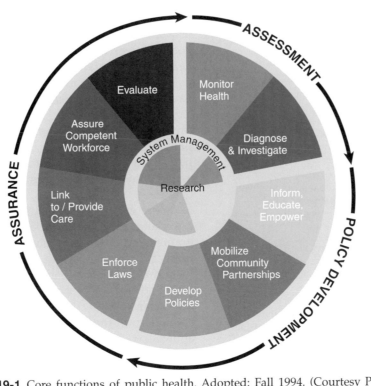

**Fig. 19-1** Core functions of public health. Adopted: Fall 1994. (Courtesy Public Health Functions Steering Committee, Members [July 1995]: American Public Health Association, Association of Schools of Public Health, Association of State and Territorial Health Officials, Environmental Council of the States, National Association of County and City Health Officials, National Association of State Alcohol and Drug Abuse Directors, National Association of State Mental Health Program Directors, Public Health Foundation, U.S. Public Health Service—*Agency for Health Care Policy and Research, Centers for Disease Control and Prevention, Food and Drug Administration, Health Resources and Services Administration, Indian Health Service, National Institutes of Health, Office of the Assistant Secretary for Health, Substance Abuse and Mental Health Services Administration.*)

---

**BOX 19-2**

## Definition of Primary Care

Primary care is the provision of integrated, accessible health care services by clinicians who are accountable for addressing most personal health care needs, developing sustained partnership with patients, and practicing in the context of family and community.[15]

---

The newer report addresses integration of public health and primary care, recognizing that the population-based function of public health and the personal care services that primary care delivers to individuals are complementary functions. The study insufficiently identifies the contributions of nonmedical primary care clinicians, such as dentists and optometrists, to pri-

mary care.[2] However, the current document does capture a succinct, workable refinement of the definition of primary care.

Primary care addresses a spectrum of personal health issues to the aging population along the continuum of health and wellness as they occur separately or in combination with other conditions over the life span of an individual. The following categories are identified as within the scope of primary care: (1) acute care, (2) chronic (long-term) care, (3) prevention and early detection, (4) coordination of referrals (Box 19-3).[16]

Public health leaders for more than a decade have been calling for an integration of population and personal health.[18] In this role as primary care providers, eye care practitioners make a significant contribution to the health

## BOX 19-3

## Categories of Primary Care

1. **Acute Care**
   a. The primary care clinician evaluates a patient with symptoms sufficient to prompt him or her to seek medical attention. Health concerns may range from an acute, relatively minor, self-limiting illness to a complex set of symptoms that could be life threatening to a mental problem. The clinician arranges for further evaluation by specialists or subspecialists when appropriate.
   b. The clinician manages acute problems or, when beyond the scope of the particular clinician, arranges for other management of the problem.

2. **Chronic (Long-Term) Care**
   a. A primary care clinician serves as the principal provider of ongoing care for some patients who have one or more chronic diseases, including mental disorders with appropriate consultations.
   b. A primary care clinician collaborates in the care of other patients whose chronic illnesses are of such a nature that the principal provider of care is another specialist or subspecialist. The primary care clinician manages intercurrent illnesses, provides preventive care (e.g., screening tests, immunizations, counseling about lifestyle), and incorporates knowledge of the family and the patient's community. An example is the management of dermatitis, hypertension, or upper respiratory infection of a patient who is under the care of a rheumatologist for rheumatoid arthritis.

3. **Prevention and Early Detection**
   The primary care clinician provides periodic health assessments for all patients, including screening, counseling, risk assessment, and patient education. Primary care must reflect an understanding of risk factors associated with these illnesses, including genetic risks, and of the early stages of disease that may be difficult to detect at its outset.

4. **Coordination of Referrals**
   The clinician coordinates referrals to and from other clinicians and provides advice and education to patients who are referred for further evaluation or treatment.[15]

and well-being of the nation. Perhaps the most significance contribution to public health is in the area of prevention and early detection.

Currently the best linkage between the personal health care system and the public health system is in the area of clinical guidelines and clinical preventive services. Clinical preventive services provide a significant link for applying the population-based perspective of public health to personal health care. To achieve the goals of increasing the span and quality of healthy life for Americans and reducing the health disparities among all Americans, the nation has adopted an approach that promotes closer working relationships among primary care, the provision of personal care, and the public health system. For the first time in the past 3 decades, the nation's public health agenda includes specific vision and eye health objectives.[26]

Before examining the nation's public health goals and objectives, a brief review of demographic and epidemiological trends and policy implications in aging that influence the shift of focus from an acute care model to long-term care and prevention will provide a greater understanding of the nation's public health agenda and the significance of vision and aging.

## PUBLIC HEALTH TRENDS IN AGING

In the United States the growing number of individuals aged 65 years or older is affecting every aspect of society, presenting challenges and opportunities to policy makers, families, businesses, and health care providers. The percentage of this population is projected to increase from just above 10% in 2000 to nearly 20% in 2030. The number of persons in this age bracket is anticipated to double, increasing from approximately 35 million in 2000 to an estimated 71 million in 2030. The number of the oldest older Americans, those individuals aged 80 years or older, is projected to increase from 9.3 million in 2000 to 19.5 million in 2030.[6]

Aging trends and predictions in the United States from 1900 to 2030 demonstrate the steady and dramatic increase in the percentage of Americans aged 65 years or older during the years 1900, 1970, 2000, and 2030 (Fig. 19-2). The pyramids highlight how the baby-boomer generation (Americans born between 1946 and 1964) contributed to this rapid increase and how more Americans are living into their 90s. The pyramids are broken into age groups for male and female populations, starting with children younger than 5 years and ending with adults aged 85 years and older. In 1900 only 4% of Americans were aged 65 years and older, but more than half were younger than 25 years. By

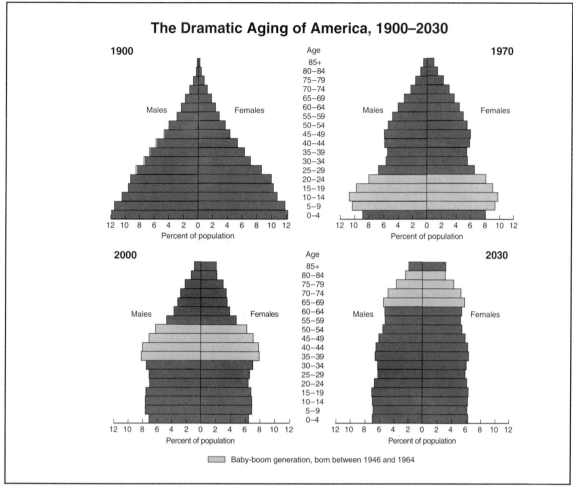

**Fig. 19-2** Aging trends in America. (Adapted from Himes CL: Elderly Americans, *Population Bulletin* 56:4, 2002.)

1970 the proportion of Americans aged 65 years or older had grown but remained small compared with younger age groups. Baby-boomers, then aged 5 to 24 years, created a bulge in the age-sex pyramid for 1970. In 2000 more than 12% of Americans were aged 65 years old or older. Baby-boomers, then aged 35 to 54 years, made up nearly 30% of the U.S. population in 2000. In 2030, when the oldest baby boomers will reach age 65 years, the U.S. population will be evenly divided across age groups. An estimated 20% of Americans will be older than 65 years. Adults aged 85 years or older will make up the fastest-growing segment of older adults populations.[12]

The most populous nine states in 1995 had the largest number of older persons. California,

Florida, Illinois, Michigan, New Jersey, New York, Ohio, Pennsylvania, and Texas each had more than 1 million persons aged 65 years of age or older.[6] The sex distribution of older U.S. residents is expected to change only moderately. Women represented nearly 60% of persons aged 65 years or older in 2000 compared with a projected estimate of 56% in 2030.[6] Larger changes in the racial/ethnic composition of persons aged 65 years or older are expected. From 2000 to 2030 the proportion of persons aged 65 years or older who are black, American Indian/Alaska Native, or Asian/Pacific Islander is expected to increase from 11.3% to 16.5%. Additionally, the proportion of the Hispanic population is expected to increase from 5.6% to 10.9%.[6]

## Demographic and Epidemiological Transition

The world is experiencing a gradual demographic and epidemiological transition. The aging of the world's population is the result of two factors: declines in fertility and increases in life expectancy.[17] A gradual demographic transition from patterns of high fertility and high mortality rates to low fertility and delayed mortality rates has occurred. The transition begins with declining infant and childhood mortality, in part because of effective public health measures.[17] Lower childhood mortality rates initially contribute to a longer life expectancy and a younger population. Declines in fertility rates generally follow, and improvements in adult health lead to an older population. At the same time the world also has experienced an epidemiological transition in the leading causes of death, from infectious disease and acute illness to chronic disease and degenerative illness. In 2001 the leading causes of death in developed countries were primarily cardiovascular diseases and cancer, followed by respiratory diseases and injuries.[6] These were the same countries that had low childhood mortality rates and delayed adult mortality rates. This epidemiological transition, combined with the demographic transition of increasing numbers of older persons, represents a challenge for public health.

### Chronic Disease

Chronic conditions such as Alzheimer's disease, arthritis, and diabetes lead to morbidity, severe disability, and increased health care costs. In the United States approximately 80% of all persons aged 65 years or older have at least one chronic condition, and 50% have at least two.[5] For example, diabetes affects approximately one in five (18.7%) persons aged 65 years or older. As the population ages, the impact of diabetes will intensify.[5] The largest increases in diabetes are expected among adults aged 75 years or older.[4] The growing number of older adults increases demands on the public health system and on health and social services. Chronic diseases, which disproportionately affect older adults, contribute to disability, diminished quality of life, and increased health and long-term care costs. (For a more comprehensive discussion of these and other chronic conditions, see Chapter 3.)

## Policy Implications: Impact on Health Care and Social Services

The increasing number of persons aged 65 years or older will potentially lead to increased health care costs. The health care cost per capita for persons aged 65 or older in the United States and other developed countries is three to five times greater than the cost for persons younger than 65 years. Additionally, the rapid growth in the number of older persons, along with continued advances in medical technology, are expected to create upward pressure on health care and long-term care spending. In 1997 the United States had the highest health care spending per person aged 65 years or older ($12,100). Other developed nations also spent substantial amounts, ranging from approximately $3600 in the United Kingdom to approximately $6800 in Canada.[1]

The demands associated with long-term care pose a tremendous challenge to personal, family, and public resources. In the United States nursing home and home health care expenditures doubled from 1990 to 2001, reaching approximately $132 billion. Of these expenses, Medicaid and Medicare paid 57% and patients or their families paid 25%.[19] In addition, from 2000 to 2020 public financing of long-term care is projected to increase by approximately 20% in the United Kingdom and the United States and by 102% in Japan.[16]

The projected growth in the number of persons aged 65 years or older and its impact on the nation's public health has been widely discussed.[17] One scenario states that if the number of working taxpayers relative to the number of older persons declines, inadequate public resources and fewer adults will be available to provide informal care to older, less-able family members and friends. However, this rationale does not account for potential increases in the numbers of persons aged 65 years or older who continue to remain in the work force and care for themselves.

Additionally, the challenge to acquire greater resources could also be mitigated if public health and primary care interventions decrease disability and enhance independence among older persons, helping them remain active and enabling them to maintain less-dependent lifestyles. Interestingly, disability among older

U.S. adults, as measured by limitations in activities of daily living (ADL), has declined since the early 1980s. Recent studies that used ADL measures have shown varied trends in disability.[8] Some studies show that the onset of disabilities can be delayed or postponed by healthier lifestyles.[13]

To address the challenges posed by an aging population, public health agencies and community organizations worldwide continue expanding their traditional scope from infectious diseases and maternal/child health to include health promotion in older adults, prevention of disability, maintenance of capacity in those with frailties and disabilities, and enhanced quality of life. In addressing prevention and aging issues, behaviors that place persons at risk for disease and disability often originate early in life.[12] Therefore the public health system also supports healthy behaviors throughout a person's lifetime. Public health also continues to develop and support better methods and systems to monitor and evaluate additional health outcomes related to older adults, such as level of function and quality of life.

If the nation is to achieve the public health goals set forth in the nation's public health agenda of increasing the span and quality of healthy life and reducing the health disparities among Americans at an affordable cost, the nation must adopt an approach that promotes closer working relationships among primary care, the provision of personal care, and public health.

## A PUBLIC HEALTH APPROACH

### The Nation's Public Health Agenda: *Healthy People 2010*

The U.S. public health system has a long history of working toward enhancing the health status of Americans. This daunting task, most recently culminating in *Healthy People 2010*, the nation's public health agenda, contains goals and objectives for the nation, including specific vision and eye care objectives. *Healthy People* goals and objectives are grounded in science, built through public consensus, and designed to measure progress. *Healthy People 2010* is the nation's health promotion and disease prevention initiative that emphasizes prevention, early diagnosis, and treatment. It brings together both the private and public health care sectors. It includes

national, state, and local government agencies; nonprofit, voluntary, and professional organizations; businesses; and communities. *HP 2010* had its beginnings nearly 3 decades earlier in the U.S. Department of Health, Education, and Welfare, known today as the Department of Health and Human Services, and continues to receive bipartisan support through both Democrat and Republican administrations. The *Healthy People* process officially began in 1979 by then Surgeon General, Julius Richmond, MD, with *Healthy People: The Surgeon General's Report on Health Promotion and Disease Prevention.*[23] In 1980 the U.S. prevention agenda was set by the document *Promoting Health/Preventing Disease: Objectives for the Nation.*[24] In the 1990s the process continued with *Healthy People 2000, National Health Promotion and Disease Prevention Objectives.*[25] *Healthy People 2010* continues the tradition to improve the nation's public health for the first decade of the twenty-first century.[26]

Many objectives focus on interventions designed to reduce or eliminate illness, disability, and premature death. Others focus on broader issues, such as improving access to quality health care, strengthening public health services, and improving the availability of health information. Objectives have a target for specific improvement to be achieved by the year 2010. The 28 focus area chapters shown in Box 19-4 contain 467 objectives.[26] Finding a focus area chapter that is not relevant to the aging process and older Americans is difficult. Chapter 28, "Focus Area of Vision and Hearing," includes 10 vision specific-objectives (Box 19-5) and a narrative (see Appendix 19-1) for improving the vision and eye health during the 2000 to 2010 decade through prevention, early detection, treatment, and rehabilitation. All the vision objectives, along with other health objectives, are designed to help a nation with dramatically changing demographics to achieve two major outcomes: to increase the quality and years of healthy life and to eliminate health disparities among different groups.[26]

New to the *Healthy People* series is a set of leading health indicators, similar to leading economic indicators, that will help individuals and communities target and track actions to improve health. The leading health indicators shown in Box 19-6 highlight major health priorities for the nation and include the individual

**BOX 19-4**

*Healthy People 2010:* **Focus Area Chapters**

1. Access to Quality Health Services
2. Arthritis, Osteoporosis, and Chronic Back Conditions
3. Cancer
4. Chronic Kidney Disease
5. Diabetes
6. Disability and Secondary Conditions
7. Educational and Community-Based Programs
8. Environmental Health
9. Family Planning
10. Food Safety
11. Health Communication
12. Heart Disease and Stroke
13. HIV
14. Immunization and Infectious Diseases
15. Injury and Violence Prevention
16. Maternal, Infant, and Child Health
17. Medical Product Safety
18. Mental Health and Mental Disorders
19. Nutrition and Overweight
20. Occupational Safety and Health
21. Oral Health
22. Physical Activity and Fitness
23. Public Health Infrastructure
24. Respiratory Diseases
25. Sexually Transmitted Diseases
26. Substance Abuse
27. Tobacco Use
28. Vision and Hearing

From U.S. Department of Health and Human Services: *Healthy People 2010, ed 2, with understanding and improving health and objectives for improving health,* 2 vols, Washington, DC, 2000, U.S. Government Printing Office.

**BOX 19-5**

*Healthy People 2010:* **Chapter 28, Vision and Hearing Objectives**

**Summary of Objectives**
The goal is to improve the visual and hearing health of the nation through prevention, early detection, treatment, and rehabilitation.

**Vision**

| | |
|---|---|
| 28-1 | Dilated eye examinations |
| 28-2 | Vision screening for children |
| 28-3 | Impairment due to refractive errors |
| 28-4 | Impairment in children and adolescents |
| 28-5 | Impairment due to diabetic retinopathy |
| 28-6 | Impairment due to glaucoma |
| 28-7 | Impairment due to cataract |
| 28-8 | Occupational eye injury |
| 28-9 | Protective eyewear |
| 28-10 | Vision rehabilitation services and devices |

**Hearing**

| | |
|---|---|
| 28-11 | Newborn hearing screening, evaluation, and intervention |
| 28-12 | Otitis media |
| 28-13 | Rehabilitation for hearing impairment |
| 28-14 | Hearing examination |
| 28-15 | Evaluation and treatment referrals |
| 28-16 | Hearing protection |
| 28-17 | Noise-induced hearing loss in children |
| 28-18 | Noise-induced hearing loss in adults |

From U.S. Department of Health and Human Services: *Healthy People 2010, ed 2, with understanding and improving health and objectives for improving health,* 2 vols, Washington, DC, 2000, U.S. Government Printing Office.

behaviors, physical and social environmental factors, and health system issues that affect the health of individuals and communities.[22]

### *Healthy People 2010* Vision and Eye Health Objectives

*Healthy People 2010* is the first *Healthy People* report to address vision objectives specifically (see Box 19-5). In previous years *Healthy People* initiatives included very few specifically vision-related objectives dispersed within the report, such as increasing dilated eye examinations for patients with diabetes. *Healthy People 2010* vision objectives highlight the importance of vision care and eye health to the nation's public health. All but two of the 10 vision objectives address objectives that are relevant to the aging population. A significant increase in the avail-

**BOX 19-6**

*Healthy People 2010:* **Leading Health Indicators Used to Describe and Assess Improvements in the Nation's Health**

Physical activity
Overweight and obesity
Tobacco use
Substance abuse
Responsible sexual behavior
Mental health
Injury and violence
Environmental quality
Immunization
Access to health care

From U.S. Department of Health and Human Services: *Healthy People 2010, ed 2, with understanding and improving health and objectives for improving health,* 2 vols, Washington, DC, 2000, U.S. Government Printing Office.

ability and access to optometric and ophthalmological services will be necessary to reduce visual impairments and reach the objectives set forth in the *Healthy People 2010*.

These national health goals and objectives will affect the provision of vision and eye care services. The objectives also influence many health care programs and the provision of health care through laws, regulations, reimbursements, and clinical guidelines enacted by federal and state agencies. Therefore primary eye care providers should understand these objectives and actively participate in the work to implement them at the national, state, and local levels. By doing this, they can help provide the services needed to reduce visual impairments and preserve the vision of aging individuals in their communities.

### Other Vision-Related Focus Area Objectives

Very few specific objectives in *Healthy People 2010* are directly related to vision and eye health outside of Chapter 28, "Vision and Hearing" (see Box 19-4). Two important ones are found in Chapter 5, "Diabetes," and in Chapter 6, "Disability and Secondary Conditions." Objective 5-13 states that adults with diabetes aged 18 years and older should have annual dilated eye examinations. Objective 6-11 states that the number of people with disabilities who do not have assistive devices should be reduced. Meeting these objectives will also increase the number of people needing eye and vision care every year.

Additionally, indirectly related objectives are scattered throughout the two-volume document in addition to focus area chapters that are relevant to public health vision and aging. Two examples of focus area chapters that are relevant include Chapter 1, "Access to Quality Health Services," and Chapter 23, "Public Health Infrastructure." Chapter 1 focuses on four components of the health care system: clinical preventive care, primary care, emergency services, and long-term and rehabilitative care. Access issues involve concerns regarding receiving health services in communities where they are already available but not provided as well as in communities where they are not available. This chapter supports the clinical preventive services provided by doctors of optometry such as blood glucose and blood pressure screening and health

education regarding modifiable risk factors such as smoking and obesity.

Clinical preventive services have a substantial impact on many of the leading causes of morbidity and mortality. People need access to preventive services that are effective in preventing disease and detecting asymptomatic disease or risk factors at early, treatable stages. The *Healthy People 2010* report is used in developing such recommendations as found in the *Guide to Clinical Preventive Services*.[10] These recommendations are widely used by the government, health-related, and managed care organizations to determine the standard of care for many diseases and disorders. For example, the Health Plan Employer Data Information Set contains measures of clinical preventive services.[20] With the *Healthy People 2010* report, the number and significance of clinical preventive services used to assess quality of health care will likely increase.

Twenty-five percent of Americans live in rural communities (populations less than 2500) where they do not have access to health care services.[26] Heart disease, cancer, diabetes, and injury rates in rural areas exceed those in urban areas. Older Americans living in rural areas are less likely to use preventive screening services, have less access to emergency and specialty services, and are more likely to be uninsured compared with people in urban areas. Because of their widespread geographical distribution, optometrists, as primary eye care providers, can make significant contributions to improving the health of rural populations and providing appropriate referrals for additional primary care services or secondary and tertiary care.[3]

Chapter 23 of *Healthy People 2010*, "Public Health Infrastructure," addresses data and information systems, workforce, public health organizations, resources, and prevention research. Understanding these areas of public health enhances the ability of eye care professionals to partner effectively within their local communities and states to enhance the health status of older members of the communities.

Also of particular interest to primary eye care providers, as well as other health professionals, is Objective 1-7 in Chapter 1. This objective calls for an increase in the number of schools of medical, nursing, and other health professional training schools whose basic curriculum for health care providers includes core competencies in health promotion and disease prevention.

*Healthy People 2010* represents an opportunity for individuals to make healthy lifestyle choices for themselves and their families. It challenges clinicians to put prevention and rehabilitation into their practices. It requires communities and businesses to support health-promoting policies. It calls for scientists to pursue new research. Above all, it encourages everyone to work together, using both traditional public health and innovative approaches, to help the American public improve its health by achieving the specific objectives.

### *Healthy Vision 2010*: Healthy Eyes, Healthy People

*Healthy Vision 2010* represents the vision community's efforts to attain the vision objectives in *Healthy People 2010*.[11] The *Healthy Vision 2010* consortium, coordinated through the National Institutes of Health and National Eye Institute (NEI), helps the vision community work together to advance vision and eye health in neighborhoods and communities by state and national programs and policy.

For example, the AOA's *Healthy Vision 2010* efforts are gathered under the auspices of their *Healthy Eyes, Healthy People* program.[11] The AOA identifies needs and develops resources and educational materials for patients and providers to raise awareness.[3] The AOA encourages the development of specific programs with state associations to address the objectives in local communities and works with employers and health care organizations to modify their benefits to include annual dilated eye examinations. The AOA continues to support vision and eye research that will reduce visual impairments caused by diabetic retinopathy, glaucoma, cataracts, macular degeneration, myopia, eye injuries, and other preventable vision disorders and also works to have vision rehabilitation services, including low vision services, and adaptive devices become well known to health providers, health care organizations, and the public. The AOA partners with other *Healthy People* consortium members to obtain their support in achieving the vision objectives set forth in *Healthy People 2010*. The AOA has developed health promotion mate-

rials for television, radio, the Internet, print media, and private practice offices to educate the public about the need for personal eye protective devices for sports and hazardous situations around the home.

The National Eye Institute (NEI) also recognizes the importance of strengthening the capacity of community-based organizations by providing resources to begin or continue vision-related health education projects. This organization provides leadership to promote health and prevent disease among Americans through management and coordination of the implementation and monitoring of the vision objectives in *Healthy People 2010*. Numerous resources have been produced, and additional new ones are being developed to help organizations, agencies, and communities achieve the *Healthy People 2010* vision objectives. The NEI also provides support through *Healthy Vision* community awards programs and nationally recognized activities, including Healthy Vision Month, that enable the vision community to come together to promote the importance of vision in promoting health for all Americans.

### Healthy West Virginia 2010

*Healthy Iowan 2010* and *Healthy West Virginia 2010* are examples of state documents that are characteristic of desirable public health planning. These state documents exemplify a public health translation of the national objectives to state and local needs. At the state and local levels public health organizations, agencies, and individuals have taken a variety of approaches in translating the national objectives to state and local initiatives. Some states have chosen to work on only 10 or 12 of the potential 28 focus areas; other states such as West Virginia have included all the focus areas. In addition, because of the significant older population, West Virginia added a chapter on "End of Life," which was not included in the federal initiative.[28] *Healthy West Virginia 2010* provides an opportunity to identify significant preventable threats to the public's health and then focus both public and private sector efforts. This enables diverse groups to combine efforts and work as a team to improve the health of the citizens of the state. West Virginia's Chapter

28, "Vision and Hearing," consists of five vision objectives. Four of the five objectives are specifically directed to vision concerns of the adult and aging population of the state. The *Healthy West Virginia 2010* document states:

> Vision and eye care are important issues in West Virginia because of its status as the oldest state in the nation. The leading causes of visual impairment are diabetic retinopathy, cataracts, glaucoma, and age-related macular degeneration. Vision and eye care services are critically important to maintaining independence and quality of life in the later years. Access to basic vision and eye health services along with specialty care in the areas of vision rehabilitative services and assistive living techniques, devices, and knowledge must be available for older adults and others with limited vision to maintain independent living.[28]

## Summary

*Healthy People 2010, Healthy Vision 2010, Healthy Eyes-Healthy People, Healthy Iowa,* and *Healthy West Virginia* all challenge individuals, communities, and professionals, in both the public and private sectors, to take specific steps to ensure that good vision, as well as good health, are enjoyed by all Americans. All these actions are important at the national and state levels. Eye care providers need to work to implement these objectives in their local communities and private practices. By understanding the *Healthy People 2010* vision objectives and knowing well the characteristics of their communities and aging patients, eye care providers can apply information and materials to reduce visual impairment and enhance quality of life in their communities. By using their own creativity and professional skills, eye care professionals can develop local programs to reduce visual impairment and enhance the vision of the older members of their communities.

Poor health, poor vision, and loss of independence are not inevitable consequences of aging. Substantial opportunities exist to improve older adults' health and quality of life. The public health challenge to vision care professionals is to incorporate the nation's public health vision and related objectives into their practices, agencies, academic institutions, industries, and associations.

## HEALTH PROMOTION AND DISEASE PREVENTION

Health promotion and disease prevention have become a major component of public health activities in enhancing and maintaining the health and well-being of the lives of older adults in society today. Moving from a focus on elementary infection control and sanitation issues, public health activities for aging Americans now center on chronic disease and quality of life issues. Concepts of the traditional medical model and disease entity are giving way to a new model of preventive health care and wellness. Eye care practitioners have tremendous potential to affect their aging patients' overall health and well-being through health promotion and disease prevention. Primary eye care providers are strategically placed within the health care system to promote prevention in the primary health care setting.

### Prevention

Prevention is generally defined as keeping from happening, averting, thwarting, hindering, or impeding. Prevention is further delineated into primary, secondary, and tertiary prevention. First, primary prevention may be thought of as increasing awareness or education. Primary prevention includes efforts to reduce the probability, severity, and duration of future illness and injury.[7] Primary prevention efforts include education on exercise, nutrition, smoking cessation, recommended intervals of care, and accident and fall prevention. Secondary prevention comes as an intervention in the form of early detection or treatment, potentially restoring the patient to a previously healthy state. Secondary prevention involves measures to detect presymptomatic disease or conditions when earlier detection will mean more effective treatment. Earlier implies a stage before the individual would normally seek treatment and usually before he or she would even be aware of the disease. Secondary prevention prevents the manifestation of illness so that health, as perceived by the patient, does not deteriorate.[7] Secondary prevention efforts include early detection of hypertension, cancer, and prediabetes, among other conditions. Many vision deficits are preventable at times if detected early and treated appropriately. Tertiary prevention works to minimize the impact of a permanent and irreversible disability. Efforts are to rehabilitate or return the individual to maximal functioning ability within the constraints of deterioration of health. Tertiary prevention involves measures to reduce the disability from existing illness and prevent it from getting worse. Tertiary prevention seeks to prevent a further fall in the health status after an initial fall in health status occurs.[7] Tertiary prevention efforts include interventions that attempt to reverse or prevent progression of the condition or illness. These interventions include vision rehabilitation services and devices for an individual who is experiencing vision loss caused by macular degeneration or glaucoma.

From a policy and implementation standpoint, the appropriate balance of resources among primary, secondary, and tertiary prevention requires an ongoing dialogue within and beyond the public health community. In addition, primary prevention efforts are challenged by a health system that is only beginning to move beyond being overwhelmingly focused on acute care.

## Eye Care Practitioners as Health Educators

Primary eye care providers include health messages regarding the health of the eye and optimal function of the visual system as a part of routine care. These practitioners provide their patients with information on tips for driving, safety eye protection and vision enhancement, the prevention of falls, good visual hygiene for computer use, and ultraviolet light protection. As a part of routine standard care for aging Americans, patient health education information is an important component of providing quality patient care.

## Hypertension

Eye care professionals realize the importance of screening their patients for hypertension through routine blood pressure measurements. When measuring a patient's blood pressure, the practitioner or a member of his or her staff has the opportunity to deliver a brief health promotion message. The eye care practitioner or staff ask patients about family history of hypertension and advise patients about the effect of hypertension on general health and well-being as well as ocular health status. The primary eye care practitioner may also provide education materials on hypertension in relation to exercise and diet or refer the patient to a general medical practitioner for further monitoring and treatment.

## Diabetes

Primary eye care professionals play an important role in screening, diagnosis, treatment, and management of diabetes. One of the goals listed in the nation's *Healthy People 2010* objectives calls for a decrease in the ocular complications of diabetes. Primary eye care practitioners have the opportunity and responsibility to be in the forefront of this challenge. Diabetes often initially presents with a shift in the patient's refractive status or fluctuation in vision, prompting the patient to seek vision care. Additionally, early detection and timely treatment can substantially reduce the risk of severe visual loss or blindness from diabetic eye disease. Many people at risk do not have their eyes examined regularly to detect problems before vision impairments occur. Knowledge alone does not create behavior change. However, the knowledge of how to access the right health care at the right time can prevent much needless human suffering and needless expenditures of both personal and societal resources.

The risk for type 2 diabetes increases with age. However, the Diabetes Prevention Program study shows that even modest weight loss of 5% to 10% through healthy eating and increased physical activity was highly effective in preventing type 2 diabetes in people older than 60 years. The latest National Diabetes Education Program, a collaboration between the Centers for Disease Control and Prevention and National Institutes of Health, uses the "It's Never Too Late" campaign to focus specifically on aging Americans who may be predisposed to diabetes. Materials are designed specifically for older adults to promote the news that diabetes prevention is "proven, possible, and powerful." These materials are available on the National Diabetes Education Web site at *www.ndep.nih.gov*.

## Fall Prevention

Many falls can be prevented and their costly risks reduced. Although exercise can reduce the risk of falling, older persons are typically not exercisers, and many persons older than 65 years do not engage in any leisure physical activity. Additionally, physicians and other health care providers are not widely practicing fall prevention and assessment strategies despite published clinical guidelines. Most of these falls are associated with one or more identifiable risk factors (e.g., weakness, unsteady gait, confusion, and certain medications). Research has shown that attention to these risk factors can significantly reduce rates of falling. Considerable evidence now documents that the most effective (and most cost effective) fall reduction programs have involved systematic fall risk assessment and targeted interventions, exercise programs, and environmental inspection and hazard reduction programs.

## ASK, ADVISE, ASSIST, ARRANGE

The "ask, advise, assist" technique, which originated at the National Cancer Institute, has been used in a variety of health promotion interventions from smoking cessation to increasing physical activity to bring about behavior change. The single most important factor influencing smoking cessation has been "a doctor's advice to stop." Smoking robs the body of vitamin A, causing decreased night vision and dry eye symptoms. Smoking may cause ocular irritation, worsen complications of systemic disease, and increase the incidence of cataract formation. *Asking* every patient about physical activity, *advising* of simple approaches to exercise for sedentary people, and *assisting* with specific guidance when asked is an approach that can be implemented easily and efficiently in most practices (Box 19-7).

The implementation of health promotional activities in a busy office setting may take less time and resources than initially considered. Teachable moments in the primary care setting provide tremendous potential to promote healthy choices among the older adult population. For example, the external ocular examination includes concern regarding detection of skin cancer lesions around the eyes and facial areas. This is an opportune time to educate patients on the use of sunscreen for prevention of skin cancer as well as self-examination for the early detection of cancerous lesions. In this role as a primary health provider the eye care professional assumes the role and responsi-

---

**BOX 19-7**

### Application of Ask, Advise, Assist, Arrange

**Hypertension**
**Ask** about family history of hypertension, stress level, diet, and exercise habits.
**Advise** about the risk of stroke or heart attack along with possible ocular health complications.
**Assist** by screening for hypertension in the office.
**Arrange** for another appointment to recheck blood pressure or make appropriate referral. Refer for stress management, nutritional, or exercise counseling to minimize risk.

**Smoking**
**Ask** about tobacco use.
**Advise** about the serious health risks involved.
**Assist** by providing educational brochures or a nicotine addiction questionnaire.
**Arrange** for referral to a support group; follow up with a physician to prescribe nicotine patches or counseling.

**Diabetes**
**Ask** about family history of diabetes.
**Advise** about the effect of diabetes on vision and ocular health.
**Assist** by providing a diabetes checklist to rate the risk for diabetes.
**Arrange** for the patient to see his or her physician if signs warrant concern.

**Exercise**
**Ask** about routine exercise levels.
**Advise** on the overall benefits of stress reduction, weight control, and improved cardiovascular fitness.
**Assist** by suggesting some activities such as walking, cycling, swimming, or taking an exercise class.
**Arrange** for the patient to consult his or her physician about starting an exercise program and setting a start date to begin exercising.

---

bilities of health educator. While providing eye care for the individual, primary eye care providers also work toward ensuring the future health of the patient, his or her family, and the community at large by delivering positive health promotion and disease prevention messages.

## REFERENCES

1. Anderson GF, Hussey PS: Population aging: a comparison among industrialized countries, *Health Affairs (Millwood)* 19:191-203, 2000.
2. Bowyer NK: Defining primary care, *J Am Optom Assoc* 68:6-9, 1997.
3. Bowyer NK: *Healthy People 2010:* the nation's health agenda, *Issues in Interdisciplinary Care* 3:207-11, 2001.

4. Boyle JP, Honeycutt AA, Narayan KM, et al: Projection of diabetes burden through 2050: impact of changing demography and disease prevalence in the US, *Diabetes Care* 24:1936-40, 2001.
5. Centers for Disease Control and Prevention National Center for Chronic Disease Prevention and Health Promotion: Chronic disease notes and reports: special focus, *Healthy Aging* 12:3, 2001.
6. Centers for Disease Control and Prevention: Public health and aging, *MMWR* 52:101-5, 2003.
7. Cohen D, Henderson, J: *Health, prevention and economics*, New York, 1988, Oxford University.
8. Freedman VA, Martin LG, Schoeni RF: Recent trends in disability and functioning among older adults in the United States: a systematic review, *JAMA* 288:3137-46, 2002.
9. *Guide to clinical preventive services*, ed 3, http://www.ahrq.gov/clinic/cps3dix.htm, accessed Aug 10, 2004.
10. *Healthy eyes, healthy people*, http://www.aoa.org, accessed Aug 10, 2004.
11. *Healthy vision 2010*, http://www.healthyvision2010.org, accessed Aug 10, 2004.
12. Himes CL: Elderly Americans, *Population Bulletin* 56:4, 2002.
13. Hubert H, Bloch DA, Oehlert JW, et al: Lifestyle habits and compression of morbidity, *J Gerontol A Biol Sci Med Sci* 57A:347-51, 2002.
14. Institute of Medicine: *The future of public health*, Washington, DC, 1988, National Academy Press.
15. Institute of Medicine: *Primary care: America's health in a new era*, Washington, DC, 1996, National Academy Press.
16. Jacobzone S: Coping with aging: international challenges, *Health Affairs (Millstone)* 19:213, 2000.
17. Kinsella K, Velkoff V: *An aging world: 2001*, Washington, DC, 2001, U.S. Census Bureau.
18. Lee PR: *Re-inventing public health*, Shattuck Lecture, Massachusetts Medical Society Annual Meeting, Boston, Mass, May 21, 1994.
19. Levit K, Smith C, Cowan C, et al: Trends in U.S. health care spending 2001. *Health Affairs (Millwood)* 22:154-64, 2003.
20. National Committee on Quality Assurance: *Health plan employer data and information set (HEDIS)*, Washington, DC, 2003, National Committee on Quality Assurance.
21. Nelson JC, Essien J, Loudermilk R, et al: *The public health competency handbook: optimizing organizational and individual performance for the public's health*, Atlanta, 2002, Emory University.
22. Public Health Functions Steering Committee: Public health in America: essential public health services, July 1995, http://www.health.gov/phfunctions/public.htm, accessed Aug 10, 2004.
23. U.S. Department of Health, Education, and Welfare: *Healthy people: the surgeon general's report on health promotion and disease prevention*, Washington, DC, 1979.
24. U.S. Department Health and Human Services: *Promoting health/preventing disease: objectives for the nation*, Washington, DC, 1980, U.S. Government Print Office.
25. U.S. Department of Health and Human Services: *Healthy people 2000: national health promotion and disease prevention objectives*, Washington, DC, 1991, U.S. Government Printing Office.
26. U.S. Department of Health and Human Services: *Healthy people 2010, ed 2, with understanding and improving health and objectives for improving health*, 2 vols, Washington, DC, U.S. Government Printing Office, November 2000.
27. Vinicor F: Is diabetes a public health disorder? *Diabetes Care* 17(suppl 1):22-6, 1994.
28. West Virginia Department of Health and Human Resources : *A healthier future for West Virginia: healthy people 2010*, Charleston, WV, 2001, Bureau for Public Health.

## SUGGESTED READINGS AND RESOURCES

*Healthy eyes, healthy people*, http://www.aoanet.org
*Healthy Iowans 2010*, http://www.idph.state.ia.us/bhpl/healthy_iowans_2010.asp
*Healthy people 2010*, http://www.healthypeople.gov
*Healthy vision 2010*, http://www.healthyvision2010.org
*Healthy West Virginia 2010*, http://www.wvdhhr.org/bph/hp2010/objective/28.htm
National Diabetes Education Program, *It's not too late to prevent diabetes*, http://ndep.nih.gov/campaigns/SmallSteps/SmallSteps_nottoolate.htm

APPENDIX 19-1*

# Healthy People 2010: *Narrative from Chapter 28, Vision and Hearing*

Goal: Improve the visual and hearing health of the nation through prevention, early detection, treatment, and rehabilitation.

*From U.S. Department of Health and Human Services: *Healthy people 2010, ed 2, with understanding and improving health and objectives for improving health*, 2 vols, Washington, DC, U.S. Government Printing Office, November 2000.

## OVERVIEW

Among the five senses, people depend on vision and hearing to provide the primary cues for conducting the basic activities of daily life. At the most basic level, vision and hearing permit people to navigate and to stay oriented within their environment. They provide the portals for language, whether spoken, signed, or read. They are critical to most work and recreation and allow people to interact more fully. For these reasons, vision and hearing are defining elements of the quality of life. Either, or both, of these senses may be diminished or lost because of heredity, aging, injury, or disease. Such loss may occur gradually, over the course of a lifetime, or traumatically in an instant. Conditions of vision or hearing loss that are linked with chronic and disabling diseases pose additional challenges for patients and their families. From the public health perspective, the prevention of either the initial impairment or additional impairment from these environmentally orienting and socially connecting senses requires significant resources. Prevention of vision or hearing loss or their resulting disabling conditions through the development of improved disease prevention, detection, or treatment methods or more effective rehabilitative strategies must remain a priority.

## VISION: ISSUES AND TRENDS

Vision is an essential part of everyday life, depended on constantly by people at all ages. Vision affects development, learning, communicating, working, health, and quality of life. In the United States, an estimated 80 million people have potentially blinding eye diseases, 3 million have low vision, 1.1 million people are legally blind, and 200,000 are more severely visually impaired. In 1981, the economic impact of visual disorders and disabilities was approximately $14.1 billion per year. By 1995, this impact was estimated to have risen to more than $38.4 billion—$22.3 billion in direct costs and another $16.1 billion in indirect costs each year.

Estimates of the number of people in the United States with visual impairment vary with its definition. Legal blindness represents an artificial distinction and has little value for rehabilitation but is a significant policy issue, determining eligibility for certain disability benefits from the federal government. Because of their reliance on narrow definitions of visual impairment, many estimates of the number of people with low vision are understated. When low vision is more broadly defined as visual problems that hamper the performance and enjoyment of everyday activities, almost 14 million persons are estimated to have low vision. Visual impairment is 1 of the 10 most frequent causes of disability in America. In children, visual impairment is associated with developmental delays and the need for special educational, vocational, and social services, often into adulthood. In adults, visual impairment may result in loss of personal independence, decreased quality of life, and difficulty in maintaining employment. Impairment may lead to the need for disability payments, vocational and social services, and nursing home or assistive living placements.

The leading causes of visual impairment are diabetic retinopathy, cataract, glaucoma, and age-related macular degeneration (AMD). People with diabetes are at risk of developing diabetic retinopathy, a major cause of blindness. Because early diagnosis and timely treatment have been shown to prevent vision loss in more than 90 percent of patients, health care practice guidelines recommend an annual dilated eye exam for all people with diabetes. Studies indicate, however, that many people with diabetes do not get an annual dilated eye exam. An estimated 50 percent of patients are diagnosed too late for treatment to be effective. People with diabetes also are more likely to have cataracts and glaucoma. Glaucoma is a major public health problem in this country. The disease causes progressive optic nerve damage that, if left untreated, leads to blindness. An estimated 3 million people in the United States have the disease and of these, as many as 120,000 are blind as a result. Furthermore, glaucoma is the number one cause of blindness in African-Americans. Treatments to slow the progression of the disease are available. However, at least half of the people who have glaucoma are not receiving treatment because they are unaware of their condition. Blindness from glaucoma is believed to impose significant costs annually on the federal government in social security benefits, lost tax revenues, and health care expenditures.

While important strides have been made in the prevention and treatment of eye disease, there is no cure for many causes of vision loss, particularly AMD. In addition to being a leading cause of blindness in the United States, AMD is a leading cause of low vision. People with low vision often cannot perform daily routine activities, such as reading the newspaper, preparing meals, or recognizing faces of friends. The inability to see well affects functional capabilities and social interactions and can lead to a loss of independence.

Myopia, or nearsightedness, is a common condition in which images of distant objects are focused in front of, instead of on, the retina. Myopia occurs in approximately 25 percent of the U.S. population. In children, myopia is found in 2 percent of those entering first grade and 15 percent of those entering high school. Many infants and young children are at high risk for vision problems because of hereditary, prenatal, or perinatal factors. These individuals need to be identified and tested early and annually to make sure their eyes and visual systems are functioning normally. Research in the 1980s and 1990s found that amblyopia, a leading cause of visual impairment in children, results from visual problems in very early life. These problems can be prevented or reversed with early detection and appropriate intervention.

While nothing medically can be done for patients with low vision, their quality of life can be greatly improved. Many low vision services and devices are available to help patients maintain their independence. Generally, devices fall into two categories: visual and adaptive. Visual devices use lenses or combinations of lenses to provide magnification. They include such aids as magnifying spectacles, hand-held magnifiers, stand magnifiers, computer monitors with large type, and closed-circuit televisions. Adaptive devices include large print reading materials (books, newspapers), check writing guides, and high-contrast watch dials. Also in this latter category are aids such as talking computers.

## DISPARITIES

More than two-thirds of visually impaired adults are over age 65 years. Although no gender differences exist in the number of older adults with vision problems, more women are visually impaired than men are because, on average, women live longer than men do. By 1999, almost 34 million persons in the United States were expected to be over age 65 years. This number is expected to more than double by the year 2030. As the population of older adults grows larger, it is estimated that the number of people with visual impairment and other aging-related disabilities will increase.

African-Americans are twice as likely to be visually impaired as are whites of comparable socioeconomic status. Studies conducted in the United States and the West Indies have shown that primary open-angle glaucoma exists in a substantially higher proportion of Caribbean blacks and African Americans than in whites.

Hispanics have three times the risk of developing type 2 diabetes as whites, and they also have a higher risk of complications. Available data suggest that visual impairment may be important public health problem in the Mexican-Hispanic population. There also is a higher rate of myopia in Asian children. Many barriers still need to be overcome in reducing vision disorders. Among the major prevention strategies are educating health care professionals and the general population about the benefits of prevention, improving access to quality health care across socioeconomic classes to decrease disparities, and gaining cooperation of families in the screening and treatment of infants and children.

## OPPORTUNITIES

Blindness and visual impairment from most eye diseases and disorders can be reduced with prevention, early detection and treatment. Most eye diseases, however, lack symptoms until vision is lost. Vision that is lost cannot be restored. Therefore early intervention through regular vision exams needs to be emphasized. Health education programs directed at groups at higher risk for eye diseases and disorders are essential in preventing blindness and visual impairments. The incorporation of vision into health education programs can be beneficial to participants and to agencies seeking to provide quality care to their clients.

The prevention of blindness and visual impairment and the promotion of eye health result in improved health status and reduced risk factors for illness, disability and death from diseases and injuries across all age groups. Translation of scientific advances can help people who are blind and visually impaired maintain their quality of life and independence.

# CHAPTER 20

# Ethical Issues in the Care of the Older Adult

R. NORMAN BAILEY

The health care professional is expected to behave in a more compassionate manner than the average businessperson. Those served by eye care professionals are frequently unable to understand fully the nature of their eye or vision problem and must trust that the professional will place patients' needs above personal interests. Ethical obligations derive from the reality that those who seek the services of health care professionals are vulnerable because of their needs.

Many older adults live independently in their communities and deserve recognition of their competence in the health care setting.[12] However, many older adults may be less able to understand clinical information because of functional decline, with dependence and vulnerability frequently accompanying them into the clinical setting. Therefore some older adults may be limited in making informed and independent health care decisions, although care must be exercised by the clinician before making that assumption. The goal of this chapter is to examine the ethical basis for the patient-clinician relationship and its importance in the care of the older adult.

The number of older patients seeking eye and vision care services from eye care professionals is expected to increase markedly over the next several years. According to the U.S. Census Bureau, the 2000 census showed an increase of 12% over the 1990 count for those aged 65 years and older, increasing from 31.2 million to 35 million. During this period, the group aged 85 years and older grew at a faster rate than the group aged 65 to 85 years. This trend is expected to shift in 2011 as the first of the baby-boomers (those born from 1946 through 1964) reach age 65 years.[15] This growth of the population older than 65 years will heighten the importance of the eye care professional's ethical obligation to behave with compassion and competence in the care of the older patient because more will be called on to serve this demographic group.

## TERMS AND CONCEPTS

The discipline of ethics has been defined as "the study and analysis of values and standards related to duty, responsibility, and right and wrong behavior."[14] Values are ideals that reflect the perceived importance or worth of people, things, activities, and social institutions; standards are typically defined expectations of behavior, or outcome performance, usually for a specific group or for a class of individuals. The practice of ethics involves reflecting on and deciding the right thing to do when faced with ethical or moral issues in practice. The ethical decision-making process may be subconscious when established attitudes and values direct behavior in the most basic of circumstances. When compelling values and standards are in conflict, the clinician must engage in a critical-thinking, decision-making process to determine the "best" action to take.

## ETHICS

Ethical issues occur regularly in clinical practice whenever questions involving ethical values or moral principles are present in decision making. However, ethical problems arise when two or more values or ethical principles conflict with each other in the clinical decision-making process. A true ethical dilemma occurs when two apparently equally compelling and mutually exclusive value-supported actions with equally powerful moral arguments come into conflict in such a way that to follow one action requires sacrificing the other.[18]

The eye care professional will often face circumstances in which important ethical norms or standards of conduct conflict when deciding the most appropriate action for a given clinical situation. The thoughtful clinician will become very aware of the judgment necessary to address these conflicts in a way that honors and gives appropriate consideration to all conflicting values. At times achieving a fully satisfactory outcome may be difficult, and more questions than answers may result from the effort.

New technologies and the ever-expanding scope of practice in the changing health care environment raise new challenges to the eye care professional's efforts to uphold professional obligations. However, clinicians are not alone in the decision-making process. Eye care professionals have obligations toward patients to honor and respect their moral and legal rights. In the modern eye care setting, the patient is not considered an object of the examination and treatment, but rather an active decision-making partner in care.[3]

The eye care professional's duty to respect patients' legal rights is obvious, but some ethical obligations extend beyond those spelled out in the law. The law is inherently reactive and cannot be expected to address the full array of ethical considerations that health care providers must honor. Eye care professionals have not fulfilled their obligations to patients by solely meeting the letter of the law. In the end, they are expected to go beyond the minimal standards of the law by following standards of behavior that will build trusting patient relationships.[9]

Optometry, as other health care professions, has a number of formal statements of ethical principles and rules for guiding the professional behavior of its members. The two primary national documents for guiding the professional conduct of optometrists are the American Optometric Association's Code of Ethics and the Optometric Oath, provided in Boxes 20-1 and 20-2. The ethical principles on which these statements are based have historically guided the behavior of health care professionals, including that of all eye care clinicians. The Code of Ethics, adopted in 1944 and amended in 2005, is a list of nine statements, including optometrists' duties to remain competent, cooperate with other health professionals, and serve society. A few of the statements relate more directly to the care of patients and charge optometrists to place patients' needs above their own, honor patient confidentiality, and work toward the goal that no person will lack needed care. The Optometric Oath, adopted in 1986, is also composed of nine statements, including duties similar to those laid out in the Code of Ethics, but written in an oath format.[3]

---

**BOX 20-1**

### Code of Ethics*

It Shall Be the Ideal, the Resolve and the Duty of the Members of The American Optometric Association:

- TO KEEP the visual welfare of the patient uppermost at all times;
- TO PROMOTE in every possible way, in collaboration with this Association, better care of the visual needs of humankind;
- TO ENHANCE continuously their educational and technical proficiency to the end that their patients shall receive the benefits of all acknowledged improvements in visual care;
- TO STRIVE TO SEE THAT no person shall lack for visual care;
- TO ADVISE the patient whenever consultation with an optometric colleague or reference for other professional care seems advisable;
- TO HOLD in professional confidence all information concerning a patient and to use such data only for the benefit of the patient;
- TO CONDUCT themselves as exemplary citizens;
- TO MAINTAIN their offices and their practices in keeping with professional standards;
- TO PROMOTE and maintain cordial and unselfish relationships with members of their own profession and of other professions for the exchange of information to the advantage of humankind.

Source: American Optometric Association, 243 N. Lindbergh Boulevard, St. Louis, MO, 63141-7881.
*Adopted in 1944.

## BOX 20-2

### The Optometric Oath*

With full deliberation I freely and solemnly pledge that:
- I will practice the art and science of optometry faithfully and conscientiously, and to the fullest scope of my competence.
- I will uphold and honorably promote by example and action the highest standards, ethics and ideals of my chosen profession and the honor of the degree, Doctor of Optometry, which has been granted me.
- I will provide professional care for those who seek my services, with concern, with compassion and with due regard for their human rights and dignity.
- I will place the treatment of those who seek my care above personal gain and strive to see that none shall lack for proper care.
- I will hold as privileged and inviolable all information entrusted to me in confidence by my patients.
- I will advise my patients fully and honestly of all which may serve to restore, maintain or enhance their vision and general health.
- I will strive continuously to broaden my knowledge and skills so that my patients may benefit from all new and efficacious means to enhance the care of human vision.
- I will share information cordially and unselfishly with my fellow optometrists and other professionals for the benefit of patients and the advancement of human knowledge and welfare.
- I will do my utmost to serve my community, my country and humankind as a citizen as well as an optometrist.
- I hereby commit myself to be steadfast in the performance of this my solemn oath and obligation.

Source: American Optometric Association, 243 N. Lindbergh Boulevard, St. Louis, MO, 63141-7881.
*Adopted in 1986 by the Association of Schools and Colleges of Optometry, the American Optometric Association, and the American Optometric Student Association.

## BOX 20-3

### Ethics

As a process, ethics may be understood more fully through the methods used to identify, define, describe, analyze, illustrate, understand, and justify the norms or moral standards set by a society for the acceptable conduct of its members in general and, more specifically, for members of subsets of society such as health professionals.[5,11,16,23] These methods may be divided into nonnormative and normative ethics.

Nonnormative ethics may be considered the more objective of these two divisions and is further divided into descriptive ethics and metaethics.[5] Descriptive ethics uses the scientific techniques of anthropology, history, psychology, and sociology to study the moral norms present in societies and the professions over time, as well as in the present, including descriptive studies of the professional codes of ethics and oaths as in optometry. Metaethics analyzes the language, concepts, and methods of reasoning in ethics.

Normative ethics, on the other hand, uses varying methods to identify and justify the moral norms that are applied to everyone in a society (general normative ethics) and to smaller subgroups such as the professions (practical or applied ethics).[5] Professional codes of ethics, for example, are a form of normative or practical ethics that use various moral theories as the tools to identify and justify their ethical values and standards of behavior. The arguments for identifying and justifying moral norms can be quite varied among the theories and, in some cases, even antagonistic to each other.

## BOX 20-4

### Morality and Moral Character of the Eye Care Professional

Some moral norms tend to be universal across societies and time and comprise the common morality, including the norms related to basic human rights such as life, liberty, and the pursuit of happiness. Other norms, such as those expressed in professional codes of ethics, are more specific to certain communities, such as the norms that comprise the professional morality or ethics of any specified group such as optometry. Codes of ethics for professions also tend to focus on professional virtues. Virtues may be thought of as the predispositions of an individual to act in certain ways. The ideal health professional will reflect many virtues, including the central virtues of compassion, discernment, trustworthiness, integrity, and conscientiousness.[5]

The goal of this chapter is to convey the ethics and values undergirding the patient-clinician relationship with older patients, which requires the development of trust. A concise theoretical overview of the primary themes and concepts in ethics is provided in Boxes 20-3 to 20-6 for those interested in more than a discussion on the application of ethical standards in the care of older patients.

### Ethical Norms Relevant to Health Care

Through moral reflection over time, ethical norms relevant to the practice of medicine and optometry have been identified and justified in

## BOX 20-5

### Ethical Theories

Ethical theories have been developed over time as methods for identifying and justifying moral conduct. The theories may be classified by their approach to this task. Some theories may appear more adequate than others, but no theory fully meets the demands of ethical discourse in all instances, regardless of attempted refinements over time.

Some theories place central emphasis on actions that bring the greatest good, placing more weight on the consequences than on the conduct that brings the good outcome. Such theories may accept withholding the truth from a patient as valid as long as the outcome produces the "greatest" benefit. In contrast, some theories place more emphasis on the duty to act in certain ways. In these theories, rightness or wrongness is determined more by the action than by the consequence of the action. This category of theory supports the need to follow the rules of conduct, such as truth telling, in an obligatory manner. Telling the truth will hold a higher imperative than less truthfulness, regardless of the goodness of the intended outcome.

Another major category of theories includes those based on individual rights. "Statements of rights provide vital protections of life, liberty, expression, and property. They protect against oppression, unequal treatment, intolerance, arbitrary invasion of privacy, and the like."[5] When the rights of one person affect the rights of another, whose rights prevail? For one to claim entitlement to a moral right, supportive justification must be present by moral principles and rules, much in the same way that claims of legal rights must be supported by legal principles and rules. As with other norms, seldom can rights be considered absolute and must be weighed and balanced with the rights of others and of the community. However, individual rights should hold and be protected except when infringement is justified by overwhelming circumstances. Blatantly violating rights is never morally justified.

In contrast to rights theories are the community-based theories, sometimes known as communitarianism.[5] Currently, this category of theory places communal norms and the needs of the community above individual rights, although obligations of the community to the individual are generally recognized. In these theories community rights are primary and can trump individual rights.

A final category of theories are relationship-based accounts that place the emphasis on "care" principles, that is, the willingness to care for those with whom one has a significant emotional commitment.[5] Historically, philosophers have promoted moral judgment as a matter of reason rather than of emotion because emotional considerations may discourage impartiality and introduce bias into the decision-making process. The emotional elements present in the patient-clinician relationship, for instance, may affect the practitioner's reflection on what should be done in any particular situation. However, awareness and acknowledgment of this relational content should enhance the clinician's rational judgment when attempting to balance considered actions that present conflicting norms. The "care" aspect may play an important advocacy role as well. Balance among all elements involved in the decision-making process is of key importance.

---

ethical theory and other reflective deliberations. Modern bioethics recognizes that even though norms of the common morality may be universal, they are not absolute and any one may be superseded by a conflicting norm under certain circumstances.

Beauchamp and Childress[5] have helped clarify several ethical norms significant to health care professions. The norms they have identified include principles that are grounded in the common morality but not exclusively supported by any one theory or doctrine. Although these principles are reflected in some form in the classical ethical theories, the acknowledgment that occasional conflicts may occur between important ethical standards should relieve expectations that following any single moral theory will be enough to prevent tension in patient care.

The ethical norms identified from the common morality in the health professions can be grouped into four clusters of principles.[5] These identified clusters include (1) the respect for autonomy, which acknowledges the individual's independent decision-making rights; (2) nonmaleficence, which requires the avoidance of harm; (3) beneficence, which weighs all factors for their potential to provide benefit; and (4) justice, which fairly distributes benefits and burdens.

This framework actually includes several classes of norms, including principles, rules, judgments, rights, virtues, and moral ideals, some of which are more specific in their application than others. Both principles and rules are general in nature; however, rules are more restrictive and specific whereas principles generally give more flexibility to judgment. Moving from principles to rules to judgments to rights

## BOX 20-6

### Ethical Reasoning

Each theory presents themes and results that meet moral convictions in some circumstances but in other instances may come into direct conflict with some most basic of beliefs. Although the various theories have different strategies, they frequently produce similar guidelines for action. This convergence contributes to the notion that when conflicts emerge, resolution should be attempted through balancing, that is, by modifying either the theories or the moral convictions to achieve equilibrium. This attempt at coherence identifies coherence theory, described as "reflective equilibrium" by John Rawls.[19] Rawls sees justification as the use of reflective testing of moral beliefs and theoretical postulates to achieve as much coherence between them as possible.

Beauchamp and Childress[5] further developed the concept of coherence through common morality theory. They identify the common morality as the source of the four clusters of ethical principles previously noted. W. D. Ross, a twentieth-century writer on common morality theory, is reported to be the most influential person on the work of Beauchamp and Childress.[5] The search for coherence, when deciding the most desirable action in cases in which ethical standards are in conflict, requires the engaged principles, rules, and rights to be weighed against each other to bring balance in the given circumstance. Principles and rules are recognized as absolute by some theories, expendable by other theories, and in a hierarchy of obligation by yet other theories. To prevent irresolvable dilemmas, principles, rules, and rights must be accepted as not absolute, yet the notion that some should be held as valid (prima facie) until more compelling norms override their position should be accepted. Therefore a prima facie obligation must be followed unless it conflicts on a particular occasion with an equal or more compelling obligation. Conflicting norms should be given relative weights to assist the process of balancing. No single method for justification is satisfactory in all cases. The decision maker, when faced with conflicting duties, has the obligation to investigate all questions and look for balance on the basis of relative weights of principles and rules to determine the best action. Care must be taken to not easily override those norms of common conviction simply for the sake of convenience.

Several conditions have been identified that restrict balancing. Stronger reasons must be present for honoring the overriding norm than protecting the infringed norm, the action directed by the stronger overriding norm must be reasonably achievable, the infringing action becomes necessary in the face of no reasonably available morally preferred alternative action, negative outcomes from the infringing action must be minimized, and impartiality toward all affected parties must be maintained.[5] No ethical theory or professional code of ethics has presented a framework of ethical norms that need no balancing at times.

and other similar norms, guidance of the norms becomes increasingly specific for more limited circumstances. The Code of Ethics of the American Optometric Association lists a number of principles and rules that, along with other moral norms, guide the eye care professional's ethical conduct in daily practice.[3]

Rules may be substantive, authoritative, or procedural.[5] Substantive rules include truth telling, confidentiality, and privacy. Authoritative rules set guidelines for who should serve as surrogate decision maker, for those given professional authority to accept or deny a patient's choice of alternative therapies, and for those with distributional authority when allocating limited resources. Procedural rules establish the process to be followed by those granted authority to make decisions. A comprehensive framework guiding moral judgment must consider individual rights, the virtues of the moral decision maker, and the emotional content of the circumstance receiving moral judgment.

### Ethical Analysis and Decision Making: The Process

As previously mentioned, most decisions made in clinical practice involve little ethical conflict. However, in traditional practice as well as in response to the advancement of technologies and expansion of the scope of practice, the eye care professional is increasingly challenged with competing ethical values and must determine the most appropriate action to balance competing obligations. Whenever the best action in a given circumstance is unclear, the clinician should use a systematic approach to analyze possible courses of action. Heitman and Bailey[14] have presented a framework for ethical analysis and decision making. Box 20-7 outlines this six-step structured framework for ethical analysis and decision making as one such approach.

### THE PATIENT-CLINICIAN RELATIONSHIP

The relationship between the eye care professional and the patient is the center of the ethical focus of optometry. Several ethical principles and related concepts are important to the ethical patient-clinician relationship, including trust, communication, truth telling, self-determination, decision-making capacity, culture and cultural competence, and vulnerability.

BOX 20-7

# Framework for Ethical Analysis and Decision Making

### Step 1: Recognize and Identify the Ethical Problem(s)

A stepwise process of ethical decision making begins with a comprehensive understanding of the problem. Remarkably, one of the hardest parts of ethical analysis is recognizing that a clinical problem involves a question of ethics. Most clinicians are trained to see problems primarily in technical terms and may believe that proper diagnosis and appropriate knowledge of treatment options are sufficient to define an acceptable course of action. Although ethical decision making is often portrayed as an unemotional, rational process, an unexpected negative emotional response to a situation is often an indication of an ethical problem. Anger, confusion, frustration, and even disgust can be signals that more careful analysis is called for.

### Step 2: Identify the Clinically Relevant Facts, Establish Important Definitions, and Gather Any Additional Necessary Information

As in clinical diagnosis, having the essential facts of the situation is important before making a judgment. Some important questions to consider include the following:

- Who are the principal parties involved in the situation, what are their relationships, and what do they think are their respective roles?
- What are the relevant clinical, social, and financial facts of the matter? Which facts (if any) are in dispute? What information is missing?
- How are the facts and definition of key concepts interpreted by the relevant parties? Why do they believe the problem exists? What do they think is the solution?
- When did events important to the situation occur, and when does a decision need to be made to address the identified problems?

Seeking more information can frequently resolve many issues, and outside advice can be as helpful in clinical ethics as in other aspects of patient care. Conferring with others can provide new perspectives and new options. However, uncertainty about some aspects of the question may be unavoidable, and the problem is likely to need a response even when knowing basic related facts is impossible.

### Step 3: Identify Relevant Professional Ethical Codes, Ethical Practice Standards, and Ethical Principles and Where Conflict May Exist among Them

Although every patient encounter is unique, much about ethical patient care can be described in general terms. Determining whether the issue in question is addressed by the American Optometric Association, in either the Code of Ethics or a resolution from the House of Delegates, or another professional organization may provide a starting point for consideration if not a definitive action plan. Similarly, relevant state and federal laws may provide some general guides for action. If formal authoritative statements on the issue in question conflict, consider the principles that the statements reflect and whether any hierarchy among them is present. How do specific standards relate to other important values and standards? That is, is any standard more important than others, and why?

### Step 4: Identify Possible Alternative Courses of Action and Their Likely Outcomes

Considering the goals that are most important to achieve and the standards of behavior that are most important to follow, outline a best case, worst case, and middle ground scenario. Determine whether the means (the actions) or the ends (the outcomes) are more important ethically in this situation. Recognition that the ideal scenario may not be possible to achieve or possible only with significant sacrifice is important. Because some alternatives may create additional conflicts for various parties, tracing out the possible consequences of potential actions may prevent new problems from arising.

### Step 5: Choose the Course Best Supported by Analysis and Act Accordingly

Not to act is to act by default. Health care professionals are held ethically accountable for the outcomes of patient care as well as for their specific actions, and it is professionally more responsible for the clinician in a difficult situation to make a reasoned choice than to leave the problem to outside forces. In a litigious environment, many clinicians may be tempted to act against their professional judgment in response to the real or imagined demands of patients and insurers. However, it is ethically preferable and better risk management for practitioners to act in a way that (1) is consistent with good clinical practice, (2) is supported by a clear process of reasoning, and (3) they believe in personally. The rationale for such ethical decisions, as well as the consequent actions, should always be carefully documented in the patient's chart.

### Step 6: Evaluate the Actions Taken and Their Subsequent Outcomes

After acting on a considered ethical decision, observe how closely what occurs matches what was predicted. By evaluating such actions and their outcomes, redirecting events that do not go as expected, as well as learning how similar decisions might work in the future, may be possible. Conscious reflection on practice gives clinicians skill in ethical analysis and decision making, which can become an almost instinctive understanding of how to proceed when an ethical issue arises. Discussing such experiences with colleagues can also provide valuable feedback, including confirmation of professional standards of care. At the organizational level, communication with others about unusual clinical ethics issues can inform the profession about problems on the horizon and permit the formulation of a policy response.

---

Adapted from Bailey RN, Heitman E, editors: *An optometrist's guide to clinical ethics*, St. Louis, 2000, American Optometric Association, pp 14-16.

## Trust

Trust is important in most human interactions but becomes essential in the therapeutic patient-clinician relationship.[2] Interactions between patient and eye care professional may be casual at times, but the trust on which the relationship depends is based on the patient's belief that the clinician upholds the highest of professional virtues and the belief that the patient will provide full disclosure of clinically important information and adhere to mutually agreed upon treatment plans. This trust is based on professional values and competence guiding the practitioner as care is delivered in a responsible manner.

The clinician's obligations toward the patient are somewhat greater than those of the patient toward the clinician, in that these relationships are of unequal power. The patient is vulnerable because of his or her health needs, and the eye care professional's obligations to protect the interests of the patient are great. Patients are often unaware of and unable to understand fully the nature of their eye and vision conditions and must trust their clinicians to assess and treat them appropriately. This is especially true of some older patients who may feel less secure in their ability to understand unfamiliar concepts and new medical terminology and, therefore, may have a greater need to trust the clinician's recommendations. The competence gap between clinician and patient must be bridged by the patient's trust in the practitioner's professional competence and commitment to placing the patient's interests above other considerations.

## Communication

Central to a trusting patient-clinician relationship is clarity and openness of all communication. The dialogue between patient and eye care professional plays a greater role in successful patient outcomes than many realize; patient-clinician communications therefore are central to professional ethics. Communication at all levels plays a major role in the development of a trusting therapeutic relationship. Adequate communication between patient and eye care professional are essential in helping the patient maintain some autonomy. In addition, the patient's medical record as well as any spoken communication among providers must be clearly communicated to prevent harm. Although the patient-clinician relationship should have good lines of communication established, good communication between multiple persons providing care to the same patient is also essential to prevent undesired outcomes and maintain positive provider relationships with the patient.[21]

Some clinicians with busy schedules may not listen intently or with compassion to what their patients say. Frequently interrupting the patient or failing to give the patient undivided attention will cause the eye care professional to appear quite rude. Such a detached attitude from patients' concerns can be harmful to the relationship with older patients, especially if they are fearful from not understanding the circumstances surrounding their health needs. Eye care professionals need to train themselves to listen to their patients with empathy. Patients have been found to complain most about clinician disrespect, disagreement with the clinician about expectations of care, inadequate information from the clinician, distrust of the clinician's motives, and perceived unavailability of the clinician.[24]

The eye care professional should, in most cases, be open and transparent in communicating with patients to give them the opportunity to participate as fully as possible in the decisions surrounding their care. The patient is most vulnerable in situations of uncertainty and is more likely to cede power to the practitioner on those occasions. Some clinicians may "mystify" their knowledge or act in ways to support uncertainty to maintain the power imbalance with the patient.[22] Deceptive reassurance should not replace truth telling and informed consent in communications with an older patient.[2]

## Truth Telling

The more specific normative rules of veracity, privacy, confidentiality, and fidelity also play important roles in a trusting patient-clinician relationship.[5] Truth telling, or veracity, is probably more central to a trusting patient-clinician relationship than any other norm. The trust of any relationship depends largely on open and honest communication that does not deceive. As for the other norms, most ethicists would hold that truth telling is prima facie binding and not absolute. That being said, this slippery-slope should not provide a blanket excuse for any less than truthful disclosure simply for convenience.

Truth telling, on first disclosure, may create anxiety for the older patient. Most now believe that although assisting the patient in understanding his or her health condition is important, disclosing certain information more gently and over time rather than fully at the time of diagnosis may be more beneficial. In some cases the older patient may be more comfortable with family members present; on other occasions the patient may wish confidentiality. Early determination in privacy (during the initial patient interview) of whom the patient would be most comfortable having present during diagnosis and treatment discussions is best. This can be confirmed later during examination if warranted.

## Self-Determination

Many clinician obligations toward the patient arise from the ethical principles that both respect and promote the patient's right to autonomy. Autonomy refers to the individual's self-determination, and respect for patient autonomy imposes significant restrictions on health care professionals' paternalism. The patient has the right to make an informed choice from among alternative treatment plans, including the acceptance of none.[2] In most cases patients will make choices that have the highest probability of beneficial outcomes. However, the need to respect the patient's autonomy does not reduce the eye care professional's obligation to use due diligence in preventing harm while expending competent effort to provide optimal patient benefits in a fair and just manner. Many older patients are quite competent to make decisions for themselves, and they may choose courses of action other than that recommended by the clinician. But the best interests of the patient are of particular concern when the patient's decision making capacity is compromised by ill health or advanced age. The eye care professional must be careful in distinguishing whether a disagreement is the result of a patient's lack of understanding, lack of capacity, or a real difference of values.

Autonomy in its purest sense assumes the informed individual has complete liberty to make choices and the competence to do so, without coercion from the clinician. In exercising this right, the patient may willingly accept community standards, religious principles, or other guidelines to direct action. Coercion results when undue external pressure is placed on the patient to respond in a certain way. For example, by not fully informing the patient or by taking a paternalistic attitude, the eye care professional may coerce the patient into accepting a treatment plan that, if otherwise fully informed and allowed to do so, he or she would not accept. However, the right to choose a treatment option does not obligate the patient to choose. The "choice" may be to ask another to assist in or actually make the treatment decision; this is still an expression of autonomy.[5] Older adults and those who are seriously ill may be more likely to ask others to make health care choices for them.[20] A lowered level of understanding or fear of the unknown may be factors that lead these individuals to seek assistance from others in making choices. However, patients should be assisted in understanding their conditions and the options for management to be empowered by this knowledge and others' support to make informed choices. If competent patients ask others to assist in their health care decisions, the request should be based on something other than inadequate information, coercion, or not having the necessary emotional support for such personal decision making.

Some have argued that the reason health care professionals should care about a patient's autonomy is because clinicians care even more for the patient's dignity.[17] Treating older adults with dignity and respect and not as if they were children is a norm contemporary Western society often forgets. Physical limitations, such as hearing impairment, should not automatically lead the clinician to believe an older patient has reduced cognitive capacities and thereby respond to the patient in a manner that disrespects his or her dignity.

## Decision-Making Capacity

To consent or withhold consent, the patient must have the cognitive capacity necessary to make health care decisions. The health care practitioner is obliged to provide the required information related to the diagnosis and treatment options to support a considered decision by a competent patient. When the patient does not have the capacity to make reasoned decisions, legal and ethical considerations must be made to determine how surrogate decision making should occur. The standards for surrogate decision making vary; the patient may have previously expressed determined choices through advance directives while competent, or an appointed surrogate may use substituted judgment to determine what the patient would have chosen. When the patient's probable wishes cannot be determined, the surrogate may seek to make decisions in keeping with the patient's perceived best interests. The line between competence and incompetence is gray. Loss of decision-making capacity does not always occur with advanced age. When they do occur simultaneously, the onset is a gradual process in most cases. Making arrangements for surrogate decision making for older patients before medical need is always helpful, but many patients and their families do not do so. When prior arrangements have not been made, and especially when disputes arise among caregivers and family members, the courts may have to determine the patient's competence and appoint a guardian for the purpose of making health care decisions.[5] Obviously, someone with decision-making authority for the patient will need to be available when the eye care professional examines or cares for an incompetent patient.

### Culture and Cultural Competence

Cultural competence has been defined as the ability of providers and organizations to deliver effective health care services that meet the social, cultural, and linguistic needs of culturally diverse patients.[6] By the year 2050 20% of the U.S. population is estimated to be aged 65 years or older, and racial and ethnic minorities will likely comprise approximately 35% or more of that demographic group.[8] Eye care professionals are increasingly challenged to recognize and attend to the cultural issues and language differences that may affect communication and interaction with patients. Clinicians who are responsive to their patients' culturally influenced views of good health care and the expected behavior of practitioners will be better able to gain and sustain their patients' trust and thus better serve their needs.

Ethnicity and cultural background, for instance, can play a major role in determining how older patients feel when making health-related decisions for themselves.[7] Older patients from some cultures often believe that families should make certain health care decisions rather than the patient. Older adults from some cultures are at more risk of developing disabling chronic health conditions than are those from other groups.[10]

Language and literacy rates can also vary significantly among cultural groups. If the patient and eye care professional speak different languages, an interpreter will need to be present. Many patients with limited English proficiency bring family members with them to help them communicate with health care professionals. However, this apparent solution to the communication gap can cause serious problems itself. No guarantee exists that the practitioner's conversation will be interpreted correctly to the patient, and the patient's interpreted comments may not be accurately conveyed. Often the translation will more likely reflect the translator's knowledge and bias, especially if a family member provides the translation. Whenever possible a third-party interpreter, such as a bilingual staff member whose fluency in both languages meets the need of clinical communication that must take place, should be used.

The need for eye care professionals to be knowledgeable of and sensitive to these and other cultural differences among patients becomes increasingly important as the U.S. population becomes culturally more diverse.

### Vulnerability and Elder Abuse

As older adults become both physically and mentally more challenged by the aging process, their vulnerability may make decision making more difficult and place them at a higher risk of being neglected or of receiving physical, emotional, financial, and other forms of abuse from others on whom they depend. Such abuse may occur at the hands of family members or other caregivers in the home or in an institutional setting. Protecting abused older patients is not unlike the ethical and legal requirements to protect children, but elder abuse is commonly underreported and is seldom mentioned by the victim. As primary health care providers, eye care professionals are often in a position to detect physical signs of abuse and neglect that others may miss or overlook. Uncovering the nature of a specific patient's abuse may be difficult, and prudence dictates caution to avoid accusing the innocent. However, the duty to the patients' interests means that clinicians should report suspicious cases to an Adult Protective Services agency when good cause is present to believe that neglect or abuse may have occurred.[1,4]

### Confidentiality and Privacy

Confidentiality and privacy are two norms of significant importance to the patient-clinician relationship. Trust is supported by a sense of loyalty or fidelity in the relationship. The patient believes that the clinician will be faithful to the relationship by maintaining confidentiality and not divulging to others private information obtained during the examination. Others may believe they have a right to sensitive patient information simply because they are the caretakers of their older parents, or because they are paying for the care and need evidence of medical necessity. The latter may occur when the patient's care is covered by Medicare or other insurance carriers. Patients have a right to have their privacy protected as much as possible and to know the limits of that protection, such as when the clinician is required to disclose some patient information to insurance carriers. Patient privacy is becoming increasingly more difficult for eye care providers to observe in the face of third-party payer demand for patients' information and the myriad issues raised by new information technologies that make the storage and exchange of patient data simple and quick. Diagnostic technologies, including genetic diagnosis, also make more information available than ever before, raising the risk that something will be inappropriately disclosed. The federal government has established legal guidelines for protecting patient privacy under certain conditions, but these guidelines are only a partial solution to a growing ethical challenge.[13]

Older patients' confidentiality may be at greater risk of compromise than that of other patients simply because they are frequently accompanied to the eye care professional's office by one or more family members or friends. Sometimes these individuals are involved in caring for the patient, but often they are simply there to provide company or transportation. Care must be taken to not disclose information to the patient's family or other companions without having first received the patient's permission to discuss their private health matters. Sensitive matters frequently need to be discussed with the patient and, to ensure open and truthful communication from the patient, not having family members present during the examination would be prudent unless permission has been granted by the patient. The patient needs to be informed that personal issues may come up for discussion during the examination, a circumstance that many do not expect to arise during a routine vision and eye examination. A better choice may be to ask family members to wait in the reception area until the conclusion of the exam.

This chapter, although covering a broad range of topics from moral theory to ethical decision making, is not intended to be comprehensive on any single topic. The chapter was designed to assist the reader in gaining an appreciation of ethical considerations important in the care of the older adult patient.

### CASES FOR REFLECTION*

A few hypothetical cases representing circumstances that may be common in the care of the older optometric patient follow. The reader may find it instructive to follow the framework for ethical analysis and decision making previously described to identify the relevant ethical principles and rules involved in each case and which of the possible alternative actions would more likely achieve an outcome with the least negative impact on the ethical norms.

**CASE #1** Dr. Wilson had just completed his examination of Mrs. Dobbs' eyes and vision and determined that she had advanced diabetic retinopathy in the periphery of both eyes. He was preparing to discuss his diagnostic findings with her when she advised him, "Whatever you have found, I do not want you to tell my daughter, she would just worry too much. If it is anything serious requiring surgery, I do not want to know anything about it. I have lived

---

*Cases 1 through 4 were adapted from Bailey RN, Heitman E, editors: *An optometrist's guide to clinical ethics*, St. Louis, 2000, American Optometric Association, pp 19, 109, 133, 147.

a long life and I don't want to spend the last of it having to deal with lots of complicated medical procedures."

**CASE #2** Mrs. Rosen is an 85-year-old widow who lives by herself in a suburban neighborhood. Her grown children live in another state. Mrs. Rosen is being treated by a geriatrician for mild hypertension. She tolerates her medications well and is otherwise in good health. However, she has progressive vision loss and has been told by her optometrist, Dr. Soileau, that she has macular degeneration. Her visual acuity is 20/200 in her right eye and 20/70 in her left. One of Mrs. Rosen's friends, who is also a patient of Dr. Soileau, confides to him that Mrs. Rosen is still driving. She is concerned that it may not be a good idea, considering Mrs. Rosen's poor vision. At Mrs. Rosen's next visit, Dr. Soileau asks her about her driving. "Of course I'm still driving," she says. "How can you survive here without a car?" She is eager to point out that she has never been in an accident, only drives to the store now and then, drives "well below the speed limit," and would "certainly be able to see anyone crossing the road." She assures the doctor that no small children are around and that she will be careful. Besides, she asserts, her side vision is "as good as ever."

**CASE #3** Mrs. Grace has slowly been losing her functional vision for 3 years as a result of glaucoma. She already has a closed-circuit television, bioptic telescopes, and a number of magnifiers, but she rarely uses any of them. In the 2 years since she first came to see him, Dr. Peng has been dismayed by Mrs. Grace's lack of goals and her husband's insistence on providing for even her most basic daily living needs. On this visit, however, Mrs. Grace seems despondent. "If I can't read I don't want to go on living," she tells Dr. Peng. Mrs. Grace is accompanied by her adult son, who tells Dr. Peng that his father recently had a stroke and will likely be confined to a wheelchair for the rest of his life. "We could probably afford to keep both my parents at home with a paid attendant," he tells Dr. Peng, "if Mother could qualify for disability benefits."

**CASE #4** Dr. Carroll looked at the boy and then at the man who had just sat down in the examination chair. The man nudged the boy. "Dile a la doctora que se me arañó el ojo ayer y que me duele. Y dile que se me quebraron los lentes y que necesito otros." ("Tell the doctor that I scratched my eye

yesterday and that it hurts. And tell her that I broke my glasses and need new ones.") The child turned to the optometrist and said shyly, "My grandfather wants glasses." Dr. Carroll had taken Spanish in high school but found it hard to work with the growing number of Spanish-speaking patients who came to her office. She was glad to see that this patient had brought his 9-year-old grandson to translate.

**CASE #5** Dr. Ramirez noticed that 78-year-old Mr. Sanchez, a new patient, hardly replied to his greeting on entering the examination room. Mr. Sanchez did smile shyly and nod his head slightly, but Dr. Ramirez was uncertain of the meaning of the weak response, only knowing from the preexamination questionnaire completed with the help of his assistant that Mr. Sanchez was diabetic and had had a slight stroke 1 year earlier. Mr. Sanchez was receiving limited financial assistance from the local Lions Club for his eye and vision care expenses. Dr. Ramirez discovered that Mr. Sanchez seemed to understand him better if he raised his voice a little; however, the patient seemed at times to be confused by the interview questions. Mr. Sanchez had a progressive hearing loss problem that had been diagnosed 6 years earlier but had been unable to afford a hearing aid. Dr. Ramirez did not have this information and erroneously assumed that the stroke had impaired Mr. Sanchez's mental capacity. Dr. Ramirez instructed his assistant to reschedule Mr. Sanchez's visit when a competent caregiver who knew his health history and needs could accompany him to the examination. Mr. Sanchez was unable to hear much of what was being said by the clinician, but he did catch the words that he was mentally incompetent, which caused him much distress.

**CASE #6** Ms. Tan presented to Dr. Patel's office with the complaint of blurred vision. She was accompanied by her younger sister, who had to lead her by the hand because of her extremely poor vision. Ms. Tan stated that she was afraid of doctors, but that her sister had insisted she come to see the eye doctor to determine if her vision could be improved with glasses. Ms Tan had received her last comprehensive eye and vision examination 10 years earlier, when she was first told that she had beginning cataract development. Ms. Tan, now 72 years old, had remembered the terrible time her mother had after cataract surgery some 30 years earlier. As a result of her mother's tragic outcomes, Ms. Tan has been fearful of cataract surgery. Dr. Patel's examination revealed mature cataracts that reduced Ms. Tan's vision to light perception. She recommended that Ms. Tan seek a consultation for possible cataract surgery from an eye surgeon. Dr. Patel believed that Ms. Tan's vision could likely be improved, thereby returning her to self-sufficiency from blindness. Ms. Tan started crying and said she would never have cataract surgery.

## ACKNOWLEDGMENTS

I thank Elizabeth Heitman, PhD, at Vanderbilt University's Center for Clinical and Research Ethics, my friend and colleague in ethics, for her thoughtful review and many significant suggestions for the final manuscript.

I would also like to thank N. Scott Gorman, OD, MS, EdD, of Nova Southeastern University College of Optometry for recommending me as the author for this chapter. I appreciate his initial suggestions for the chapter as well as his review and comments on the manuscript.

## REFERENCES

1. Ahmad M, Lachs MS: Elder abuse and neglect: what physicians can and should do, *Cleve Clin J Med* 69:801-8, 2002.
2. Bailey RN, Heitman E: Communicating with patients in the doctor-patient relationship. In Bailey RN, Heitman E, editors: *An optometrist's guide to clinical ethics*, St. Louis, 2000, American Optometric Association. Available at http://www.aoa.org/documents/book.pdf.
3. Bailey RN, Heitman E: Ethics in clinical optometry. In Bailey RN, Heitman E, editors: *An optometrist's guide to clinical ethics*, St. Louis, 2000, American Optometric Association. Available at http://www.aoa.org/documents/book.pdf.
4. Baron S, Welty A: Abuse and neglect of older persons, *J Gerontol Social Work* 25:33-57, 1996.
5. Beauchamp TL, Childress JL: *Principles of biomedical ethics*, ed 5, New York, 2001, Oxford University.
6. Betancourt JR, Green AR, Carrillo JE: *Cultural competence in health care: emerging frameworks and practical approaches*, New York, 2002, The Commonwealth Fund.
7. Blackhall LJ, Murphy ST, Frank F, et al: Ethnicity and attitudes toward patient autonomy, *JAMA* 274:820-25, 1995.
8. Day JC: *Population projections of the United States by age, sex, race, and Hispanic origin: 1995 to 2050* (U.S. Bureau of the Census, Current Population Reports, 25-1130), Washington, DC, 1996, U.S. Government Printing Office.
9. Flores A: *Professional ideals*, Belmont, CA, 1988, Wadsworth.
10. Fried VM, Prager K, MacKay AP, et al: *Health, United States, 2003: chartbook on trends in the health of Americans*, Hyattsville, MD, 2003, National Center for Health Statistics.
11. Giersson H, Holmgren M: *Ethical theory: a concise anthology*, Orchard Park, NY, 2002, Broadview.
12. Gorman NS: The elderly. In Bailey RN, Heitman E, editors: *An optometrist's guide to clinical ethics*, St. Louis, 2000, American Optometric Association. Available at http://www.aoa.org/documents/book.pdf.
13. The Health Insurance Portability and Accountability Act of 1996 (HIPAA), Washington, DC, 2002, Centers for Medicare and Medicaid Services. Available at http://www.cms.hhs.gov/HIPAAGenInfo/.
14. Heitman E, Bailey RN: Ethical decision making in clinical practice. In Bailey RN, Heitman E, editors: *An optometrist's guide to clinical ethics*, St. Louis, 2000, American Optometric Association. Available at http://www.aoa.org/documents/book.pdf.
15. Hetzel L, Smith A: *The 65 years and over population: 2000*, Washington, DC, 2001, U.S. Census Bureau. Available at http://www.census.gov/population/www/socdemo/age.html#bb
16. Mappes T, DeGrazia D: *Medical ethics*, ed 5, New York, 2001, McGraw-Hill.
17. Moody HR: The cost of autonomy, the price of paternalism, *J Gerontol Social Work* 29:111-27, 1998.
18. Purtilo R: *Ethical dimensions in the health professions*, Philadelphia, 1993, W.B. Saunders.
19. Rawls J: *A theory of justice*, Cambridge, MA, 1971, Harvard University.
20. Schneider CE: *The practice of autonomy: patients, doctors, and medical decision*, New York, 1998, Oxford University.
21. Sutcliffe KM, Lewton E, Rosenthal MM: Communication failures: an insidious contributor to medical mishaps, *Acad Med* 79:186-94, 2004.
22. Waitzkin H, Stoeckle JD: The communication of information about illness, *Adv Psychosomat Med* 8:185-9, 1972.
23. Waluchow WJ: *The dimensions of ethics*, Orchard Park, NY, 2002, Broadview.
24. Wofford MM, Wofford JL, Bothra J, et al: Patient complaints about physician behaviors: a qualitative study, *Acad Med* 79:134-8, 2004.

# CHAPTER 21

# The Vision Rehabilitation Field and the Aging Network

**ALBERTA L. ORR**

*Although the world is full of suffering,*
*it is full also of the overcoming of it.*
HELEN KELLER

For older patients experiencing age-related vision loss, eye care professionals are the most important referral source to the field of vision rehabilitation where vision rehabilitation professionals can provide instruction in adaptive ways of carrying out routine daily activities. Such instruction makes a significant difference in the life of older adults who are visually impaired by increasing their level of independence. Local vision rehabilitation agencies and eye care professionals can work in partnership to ensure that this population receives the vision-related services that can enable them to continue to live independent and productive lives. The eye care professional's role in making referrals is key to the older person's best level of independent functioning. This chapter describes how eye care professionals and vision rehabilitation agencies can partner on behalf of the older consumer population experiencing age-related vision loss.

Much has already been said about the growing number of older people experiencing vision loss, but some of it bears repeating. More than 2 million people celebrated their sixty-fifth birthday in 2003, when 35.6 million older people were already aged 65 and older in the United States.[1] This number represents 12.4% of the overall U.S. population, or 1 in every 8 Americans. By 2030 the population of older people will more than double, reaching 71.5 million and growing at a faster pace than American society has ever experienced. At that time, the 65 years and older age group will represent 20% of the overall population. On January 1, 2006, the oldest of the baby boomers reached age 60 years, making them eligible for services funded by the Older Americans Act, such as Meals on Wheels.

Currently approximately 6.5 million people aged 55 years and older are experiencing age-related vision loss, as are 5 million aged 65 years and older—and these numbers are expected to double by the year 2030, when the last of the baby-boom generation reaches its senior years. This means that approximately 20% of the overall aging population experiences vision loss sufficient enough to interfere with the ability to carry out routine daily tasks. These demographics bear repeating because many people outside the aging and vision field cannot conceptualize the enormity of this population's current and future needs for services. Most are unaware of the vision rehabilitation service delivery system and its functioning and the eligibility of those aged 55 years and older for its services. Most older persons and their family members have never heard of the vision rehabilitation field or independent living skills training specifically targeted for older people who are experiencing vision problems severe enough to interfere with their ability to carry out routine daily tasks. They have also never heard of a low vision evaluation, low vision devices, or low vision rehabilitation services.

Although the vision rehabilitation field has worked quite hard to educate various target groups to be effective referral sources to its field, many more efforts are needed in this area to assist older people who are visually impaired to get the services they need. Eye care professionals are key to this effort.

## ROLE OF EYE CARE PROFESSIONALS IN VISION REHABILITATION

Eye care professionals who are familiar with local vision rehabilitation agencies can play the most significant role in ensuring that older patients know about these services and making referrals. Unfortunately, many eye care professionals are not fully informed about the services available in their communities or the eligibility criteria, particularly as they relate to older people. The term eye care professional is used here because the need to refer older patients for a low vision exam and to vision rehabilitation services rests on both the optometrist and the ophthalmologist. If the clinician is unsure that a referral for such services has already been made by another eye care professional, making another referral is best. The vision rehabilitation agency can easily check to make sure a referral has already been made and, in this way, the eye care professional can ensure that the older patient does not fall through the cracks.

The essential point is just how critical that referral is and how important the role of the eye care professional is in making sure that patients have access to all the vision-related services available to them and for which they are eligible. Therefore knowledge about the vision rehabilitation agencies in the community, what services they offer, their eligibility criteria, and whether they have a waiting list is important. An example of how one agency worked to create an effective referral process follows.

### Outreach to Physicians

In 2000, the Kansas Division of Services for the Blind embarked on a program to increase referrals to their agency by working with a former client, Dr. S, a cardiologist, who has degenerative myopia and has lost vision to the point that he could not continue his practice. Although the cardiologist saw several ophthalmologists over

a several-year period, not one mentioned a vision rehabilitation program to him. Instead, he found out about the Kansas Rehabilitation Center for the Blind through a friend. He completed the vision rehabilitation program at the rehabilitation center and was able to go back to work part time in a teaching position. After Dr. S completed his training, the administrator of the Kansas Division of Services for the Blind talked to him about the lack of referrals from physicians in Kansas and requested his help in starting an outreach program to this group.

The Kansas agency serves older consumers who are visually impaired by providing intensive vision rehabilitation programs throughout the state. Dr. S and the administrator decided to target ophthalmologists, optometrists, and physicians of internal medicine in the areas in which these programs would be held to get referrals for the classes in the vision rehabilitation intensives. During an 18-month period, the team was able to reach 21 cities in Kansas, and referrals to the agency have increased to the point a waiting list has been established for services for all age groups.

### The Approach

Dr. S makes a personal phone call to each physician, requesting a 15-minute appointment. Dr. S and other members of the Kansas outreach team meet with the clinician in his or her office. Dr. S explains his vision problem and what the vision rehabilitation program has meant to him and asks the practitioner to refer patients to the program. Often the practitioner invites office staff to attend the meeting and extends the appointment from 15 minutes to as much as 45 minutes to an hour. Dr. S invites the office staff to sit in on the intensive that will be offered in their area so they can learn more about the vision rehabilitation training programs.

Educating office staff can be an effective strategy because the eye care professional may feel he or she does not have the time to be involved in making referrals. Vision rehabilitation agencies can develop materials specific to their programs and make them available to office staff, including materials that can be handed out to patients. In addition to the personal approach, Dr. S and the staff have developed a brochure written in conversational language to hand out at their appointments. They also use an effective tool: they leave a 15-minute video about the Kansas Rehabilitation Center for the clinician and staff to view and to show to patients.

## Recommendations for Starting Similar Programs

Dr. S and the administrator strongly recommend the personal approach to clinicians and their staff. The agency administrator credits Dr. S's credentials as a physician and his ability to approach the medical community on their terms as a key to the success of the program. Dr. S uses personal experiences to lend credibility to the Kansas rehabilitation program. He states that clinicians are ethically unable to refer their patients to a vision rehabilitation program they know nothing about and may also not understand that the full breadth of vision rehabilitation services and what they can do for people, regardless of the degree of vision loss. Thus, to feel comfortable in making referrals, the eye care professional needs to know essential information about local vision rehabilitation programs. The eye care professional must be committed to the fact that services beyond optometry and ophthalmology exist, and that these vision rehabilitation services can make a difference in the lives of their patients.

## VISION REHABILITATION FIELD

Patients rely on their eye care professionals to tell them about what to do about their eyes, even if nothing more can be done medically for the patient. Because of this reliance on their expertise, eye care professionals are more often than not the key to older persons and their family members finding out about and using needed services. Therefore eye care professionals should know about the service delivery system available specifically for older people who are blind or visually impaired. This is particularly important because a majority of older people who are patients will have little or no knowledge about the vision rehabilitation services or that they are eligible. Accompanying family members will also be unfamiliar about the vision rehabilitation field and therefore will not know to ask questions. They will look to the clinician to inform them about appropriate services and assume they will be told everything they need to know about services available in their immediate areas.

More opportunities must be created at the national, state, and local levels to bring the vision rehabilitation field to the forefront. The need for vision rehabilitation services was recently recognized by the addition of a vision component to the Department of Health and Human Services *Healthy People 2010* initiative. This initiative includes the following objectives: (1) increase the use of vision rehabilitation services by people with visual impairments and (2) increase the use of adaptive devices by people with visual impairments. (See Chapter 19 for further discussion of public health aspects of older adult patient care.)

The National Eye Institute, National Institutes of Health, is responsible for implementing this initiative and has developed a number of activities such as publications and community efforts to ensure that individuals receive appropriate and timely vision rehabilitation services (*http://www.healthyvision2010.org/ rehabilitation/index.asp*). The vision rehabilitation system is composed of both private and public (state) agencies. Of most significance is the portion of the Rehabilitation Act of 1973 that is specifically earmarked for older people with vision loss: Title VII Chapter 2 of the act, "Independent Living Services for Older Individuals Who Are Blind." The program started in 1986 with a funding level of $5 million. Through strong advocacy efforts initiated by the American Foundation for the Blind, soon joined by the National Council of State Agencies for the Blind, and individual advocates—both vision rehabilitation professionals and older consumers—the funding has been increased to $32 million, a figure still not even close to an adequate level for a national service delivery program.

The Title VII Chapter 2 funds are administered by the Rehabilitation Services Administration, Department of Special Education and Rehabilitation Services, U.S. Department of Education. The funds are distributed to state vocational rehabilitation agencies on the basis of the number of older persons in each state. Therefore some states receive the baseline funding level of $225,000, whereas states such as California, with the largest number of older people in the country, receive more than $3 million. Florida and New York are the second and third largest recipients, respectively.

## DELIVERY OF VISION REHABILITATION SERVICES

Once referred to a local vision rehabilitation services provider, the older consumer will be evaluated for the types of vision rehabilitation services needed. A plan of service will be developed and services provided in a variety of settings: in the home, in an agency setting, or in an outreach setting such as that described in the Kansas example. Each state's model of service delivery varies. Some state agencies provide services through their own staff, others subcontract with private agencies, and others use both models. Some agencies maintain waiting lists because of the high demand for services and low funding. Eligibility for services varies from state to state. Some states provide services for individuals who have low vision, and others require legal blindness. A state with very little money or one with so many older people with vision loss may need to impose the criteria of legal blindness because it cannot afford to serve the larger group with low vision.

If unsure of how to find the appropriate local resource for patients, the eye care professional can contact the American Foundation for the Blind's information line. The Foundation also maintains a national directory of services. This directory can be accessed online at *www.afb.org*. The older patients whom the eye care professional sees are typically an extremely diverse group (Box 21-1).

The professional disciplines in the vision rehabilitation field who work with these individuals are the vision rehabilitation therapist (aka rehabilitation teachers), orientation and mobility specialist, and the low vision therapist. The three disciplines are credentialed through the Academy for Certification of Vision Rehabilitation and Education Professionals. However, these professional disciplines are not licensed. Some states such as New York are pursuing licensure as a positive step toward third-party reimbursement. Currently, they are not reimbursable through Medicare.

The vision rehabilitation therapist teaches consumers (the nomenclature used in the vision rehabilitation field is consumer or client rather than patient) independent living skills and adaptive techniques for carrying out routine daily activities (often referred to as instrumental activities of daily living) such as preparing a meal, managing medications, managing household tasks, and organizing cabinets and closets to find items easily. These activities are distinguished from activities of daily living, such as bathing, transferring from bed or chair, toileting, eating, and dressing, the most basic tasks

---

**BOX 21-1**

### Examples of Older Patients

- The preretirement patient, a still-employed individual who will be able to remain in the workforce if he or she is referred for independent living skills training and vocation rehabilitation rather than being encouraged to retire.
- The 71-year-old woman who takes care of her mother who is 90 years old and may be helped to continue assisting her mother so they can both stay at home if she receives adaptive skills training for routine daily tasks.
- The 69-year-old man who has never cooked or maintained the household who will learn to do these tasks for himself if he is referred to the vision rehabilitation agency.
- The 80-year-old woman who wanted to be able to take care of herself so her daughter will not worry about her and so she will be able to remain at home and age in peace.

---

of independent living that vision loss, in most cases, does not affect.

The orientation and mobility specialist orients the consumer to the environment and provides instruction on how to travel outdoors with confidence by using the white cane. They also teach travel techniques to enable persons with significant vision loss to walk comfortably and safely with a sighted person, such as a spouse.

The low vision therapist supports the instructional activities of the optometrist or ophthalmologist who provides low vision services. The therapist's job is to instruct the patient in the use of low vision devices in various environments and ensure that appropriate lighting is used. Often older consumers will have "upper drawer syndrome" if not properly instructed about how to use a low vision device in the home environment. In other words, they put the device away, thinking it does not work at home or is too hard to use.

## IMPACT OF THE TITLE VII CHAPTER 2 PROGRAM

### Mrs. W

Mrs. W is a 64-year-old woman who lives alone and has comorbidities, including diabetes, hearing and vision loss, heart failure, a history of minor stroke, transient ischemic attacks, neuropathy, and bipolar disorder. She provides child care for two of her grandchildren. She wanted to become as independent and functional as possible.

The low vision evaluation provided her with magnification corrections that allow her to read cooking directions on packages so that she can resume some cooking. Cooking instruction and many cooking aids such as a clip-on lamp, black-and-white cutting board, large-print measuring cups and spoons, large-print timer, a liquid level indicator that beeps when nearing the top of a cup or glass when pouring, and oven mitts were provided. Markings on her oven, microwave, and thermostat were tactile. She can now prepare healthy recipes and meals for herself and her grandchildren. She has also learned kitchen safety techniques. An electronic magnification device allows her to read her mail and pay bills. She can read her medicine bottles with her magnifier and does not have to ask someone for assistance. She was given, and instructed in the use of, a talking glucometer to assist her in managing her blood sugar levels, resulting in more control of her diabetes. A talking blood pressure monitor was provided to her to keep track of her blood pressure as directed by her physician. A talking scale was provided so that she could monitor her weight. A talking oral thermometer was also provided. She was also given instruction in orientation and mobility and can travel short distances safely with a combination of a long cane and a support cane. Sunglasses and a visor assist her with glare when traveling. For winter mobility she was given snow grabbers for her shoes and an ice spike for her cane. As a result of all these services, Mrs. W is now able to continue to live an independent life and care for her grandchildren.

### Mrs. N

Mrs. N has had macular degeneration for many years. She went to many clinicians over the years looking for a miracle cure but finally realized that the condition has no cure. She contacted a vision rehabilitation agency for low vision and rehabilitation services. When she came to the Mini Center for a low vision evaluation, she was using a small jeweler's loop for reading the newspaper. Because the loop was so small, she was only able to read one word at a time, but she was accustomed to it and read the newspaper fairly well with it. The importance of proper use of lighting was discussed and various types of lamps were demonstrated. She came to realize how much adjustable lighting improved her reading ability.

She also underwent a low vision examination by an optometrist with a specialization in low vision and is now using 8× magnifying spectacles to read the newspaper. The reading spectacles have a distortion-free aspheric lens for her right eye, which provides a wider view. As a result, her reading speed has significantly improved. A swing-arm lamp with a weighted base was provided so light could be adjusted to shine directly on her reading material. Dials and buttons on her appliances were marked with a quick-drying substance called "hi marks," which produces a raised tactile marking so that she is able to apply tactual techniques to locate the appropriate settings and functions.

As a result of Chapter 2 funding, all necessary services and equipment in these cases were provided at no cost. Sometimes, however, the older person is asked to contribute to the cost. These vision rehabilitation services and professionals are not reimbursable through Medicare or private insurances at this time. The Chapter 2 program described earlier remains the only national program available to fund such services. However, progress has been made with regard to securing Medicare reimbursement of vision rehabilitation services.

## COVERAGE FOR VISION REHABILITATION SERVICES AND PERSONNEL: CURRENT STATUS

The most common source of funding or reimbursement for many medical services for older Americans is Medicare. Family members, older people, and even professionals may assume that Medicare covers vision rehabilitation services and adaptive devices related to vision loss, just as it does for other conditions requiring physical rehabilitation. Most also assume that the professionals providing these services are reimbursed by Medicare just as their counterparts in physical rehabilitation (occupational therapists and physical therapists) are. Parallels do exist; if a patient breaks a hip, or her hip is not functioning, her physical rehabilitation is covered by Medicare. But if a patient loses vision because of an eye condition such as macular degeneration or diabetic retinopathy, the medical aspects would be covered, but vision rehabilitation services and specialists providing instruction are not. How can one be covered and the other not?

One answer is that the vision rehabilitation field grew out of an educational model, one of instruction rather than one of medically based intervention or therapy within the medical model. Also, state licensure does not exist in most states for vision rehabilitation services, and vision rehabilitation services have not been traditionally "ordered" by physicians because they do not fall under the medical services rubric. Since 1998 national efforts have been underway to secure third-party reimbursement for vision rehabilitation professionals—vision rehabilitation therapists, orientation and mobility specialists, and low vision therapists—through Medicare, but legislation has not yet made this a reality. Congress has authorized the Secretary of Health and Human Services to carry out a nationwide outpatient vision rehabilitation services demonstration project. The purpose of this 5-year demonstration project is to examine the impact of standardized national coverage for vision rehabilitation services in the home by physicians, occupational therapists, and certified vision rehabilitation therapists.

The Low Vision Rehabilitation Demonstration locales include New Hampshire; all five boroughs of New York City; Atlanta, Georgia; North Carolina; Kansas; and Washington State. Eligible beneficiaries—those diagnosed with moderate to severe visual impairment—in these areas will receive medical eye care from an ophthalmologist or optometrist who practices in these areas and will be covered for up to 9 hours of rehabilitation services provided in an appropriate setting, including the older person's home.

The vision rehabilitation services must be prescribed by a qualified physician and administered under an individualized, written plan of care developed by a physician or occupational therapist in private practice. The rehabilitation services will be provided on a one-to-one, face-to-face manner by an occupational therapist, or by a low vision therapist, orientation and mobility specialist, or vision rehabilitation therapist certified by the Academy for Certification of Vision Rehabilitation Professionals (ACVREP). Group services will not be covered.

## AGING NETWORK SERVICES

Eye care professionals should also know about the services available to older people through the aging network. Just as vision rehabilitation services are funded through the Rehabilitation Act, services from the aging network are funded by the Older Americans Act of 1965. The Administration on Aging at the federal level filters funds to the State Units on Aging at the state level, and then to the Area Agency on Aging (AAA) at the local level. AAAs have different names, such as the New York City Department for the Aging or the First Tennessee AAA. The AAAs subcontract with private agencies serving older people in the communities. Some AAAs also provide services directly. Services such as congregate meals in senior centers and home-delivered meals (e.g., Meals on Wheels) are funded. Local services in each state can be located by an easy system the Administration on Aging developed in 1991 called the Eldercare Locator, a nationwide toll-free service. The toll-free Eldercare Locator service operates Monday through Friday, 9 AM to 8 PM Eastern time and can be reached at 800-677-1116. The online service can be accessed at *http://www.eldercare.gov.*

Many older consumers who are visually impaired, their family members, and professionals frequently do not know what to look for regarding various service needs. For example, although assistance with home-delivered meals is provided through the aging network for older people, a family member may call an agency serving the visually impaired because the family member is visually impaired.

Unfortunately, some professionals in the aging arena may not be aware of vision rehabilitation services available in their area, although collaborative efforts have increased over the years. Early in the establishment of the Title VII Chapter 2 program, many Chapter 2 project directors prioritized getting to know their counterparts in the aging field and educating them about the services available to older people with visual impairments through Chapter 2 funds. As relationships developed, many program managers invited aging network staff to serve on their advisory committees, and in this way their knowledge grew. Nevertheless, some service providers in the aging network are still less aware of vision rehabilitation services so they are not always able to be an effective referral source. This situation increases the key role that eye care professionals play in connecting older persons and their families to services. Throughout the country, many excellent examples exist of how the vision field and the aging network have worked together to ensure that older consumers who are visually impaired will not get lost in the system. Many professionals in the aging field now recognize that the older individual who is visually impaired is a mutual consumer of both the aging and vision rehabilitation service delivery systems.

## NATIONAL AGENDA ON VISION AND AGING

Eye care professionals should also be aware of some of the critical issues confronting older people experiencing age-related vision loss and the vision rehabilitation field as a whole, as well as how these issues have been addressed by the National Agenda on Vision and Aging. Beginning in 1997, national aging program staff at the American Foundation for the Blind began to identify some of the most pressing trends and service needs of the growing number of older people experiencing age-related vision loss. With a survey of key leadership and colleagues in the vision rehabilitation field, seven of the most critical issues were identified for collaborative work and became the substance of the National Agenda on Vision and Aging.

The purpose of the National Agenda on Vision and Aging is to shape public policies and public attitudes that enable individuals aged 55 years and older who are blind or visually impaired to participate fully in all aspects of society. The purpose of the National Agenda will be accomplished through the goals listed in Box 21-2. Approximately 140 professionals and a number of older consumers worked in working groups to achieve the outcomes of the seven goals. A final report is now available from

---

**BOX 21-2**

### Goals of the National Agenda

1. Develop self-advocacy awareness and skills of older persons who are blind or visually impaired and their family members.
   - A training curriculum, *Self-Advisory Skills Training for Older Individual Who Are Visually Impaired* by Alberta L. Orr and Priscilla Rogers, was developed and published by AFB Press.
2. Increase public awareness and promote positive attitudes about the needs and capabilities of older individuals who are blind or visually impaired.
   - Public education campaigns were carried out to encourage older people to get an eye examination and to request a referral to a low vision specialist when told they are experiencing age-related vision loss. Campaigns in English and Spanish were carried out in partnership with the National Eye Institute about low vision.
3. Increase the availability of and access to vision rehabilitation services through adequate public funding. (Title VII Chapter 2 of the Rehabilitation Act of 1973, "Independent Living Services for Older Individuals Who Are Blind" program).
   - Extensive legislative advocacy efforts were carried out, and federal funds for the independent living program stood at $32 million for fiscal year 2004.
4. Increase the supply of qualified personnel to meet the needs of older persons who are blind or visually impaired.
   - A curriculum for service providers entering the vision rehabilitation field was developed and is available online at the website of the American Foundation for the Blind at *www.afb.org*.
5. Expand access to information and community resources such as employment opportunities.
   - A training curriculum for rehabilitation counseling professionals was developed and is online at the website of Mississippi State University's Rehabilitation Research and Training Center.
6. Promote the coordination of data collection and outcome measurement efforts that support the targeted goals of increased consumer self-advocacy, greater public awareness of vision rehabilitation services, sufficient funding for services, an increased supply of qualified personnel, and expanded access to information and community resources.
   - An Internet-based Nationally Standardized Minimum Dataset (NSMD) has been developed through federal funds from the National Institute on Disability and Rehabilitation Research for use by the Title VII Chapter 2 independent living programs. The data collection instrument includes preservice and postservice data and a functional assessment instrument. A program participant interview is conducted to determine the older person's perceptions of functional status after services have been received.
7. Support the efforts toward Medicare reimbursement of vision rehabilitation services.
   - National Agenda on Vision and Aging activities have supported the efforts to secure Medicare reimbursement for vision rehabilitation services currently underway in 2004.

AFB entitled "National Agenda on Vision and Again 1998-2005: A Report to the Field."

In summary, the eye care professional is responsible for taking a proactive role in learning about vision rehabilitation services in the local geographic area and referring patients for these services. In most cases, the patient and family members rely on the eye care professional for guidance, support, critical information, and next steps. A delay in finding out about such services can mean years of frustration for the older person and family members who think that life is over and that independence and productivity are no longer part of their reality. Through vision rehabilitation services, older people who are experiencing vision loss can be productive and contributing members of their families and communities.

## REFERENCE

1. Administration on Aging: *A profile of older Americans*, Washington, DC, 2004.

# *Index*

## A

Abbreviations, medical, 355*t*
Abducens nerve, 83
Absorption of drugs, 189, 192*t*
Abuse of elders, 21-22, 391-392
Accessory or nonoptical devices, 275-277
Accommodative convergence, 43-44
Acetaminophen, 195
Acquired diplopia, 129-130
Acquired lesions of lids, 94-95
Actinic keratosis, 96
Acuity. *See* Visual acuity
Acute care, 368*b*
Acuvue Bifocal lens
    design, 227*f*
    problem solving, 228*b*
Adaptation. *See also* Dark adaptation
    to combined hearing and vision loss, 184-185
    sensory, training, 260-262
Advance history form, 353*f*
Adverse effects
    as cause of iatrogenic illness, 189
    of frequently prescribed medications, 190*t*-192*t*
    of hypertension drugs, 52
Advice offered by optometrist, 160-161
Age-Related Eye Disease Study, 280-281, 336
Age-related maculopathy, 305-306
Aging
    definition of, 2-3
    and driving, 303
    effects on nutritional requirements, 334-335
    hearing loss from, 180-183
    immunocompetence theory of, 340-341
    normal, physical changes associated with, 268*b*
    and nutritional impact, 336-337
    primary, 4-5
    as public health concern, 366
    public health trends in, 368-371
    secondary, 5
    successful, 19
Aging and vision
    crystalline lens changes, 304-305
    diabetic retinopathy, 306
    glaucoma, 306
    national agenda on, 401-402
    normal and diseased state, 303-304
    ocular melanoma, 306
    retinal changes, 305-306
    retinitis pigmentosa, 306
Aging network services, 398-399

Alcohol
    drug interactions, 197*t*, 198
    recommended limits, 16
Alpha-2 adrenergic agonists, 199
Alpha-1 inhibitors, 51
Alternating vision bifocal contact lenses, 221-222
    gas-permeable, 223-226
Alzheimer's disease, 130, 347
    demographics, 14-15
    driving and, 308
    stages of, 15
Amaurosis fugax, 79, 126
Ambulatory patients, eye exam and, 166
American drivers, 303
American Foundation for the Blind, 398
Americans with Disabilities Act (1990), 312-313
Amplitude of accommodation, 37
Amsler grid, 146
Anemia, 8
    macrocytic, 69-70
    microcytic, 68-69
    normocytic, 69
Aneurysm
    berry, 83
    microaneurysms in diabetes, 123
Angina pectoris, 56
Angiotensin-converting enzyme (ACE) inhibitors, 50-51,
        57, 190*t*, 195
Aniseikonia, 262
Anisometropia, 143, 211-212, 219, 262
Antacids, interactions with drugs, 197*t*
Anterior chamber, age-related changes, 35
Anterior ischemic optic neuropathy, 76-77
Anterior segment diseases
    ciliary body, 102
    conjunctiva, 98-99
    cornea, 99-101
    eyelids, 93-98
    iris, 101
    lacrimal gland and tear drainage system, 98
    lens and zonules, 102-103
    trabecular meshwork, 102
Anterior segment screening, 168-169
Anticholinergic drugs, 196-197
Anticoagulation
    drugs, 190*t*-191*t*
    and hypercoagulability, 53-54
Antidepressants, 191*t*
Antihistamines, 196
Antimicrobial drugs, 197
Antioxidants, cataracts and, 339-340
Antipsychotic agents, 196
Antireflective coatings, 207-208
Apathetic thyrotoxicosis, 6

Page numbers followed by *f* indicate figures; *t*, tables;
*b*, boxes.

Aphakia, 10
  aniseikonia and anisometropia, 262
  convergence requirements, 261-262
  intraocular lens implants, 262
  rehabilitation, 260-261
  spectacle corrections, 149
Aplastic anemia, 69
Apnea, 9
Arc perimeter test, 247-248
Arcus senilis, 100-101
Area Agency on Aging, 400
Arteriosclerosis, posterior segment manifestations of, 120-122
Ask, Advise, Assist technique, 378
Aspheric contact lens design
  bifocal, 221
  gas-permeable bifocal, 222-223
Aspirin, 54, 195
  drug interactions, 197t
Assistive listening devices (ALDs), 185, 296-297
Astigmatism
  against-the-rule, 32-34
  determination of, 137, 139
  residual, 219
  and soft bifocals, 229f
  unwanted, 204-205
Atherosclerosis
  diagnosis and treatment, 55
  risk factors, 54-55
  symptoms and signs, 55
Atrophy
  muscle, 7
  optic, 118
Attention, age-related changes in, 41
Attention window (useful field of view), 307, 321-322
Attitudes regarding older people, 271
Auditory impairment. See Hearing impairment.
Autorefraction, 175
  portable keratometer, 352f

**B**

Bacterial infection, tear film, 99-100
Balance, 8-9
Barbiturates, 194b
Basal cell carcinoma of lids, 97
Base-down prism effect, 207f
Basilar-vertebral artery, ischemic stroke, 87-89
B cells, 341
Bedridden patients, eye exam and, 166
Bedside vision testing, in neurologically impaired patients, 84-85
Behavioral factors, and vehicle crashes, 308-309
Behavioral signs of hearing loss, 183b
Benign lesions of lids, 95-96
Benzodiazepines, 194b, 196
Beta-blockers, 56, 190t, 194b, 195
Bifocal add flippers, 176
Bifocal and trifocal lens segments, 11, 148-149, 203-204, 206-207
Bifocal contact lenses
  alternating vision, 221-222
  gas-permeable, 222-226
  and multifocals: fitting guidelines, 231b
  simultaneous vision, 220-221
  use, 220
Bifocal dissimilar segments, 212-213
Binocular telescopes, 151
Binocular vision assessment, 142-143
BIO-20D loupe, 169f
Biomicroscopy, 107-108
Bioptic telescopes, 152
Blepharitis, 94-95
Blepharoptosis of lids, 93-94
Blindness
  prevention of, 381
  in temporal arteritis, 75
Blood pressure
  and hearing impairment, 181t, 183
  monitoring, 5
Blur
  area of blended segment, 206
  monocular, 219
Bobbing, ocular, 90
Bone, changes in, 7
Bowl perimeter examination, 145
Bowman's layer, 100
Bracketing, 138-139, 173-174
Brown's superior oblique tendon sheath syndrome, 243
Brunescence, 12
Bulbar conjunctiva disease, 99

**C**

Calcarine cortex infarction, 80-81
Calcium channel blockers, 190t, 195
Camera systems for video magnifiers, 157
Cancer
  eyelids, 97-98
  skin, 7
Capillary permeability, in diabetic retinopathy, 123
Carbohydrates, free radical effects, 338
Cardiac glycosides, 190t, 195
Cardiovascular system, 5
  drugs for, 194-195
Caregivers, 20-21, 361
Care regimen for contact lenses, 233-234
Carotid artery distribution, ischemic stroke, 84
Case history, 18, 128
  advance history form, 353f
  complex, eye exam and, 166
  in diagnosis of oculomotor dysfunctions, 242
  interview, 272-273
  nutritional screening, 344b
  in optometric examination, 133-135
Case studies regarding ethical principles, 390-392
Cataracts, 12, 102, 305
  antioxidants and, 339-340
  effect on subjective refraction, 173f
Catecholamines, 51
Center-distance lens design, 227-229
Center-near lens design, 229
Central artery occlusion, 113-114
Central fields, evaluation of, 107
Central nervous system agents, 191t, 196

Central retinal vein occlusion, 114-115
Central suppression
    rehabilitative management of, 252-253
    vergence training for, 257b
Cephalosporins, 194b
Cerebrovascular disease, 58-61
    manifestations of, 79-80
Cerebrovascular disorders
    calcarine cortex infarction, 80-81
    intracranial hemorrhage, 89-90
    ischemic cranial neuropathy, 81-89
Chalazion, 95f
Charts
    lightbox for, 357f
    logMAR, 172
    in near vision assessment, 141-142
    Pelli-Robson, 147, 321
    in visual acuity measurement, 139-140
Cholesterol emboli, retinal arteriolar, 80f
Choroid, 105
Choroidal melanoma, 110, 306
Choroidal neovascularization, 112-113
Chronic disease trends, 370
Chronic immune thyroiditis, 66
Chronic obstructive pulmonary disease (COPD), 67-68
Ciliary body, changes in, 102
Ciliary muscle, 37
Clinical evaluation
    essential skills for, 272-280
    of posterior segment, 106-109
Closed-circuit television (CCTV), 293-294
Coatings, antireflective, 207-208
Code of ethics, 382b
Coding for eye examination, 359t
Cognitive function, technology and, 287-288
Cognitive impairment, eye exam and, 164-165
Collagen fibers, Bowman's layer, 100
Color insensitivities, 10, 36-37, 39, 276
Color vision testing, 146
Comanagement, 3
Comitant deviations
    binocular rehabilitation, 249-253
    cover tests, 243-244
    fixation disparity testing
        lateral vergence range and, 244-246
        vertical heterophoria and, 246
Comitant strabismus, 242-243
Commercial-to-custom technology, 286-287
Communication
    between clinician and patient, 389
    with hearing impaired, 164b, 186b
    optimization through technology, 185
    privileged communications, 315-316
Community service agency setting, 360-361
Complications
    of diabetes mellitus, 63
    impacting eye examination, 163-177
    of temporal arteritis, 74-75
    of therapeutic contact lenses, 237
Computers, 157-158, 286-287
    accessibility options, 294-295
    geriatric accessibility features, 276

larger monitors, 295
    software, 295-296
    vision problems with, 205b
Concentric/annular contact lens design, 221
    gas-permeable, 223-224
Cone density, 37-38
Confidentiality, ethics and, 392
Confrontation visual field testing, 84-85, 170-172
Congenital palsy, uncompensated, 243
Congestive heart failure
    definition, 57
    treatment, 58
Conjuctiva, and contact lens use, 217
Conjugate gaze, disorders of, 88-89
Conjunctiva, diseases of, 98-99
Conjunctival melanoma, 99
Connective tissue changes in eyelids, 93-94
Consent form, 354f
Contact lenses
    anatomical and physiological changes and, 216-219
    bifocal, 220-222
    gas-permeable designs, 222-226
    in gonioscopy, 109
    lens selection
        factors important to patient success, 230-231
        success rates, 230
    for low-vision patients, 158-159
    monovision, 219-220
    patient education and lens care, 231-234
    patient selection, 215-216
    single-vision, and reading glasses, 219
    soft bifocal/multifocal designs, 226-230
    therapeutic (bandage), 234-237
Contracture prevention, 256
Contrast sensitivity
    age-related changes in, 40-41
        and contact lens use, 218
    in evaluating acuity, 106
    measurement of, 146-147, 172-173
    tests, 321
Convergence
    accommodative and proximal, 43-44
    free fusion rings, 253f
    requirements, aphakia and, 261-262
Cornea, age-related changes in, 32-34
    and contact lens use, 217-218
Corneal anesthesia, 128
Corneal disease
    Bowman's layer, 100
    decrease in corneal sensitivity, 99
    endothelium and Descemet's membrane, 101
    epithelium, 100
    stroma, 100-101
    tear film, 99-100
Coronary artery disease, 5
    definition and epidemiology, 55
    diagnosis, 55-56
    syndromes, 56-57
Corticosteroids, for treatment of vasculitic syndromes, 71-72
Cotton wool spots, 111f, 120, 122, 123
Cough and cold preparations, 197-198

Counseling, practitioner's role in, 279-280
Cover tests, for comitant deviations, 243-244
Cranial arteritis, 126
Cranial nerve palsy, in ischemic cranial neuropathy, 82-83
Cranial nerves, in posterior circulation strokes, 87-89
C-reactive protein, 74
Creatinine clearance, 193
CR-39 lenses, 203
Cultural competence, 389
Cupping, glaucomatous, 118f
Curvature
    cornea, 32-34
    lens, 35-36
Cutaneous horns on lids, 96
Cyclovertical muscle, 248t
Cysts, in pars plana, 102

**D**

Dark adaptation, 12, 40, 147
Decision making
    capacity for, 388-389
    ethical analysis and, 385, 386b
Degrees of hearing loss, 182, 183t
Delivery of vision rehabilitation services, 396
Dementia, 8, 13, 130-131
    driving and, 308
    signs of, 165b
Demographics, 1-2, 395
    of Alzheimer's disease, 14-15
    of older workers, 19
    and traffic safety, 301-303
    transitional state of, 370
Depression
    eye exam and, 165
    misdiagnosed, 196
    other problems caused by, 14
    role of optometrist, 271
    suicide and, 16
    triggers of, 17
Depth perception tests, 320
Descemet's membrane, 101
Detachment
    retinal, 110-111, 115-116
    serous choroidal, 110
Diabetes mellitus
    complications, 63
    diagnosis, 63
    education regarding, 377
    glucose surveillance, 63
    pathogenesis, 62
    posterior segment manifestations of, 123-124
    symptoms and signs, 62
    treatment, 64-66
Diabetic retinopathy, 123, 306
Diagnosis
    COPD, 67-68
    coronary artery disease, 55-56
    diabetes mellitus, 63
    oculomotor dysfunctions, 242-243
    peripheral arterial disease, 61

Diet manipulation, 335-336
Diffractive contact lens design, 221
    soft bifocal/multifocals, 229-230
Digoxin, 194b, 195
Diminished capacity for driving, 301-302
Diminished quality of vision, eye exam and, 166-167
Diplopia
    acquired, 129
    causes of, 242-243
    in cranial nerve palsy, 83
    representative fields, 249f
Dipping, ocular, 90
Disability glare, 208-209, 276
    tests of, 147
Disc edema, 116-117
Disease prevention, health promotion and, 375-377
Display screens for video magnifiers, 157
Dissimilar bifocal segments, 212-213
Distance esophoria, 251-252, 254b
Distance exophoria, 251b-252b
Distance heterophoria, 43
Distance vision
    decline in, 270
    magnification for: telescopes, 149-152
    taking history for, 134
Distribution of drugs, 192t, 193
Diuretics, 51, 190t, 194-195
Double aperture rule trainer, home vision therapy, 255f-256f
Double-elevator palsy, 127
Drivers license
    administration of tests and types of vision tests, 319-320
    relicensing policies, 316
    renewals, 311, 318-319
    uneven application of policies, 318
    vision screening, 317-322
Driving
    Americans with Disabilities Act, 312-313
    changes in visual function and, 45
    demographics and traffic safety, 301-303
    diminished ability for, 270
    financial impact of vehicle crashes, 300
    glare and, 210
    legal and ethical issues, 313-314
    nondriver crash-related factors, 309-312
    nonvision function and crashes, 307-309
    policy-related studies, 322-324
    public health-related
        duty to warn, 314-315
        privileged communications, 315-316
        public policy and traffic safety, 316-317
    U.S. traffic crash trends, 299-300
    vision and aging, 303-306
    vision function and crashes, 306-307
    vision screening, 317-322
Drugs. See also specific drugs and drug classes.
    absorption, 189, 192t
    in COPD, 68t
    depression in relation to, 17
    diabetic, oral, 64t
    distribution, 192t, 193

drug-receptor interactions, 194
elimination, 192*t*, 193-194
environmental factors, 194
and hearing loss, 181
in hypertension treatment, 51-52*t*
metabolism, 192*t*, 193
multiple medication use, 189
protein binding, 193
Drusen, in age-related macular degeneration, 113*f*
Dry eye syndromes, 11, 98
Duty to warn, regarding driving, 314-315
Dyspnea, in COPD, 67

**E**
Ear
    anatomy of, 181-182
    inner, structural changes to, 181
Early pupil dilation, 167
Eccentric viewing, 140
Echelon soft bifocal contact lens, 229*f*
Economic considerations
    health service costs, 20
    of traffic crashes, 300
Economic status, 18-19
Ectropion, 94*f*
Edema
    in anterior ischemic optic neuropathy, 77
    diabetic macular, 111*f*
    disc, 116-117
    retinal, 78-79, 111
Educational issues
    patient education regarding health, 17-18
    training in geriatric medicine, 17
Ejection fraction, 57
Elder abuse, 21-22, 389-390
Elder care, 20-21
    toll-free locator service, 398
Electronic display systems, 156
Elimination of drugs, 192*t*, 193-194
Elschnig spots, healed, 121*f*
Endocrine system, 6
    drugs for, 192*t*
Endothelial cells
    corneal, 101
    trabecular meshwork, 102
Entropion, 94*f*
Environmental factors. *See also* Home environment
    affecting drug metabolism, 194
    geriatric-friendly office, 272*b*
    interior safety checks, 277*b*
    and vehicle crashes, 309-311
Epidemiology, transitional state of, 370
Epithelium, corneal, 100
Equipment
    for on-site vision care, 350-351
    in out-of-office examinations, 355*b*
Equivalent viewing distance (EVD), 152-157
Ergonomic positioning, 289-290
Erythrocyte sedimentation rate, 126
Esophoria, rehabilitative management of, 251-252

Ethical issues
    case studies pertaining to, 390-392
    ethical analysis and decision making, 385, 386*b*
    ethical norms relevant to health care, 383-385
    patient-clinician relationship
        communication, 387
        confidentiality and privacy, 390
        culture and cultural competence, 389
        decision-making capacity, 388-389
        self-determination, 388
        trust, 387
        truth telling, 387-388
        vulnerability and elder abuse, 389-390
    regarding driving, 313-314
    respecting patients' legal rights, 382
    terms and concepts in ethics, 381
Ethical reasoning, 385*b*
Ethical theories, 384*b*
Examination form, 356*f*-357*f*
Exercise, regular programs of, 4
Exit pupil of telescope, 150-151
Exophoria, rehabilitative management of, 250-251
Exotropia, 243
Extraocular muscles
    abnormal head posture and, 247*t*
    and their fields of action, 248*t*
Exudates, soft and hard, 111
Eye
    fixing, 259*b*
    movement disorders
        with anterior circulation strokes, 85-87
        with posterior circulation strokes, 87-89
    physical parameters, biometric data of, 42*t*
    protecting from glare and UV radiation, 210-211
    vergence movements, 241-242
    version movements, 43, 142
Eye care practitioners. *See also* Health care providers;
        Optometrists.
    as health educators, 376
    relationship with patient, 385-390
    role in vision rehabilitation, 396-397
Eye care services consent form, 354*f*
Eyedrops, mydriatic: combining, 170
Eye examination, 135-136
    complicating factors
        cognitive impairment, 164-165
        complex medical/ocular history, 166
        depression, 165
        diminished quality of vision, 166-167
        examination procedures, 167-177
        hearing impairment, 163-164
        limited mobility/examination environment, 166
    for low vision, 273-274
    in nontraditional settings, recommended sequence of,
        353, 355, 357-358
Eyelids
    acquired lesions of, 94-95
    age-related changes, and contact lens use, 216-217
    benign lesions of, 95-96
    blepharoptosis, 93-94
    malignant lesions of, 97-98
    and proper use of contact lenses, 231-232

# F

Facility staff, interactions, 349-350
Falls, 9-11
    benzodiazepines and, 196
    head trauma from, 60
    prevention of, 377-378
Farnsworth Panel D-15 test, 146
Feinbloom chart, 140
Fibrinolytic agents, 54
Filters
    light, 293
    for near-vision magnification systems, 158
Financial impact of traffic crashes, 300
Finger count confrontation field technique, 171f
Fitting
    of annular/concentric GP lenses, 224
    guidelines for bifocal/multifocal contact lenses, 231b
    of hydrogel contact lenses, principles of, 235-236
    of monovision contact lenses, 220b
Fitting height comparison, for progressive lenses, 204f
Fixation disparity
    binocular rehabilitation, 252-253
    testing
        lateral vergence range and, 244-246
        vertical heterophoria and, 246
Fixed-focus stand magnifiers, 155
Flashes and floaters, 115
Flickering grating, 144
Fluorescein angiography, 112
Fluorescent lighting, 271, 292
Focus Progressive multifocal lens design, 229f
Folate deficiency anemia, 70
Follow-up to optometric exam, 359
Forced vergence fixation disparity curves, 244, 246
Fourth cranial nerve palsy, 83
Fovea, in retinal artery occlusion, 78-79
Fractures, 7
    hip, 10
Frames
    materials and shapes of, 211
    trial, 175-177
Free fusion rings, home vision therapy, 253f
Free radicals
    defense against, nutritional manipulation of, 339-340
    effects on molecules, 338-339
    nitrogen species, 338
    oxidation, protection from, 339
    oxygen species, 337-338
Frequency doubling perimetry, 144, 172
Frequency 55 Multifocal lens design, 228-229
Fresnel prism, 211-212
Fuch's dimples, 100
Functional implications
    of hearing loss, 183
    of low vision, 269-271
Fundus
    clinical evaluation of, 108
    in retinal artery occlusion, 77-79
    suspected mass in, 110
Furrow degeneration, 101
Fusional (disparity) vergence, 43
Fusional disturbances, 242

# G

Gas-permeable bifocal designs, 222-226
Gastrointestinal system, 5-6
    drugs for, 191t
Gaze, conjugate, disorders of, 88-89
Gender ratio, 2
Geriatrics
    geriatric medicine as academic study, 17, 23
    geriatric patient care, 269b
    primary vision care in, 1-24
Giant cell (temporal) arteritis, 70-72
    posterior segment manifestations of, 124-126
Glare
    control, 291-292
        for near-vision magnification systems, 158
    disability, 208-209, 276
        tests of, 147
    intolerance, 10
    problems with, 270
    protecting eye from, 210-211
    recovery from, 40
Glaucoma, 11-12
    and changes in trabecular meshwork, 102
    early detection of, 144
    groups at high risk for, 306
    low-tension, 117
    risk factors, 119
Glucose surveillance, 63
Goldmann visual field charts, 76f, 81f, 82f
Gonioscopy, 108-109
Government role in public health, 365
Grating
    flickering, 144
    in measurement of contrast sensitivity, 147
Graves' disease, 66-67, 127
Guidelines
    for bifocal/multifocal contact lens fitting, 231b
    for drug use, 194b

# H

Halogen light, 271, 292
Haloperidol, 196
Handheld magnifiers, 154
Hashimoto's disease, 66-67
H₁-blocking agents, 196
H₂-blocking agents, 196
Headache, with neuro-ophthalmic disorders, 128
Head-mounted loupes, 155-156
Head trauma from falls, 60
Health care
    costs, 20, 370-371
    ethical norms relevant to, 385-387
Health care providers. See also Eye care practitioners;
        Optometrists.
    assessment of patient nutritional status, 342-343
    need for, 22-23
    role in delivery of low vision care, 281-282
Health history, 134
Health Insurance Portability and Accountability Act
        (HIPAA), 23-24
Health status, and vehicle crashes, 308

*Healthy People 2010,* 371-374
  *Vision and Hearing*
    disparities, 380
    issues and trends, 379-380
    objectives, 372*b*
    opportunities, 380
    overview, 379
*Healthy West Virginia 2010,* 374-375
Hearing aids, 185, 296-297
Hearing impairment
  accommodating for hearing plus vision loss,
      184-185
  anatomy of ear, 181-182
  dual sensory loss and independence, 184
  eye exam and, 163-164
  hearing loss, 180-183
    interacting with individual with, 185-186
  optimizing communication through technology, 185
  prevalence data overview, 179-180
Hematoma, subdural, 60-61
Hemianopic mirrors, 159-160
Hemianopsia, 85
  right and left, 263-264
Hemispheric stroke, 59
Hemolytic anemia, 69
Hemorrhage
  intracranial, 89-90
  retinal, 111
Hemorrhagic stroke, 60-61
Heparin, 53-54, 61
Herpes zoster, 8
Heterophoria
  distance, 43
  measurement of, 143
  vertical, and fixation disparity testing, 246
High technologies, 286
Hip fractures, 10
History. *See* Case history
Home environment
  interior safety checks, 277*b*
  modifications to, 11
  optical aids, 18
  setting for optometric examination, 361
Home vision therapy
  double aperture rule trainer, 255*f*-256*f*
  free fusion rings, 253*f*
  television trainer, 258*f*
Homocysteine, 55
Hordeolum, external, 94*f*
Horizontal conjugate gaze, 88
Horizontal strabismus, A and V patterns, 243
Hospital setting, 360
Housing continuum, 348
Hudson-Stähli line, 100
Hydrogel contact lenses
  benefits, 234*b*
  contraindications for, 237
  fitting principles, 235-236
  indications for, 236*b*-237*b*
Hydrogen peroxide, 338
Hypercoagulability, and anticoagulation, 53-54
Hyperglycemia, 63

Hypertension, 5, 377
  adverse effects, 52-53
  definition and epidemiology, 49
  pathogenesis, 50
  posterior segment manifestations of, 122
  risk factors, 49-50
  signs and symptoms, 50
  treatment, 50-51
Hyperthyroidism, 6, 66
Hypnotics, 191*t*
Hypoglycemia, 65
Hypotension, 52
Hypothyroidism, 66


**I**

Idiopathic cold agglutinin disease, 69
Illumination
  and color discrimination, 39
  and contact lens use, 218
  devices for, 291-292
  in measuring visual acuity, 139-140
  in near vision assessment, 141
  for near-vision magnification systems, 158
  requirements for, 271
  of typical environments, 209*t*
  and vehicle crashes, 310-311
Image jump, 207*f*
Immune function, age-related changes in, 341
Immune response, nutrional modulation of, 341-342
Immunocompetence theory of aging, 340-341
Immunological system, 6
Incandescent lighting, 271, 292
Incarcerated inmates, 2
Independence
  dual sensory loss and, 184
  independent living statistics, 268*b*
  optimization through technology, 185
Index of refraction, 37, 42
Individual role in public health, 366
Infarction
  calcarine cortex, 80-81
  myocardial, 56-57
Infarcts
  lacunar, 60
  retinal, 111
Inflammation, optic nerve, 116
Injury
  to optic nerve, 118
  prevention strategies regarding driving, 317
Inner ear
  anatomy, 182
  structural changes to, 181
Instruction manuals for contact lens use, 232-233
Instrumentation for on-site vision care, 350-351
Insulin, 6
  kinds used in U.S., 65*t*
Interactions
  drug, 190*t*-192*t*
  drug-receptor, 194
  with $H_2$-blocking agents, 196
  OTC drugs, 197*t*

Interior safety checks, 277*b*
Internuclear ophthalmoplegia, 89
Intracranial hemorrhage, 89-90
Intraocular lens implants, 262
Intraocular tension readings, 107
Iris
   age-related changes, 35
   diseases of, 101
   new vessels, in diabetes, 123
Iron, superoxide anion and, 338
Ischemic cranial neuropathy, 81-89
   anterior circulation ischemic stroke, 84
   bedside vision testing, 84-85
   disorders of conjugate gaze, 88-89
   eye movement disorders
      with anterior circulation strokes, 85-87
      with posterior circulation strokes, 87-88
   fourth cranial nerve palsy, 83
   sixth cranial nerve palsy, 83
   third cranial nerve palsy, 82-83
Ischemic optic neuropathy, 118
Ischemic stroke, 58
   anterior circulation, 84
   posterior circulation, 87-89
Isolation, feelings of, 15

**J**

Jackson Cross Cylinder, 139, 174
Jaeger notation, 142
Jaw claudication, 73-74

**K**

Kansas Division of Services for the Blind, 396-397
Keplerian telescopes, 151-152
Keratoacanthomas of lids, 95-96
Kidney function, 6

**L**

Labyrinth disease, 128
Lacrimal gland diseases, 98
Lacunar infarcts, 60
Large print, 290-291
Laser panretinal photocoagulation, 124*f*
Lateral vergence range, and fixation disparity testing,
    244-246
Laxatives, 198
Legal issues
   and privileged communications, 315-316
   regarding driving, 313-314
Lens. *See also* Aphakia.
   age-related changes in, 35-37, 304-305
   intraocular implants, 262
   structural and biochemical changes in, 102-103
Lenses
   antireflective coatings, 208
   appearance, performance, and weight, 206-207
   contact. *See* Contact lenses
   glare, 208-209
   materials and designs, 203-205

   photochromic, 209
   polarized, 209-210
   tints and coatings, 207-208
   trial, 137
Life expectancy, 375-376
Lifestyle changes
   for diabetes mellitus treatment, 64
   questionnaire regarding, 201, 202*f*
   taking history for, 134
Light
   absorption by lens, 36, 103
   filters, 293
   perception, absence of, 106
   sensitivity, 12
   transmission, reduction by lenses, 207*t*
Lipids, free radical effects, 339
Liver, diminishment of function, 6
Locale of nontraditional on-site vision care, 350-351
Locomotion, 9-11
Long-term care setting, 359-360, 368*b*
Loupes
   head-mounted, 155-156
   illuminated, 169*f*
Low technologies, 286
Low-tension glaucoma, 117
Low vision, patients with. *See* Patients with low vision.

**M**

Macrocytic anemias, 69-70
Macula, clinical evaluation of, 108
Macular degeneration, 112-113
Maculopathy, age-related, 305-306
Magnification, 185, 399
   for distance vision: telescopes, 149-152
   electronic
      CCTV, 293-294
      computers, 294-296
   for near vision, 152-160
   stand magnifiers, 274
Major organ systems, as primary care issue, 5-9
Malignant lesions of lids, 97-98
Malnutrition, 343-344
Mandell Seamless Bifocal, 224*f*
Marcus Gunn pupil, 107
Medial longitudinal fasciculus, syndrome of, 89
Medical abbreviations, 355*t*
Medicine, taking of, 10
Meibomian gland dysfunction, 95
Melanoma
   choroidal, 110, 306
   conjunctival, 99
   iris, 101
Memory loss
   with Alzheimer's disease, 15-16
   with anticholinergic drugs, 196-197
Menière's disease, 128
Mental health status, and vehicle crashes, 308
Metabolic disease, 8
Metabolism of drugs, 192*t*, 193
Methylprednisolone, 75
Microaneurysms, in diabetes, 123

Microcytic anemia, 68-69
Microvascular complications of diabetes mellitus, 63
Middle ear, 182
Minerals, RDA, 336*t*
Minority populations, ocular dysfunction, 9, 381
Mirrors
    binocular and monocular, 263
    hemianopic, 159-160
Misoprostol, 196
Mobile clinic setting, 362
Mobile eye care equipment, 351*f*-352*f*
Mobility, eye exam and, 166
Monitoring
    blood pressure, 5
    rehabilitative therapy, 264
Monocularity, 260
Monovision contact lens correction, 219-220
Motor systems
    age-related changes, 43-44
    control, technology and, 288-289
Multifocal contact lens designs, 226-230
    guidelines for fitting, 231*b*
Musculoskeletal system, 7-8
Myasthenia gravis, 130
Mydriatic eyedrops, combining, 170
Myocardial infarction, 56-57
Myopia, 380

**N**

National Agenda on Vision and Aging, 399-400
Near exophoria, 250*b*-251*b*
Near vision
    assessment of, 141-142
    taking history for, 134
Near vision: magnification
    computers, 157-158
    determining EVD required, 153-154
    determining magnification requirements, 152-153
    electronic display systems, 156
    nonmagnifying aids to vision, 158-160
    selecting magnifying aid, 154-156
    video magnifiers, 156-157
Neglect, 21-22
Neovascularization, choroidal, 112-113
Neural connections, age-related changes, 37-40
Neuralgia, trigeminal, 128
Neuritis, optic, 108
Neurological diseases
    anterior ischemic optic neuropathy, 76-77
    cerebral vascular disorders, 79-90
    retinal artery occlusion, 77-79
    temporal arteritis, 73-75
Neurological function, 8-9
Neuronal synapses, establishment of, 16
Neuro-ophthalmic disorders, 128-131
Neuropathy
    diabetic, 63, 124
    ischemic cranial, 81-89
    ischemic optic, 118
        anterior, 76-77
Niacin, 198

Night vision, lenses and, 209
Nitrogen species, 338
Nitroglycerin, 190*t*
Noncomitant deviations
    rehabilitative management of, 254-257
    tests and measurements for, 246-248
Noncompliance, patient, 279
Nonoptical devices
    for ergonomic positioning, 289-290
    relative size devices, 290-291
Nonsteroidal antiinflammatory drugs (NSAIDs), 191*t*,
        194*b*, 195-196
Normal vision changes
    anterior chamber, 35
    attention factors, 41
    contrast sensitivity, 40-41
    cornea, 32-34
    dark adaptation, 40
    iris, 35
    lens, 35-37
    motor systems, 43-44
    and prescribing spectacles for the normally sighted,
        147-149
    recovery from glare, 40
    refractive error, 42
    retinal and neural connection, 37-40
    temporal and spatial interactions, 41
    variability in visual performance, 44-45
    visual acuity, 31-32, 41-42
    vitreous, 37
Normocytic anemia, 69
Nucleic acids, free radical effects, 338
Nutrients
    affecting drug metabolism, 194
    aging effects on nutritional requirements, 334-335
    assessment of patient nutritional status, 342-343
    and diet manipulation, 335-336
    malabsorption of, 5-6
    in modulating immune response, 341-342
    in protecting against free radical oxidation, 339-340
    risk factors for malnutrition, 343, 344*b*
    theories of aging and impact of nutrition, 336-337

**O**

Obesity, 333-334
Objective cover tests, 244
Objective refraction, 136
Objectives of *Healthy People 2010*, 372-374
Observation distance, 137, 139-140, 150
Occluder flipper, 167*f*-168*f*
Occlusion, sector, 256, 259*f*
Occlusive disease of retinal circulation, 113-115
Ocular disease, posterior segment manifestations of,
        109-120
Ocular health examination, 135-136
Ocular pursuit system, 86-87
Oculomotor dysfunctions
    diagnosis, 242-243
    rehabilitation, 248-257
Oculus Easyfield, 172
"Old" cohort, 2

Open-angle glaucoma, 11-12, 119
Ophthalmodynamometry, 127
Ophthalmopathy, thyroid, 127-128
Opioid analgesics, 194*b*
Optical aids, training in use of, 160
Optic disc
    in anterior ischemic optic neuropathy, 76*f*
    changes in glaucoma, 119-120
Optic nerve
    degenerative changes in, 105
    diseases of, 116-118
Optometric care, effective, 268-272
Optometric examination
    advice and recommendations, 160-161
    binocular vision assessment, 142-143
    case history, 133-135
    color vision testing, 146
    contrast sensitivity measurement, 146-147
    dark adaptation testing, 147
    disability glare tests, 147
    near vision assessment, 141-142
    in nontraditional settings, 357-358
    ocular health, 135-136
    prescribing spectacles for patients
        with low vision, 149-160
        with normal sight, 147-149
    refraction, 136-139
    visual acuity measurement, 139-141
    visual field measurement, 143-146
Optometric Oath, 383*b*
Optometrists. *See also* Eye care practitioners; Health care
        providers.
    advice offered by, 160-161
    privileged communications, 315-316
    role in patient depression, 271
Organ systems, as primary care issue, 5-9
Outer ear, 182
Outreach to physicians, by eye care professionals, 396
Overrefraction, 137-138
Overspectacles, 219
Over-the-counter drugs, 197-198
Oxidative stress, free radicals and, 337-340
Oxygen species, 337-338

**P**

Pain, in ischemic cranial neuropathy, 81-82
Pallid edema, 77
Palpebral conjunctiva disease, 99
Papilledema, 89-90
    with neuro-ophthalmic disorders, 129
Paretic muscle, and eye fixing, 259*b*
Partial prisms, 159
Pathogenesis
    diabetes mellitus, 62
    hypercoagulability and anticoagulation, 53
    hypertension, 50
    TIA, 126
Patient care, public health aspects of, 365-378
Patient-clinician relationship
    communication, 387
    confidentiality and privacy, 390

culture and cultural competence, 389
    decision-making capacity, 388-389
    self-determination, 388
    trust, 387
    truth telling, 387-388
    vulnerability and elder abuse, 389-390
Patient education
    contact lenses
        care and handling of, 231-232
        care regimen, 233-234
        educational methods, 232-233
    instructions for home vision therapy, 253*f*, 255*f*-256*f*, 258*f*
    and patient compliance, 278-279
    practitioner's role in, 279-280
    in rehabilitative management, 264-265
Patient rights, 23*b*
Patient selection
    for contact lenses, 215-216
    for rehabilitative therapy, 264-265
Patient success with contact lenses, 230-231
Patients with low vision
    contact lenses for, 158-159
    devices for, 380-381
    management of, 277-278
    prescribing spectacles for, 149-160
    psychological and functional effects of low vision,
        269-271
    psychological set, 271-272
    refraction examination, 137-138
    talking devices, 399
    vision care, 267-268, 280-282
    visual acuity measurement, 139-141
    visual field measurement, 145-146
Patients with normal sight, prescribing spectacles for,
        147-149
Penicillin, 194*b*
Perceptual function, technology and, 287
Perceptual rehabilitation, 260
Perimetry
    automated devices, 144-145
    clinical evaluation of, 107
    in neuro-ophthalmic diagnosis, 129
Peripheral arterial disease, 61-62
Peripheral field loss, 275, 307
Peripheral localization ability, 41
Peripheral vision, and driving, 320
Personal demographics and driving experience, 302-303
Phagocytosis, 341
Pharmacotherapy, for diabetes mellitus treatment, 64-66
Phenylephrine, 197*t*
Phenytoin, 194*b*
Phorias, measurement of, 142-143
Photochromic lenses, 209
Physiological factors affecting drug action, 192*t*
Pigments
    dispersion, 112
    lens, 36
Plasma, oxidative events in, 339
Platelet antagonists, 54
Pocketalker, 164*f*
Polarized lenses, 209-210
Polycarbonate lenses, 203

Polymyalgia rheumatica, 70-72, 74-75
Pontine hemorrhage, 90
Population density, and traffic fatalities, 311-312
Posterior segment
    anatomical changes in, 105
    clinical evaluation of, 106-109
    manifestations of
        ocular disease, 109-120
        systemic disease, 120-131
Postherpetic neuralgia, 8
Postoperative diplopia, 242
Power, changing, 141
Prednisone, 75
Preretinal macular gliosis, 116
Presbycusis, 180, 183
Presbyopia
    correction for, 148, 203
        with contact lenses, 216, 218-219
    and segmented translating designs, 226
Prevalence data on auditory impairment, 179-180
Prevention of disease, 376-377
Primary aging, 4-5
Primary care issues
    acute and chronic care, 368b
    comanagement of health problems, 3
    major organ systems, 5-9
    primary aging, 4-5
    public health, 366-368
    secondary aging, 5
    vision, balance, and locomotion, 9-11
Primary vision care in geriatrics
    changes to eye and periorbital tissues, 11-13
    demographics, 1-2
    economic considerations, 20
    educational issues, 17-18
    elder abuse, 21-22
    elder care, 20-21
    health care providers needed, 22-23
    HIPAA, 23-24
    primary care issues, 3-11
    psychological issues, 13-17
    social issues, 18-20
    terminology, 2-3
Print size
    in near visual acuity measurement, 141-142
    relative size devices and, 290-291
Prisms, 143
    and contracture prevention, 256
    Fresnel, 211-212
    for fusion, 257
    partial, 159
    in rehabilitation of visual field defects, 263-264
    vertical, 246
Privacy, ethics and, 392
Privileged communications, 315-316
Prognosis, vision therapy, 257, 259-260
Progressive addition lenses, 148, 203-205
Proliferative diabetic retinopathy, 123, 124f
Protein binding drugs, 193
Proteins, free radical effects, 338
Proximal convergence, 43-44
Pseudoephedrine, 197t

Pseudohypertension, 52-53
Psychological issues
    Alzheimer's disease, 14-16
    dementia, 13
    depression, 16-17
    regarding low vision, 269-271
Psychosocial functioning, technology and, 288
Public health
    aging as public health concern, 366
    ask, advise, assist technique, 378
    and driving
        duty to warn, 314-315
        privileged communications, 315-316
        public policy and traffic safety, 316-317
    government role in, 365
    health promotion and disease prevention, 375-377
    *Healthy People 2010*, 371-374, 378-380
    *Healthy West Virginia 2010*, 374-375
    individual role in, 366
    and the law
        Americans with Disabilities Act (1990), 312-313
        legal and ethical issues regarding driving, 313-314
    and primary care, 366-368
    trends in aging, 368-371
    vision-related focus area objectives, 373-374
Public policy
    and traffic safety, 316-317, 322-324
    and vision care in nontraditional settings, 362
Pulmonary diseases, 6
Pupil
    clinical evaluation of, 107
    diameter, 35
    early dilation, 167
    exit pupil of telescope, 150-151
    in third cranial nerve palsy, 82-83
Pupillary reflexes, 107

**Q**

Questions for case history interview, 273b

**R**

Reading glasses, and single-vision contact lenses, 219
Reading problems, 263-264
Reading stands, 289f
Recommended Dietary Allowance (RDA)
    for minerals, 336t
    for vitamins, 335t
Reflections, lens surface, 207-208
Refraction
    examination procedures, 138-139, 357-358
    objective, 136
    of patients with low vision, 137-138
    subjective, 136-137, 173-175
    trial frame, 176b, 177
Refractive error, 42
    high: correction for, 148-149
Refractive status, 9, 12-13
Rehabilitation
    aphakic, 260-262
    of oculomotor dysfunctions, 248-257

Rehabilitation (*Continued*)
  oculomotor functions and, 241
  patient education, monitoring, and selection for, 264-265
  perceptual, 260
  prognosis and, 257, 259-260
  sensory adaptation training, 260-262
  tests and measurements, 243-248
  vergence eye movements, 241-242
  vision
    coverage for services, 399-400
    delivery of services, 398
    field of, 397-398
    role of eye care practitioners, 396-397
  vision and hearing, 184
  visual field defects, 262-264
Renal system, 6
Resistance exercise, 4
Resolution goal, 153
Respiratory system, 6
Restrictive syndromes, 247
Retina
  age-related changes in, 305-306
  aging of, 105
  diseases of, 110-116
  and neural connection changes, 37-40
Retinal artery occlusion, 77-79, 120, 122
Retinal detachment, 110-111, 115-116
Retinal illuminance, 38, 40
Retinitis pigmentosa, 306
Retinoscopy, 175
Retirement, 19
Reversed telescopes, 159
Reverse slab-off lenses, 213*f*
Rhegmatogenous retinal detachment, 115-116
Risk factors
  for atherosclerosis, 54-55
  for glaucoma, 119
  for hypertension, 49-50
  for malnutrition, 343, 344*b*
  for peripheral arterial disease, 61
  social and medical, 343*b*
Rubeosis iridis, 125*f*
Rural populations, 373

**S**
Saccades, 86-87
Safety
  home interior, checks for, 277*b*
  traffic, 301-303, 314-317, 320-324
Sample progress note, 359*f*
Scaling, in chart design, 139-140
Scattering, lens, 103
Schlemm's canal, 102
Scotomas, central or paracentral, 140-141
  functional field loss with, 274-275
Screening
  anterior segment, 168-169
  population-based, 323
  vision, at driver license renewal, 317-322
  visual acuity, 167
  visual field, 172

Seat belt use, 309
Sebaceous gland carcinoma of lids, 97-98
Seborrheic keratosis, 95, 96*f*
Secondary aging, 5
Sedatives, 191*t*
Segmented gas-permeable contact lens design,
    224-226
Self-determination, 390
Self-restriction with driving, 302-303
Senile miosis, 12, 35, 101
Sensitivity. *See also* Color insensitivities.
  contrast, 40-41, 106, 146-147, 172-173, 218, 321
  corneal, 99, 218
  light, 12
Sensory adaptation training
  aphakia
    aniseikonia and anisometropia, 262
    convergence requirements, 261-262
    intraocular lens implants, 262
    rehabilitation, 260-261
  monocularity, 260
  perceptual rehabilitation, 260
Sensory loss, dual, 184-185
Sensory perception, 8
Serous choroidal detachment, 110
Short-term memory loss, 15
Sign language, 185
Signs and symptoms
  atherosclerosis, 55
  diabetes mellitus, 62
  hypertension, 50
  peripheral arterial disease, 61
  TIA, 59
  vasculitic syndromes, 71
Simultaneous vision
  bifocal contact lenses, 220-221
  gas-permeable bifocal designs, 222-223
Single-vision contact lenses, and reading glasses, 219
Sixth cranial nerve palsy, 83
Skin, changes in, 6-7
Slab-off lenses, 213
Sleep disorders, 8-9
Slit lamp examination, 169, 352*f*
Smoking
  atherosclerosis and, 55
  COPD and, 67
  effect on drug metabolism, 194
Snellen acuity, 12
Social issues
  antiaging pseudoscience, 19-20
  economic status, 18-19
  employment and retirement, 19
  policy implications of growing numbers of older adults,
    370-371
Socialization of sensory-impaired adults, 185-186
Socioeconomic status, and vehicle crashes, 308-309
Soft bifocal/multifocal designs
  center-distance design, 227-229
  center-near design, 229
  diffractive bifocals, 229-230
  quality of vision, 226
Software, 295-296

Solutions Bifocal lens, 225*f*
Sound eye fixing, 259*b*
Spatial interaction changes, 41
Spectacles. *See also* Lenses.
   changes in prescription, 201, 203
     prescribing for
       the normally sighted, 147-149
       patients with low vision, 149-160
Speech distortion, 183
Sphere/cylinder flipper, 174*f*
Spherical refractive error, 138-139
Squamous cell carcinoma of lids, 97
Squamous papilloma of lids, 95*f*
Stand magnifiers, 154-155, 274-275
Staphylococcal blepharitis, 94*f*
Statins, 55
Stem cells, 341
Stereopsis
   reduced, 219
   training
     for central suppression and fixation disparity, 257*b*
     for distance esophoria, 254*b*
     for distance exophoria, 252*b*
Stereoscopic vision test, 320
Strabismus, comitant, 242-243
Stroke
   anterior circulation, 85-87
   hemispheric, 59
   hemorrhagic, 60-61
   ischemic, 58, 84, 87-89
   neuro-ophthalmological manifestations, 79-80
Stroma, changes in, 100-101
Subdural hematoma, 60-61
Subjective cover tests, 244
Subjective refraction, 136-137, 173-175, 358
Success rates for contact lenses, 230
Sudden-onset comitant strabismus, 243
Suicide, 16
Superoxide anion, 338
Support service provider, 185
Surgery
   cataract, 12
   vitreoretinal, indications for, 125*f*
Sweat glands, 7
Swinging flashlight test, 169*f*
Syndrome of the medial longitudinal fasciculus, 89
Syndromes of coronary artery disease, 56-57
Systemic disease
   anemia, 68-70
   atherosclerosis, 54-55
   cerebrovascular disease, 58-61
   congestive heart failure, 57-58
   COPD, 67-68
   coronary artery disease, 55-57
   diabetes mellitus, 62-66
   hypercoagulability and anticoagulation, 53-54
   hypertension, 49-53
   peripheral arterial disease, 61-62
   posterior segment manifestations of, 120-131
   thyroid disorders, 66-67
   vasculitic syndromes, 70-72
Systemic effects of topical ophthalmic agents, 198-199

**T**
Tactile markers, 185
Talking devices, 399
Tangent screen, 145
   in evaluating noncomitance, 247-248
Tangent Streak trifocal design, 224*f*-225*f*
T cells, 341
Tear drainage system diseases, 98
Tear film, 99-100
   and contact lens use, 217
Technology
   for accessory or nonoptical devices, 275-276
   assistive or educational, 285-286
   commercial to custom, 286-287
   electronic magnification, 293-296
   ergonomic positioning, 289
   general, 286
   hearing aids and ALDs, 296-297
   low to high, 286
   for motor control, 288-289
   nonoptical devices, 289-293
   optimization of communication through, 185
   for perceptual and cognitive function, 287-288
   for psychosocial functioning, 288
   for visual function, 287
Telescopes, 149-152, 185
   achieving required acuity, 150-151
   hand-held monocular, 274
   near-vision, 156
   reversed, 159
   selection of, 151-152
Television trainer, home vision therapy, 258*f*
Temporal arteritis, 73-75
Temporal interaction changes, 41
Tests and measurements
   for comitant deviations, 243-246
   for drivers license renewal, 319-320
   for noncomitant deviations, 246-248
Tetracyclines, 197
Thalamic hemorrhage, 90
Thalassemia minor, 69
Theories of aging
   immunocompetence theory, 340-341
   and the nutritional impact, 336-337
Therapeutic approaches to low vision care, 280-281
Therapeutic (bandage) contact lenses
   available designs, 235
   collagen shields, 237
   complications, 237
   hydrogel
     benefits, 234*b*
     contraindications for, 237
     fitting principles, 235-236
     indications for, 236*b*-237*b*
   success of, 237
Thickness, lens, 36*f*
Third cranial nerve palsy, 82-83
Thyroid disease, 6, 66-67
Thyroid ophthalmopathy, 127-128
Tiered approach to nutritional screening, 342-343
Tinnitus, 183
Title VII Chapter 2 of the Rehabilitation Act of 1973, 397, 399

Tonic vergence, 43
Tonometry, 169-170
Topical ophthalmic agents, systemic side effects of, 198-199
Total vergence, 43
Toxicity of anticholinergic drugs, 196-197
Toxic labyrinthitis, 128
Toxic optic neuropathies, 118
Trabecular meshwork, changes in, 102
Traffic crash trends in U.S., 299-300
Traffic safety
    demographics and, 301-303
    and duty to warn, 314-315
    policy-related studies, 322-324
    public policy and, 316-317
    and vision screening, 320-322
Training
    sensory adaptation, 260-262
    stereopsis, 252*b*, 254*b*, 257*b*
    in use of optical aids, 160
    vergence, 250*b*, 254*b*, 257*b*
Transient diplopia, 130
Transient ischemic attack (TIA), 59-60
    posterior segment manifestations of, 126-127
Translating gas-permeable lenses, 226
Transparency of lens, 305
Transpupillary thermal therapy, 110
Treatment
    cerebrovascular disease, 61
    congestive heart failure, 58
    COPD, 68
    coronary artery disease, 56-57
    diabetes mellitus
        lifestyle changes, 64
        pharmacotherapy, 64-66
    hypertension, 50-51
    peripheral arterial disease, 61-62
    thyroid disorders, 66-67
    vasculitic syndromes, 71-72
Trends
    in aging, 368-371
    discussed in *Healthy People 2010: Vision and Hearing*,
        380-381
Trial frames, 175-177
Trial lenses, 137
Trifocals. *See* Bifocal and trifocal lens segments; Multifocal
        contact lens designs.
Trigeminal nerve disease, 128
Trivex lenses, 203
Trochlear nerve, 83
Trust, 387, 389
Truth telling, in clinician-patient relationship, 389-390
Tuberculosis, 6
Tumbling E confrontation field technique, 171*f*
TypeWell Educational Transcription System, 185
Typoscope, 158, 292


**U**

Ultraviolet radiation
    cataracts and, 340
    protecting eye from, 210-211
Uncompensated congenital palsy, 243

Undernutrition, 336
Unilateral cover test, 244
United States
    aging trends in, 369*f*
    kinds of insulin used in, 65*t*
    public health in, 366*b*
    traffic crash trends in, 299-300
Useful field of view (attention window), 307, 321-322
Uveal tract diseases, 109-110
Uveitis, 101
    posterior, 109-110


**V**

Variability in visual performance, 44-45
Variable focus lenses, 205
Vascular ischemic attacks, 127
Vasculitic syndromes, 70-72
Vergence eye movements, 241-242
Vergences, 43
Vergence training
    for central suppression and fixation disparity, 257*b*
    for distance esophoria, 254*b*
    for near exophoria, 250*b*
Vernier acuity, 39
Vernier alignment thresholds, 39
Version eye movements, 43, 142
Vertical heterophoria, and fixation disparity testing, 246
Vertigo, 128
Video magnifiers, 156-157
Virchow's triad, 53*b*
Vision and aging
    crystalline lens changes, 304-305
    diabetic retinopathy, 306
    glaucoma, 306
    national agenda on, 399-400
    normal and diseased state, 303-304
    ocular melanoma, 306
    retinal changes, 305-306
    retinitis pigmentosa, 306
Vision care
    effective optometric care, 268-272
    essential clinical skills and understanding in, 272-280
    for patients with low vision, 267-268, 280-282
    primary, 1-24
Vision care in nontraditional settings
    coding, 359
    community service agency setting, 360-361
    future trends in, 362
    history and consent forms, 351, 353
    hospital setting, 360
    instrumentation, equipment, and locale, 350-351
    key staff interactions, 349-350
    long-term care setting, 359-360
    mobile clinic setting, 361-362
    outreach services, 348-349
    private home setting, 360-361
    recommended examination sequence, 353, 355, 357-359
    reporting and follow-up, 359
Vision changes: normal age-related
    anterior chamber, 35
    attention factors, 41

contrast sensitivity, 40-41
cornea, 32-34
dark adaptation, 40
iris, 35
lens, 35-37
motor systems, 43-44
recovery from glare, 40
refractive error, 42
retinal and neural connection, 37-40
temporal and spatial interactions, 41
variability in visual performance, 44-45
visual acuity, 31-32, 41-42
vitreous, 37
Vision corrections
 for anisometropia patients, prescribing strategies for, 211-212
 antireflective coatings, 208
 dissimilar bifocal segments, 212-213
 frame considerations, 211
 glare, 208-209
 lens appearance, performance, and weight, 206-207
 lens materials and designs, 203-205
 lifestyle changes, 201
 lifestyle questionnaire, 202*f*
 photochromic lenses, 209
 polarized lenses, 209-210
 protecting eye from glare and UV radiation, 210-211
 slab-off, 213
 spectacle prescription changes, 201, 203
 tints and coatings, 207-208
 variable focus lens, 205
Vision function and vehicle crashes, 306-307
Vision loss
 combined with hearing loss, 184-185
 fears regarding, 134-135
 leading causes of, 267-268
 nutrition effects, 344*b*
 peripheral field, 146
Vision rehabilitation
 coverage for services, 397-398
 delivery of services, 395-396
 field of, 395-396
 role of eye care professionals, 394-395
Vision screening, at drivers license renewal, 317-322
Visual acuity
 bedside testing, in neurologically impaired patients, 84
 changes in, 9, 12
 clinical evaluation of, 106-107
 corrected, 31-32, 38
 dynamic, testing for, 321
 dynamic changes with age, 41-42
 measurement, 172
  in low vision patients, 139-141
 near, 141-142

required, prescribing telescopes and, 150-151
 screening, 167
 static, 319-320
Visual field
 changes, in glaucoma, 120
 confrontation testing, 170-172
  at bedside, 84-85
 functional field loss with scotomas, 274-275
 measurement of, 143-146
 no demonstrable field loss, 274
 peripheral field loss, 275, 307
Visual field defects
 in calcarine cortex infarction, 80-81
 optical devices for, 159
 rehabilitation, 262-264
Visual performance
 assessment of, 280
 clinical evaluation of, 106-107
 limitations, technology and, 287
 variability in, 44-45
Vitamin B$_{12}$ deficiency, 6, 8
 anemia, 70
Vitamin C, 340, 342
Vitamin E, 339-340
Vitamins
 excessive intake of, 198
 high doses of, 112
 RDA, 335*t*
Vitreoretinal surgery, indications for, 125*f*
Vitreous
 age-related changes, 37
 hemorrhage, 125*f*
Vulnerability, decision making in light of, 391-392


**W**

Warfarin, 54
Water content of hydrogel lenses, 235-236
Wax, ear, 181
Wet macular degeneration, 112-113
Wheelchair patients, eye exam and, 166
Women
 as caregivers, 20-21
 and driving, 302
Workers, demographics, 19


**X**

Xanthelasma, 96


**Z**

Zinc, 342
Zonules, structural and biochemical changes in, 102-103